Recent Progress in Neuropsychopharmacology

Recent Progress in Neuropsychopharmacology

Editor: Christopher Green

AMERICAN
MEDICAL PUBLISHERS
www.americanmedicalpublishers.com

AMERICAN
MEDICAL PUBLISHERS
www.americanmedicalpublishers.com

Cataloging-in-Publication Data

Recent progress in neuropsychopharmacology / edited by Christopher Green.
p. cm.
Includes bibliographical references and index.
ISBN 978-1-63927-557-1
1. Neuropsychopharmacology. 2. Neuropharmacology. 3. Psychopharmacology. I. Green, Christopher.
RM315 .R43 2022
615.78--dc23

American Medical Publishers,
41 Flatbush Avenue,
1st Floor, New York,
NY 11217, USA

ISBN 978-1-63927-557-1 (Hardback)

Contents

Preface

It is often said that books are a boon to mankind. They document every progress and pass on the knowledge from one generation to the other. They play a crucial role in our lives. Thus I was both excited and nervous while editing this book. I was pleased by the thought of being able to make a mark but I was also nervous to do it right because the future of students depends upon it. Hence, I took a few months to research further into the discipline, revise my knowledge and also explore some more aspects. Post this process, I begun with the editing of this book.

Neuropsychopharmacology is the interdisciplinary science which overlaps psychopharmacology and neuroscience. It attempts to develop and understanding about the impact of drugs on neural mechanism that influence behavior. It encompasses the research of mechanisms of neuropathology, pharmacodynamics, psychiatric illnesses, and states of consciousness. Studies comprising neurotransmission/receptor activity, biochemical processes, and neural circuitry are also conducted within this field. The clinical aspect of this field encompasses psychiatric as well as neurologic pharmacology-based treatments. This book traces the progress of this field and highlights some of its key concepts. Research in this field has an impact on the study of various disorders such as anxiety disorders, affective disorder, psychotic disorder, etc. It is a valuable compilation of topics, ranging from the basic to the most complex advancements in this field. This book will help the readers in keeping pace with the rapid changes in the field of neuropsychopharmacology.

I thank my publisher with all my heart for considering me worthy of this unparalleled opportunity and for showing unwavering faith in my skills. I would also like to thank the editorial team who worked closely with me at every step and contributed immensely towards the successful completion of this book. Last but not the least, I wish to thank my friends and colleagues for their support.

Editor

Preface

1

Antidepressant activity: contribution of brain microdialysis in knock-out mice to the understanding of BDNF/5-HT transporter/5-HT autoreceptor interactions

Alain M. Gardier*

EA 3544 "Pharmacologie des troubles anxio-dépressifs et Neurogenèse", Faculté de Pharmacie, Université Paris-Sud, Chatenay-Malabry, France

Edited by:
Laurence Lanfumey, Institut National de la Santé et de la Recherche Médicale, France

Reviewed by:
Laurence Lanfumey, Institut National de la Santé et de la Recherche Médicale, France

***Correspondence:**
Alain M. Gardier, EA 3544 "Pharmacologie des troubles anxio-dépressifs et Neurogenèse", Faculté de Pharmacie, Université Paris-Sud, 5, rue J-B Clement, Tour D1, 2e etage, F-92296 Chatenay-Malabry Cedex, France
e-mail: alain.gardier@u-psud.fr

Why antidepressants vary in terms of efficacy is currently unclear. Despite the leadership of selective serotonin reuptake inhibitors (SSRIs) in the treatment of depression, the precise neurobiological mechanisms involved in their therapeutic action are poorly understood. A better knowledge of molecular interactions between monoaminergic system, pre- and post-synaptic partners, brain neuronal circuits and regions involved may help to overcome limitations of current treatments and identify new therapeutic targets. Intracerebral *in vivo* microdialysis (ICM) already provided important information about the brain mechanism of action of antidepressants first in anesthetized rats in the early 1990s, and since then in conscious wild-type or knock-out mice. The principle of ICM is based on the balance between release of neurotransmitters (e.g., monoamines) and reuptake by selective transporters [e.g., serotonin transporter for serotonin 5-hydroxytryptamine (5-HT)]. Complementary to electrophysiology, this technique reflects pre-synaptic monoamines release and intrasynaptic events corresponding to ≈80% of whole brain tissue content. The inhibitory role of serotonergic autoreceptors infers that they limit somatodendritic and nerve terminal 5-HT release. It has been proposed that activation of 5-HT_{1A} and 5-HT_{1B} receptor subtypes limits the antidepressant-like activity of SSRIs. This hypothesis is based partially on results obtained in ICM experiments performed in naïve, non-stressed rodents. The present review will first remind the principle and methodology of ICM performed in mice. The crucial need of developing animal models that display anxiety and depression-like behaviors, neurochemical and brain morphological phenotypes reminiscent of these mood disorders in humans, will be underlined. Recently developed genetic mouse models have been generated to independently manipulate 5-HT_{1A} auto and heteroreceptors and ICM helped to clarify the role of the pre-synaptic component, i.e., by measuring extracellular levels of neurotransmitters in serotonergic nerve terminal regions and raphe nuclei. Finally, we will summarize main advantages of using ICM in mice through recent examples obtained in knock-outs (drug infusion through the ICM probe allows the search of a correlation between changes in extracellular neurotransmitter levels and antidepressant-like activity) or alternatives (infusion of a small-interfering RNA suppressing receptor functions in the mouse brain). We will also focus this review on post-synaptic components such as brain-derived neurotrophic factor in adult hippocampus that plays a crucial role in the neurogenic and anxiolytic/antidepressant-like activity of chronic SSRI treatment. Limitations of ICM will also be considered.

Keywords: knock-out mice, antidepressants, autoreceptors, serotonin, BDNF, microdialysis

INTRODUCTION

Most of the antidepressants such as selective serotonin reuptake inhibitors (SSRIs) act as indirect agonists of monoamine receptors. While SSRI drugs produce relatively rapid blockade of serotonin [5-hydroxytryptamine (5-HT)] transporters (SERTs) *in vitro*, the onset of clinical benefits usually takes several (4–6) weeks to occur (Blier et al., 1987). This gap in timing between SSRI near-immediate effect on neurotransmitter systems and the slow symptomatic recovery is a paradox that has not been completely solved yet. At pre-synaptic level, SSRI-induced blockade of SERT results in a rapid suppression of the firing activity of 5-HT neurons in the brainstem (Blier, 2001): these results have been obtained by using an electrophysiological technique in anesthetized animals.

MICRODIALYSIS: PRINCIPLE AND METHODOLOGY IN MICE

The principle of microdialysis technique is based on the balance between the release of neurotransmitters (e.g., 5-HT) and its reuptake (e.g., by SERT). Usually, male 3- to 4-month-old wild-type (WT) or mutant mice (25–30 g in body weight) are used for microdialysis experiments.

Conventional intracerebral in vivo microdialysis

Whole brain tissue measurements represent a mixture of the intracellular (≈20%) and extracellular (≈80%) content. To obtain a measurement more directly related to synaptic transmission, it is interesting to sample specifically the content of the extracellular space, which is the site of exchanges between neurons, glial cells, and blood vessels (Zetterström et al., 1983). It contains various monoamines, excitatory and inhibitory amino acids, neuropeptides and their metabolites as well as precursors of these neurotransmitters. In the mid-1980s, the development of very sensitive analytical techniques such as liquid chromatography and electrochemical detection (LC-ED) had made possible to perform *in vivo* microdialysis first in anesthetized rodents, then in awake, freely moving animals.

In vivo microdialysis technique, in anesthetized or awake animals, was developed by the group of Delgado et al. (1972) in monkeys and then improved in rats by the group of Ungerstedt (Zetterström et al., 1983) in the early 1980s. It is based on the law of passive diffusion of low molecular-weight compounds through a porous membrane from the compartment with the highest concentration of neurotransmitters (the synaptic extracellular space) to the less concentrated compartment (i.e., the dialysis probe perfused with a buffer solution at physiological pH that does not contain neurotransmitters; **Figure 1**). This technique, now currently applied in our laboratory in awake, freely moving WT control or knock-out (KO) adult mice, allows the collection of samples (named "dialysates") every 10 or 20 min with a flow rate from 0.5 to 1.5 μl/min depending on the experimental protocol and the brain region studied. These samples contain, among other molecules, serotonin, its major metabolite (5-HIAA) and norepinephrine (NE), dopamine (DA), and their metabolites. These molecules are then quantified by using high-performance LC coupled to an amperometric detector (e.g., 1049A, Hewlett-Packard, Les Ulis, France). The limit of sensitivity for 5-HT is ~0.5 fmol/sample (signal-to-noise ratio = 2).

The concentrations of neurotransmitters reflect the physiological balance between the calcium-dependent neurotransmitter release and its reuptake by SERT located on the membrane of pre-synaptic neurons. A comprehensive study of intracerebral microdialysis has four phases: (1) surgical stereotaxic implantation of the probe under anesthesia, (2) the collection of dialysates (first to measure baseline value of extracellular neurotransmitter levels before and 2–3 h after drug treatment), (3) the collection of brains for the accurate verification of the implantation site of the microdialysis membrane, and (4) of chromatographic analysis of dialysate samples (see Malagié et al., 2001; Guiard et al., 2004 for details).

Drug administration by reverse microdialysis

A major advantage of the microdialysis technique is to infuse a drug locally into the brain to confirm central effects on dialysates first measured following a peripheral injection of the drug. Thus, drugs with a high molecular weight can be dissolved in artificial cerebrospinal fluid (aCSF) and administered locally, for example, into the ventral hippocampus *via* a silica catheter glued to the microdialysis probe (flow rate: 0.2 μl/min for 2 min), at the dose of 10–100 ng (Guiard et al., 2007; Deltheil et al., 2008). For each experiment, a control group must receive the appropriate vehicle.

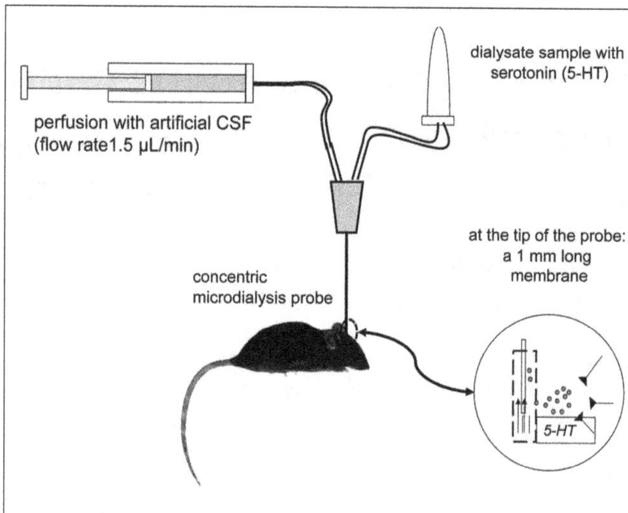

FIGURE 1 | Principle of intracerebral microdialysis in awake, freely moving mice.

Zero net flux method of quantitative* intracerebral microdialysis

The zero net flux method of quantitative microdialysis is used to quantify basal extracellular neurotransmitter concentrations and the extraction fraction (E_d) of this neurotransmitter, which provides an index of the functional status of the neurotransmitter uptake *in vivo*. Usually, four samples are collected to determine basal hippocampal 5-HT levels (as in David et al., 2004 in NK1 receptor KO mice), before local perfusion of increasing concentrations of 5-HT (0, 5, 10, and 20 nM). The dialysate 5-HT concentrations (C_{out}) obtained during perfusion of the various concentrations of 5-HT (C_{in}) are used to construct a linear regression curve for each animal (Guiard et al., 2008). The net change in 5-HT (C_{in}-C_{out}) is plotted on the *y*-axis against C_{in} on the *x*-axis. Extracellular 5-HT levels ($[5\text{-HT}]_{ext}$) and the extraction fraction of the probe (E_d) are determined as described by Parsons et al. (1991). The concentration of 5-HT in the extracellular space is estimated from the concentration at which C_{in}-C_{out} = 0 and corresponds to a point at which there is no net diffusion of 5-HT across the dialysis membrane. The extraction fraction (E_d) is the slope of the linear regression curve and has been shown to provide an estimate of changes in transporter-mediated 5-HT uptake (Parsons et al., 1991; Gardier et al., 2003).

As an example of the relevance of the zero net flux method of quantitative microdialysis, we have recently shown the critical impact of a neuropeptide, brain-derived neurotrophic factor (BDNF) on serotonergic neurotransmission under basal conditions and following SSRI treatment. In a series of experiments, we examined the consequences of either a constitutive decrease (Guiard et al., 2008) or increase in brain BDNF protein levels (Benmansour et al., 2008; Deltheil et al., 2008, 2009) on hippocampal extracellular levels of 5-HT in conscious mice. The no net flux method allows unveiling differences in basal extracellular 5-HT levels in heterozygous BDNF$^{+/-}$ mice (Guiard et al., 2008). Indeed, this neurotrophic factor is known to play a role in mood disorders and the mechanism of action of antidepressant drugs. However, the relationship between BDNF and serotonergic signaling is poorly understood. BDNF$^{+/-}$ mice were used to investigate the influence of BDNF on the 5-HT system and the activity of SERT in the hippocampus. The zero net flux method revealed that these mutants have increased basal extracellular 5-HT levels in the hippocampus and decreased 5-HT reuptake capacity. These results are coherent with the lack of effect of paroxetine to increase hippocampal 5-HText levels in BDNF$^{+/-}$ mice, while it produced robust effects in WT littermates. As expected, *in vitro* autoradiography and synaptosome techniques in BDNF$^{+/-}$ mice revealed a significant decrease in [3H]citalopram-binding-site density in the CA3 subregion of the ventral hippocampus and a significant reduction in [3H]5-HT uptake in hippocampal synaptosomes. Taken together, these results provide evidence that constitutive reductions in BDNF modulate SERT function reuptake in the hippocampus.

Statistical analysis and expression of results of microdialysis experiments in KO mice

Usually, microdialysis data are reported as means ± SEM. For conventional microdialysis experiments, we used to perform statistical analyses on areas under the curve (AUC) values for the amount of 5-HT outflow collected during the 0–120 min post-treatment period. To compare different AUC values in each group of mice, a two-way ANOVA with genotype factor and treatment factor is performed. We used to present microdialysis data as histograms because statistical analysis on AUC values better reflects the pharmacological properties of a compound than the kinetics. We strongly believe that the interpretation of these data is more appropriate when performed on AUC values in dialysate 5-HT levels (Guilloux et al., 2011; Nguyen et al., 2013) as well as for DA levels (Maskos et al., 2005; Reperant et al., 2010) when changes induced by drugs are compared between WT versus KO mice.

Using intracerebral microdialysis in the hippocampus and cortex in mice, measuring statistically significant changes in dialysate 5-HT levels induced, for example, by a given drug between t_{30} min and t_{45} min offers little interest. We feel that these information make the message more difficult to interpret and do not fundamentally improve the study. These time courses are strongly dependent on the experimental conditions and consequently not reproducible between laboratories. By contrast, our experience reveals that comparable results from distinct laboratories can be obtained from the analysis of AUC values. The inclusion of the data showing the time course for the microdialysis is often superfluous. Microdialysis is a neurochemical technique, not sensitive enough to explore precisely (i.e., sample-by-sample) the time course of drug effects.

However, in some cases, it is interesting to show the time course analysis of the microdialysis data:

(1) when we need to express time course data in microdialysis experiments as concentrations (in fmol/sample, not as % changes) because the baseline dialysate levels of the neurotransmitter are statistically different between two groups of mice, i.e., in Table 1 and Figures 2 and 3 in Guiard et al. (2008): heterozygous BDNF$^{+/-}$ mice had a higher basal 5-HText levels in the hippocampus compared to WT mice. See also in Table 1 and Figure 6 in Guilloux et al. (2011), in which double 5-HT$_{1A}$/1B$^{-/-}$ mice display a higher basal 5-HText levels in the frontal cortex and dorsal raphe nucleus (DRN) compared to WT mice.

(2) when it is sometimes important to collect some pharmacokinetic information about the short-term or long-lasting effect of a new drug in rodents. The AUC analysis of microdialysis data disregards information about differences in C_{max} and duration of the drug effects.

(3) when a gray line (Figure 3 in Guilloux et al., 2006; Figures 1 and 2 in Nguyen et al., 2013) indicates the duration time of the forced swim test (FST, i.e., 6 min), which was performed, in a separate group of animal, at the maximum effect of the antidepressant on cortical extracellular 5-HT levels in mice. It emphasizes that microdialysis and behavioral experiments were carried out by using the same experimental protocol.

INTRACEREBRAL *IN VIVO* MICRODIALYSIS IN RODENTS

Another technique has provided complementary information about the mechanism of action of SSRIs: intracerebral *in vivo* microdialysis (ICM) performed in awake, freely moving animals (first in rats, now in mice). Information included in this chapter was drawn from our own experience in this field and relevant publications from other investigators.

FIRST IN RATS

When it was first used in rat brain in the mid-1980s, this technique measured, for example, extracellular concentrations of monoamines such as serotonin (5-HText), which reflect presynaptic release of 5-HT and intrasynaptic events. With its coupling to very sensitive analytical techniques, it has provided much information regarding changes in the local pre-synaptic release of monoamines following acute drug administration. Thus, it has been possible to obtain two major arguments supporting the hypothesis that somatodendritic 5-HT$_{1A}$ autoreceptors located in the raphe nuclei play an important role in the mechanism of action of SSRIs in rats (Gardier et al., 1996). At first, we have learned that a single administration of SSRIs at low doses comparable to those used therapeutically increased 5-HText in the vicinity of the cell body and the dendrites of serotoninergic neurones of the DRN (Malagié et al., 1995). This effect was more pronounced than that observed in regions rich in nerve endings (frontal cortex, ventral hippocampus; Malagié et al., 1996), probably due to a higher SERT density (Hrdina et al., 1990). Hence, the magnitude of the activation of the serotonergic neurotransmission depends on the brain area studied and the dose of the SSRIs administered to rats. This difference has been attributed to the activation of somatodendritic 5-HT$_{1A}$ autoreceptors by endogenous 5-HT in the raphe nuclei, thereby limiting the corticofrontal effects of the antidepressant. Microdialysis technique demonstrated that despite SSRI-induced 5-HT reuptake inhibition also taking place at nerve terminals, there is a decrease in 5-HT release *via* activation of 5-HT$_{1A}$ (somatodendritic) or 5-HT$_{1B}$ (nerve terminal) autoreceptors (Rutter et al., 1995). Thus, depending on the terminal 5-HT brain area, only a small increase or no change at all in the synaptic availability of 5-HT occurs (Malagié et al., 1996; Romero et al., 1996). These microdialysis results obtained in rats have then been extended to measure SSRI-induced changes in DRN 5-HText in awake, freely moving KO mice (Bortolozzi et al., 2004; Guiard et al., 2004).

Next, we have learned from microdialysis performed in rats that SSRIs cause a larger increase in 5-HText at nerve endings following an acute treatment *versus* a chronic one. As the treatment is prolonged, a robust and time-dependent downregulation of SERT was observed (Pineyro et al., 1994; Benmansour et al., 2002), while 5-HT_{1A} autoreceptors gradually desensitize leading to a progressive recovery to normal of the firing rate of 5-HT neurons (Blier et al., 1986; Chaput et al., 1986; El Mansari et al., 2005). However, these molecular events seem to depend on 5-HT_{1A} autoreceptor internalization (Popa et al., 2010). Indeed, we studied the function of the 5-HT system in the raphe nuclei and hippocampus by using repeated *in vivo* microdialysis sessions in awake, freely moving mice. We assessed the degree of 5-HT_{1A} autoreceptor desensitization by using a local infusion of the 5-HT_{1A} receptor antagonist, WAY 100635, in the raphe *via* reverse microdialysis. We found that the anxiolytic-like effects of fluoxetine correlate in time and amplitude with 5-HT_{1A} autoreceptor desensitization, but neither with the basal extracellular levels of 5-HT in the raphe nuclei, nor in the hippocampus. These results suggests that the beneficial anxiolytic/antidepressant-like effects of chronic SSRI treatment depend on 5-HT_{1A} autoreceptor internalization, but do not require a sustained increase in extracellular 5-HT levels in a territory of 5-HT projection such as hippocampus. Several studies of patients with depression appear to confirm these experimental results, suggesting that co-administration of a 5-HT_{1A} autoreceptor antagonist (pindolol) and an SSRI accelerated the onset of the antidepressant effect (Portella et al., 2011). However, given the complex pharmacology of pindolol, new drug developments may help to discover either selective and silent 5-HT_{1A} receptor antagonists to be prescribed in combination with SSRIs, or dual action agents (SSRI + 5-HT_{1A} receptor antagonists; Artigas et al., 2006).

NEXT IN WILD-TYPE AND KNOCK-OUT MICE

The use of pharmacological tools in mice

Changes in the amount of neurotransmitters (mainly monoamines such as 5-HT, NE, and DA) in synapses can be viewed as near-immediate effects of SSRI on brain neurotransmitter systems. *In vivo* brain microdialysis allows to measure basal extracellular levels of these neurotransmitters giving an idea of neurochemical events occurring at nerve terminals in brain regions of awake, freely moving rodents. In our laboratory, we extensively applied this technique in genetic and pharmacological studies aimed at investigating the relationship between neurotransmitters and brain regions, or between neurochemical changes and animal behaviors (see examples below). Among the main interests of microdialysis application is the infusion of drugs through the microdialysis probe (reverse dialysis) in conscious KO mice as well as in WT mice used as controls in these pharmacological experiments (e.g., intra-raphe perfusion of substance P in Guiard et al., 2007; BDNF in Deltheil et al., 2009).

As already mentioned, most prescribed serotonergic antidepressants show limited efficacy and delayed onset of action, partly due to the activation of somatodendritic 5-HT_{1A} autoreceptors by the excess extracellular 5-HT produced by SSRI in the raphe nuclei. A group of scientists in Spain recently addressed this problem using an original strategy. Bortolozzi et al. (2012) administered a small-interfering RNA (siRNA) to suppress acutely 5-HT_{1A} autoreceptor-mediated negative feedback mechanisms in the mouse brain. They developed a conjugated siRNA (C-1A-siRNA) by covalently binding siRNA targeting 5-HT_{1A} receptor mRNA with the SSRI sertraline in order to concentrate it in serotonin axons, rich in SERT sites. The intracerebroventricular (I.C.V.) infusion of C-1A-siRNA to mice resulted in its selective accumulation in serotonin neurons. This was associated with antidepressant-like effects in the forced swim and tail suspension tests, but did not affect anxiety-like behaviors in the elevated plus-maze. In addition, C-1A-siRNA administration markedly decreased 5-HT_{1A} autoreceptor expression and suppressed 8-OH-DPAT [7-(dipropylamino)-5,6,7,8-tetrahydronaphthalen-1-ol]-induced hypothermia (a pre-synaptic 5-HT_{1A} receptor effect in mice) without affecting post-synaptic 5-HT_{1A} receptor expression in the hippocampus and prefrontal cortex. Moreover, I.C.V. C-1A-siRNA infusion augmented the increase in cortical dialysate 5-HT levels induced by fluoxetine to the level measured in 5-HT_{1A} receptor KO mice. Hence, C-1A-siRNA represents a new approach to treat mood disorders as monotherapy or in combination with SSRI.

To learn whether or not the *in vitro* affinity of SSRIs toward monoamine transporters can predict *in vivo* microdialysis data, we studied whether a single administration of a range of doses [1, 4, and 8 mg/kg, given intraperitoneally (i.p.)] of paroxetine, citalopram, or venlafaxine may simultaneously increase dialysate 5-HText and norepinephrine (NEext) by using *in vivo* microdialysis in the frontal cortex of awake, freely moving mice (David et al., 2003). We found that citalopram and paroxetine have the highest potency to increase cortical 5-HText and NEext, respectively. In addition, the rank of order of efficacy of these antidepressant drugs to increase cortical 5-HText *in vivo* in mice was as follows: venlafaxine > citalopram > paroxetine, while the efficacy to increase cortical NEext in mice of paroxetine and citalopram is similar, and greater than that of venlafaxine. Thus, the highest doses of the very selective SSRI citalopram and the very potent SSRI paroxetine were able to increase cortical NEext. Surprisingly, the serotonin-norepinephrine reuptake inhibitor (SNRI) venlafaxine increased cortical 5-HText to a greater extent rather than NEext in the range of doses studied in mice.

We recently confirmed these data with escitalopram, the *S*(+)-enantiomer of citalopram. To analyze the mechanisms by which SSRIs activate noradrenergic transmission in the brain, we compared the effects of escitalopram on both 5-HText and NEext in the frontal cortex of WT versus mutant mice lacking the 5-HT transporter ($SERT^{-/-}$; Nguyen et al., 2013). In particular, the possibilities that escitalopram enhances NEext either by a direct mechanism involving the inhibition of the low- or high-affinity NE transporters or by an indirect mechanism promoted by 5-HText elevation were explored. The FST was used to investigate whether enhancing cortical 5-HText and/or NEext affected the antidepressant-like activity of escitalopram. As expected, a single systemic administration of escitalopram increased cortical 5-HText and NEext in WT mice. However, escitalopram failed to increase cortical 5-HText in SERT$^{-/-}$ mice, whereas its neurochemical effects on NEext persisted in these mutants. In WT mice, these neurochemical changes induced by escitalopram were associated with increased swimming parameter in the FST. Finally, escitalopram, at relevant concentrations, failed to inhibit cortical NE and 5-HT uptake mediated by low-affinity monoamine transporters (i.e., organic cation transporters such as OCT1, 2, or 3). These experiments suggest that escitalopram enhances, although moderately, cortical NEext *in vivo* by a direct mechanism involving the inhibition of the high-affinity NE transporter (NET). Such *in vivo* effects of SSRIs could not be predicted by measuring the *in vitro* affinity of SSRIs toward SERT and NET in brain synaptosomes.

These results are not surprising. Indeed, experimental conditions (rat versus mice; whole brain versus cortical membranes; cell bodies versus nerve terminal regions; etc.) highly influence the values of binding parameters of ligands to neurotransmitter receptors or transporters measured *in vitro* (B_{max}, K_D, GTP-gammaS binding, etc.). The potency and selectivity of SSRIs as determined *in vitro* do not take into account noradrenergic projections and others, which obviously interfere *in vivo*, but not *in vitro*. Thus, function of monoamines transporters are much more complex than previously thought. *In vivo* experiments help to depict this complexity when it is possible to measure correlation between neurochemical parameters and behavior paradigms.

The use of mutated mice

The mouse genome can be specifically manipulated to produce the targeted deletion, replacement of genes, or down-/over-expression of related proteins in the brain (Sotnikova and Gainetdinov, 2007). This was first obtained in embryonic stem (ES) cells, but more recently, temporal and spatial controls of gene expression were possible in adult mice. In the field of anxiety and depression, preclinical studies such as those described above, have been mostly performed in healthy, "not depressed" animals. In the mid-1990s, genetically manipulated mice became available. It complicated the experimental protocol because it was necessary to include littermates as WT control mice. Great hopes were placed in mutant lines, some of them being considered as putative animal models of anxiety or depression. Several lines of transgenic (Tg) mice (carrying a human gene) or KO mice (i.e., homozygous mice lacking the two copies of a gene coding for a receptor or transporter of neurotransmitter or neuropeptide) were generated between 1994 and 1998. The first KO mice were generated by homologous recombination in the laboratory of S. Tonegawa at MIT (Silva et al., 1992).

The mouse is a model organism of choice in the field of neurosciences because (i) numerous genes have a human equivalent, (ii) many biological and biochemical functions of the mouse are similar to those of humans, and (iii) the genome mouse is easily manipulated by homologous recombination. This technique allowed the creation of animal-related patterns of human brain pathologies. The genetic background is a fundamental parameter for analyzing the phenotype of KO mice. Historically, the mutant mice were established using ES line 129/Sv. However, creating new lines of mutant mice on a genetic background C57BL/6 is now preferred, although there are limits on the use of this strain in some behavioral tests (see Gardier, 2009 for a review).

At that time, the procedure of ICM needed to be quickly adapted to perform experiments in an animal model having a smaller brain size than rats. Microdialysis experiments were first performed in tyrosine hydroxylase Tg mice by Nakahara et al. (1993). Then, it was applied to 5-HT$_{1B}$ receptor KO mice (Saudou et al., 1994; Trillat et al., 1997), to DA transporter (DAT) KO mice (Gainetdinov et al., 1997), and so on. Of course, at the end of the experiments, the precise location of the microdialysis probe must be macroscopically verified according to the stereotaxic coordinates given by the mouse brain atlas (Paxinos and Franklin, 2001).

Regarding the pharmacological knowledge of antidepressants, the choice of KO mice as experimental models of anxiety–depression was remarkably appropriate because it is now well recognized that major depressive disorders result from a combination of genetic and environmental factors. In addition, knowing that anxiety and depression have a high co-morbidity (Gorman and Coplan, 1996; Leonardo and Hen, 2006), it is critical for basic research to develop animal models that present behavioral, neurochemical, and brain morphological phenotypes reminiscent of depression and anxiety. Some "serotonergic" KO mice display important changes in their basal phenotype. For example, constitutive 5-HT$_{1A}$ receptor KO mice were simultaneously described by three different laboratories as an animal model of anxiety-related disorder (Heisler et al., 1998; Parks et al., 1998; Ramboz et al., 1998). They display decreased exploratory activity and increased fear of aversive environments and exhibited a decreased immobility in the FST, an effect commonly associated with antidepressant treatment. Brain microdialysis performed in 5-HT$_{1A}$ receptor KO mice have proven to be a valuable technique to address key questions regarding the mechanism of action of antidepressants. One of the most interesting applications of microdialysis is to allow the study of basal extracellular levels of neurotransmitters, for example, in 5-HT$_{1A}$ receptor KO mice. While conventional microdialysis does not allow reliable measurements of these basal levels (see Conventional Intracerebral *In Vivo* Microdialysis) the no net flux (or zero net flux) method of quantitative microdialysis in mutants allows the direct and accurate determination of basal extracellular levels of neurotransmitters (see Zero Net Flux Method of Quantitative* Intracerebral Microdialysis) The DRN is a brain region where 5-HText is known to regulate serotonergic transmission through activation of 5-HT$_{1A}$ autoreceptors. When microdialysis was performed in the DRN, it was found that baseline DRN 5-HText did not differ between WT control and KO mice. This result suggests a lack of tonic control of 5-HT$_{1A}$ autoreceptors on DR 5-HT release (Bortolozzi et al., 2004; Guilloux et al., 2006).

Furthermore, microdialysis helped to decipher the brain region-dependent effects of antidepressants. Both a saline injection and handling for 3 min increased DRN 5-HText in 5-HT$_{1A}$ receptor KO mice, but not in control mice. Fluoxetine, a serotonergic antidepressant, induced a dose-dependent increase in DRN 5-HText in both genotypes, but this effect was markedly more pronounced in 5-HT$_{1A}$ KO mice. These results suggest that the increased responsiveness of dialysate 5-HText in the DRN of

5-HT_{1A} receptor KO mice at least in part explain the anxious phenotype of these mutants. Such information can help to define a better treatment of anxiety-related disorders.

The inhibitory 5-HT_{1A} receptor exists in two separate populations with distinct effects on serotonergic signaling, i.e., an autoreceptor that limits 5-HT release throughout the brain and a heteroreceptor that mediates inhibitory responses to release 5-HT. Traditional pharmacologic and Tg strategies have tried to separate the distinct roles of these two receptor populations. Recently, Richardson-Jones et al. (2010) developed a new strategy to manipulate pre-synaptic 5-HT_{1A} autoreceptors in serotonergic raphe neurons without affecting 5-HT_{1A} heteroreceptors, generating mice with higher (1A-High) or lower (1A-Low) autoreceptor levels. In this latter line, it was thus possible to examine the brain 5-HT system by partially turning off 5-HT_{1A} autoreceptors at a specific time point and to study correlations between changes in 5-HT transmission and antidepressant-like activity of SSRIs in various behavioral tests. This strategy robustly affects raphe firing rates, but has no effect on either basal extracellular 5-HT levels as measured by *in vivo* microdialysis in the frontal cortex and ventral hippocampus. Interestingly, following 8 days of fluoxetine treatment, a difference in 5-HT levels was found in the hippocampus, with higher levels in the 1A-Low mice. In addition, 1A-Low mice displayed a larger increase in 5-HT in response to an acute challenge of fluoxetine in both brain regions. Together with electrophysiology data showing an increased spontaneous neuronal activity in the dorsal raphe of 1A-Low mice under stressful conditions, the microdialysis results were consistent with an increased serotonergic tone in these animals in response to an SSRI. Compared to 1A-Low mice, 1A-High mice show a blunted physiological response to acute stress, increased behavioral despair, and no behavioral response to antidepressant, thus modeling what we can find in patients with the 5-HT_{1A} risk allele. Indeed, human studies implicate a polymorphism in the promoter of the 5-HT_{1A} receptor gene in increased susceptibility to depression and decreased treatment response (Lemonde et al., 2003). These mice may thus, be conceived as a human equivalent to SSRI response (1A-Low) and resistance (1A-High; Blier, 2010). These results establish a causal relationship between 5-HT_{1A} autoreceptor levels and response to antidepressants.

The same group of researchers used a recently developed genetic mouse system to independently manipulate 5-HT_{1A} autoreceptor and heteroreceptor populations. They found that 5-HT_{1A} autoreceptors affect anxiety-like behavior, while 5-HT_{1A} heteroreceptors affect responses to forced swim stress, without effects on anxiety-like behavior (Richardson-Jones et al., 2011). These results establish distinct roles for the two receptors' populations, providing evidence that signaling through endogenous 5-HT_{1A} autoreceptors is necessary and sufficient for the establishment of normal anxiety-like behavior.

Taken together, these data obtained in KO mice brought a lot of information about the pathophysiology of psychiatric disorders and their treatments.

Thus, in 2012, we have at our disposal a large number of genetically engineered mice, some of them being interesting animal models of anxiety and depression. These mice are very helpful to discover the underlying pathological mechanisms that limit the effects of current treatments of major depressive episodes and to identify the nature of the molecular cascades leading to the installation of disorders such as anxiety and depression. In addition, KO mice help to study the effects of acute and chronic treatment with antidepressants.

Recent advances in experimental approaches using genetically manipulated mice have already been summarized in the literature (Sotnikova and Gainetdinov, 2007). Knowing the large number of KO mice generated to date, it is not possible to detail the findings of each putative model interesting in the anxiety and depression field of research ($\text{SERT}^{-/-}$ mice, Bengel et al., 1998; NK1 receptor KO mice, Froger et al., 2001; Guiard et al., 2004; β-arrestin 2 KO mice, Beaulieu et al., 2008). Therefore, the remainder of the present chapter will only describe some examples, which explain these statements.

ADVANTAGES AND LIMITATIONS OF USING MICRODIALYSIS IN KO MICE

Depressive disorders result from a combination of genetic and environmental factors. To date, several genes appear to have in humans and animals, a greater influence than the other and emerge from the literature. Among them, the presence of a polymorphism of either SERT (Bengel et al., 1998; Kuzelova et al., 2010), 5-HT_{1A} receptor (Lemonde et al., 2003), the tryptophan hydroxylase type 2 (TPH-2; Invernizzi, 2007), or BDNF (Chen et al., 2006) is associated with the occurrence of depression related to stress, or to a response to behavioral tests predictive of the antidepressant-like activity of a molecule (Porsolt et al., 1977; Steru et al., 1985).

ADVANTAGES

In these KO mice, we can measure, for example, the paradigms of stress to predict the antidepressant potential of a molecule and the selectivity of behavioral responses in comparison with non-mutated control animals: if these responses are diminished or absent in KO mice deprived of a gene encoding a neurotransmitter receptor, we may conclude that this receptor plays a major part either in the antidepressant-like effect and/or of the molecule. Regarding microdialysis, changes in dialysate levels of neurotransmitters following acute (Malagié et al., 2001) or chronic (Gardier et al., 2003) SSRI treatment can highlight the mechanism of action of these drugs.

Thus, we combined KO mice and receptor antagonist strategies to investigate the contribution of the 5-HT_{1B} receptor subtype in mediating the effects of an SSRI, paroxetine in mice (Malagié et al., 2001). Using microdialysis, we found that a single systemic administration of paroxetine (1 or 5 mg/kg by the i.p. route) increased 5-HText in the ventral hippocampus and frontal cortex of WT control and mutant mice. However, in the ventral hippocampus, the SSRI induced a larger increase in dialysate 5-HT levels in KO 5-HT_{1B} mice than in control mice. In addition, either the absence of the 5-HT_{1B} receptor (in KO 5-HT_{1B} mice) or its pharmacological blockade with the mixed 5-HT_{1B}/1D receptor antagonist, GR 127935 (in WT mice) potentiated the effect of a single administration of paroxetine on extracellular 5-HT levels in the ventral hippocampus. Thus, these data underline several points:

(a) complementary results were obtained by combining KO mice and receptor antagonist strategies.
(b) there were already *in vitro* studies showing the role of terminal 5-HT_{1B} autoreceptors *in vivo* to control 5-HT release and reuptake (in slices; Pineyro et al., 1995). Our microdialysis data in KO 5-HT_{1B} mice brought additional information by suggesting that 5-HT_{1B} autoreceptors limit the effects of SSRIs on dialysate 5-HT levels at serotonergic nerve terminals and revealed the importance of a particular brain region, the ventral hippocampus. It is interesting to notice that recently, many experimental arguments have accumulated to suggest that antidepressants exert their behavioral activity in adult rodents, at least in part, by inducing of cellular and molecular changes in the adult hippocampus (David et al., 2010).

By using microdialysis, we can also study changes in dialysate 5-HT levels in the DRN (see Introduction). Data described above in 5-HT_{1A} receptor KO mice illustrated this important contribution. This experiment can give further information when combined with measurements of the electrical activity of 5-HT neurons. Again, the comparison of results between a KO mice model and WT mice is very informative.

Neurochemical changes as measured by using microdialysis can have functional consequences since they correlated with behavioral data obtained, for example, in the FST. Three examples can illustrate these benefits.

Example 1, in WT mice: intra-hippocampal BDNF infusion can potentiate paroxetine-induced increase in 5-HText in the hippocampus (**Figure 2A**). The antidepressant-like activity of paroxetine as measured on swimming behavior was potentiated by BDNF (**Figure 2B**). These data suggest an interesting synergy between BDNF and SSRI on 5-HT neurotransmission; thus, such a co-administration improved the antidepressant-like activity of the SSRI (Deltheil et al., 2008, 2009).

Example 2, in 5-HT_{1A} receptor KO mice: as described in Guilloux et al. (2006), paroxetine (1 and 4 mg/kg) dose-dependently increased cortical 5-HText in both WT and KO genotypes, but the effects were greater in mutants (**Figure 3A**). Paroxetine administration also dose-dependently decreased the immobility time in both strains of mice, but the response was much greater in $5HT_{1A}{}^{-/-}$ mice (**Figure 3B**). Overall these results suggest that the genetic inactivation of 5-HT_{1A} receptors, abolished the inhibitory feedback control exerted by somatodendritic 5-HT_{1A} autoreceptors, thus enhancing the response of mutant mice to stressful conditions such as the FST. Thus, following SSRI administration, an indirect activation of pre-synaptic 5-HT_{1A} receptors by endogenous 5-HT may limit its antidepressant-like effects in the FST in WT mice.

Example 3, in $SERT^{-/-}$ mice: another interest of brain microdialysis is to allow the measurement of several neurotransmitters in the same sample. Thus, we recently examined the effects of the S(+)-enantiomer of citalopram, escitalopram (ESC) on both [5-HT]ext and extracellular levels of [NE]ext in the frontal cortex (FCx) of freely moving WT and mutant mice lacking $SERT^{-/-}$ by using ICM (Nguyen et al., 2013). In WT mice, a single systemic administration of escitalopram produced a significant increase in cortical [5-HT]ext and [NE]ext (**Figure 4**). As expected, escitalopram failed to increase cortical [5-HT]ext in $SERT^{-/-}$ mice, whereas its neurochemical effects on [NE]ext persisted in these mutants. In addition, in WT mice submitted to the FST, escitalopram increased swimming parameter without affecting climbing behavior (Nguyen et al., 2013).

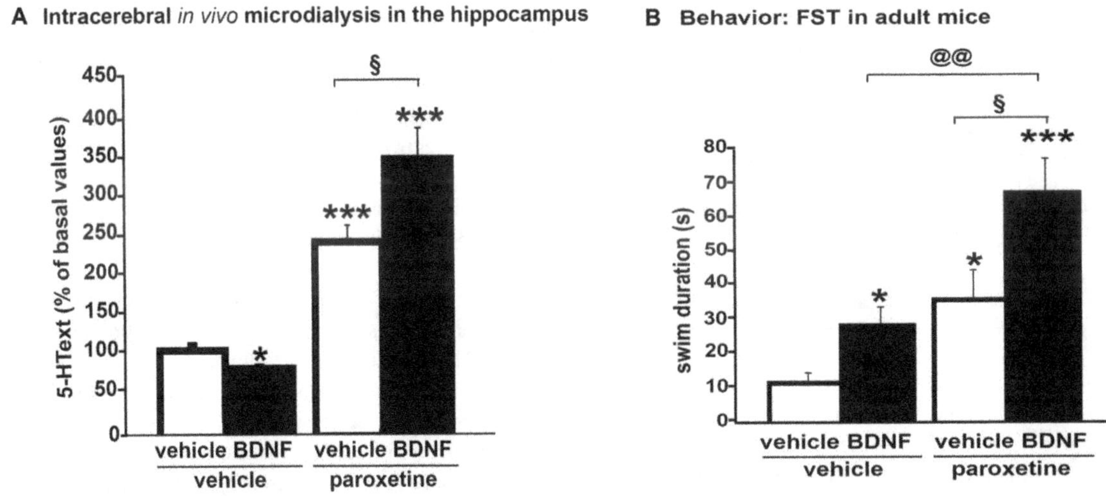

FIGURE 2 | (A) Microdialysis data showing that an acute intra-hippocampal injection of BDNF (100 ng) potentiated the effects of the systemic administration of an SSRI, paroxetine (4 mg/kg; i.p.) on dialysate 5-HText in the hippocampus of freely moving wild-type mice. Results are expressed as AUC values (means ± SEM) calculated for the amount of 5-HText collected during the 0–120 min post-treatment period. **(B)** Antidepressant-like activity of paroxetine as measured on swimming behavior in the forced swim test (FST) was potentiated by BDNF. Thus, neurochemical changes correlated with behavioral data in this protocol, suggesting that a BDNF + SSRI combination may offer new alternatives to treat mood disorders (from Deltheil et al., 2009). *$p < 0.05$, ***$p < 0.001$ when compared to the vehicle-treated group; $^{§}p < 0.05$ when compared to the paroxetine/vehicle-treated group and paroxetine/BDNF-treated group; $^{@@}p < 0.01$ when compared to the BDNF/vehicle-treated group and BDNF/paroxetine-treated group (two-way ANOVA, Fisher's PLSD *post hoc* test).

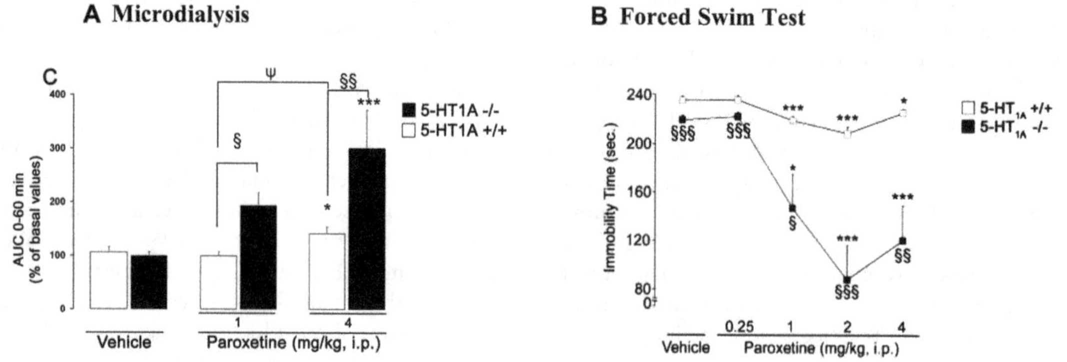

FIGURE 3 | (A) Microdialysis data showing the effects of paroxetine on cortical 5-HText in 5-$HT_{1A}{}^{+/+}$ wild-type and 5-$HT_{1A}{}^{-/-}$ mice. Results are expressed as AUC values (means ± SEM) calculated for the amount of 5-HText collected during the 0–60 min post-treatment period. **(B)** Antidepressant-like effects of paroxetine on the immobility time in the mouse forced swimming test (FST) in 5-$HT_{1A}{}^{+/+}$ and 5-$HT_{1A}{}^{-/-}$ mice. FST and microdialysis experiments have been performed separately. Microdialysis and behavioral experiments were carried out by using the same experimental protocol. The duration time of the FST was 6 min, performed at the maximum effect of paroxetine on dialysate 5-HText, i.e., 30 min after its administration (from Guilloux et al., 2006). **(A)** $^{*}p < 0.05$; $^{***}p < 0.001$ when compared to the appropriate vehicle-treated group; $^{\S}p < 0.05$; $^{\S\S}p < 0.01$ when compared to 5-$HT_{1A}{}^{+/+}$ control mice; $^{\Psi}p < 0.05$ when compared to the paroxetine 1 mg/kg-treated group (two-way ANOVA followed by a PLSD *post hoc* *t*-test). **(B)** $^{*}p < 0.05$; $^{***}p < 0.001$ when compared to the appropriate control group; $^{\S}p < 0.05$; $^{\S\S}p < 0.01$; $^{\S\S\S}p < 0.001$ when compared to 5-$HT_{1A}{}^{+/+}$ mice. Statistical analysis was carried out using a two-way ANOVA followed by Fisher's PLSD *post hoc* *t*-test.

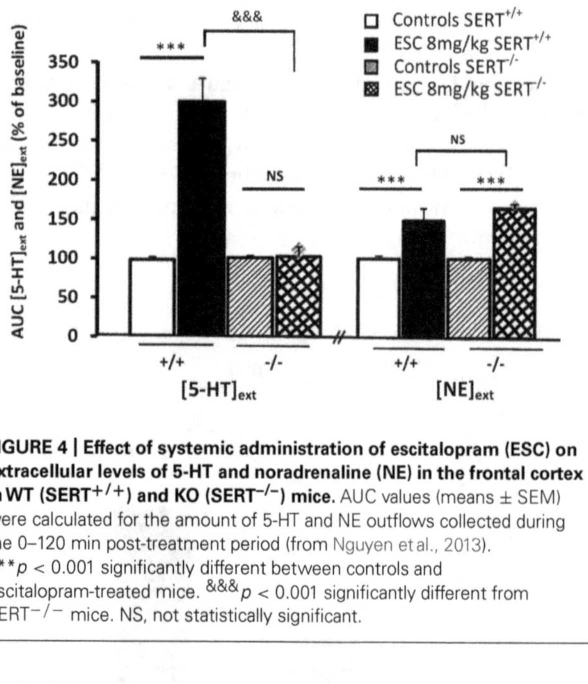

FIGURE 4 | Effect of systemic administration of escitalopram (ESC) on extracellular levels of 5-HT and noradrenaline (NE) in the frontal cortex in WT ($SERT^{+/+}$) and KO ($SERT^{-/-}$) mice. AUC values (means ± SEM) were calculated for the amount of 5-HT and NE outflows collected during the 0–120 min post-treatment period (from Nguyen et al., 2013). $^{***}p < 0.001$ significantly different between controls and escitalopram-treated mice. $^{\&\&\&}p < 0.001$ significantly different from $SERT^{-/-}$ mice. NS, not statistically significant.

LIMITATIONS

There are also limits regarding the use of constitutive KO mice. Compensatory events may occur when mice are generated by homologous recombination (Gardier, 2009). For example, 5-HT_{1B} receptor KO mice exhibit a higher efficacy of 8-OH-DPAT-induced hypothermia suggesting that an adaptive thermoregulatory process involving the functional activity of somatodendritic 5-HT_{1A} receptors is altered in 5-HT_{1B} receptor KO mice (Gardier et al., 2001). By contrast, Bouwknecht et al. (2002) found no indications for adaptive changes in pre-synaptic 5-HT_{1A} receptor function in 5-HT_{1B} receptor KO mice as measured telemetrically on body temperature and heart rate responses.

Indeed, to study the direct consequences of alterations in the targeted gene, constitutive KO mice are very valuable tools because of compensatory processes that have taken place in reaction to life-long changes in gene expression (Groenink et al., 2003). The constitutive deletion of the NET, for example, induced an up-regulation of two other monoamine transporters DAT and SERT (Solich et al., 2011). An increase in the binding of [^{3}H]paroxetine to the SERT and [^{3}H]GBR-12935 to the DAT was observed in various brain regions of NET-KO mice, without alterations of mRNA encoding these transporters, as measured by in situ hybridization. This important finding obviously impacts the interpretation of previous data. Similarly, in $SERT^{-/-}$ mice, Zhou et al. (2002) reported that 5-HT was found in DA neurons of homozygous (−/−), but not of heterozygous (+/−) mutant mice. DA neurons containing 5-HT have been observed in the substantia nigra and ventral tegmental area (VTA), but not in other brain areas of $SERT^{-/-}$ mice. To verify the role of the DA transporter in such ectopic uptake, $SERT^{-/-}$ mice were treated with DA uptake blocker GBR-12935: ectopic 5-HT in DA neurons was disappeared. These data indicate that 5-HT can be taken into DA neurons in rodents when SERT is not functionally adequate to remove extracellular 5-HT levels, and (c) the DA transporter is responsible for the 5-HT uptake into DA neurons. Thus, cross neuronal type uptake exists and serves as a compensatory backup when a specific transporter is dysfunctional. Thus, when using mice lacking an important protein from the earliest period of their existence, one has to be aware that compensatory alterations may occur in the brain as well as at the periphery. This point must be considered when it comes to interpretation of the experimental results.

Table 1 summarizes the main advantages as well as some critical points of the intracerebral microdialysis technique.

CONCLUSION

These past 25 years, different strains of KO mice became extremely valuable tools in Neuropharmacology. They help to identify in

Table 1 | Summary of the main advantages and some critical points of the intracerebral microdialysis technique in freely moving mice.

Main advantages of using microdialysis in WT and KO mice*	Some limitations of using microdialysis in WT and KO mice
– *In vivo* pre-synaptic test to study consequences of autoreceptor of transporter blockade on release and reuptake of neurotransmitters. – Direct access of exogenous molecules into the brain tissue, with minimal damage: an ideal approach to confirm brain effects observed following a systemic administration. Even more interesting when the drug does not cross easily the blood brain barrier [such as molecules with a high molecular weight: neurotrophic factors, e.g., BDNF (Benmansour et al., 2008; Deltheil et al., 2009); substance P (Guiard et al., 2007)] – *To validate the KO animal model: – *Possibility to implant two probes in the same mouse: a probe at the vicinity of cell bodies (e.g., raphe nuclei when studying the neuronal 5-HT system), and a probe at serotonergic nerve terminals (hippocampus, frontal cortex), thus evaluating a neural circuit – *Possibility of measuring several neurotransmitters in the same dialysate sample of WT and KO mice (Nguyen et al., 2013). – *The same of WT or KO mouse can be studied for two consecutive days, e.g., on day 1 following administration of the vehicle in the control group, and on day 2 following the novel pharmacological treatment – *Chronic microdialysis: when using a guide cannula, it is possible to collect samples once a week for several weeks in the same WT or KO mouse (Popa et al., 2010) – When applied in awake, freely moving animals, functional consequences of SSRI-induced increases in extracellular neurotransmitter levels can be studied, e.g., correlation between changes in brain 5-HText and behavioral data (the swimming time in the FST, for example (Deltheil et al., 2009; Nguyen et al., 2013)	– Compared to electrophysiology, technique of reference: o Large outer diameter of microdialysis probe (0.2 mm) o During microdialysis experiments, the samples are collected every 15–20 min (in the hippocampus and frontal cortex), every 10 min in raphe nuclei. This is due to the slow flow rate of the perfusion medium (≈ 1 μl/min), which leads to a poor temporal resolution compared to electrophysiology (400 ms) – Time consuming: o One experimenter, two mice, 1 day; 10–12 animals per group; delayed results (HPLC). Possible improvement with more sensitive analytical methods such as capillary electrophoresis coupled to a laser-induced fluorescence detection (Parrot et al., 2007; Denoroy et al., 2008), but it remains a very complex technique. o 3–6 months to complete an experiment, i.e., to evaluate the effects of several doses of an agonist-antagonist compared to mice treated with the vehicle or in WT controls. Even longer when using Tg or KO mice (breeding, genotyping, selection of age, sex, and so on...). – Delicate animal handling, to avoid effects of stress, thus requiring an experienced experimenter to perform *in vivo* microdialysis in freely moving mice. – Absolute need to check the exact location of the probe, macroscopically on brain coronal sections at the end of the experiment. Especially in mice (Bert et al., 2004) – Poor prognostic value of *basal* extracellular concentrations of 5-HT, DA, and NA. – Extracellular concentrations of metabolites in dialysates (e.g., 5-HIAA, the main metabolite of 5-HT): o *Under basal conditions*: it reflects intracellular metabolism of 5-HT (MAO A activity), and not its release or utilization (Wolf et al., 1985; Bel and Artigas, 1996) o *Following pharmacological treatment:* it has little interest because dialysate 5-HIAA levels decrease, independently of the dose of the indirect 5-HT receptor agonist administered. These changes are not related to the neuronal activity (Malagié et al., 1995; Rocher et al., 1996).

**Some advantages of this technique are very interesting in KO mice knowing the difficulties to breed most of them.*

animals susceptibility genes and proteins involved in the pathological processes leading to anxiety and depression. These biological markers could then be helpful to pose the diagnosis of the disease in human. They also give information on their functional role, thus offering opportunities to develop new drug treatments. When performed in KO mice, and together with other techniques, brain microdialysis was very useful to define central monoaminergic dysfunctions having behavioral consequences similar to those associated with endogenous depression in humans. Some KO mice with mutations of serotonin targets (e.g., the 5-HT transporter SERT, 5-HT_{1B}, 5-HT_{1A}, and 5-HT4 receptors) display changes in phenotypes similar to those induced by chronic treatment with antidepressants in WT control mice.

Chronic antidepressant treatment may regulate the expression of neurotrophic factors such as BDNF and stimulate the process of adult neurogenesis in the dentate gyrus of the hippocampus in rats (Malberg et al., 2000) and adult mice (Santarelli et al., 2003; David et al., 2009). Changes in adult neurogenesis are only seen after chronic, but not acute, antidepressant treatment. Microdialysis studies in heterozygous mice for BDNF (Szapacs et al., 2004; Deltheil et al., 2008, 2009; Guiard et al., 2008) contributed to this knowledge by exploring the relationship between the hippocampal 5-HT system (i.e., the function of its transporter, one of the main targets of antidepressants) and brain BDNF levels.

In the future, our efforts to understand the pathophysiology of mood disorders, especially anxiety/depression, will focus on the antidepressant responses, especially in non-stressed and stressed rodents. Microdialysis technique in young or adult KO mice will continue to decipher region-dependent relationships between brain neurotransmitters and circuits involved in the mechanism of action of an antidepressant drugs' polytherapy, soon available on the market. Furthermore, original strategies are now available to rescue the expression of a particular receptor subtype in a tissue-specific and temporally controlled manner in mice. For example, it is well known that agonists of the 5-HT_{1A} receptor such as buspirone have anxiolytic properties, and KO mice lacking this receptor show increased anxiety-like behavior (as indicated above). However, the relevant brain regions involved in anxious phenotype have not been delineated. Using such a tissue-specific, conditional rescue strategy for the 5-HT_{1A} receptor, Gross et al. (2002) engineered mice in which the expression of the 5-HT_{1A} receptor gene was under the control of the antibiotic doxycycline. The gene of interest was switched off when the mice were fed with the antibiotic. They used autoradiography to demonstrate that high levels of post-synaptic 5-HT_{1A} receptor expression in the hippocampus and cortex of the rescue mice, but the pre-synaptic 5-HT_{1A} autoreceptor, was undetectable in the raphe nuclei. By using mice in which the 5-HT_{1A} receptor can be knocked out at will, they show that the absence of the receptor in newborns lead to anxiety-like behavior, whereas its knock-out during adult life has no effect. In addition, they found that postnatal developmental processes help to establish adult anxiety-like behavior. Generating such a rescue mice is a long-lasting process, but each animal can be used as its own control.

Another strategy can be used to rescue a gene of interest, in which the KO mice line previously generated was used as the control group. A gene of interest is re-expressed into the midbrain of KO mice by stereotaxically injecting a lentiviral vector carrying this gene coding for a receptor to test for the selectivity of behavioral effects. This strategy was recently applied to study the role of beta2-subunit of the nicotinic acetylcholine receptor (nAChR; Maskos et al., 2005) in mediating the reinforcement properties of nicotine. In this example, microdialysis experiments were performed to confirm the rescue of nicotine effects in the vectorized line of mice compared to WT and KO lines. Regarding the serotonin field of research, global disruption of 5-HT2A receptor signaling in mice reduces inhibition in conflict anxiety paradigms without affecting depression-related behaviors. Selective rescue of 5-HT2A receptor in the cortex normalized conflict anxiety behaviors (Weisstaub et al., 2006). These findings indicate a specific role for cortical 5-HT2A receptors in the modulation of anxiety. These techniques allow greater precision and flexibility to generate KO rodents for understanding neurotransmitter function. No doubt that such novel and powerful tools, together with techniques of knock-in or SiRNA recently applied to the field of 5-HT receptors, will continue to give unexpected information on molecular and cellular mechanisms involved in mood disorders and their treatments.

REFERENCES

Artigas, F., Adell, A., and Celada, P. (2006). Pindolol augmentation of antidepressant response. *Curr. Drug Targets* 7, 139–147. doi: 10.2174/138945006775515446

Beaulieu, J. M., Marion, S., Rodriguiz, R. M., Medvedev, I. O., Sotnikova, T. D., Ghisi, V., et al. (2008). A beta-arrestin 2 signaling complex mediates lithium action on behavior. *Cell* 132, 125–136. doi: 10.1016/j.cell.2007.11.041

Bel, N., and Artigas, F. (1996). Reduction of serotonergic function in rat brain by tryptophan depletion: effects in control and fluvoxamine-treated rats. *J. Neurochem.* 67, 669–676. doi: 10.1046/j.1471-4159.1996.67020669.x

Bengel, D., Murphy, D. L., Andrews, A. M., Wichems, C. H., Feltner, D., Heils, A., et al. (1998). Altered brain serotonin homeostasis and locomotor insensitivity to 3, 4-methylenedioxymethamphetamine ("Ecstasy") in serotonin transporter-deficient mice. *Mol. Pharmacol.* 53, 649–655.

Benmansour, S., Deltheil, T., Piotrowski, J., Nicolas, L., Reperant, C., Gardier, A. M., et al. (2008). Influence of brain-derived neurotrophic factor (BDNF) on serotonin neurotransmission in the hippocampus of adult rodents. *Eur. J. Pharmacol.* 587, 90–98. doi: 10.1016/j.ejphar.2008.03.048

Benmansour, S., Owens, W. A., Cecchi, M., Morilak, D. A., and Frazer, A. (2002). Serotonin clearance in vivo is altered to a greater extent by antidepressant-induced downregulation of the serotonin transporter than by acute blockade of this transporter. *J. Neurosci.* 22, 6766–6772.

Bert, L., Favale, D., Jego, G., Greve, P., Guilloux, J.-P., Guiard, B. P., et al. (2004). Rapid and precise method to locate microdialysis probe implantation in the rodent brain. *J. Neurosci. Methods* 140, 53–57. doi: 10.1016/j.jneumeth.2004.04.042

Blier, P. (2001). Pharmacology of rapid-onset antidepressant treatment strategies. *J. Clin. Psychiatry* 15, 12–17.

Blier, P. (2010). Altered function of the serotonin 1A autoreceptor and the antidepressant response. *Neuron* 65, 1–2. doi: 10.1016/j.neuron.2009.12.028

Blier, P., de Montigny, C., and Azzaro, A. J. (1986). Modification of serotonergic and noradrenergic neurotransmissions by repeated administration of monoamine oxidase inhibitors: electrophysiological studies in the rat central nervous system. *J. Pharmacol. Exp. Ther.* 237, 987–994.

Blier, P., de Montigny, C., and Chaput, Y. (1987). Modifications of the serotonin system by antidepressant treatments: implications for the therapeutic response in major depression. *J. Clin. Psychopharmacol.* 7(Suppl.), 24S–35S.

Bortolozzi, A., Amargós-Bosch, M., Toth, M., Artigas, F., and Adell, A. (2004). In vivo efflux of serotonin in the dorsal raphe nucleus of 5-HT1A receptor knockout mice. *J. Neurochem.* 88, 1373–1379.

Bortolozzi, A., Castañé, A., Semakova, J., Santana, N., Alvarado, G., Cortés, R., et al. (2012). New antidepressant strategy based on acute siRNA silencing of 5-HT(1A) autoreceptors. *Mol. Psychiatry* 17, 567. doi: 10.1038/mp.2012.52

Bouwknecht, J. A., Hijzen, T. H., van der Gugten, J., Maes, R. A., Hen, R., and Olivier, B. (2002). 5-HT(1B) receptor knockout mice show no adaptive changes in 5-HT(1A) receptor function as measured telemetrically on body temperature and heart rate responses. *Brain Res. Bull.* 57, 93–102. doi: 10.1016/S0361-9230(01)00640-2

Chaput, Y., Blier, P., and de Montigny, C. (1986). In vivo electrophysiological evidence for the regulatory role of autoreceptors on serotoninergic terminals. *J. Neurosci.* 6, 2796–2801.

Chen, Z. Y., Jing, D., Bath, K. G., Ieraci, A., Khan, T., Siao, C. J., et al. (2006). Genetic variant BDNF (Val66Met) polymorphism alters anxiety-related behavior. *Science* 314, 140–143. doi: 10.1126/science.1129663

David, D. J., Bourin, M., Jego, G., Przybylski, C., Jolliet, P., and Gardier, A. M. (2003). Effects of acute treatment with paroxetine, citalopram and venlafaxine in vivo on noradrenaline and serotonin outflow: a microdialysis study in Swiss mice. *Br. J. Pharmacol.* 140, 1128–1136. doi: 10.1038/sj.bjp.0705538

David, D. J., Froger, N., Guiard, B., Przybylski, C., Jego, G., Boni, C., et al. (2004). Serotonin transporter in substance P (neurokinin 1) receptor knock-out mice. *Eur. J. Pharmacol.* 492, 41–48. doi: 10.1016/j.ejphar.2004.03.016

David, D. J., Samuels, B. A., Rainer, Q., Wang, J. W., Marsteller, D., Mendez, I., et al. (2009). Neurogenesis-dependent and -independent effects of fluoxetine in an animal model of anxiety/depression. *Neuron* 62, 479–493. doi: 10.1016/j.neuron.2009.04.017

David, D. J., Wang, J., Samuels, B. A., Rainer, Q., David, I., Gardier, A. M., et al. (2010). Implications of the functional integration of adult-born hippocampal neurons in anxiety-depression disorders. *Neuroscientist* 16, 578–591. doi: 10.1177/1073858409360281

Delgado, J. M., DeFeudis, F. V., Roth, R. H., Ryugo, D. K., and Mitruka, B. M. (1972). Dialytrode for long term intracerebral perfusion in awake monkeys. *Arch. Int. Pharmacodyn. Ther.* 198, 9–21

Deltheil, T., Guiard, B. P., Cerdan, J., David, D. J., Tanaka, K. F., Repérant, C., et al. (2008). Behavioral and serotonergic consequences of decreasing or increasing hippocampus brain-derived neurotrophic factor protein levels in mice. *Neuropharmacology* 55, 1006–1014. doi: 10.1016/j.neuropharm.2008 08.001

Deltheil, T., Tanaka, K., Reperant, C., Hen, R., David, D. J., and Gardier, A. M. (2009). Synergistic neurochemical and behavioural effects of acute intrahippocampal injection of brain-derived neurotrophic factor and antidepressants in adult mice. *Int. J. Neuropsychopharmacol.* 12, 905–915. doi: 10.1017/S1461145709000017

Denoroy, L., Parrot, S., Renaud, L., Renaud, B., and Zimmer, L. (2008). In-capillary derivatization and capillary electrophoresis separation of amino acid neurotransmitters from brain microdialysis samples. *J. Chromatogr. A* 1205, 144–149. doi: 10.1016/j.chroma.2008.07.043

El Mansari, M., Sánchez, C., Chouvet, G., Renaud, B., and Haddjeri, N. (2005). Effects of acute and long-term administration of escitalopram and citalopram on serotonin neurotransmission: an in vivo electrophysiological study in rat brain. *Neuropsychopharmacology* 30, 1269–1277. doi: 10.1038/sj.npp.1300686

Froger, N., Gardier, A. M., Moratalla, R., Alberti, I., Lena, I., Boni, C., et al. (2001). 5-hydroxytryptamine (5-HT)1A autoreceptor adaptive changes in substance P (neurokinin 1) receptor knock-out mice mimic antidepressant-induced desensitization. *J. Neurosci.* 21, 8188–8197.

Gainetdinov, R. R., Fumagalli, F., Jones, S. R., and Caron, M. G. (1997). Dopamine transporter is required for in vivo MPTP neurotoxicity: evidence from mice lacking the transporter. *J. Neurochem.* 69, 1322–1325. doi: 10.1046/j.1471-4159.1997.69031322.x

Gardier, A., Malagié, I., Trillat, A.-C., Jacquot, C., and Artigas, F. (1996). Role of 5-HT1A autoreceptors in the mechanism of action of serotoninergic antidepressant drugs: recent findings from in vivo microdialysis studies. *Fundam. Clin. Pharmacol.* 10, 16–27.

Gardier, A. M. (2009). Mutant mouse models and antidepressant drug research: focus on serotonin and brain-derived neurotrophic factor. *Behav. Pharmacol.* 20, 18–32. doi: 10.1097/FBP.0b013e3283243fcd

Gardier, A. M., David, D. J., Jego, G., Przybylski, C., Jacquot, C., Durier, S., et al. (2003). Effects of chronic paroxetine treatment on dialysate serotonin in 5-HT1B receptor knockout mice. *J. Neurochem.* 86, 13–24. doi: 10.1046/j.1471-4159.2003.01827.x

Gardier, A. M., Trillat, A. C., Malagié, I., David, D., Hascoët, M., Colombel, M. C., et al. (2001). 5-HT1B serotonin receptors and antidepressant effects of selective serotonin reuptake inhibitors. *C. R. Acad. Sci. III* 324, 433–441.

Gorman, J. M., and Coplan, J. D. (1996). Comorbid depression and anxiety spectrum disorders. *J. Clin. Psychiatry* 57, 34–41.

Groenink, L., Pattij, T., De Jongh, R., Van der Gugten, J., Oosting, R. S., Dirks, A., et al. (2003). 5-HT1A receptor knockout mice and mice overexpressing corticotropin-releasing hormone in models of anxiety. *Eur. J. Pharmacol.* 463, 185–197. doi: 10.1016/S0014-2999(03) 01281-0

Gross, C., Zhuang, X., Stark, K., Ramboz, S., Oosting, R., Kirby, L., et al. (2002). Serotonin1A receptor acts during development to establish normal anxiety-like behaviour in the adult. *Nature* 416, 396–400. doi: 10.1038/416396a

Guiard, B. P., David, D. J., Deltheil, T., Chenu, F., Le Maître, E., Renoir, T., et al. (2008). Brain-derived neurotrophic factor-deficient mice exhibit a hippocampal hyperserotonergic phenotype. *Int. J. Neuropsychopharmacol.* 11, 79–92.

Guiard, B. P., Guilloux, J. P., Reperant, C., Hunt, S. P., Toth, M., and Gardier, A. M. (2007). Substance P neurokinin 1 receptor activation within the dorsal raphe nucleus controls serotonin release in the mouse frontal cortex. *Mol. Pharmacol.* 72, 1411–1418. doi: 10.1124/mol.107.040113

Guiard, B. P., Przybylski, C., Guilloux, J. P., Seif, I., Froger, N., De Felipe, C., et al. (2004). Blockade of substance P (neurokinin 1) receptors enhances extracellular serotonin when combined with a selective serotonin reuptake inhibitor: an in vivo microdialysis study in mice. *J. Neurochem.* 89, 54–63. doi: 10.1046/j.1471-4159.2003.02304.x

Guilloux, J. P., David, D. J., Guiard, B. P., Chenu, F., Repérant, C., Toth, M., et al. (2006). Blockade of 5-HT1A receptors by (+/−)-pindolol potentiates cortical 5-HT outflow, but not antidepressant-like activity of paroxetine: microdialysis and behavioral approaches in 5-HT1A receptor knockout mice. *Neuropsychopharmacology* 31, 2162–2172. doi: 10.1038/sj.npp.1301019

Guilloux, J. P., David, D. J., Xia, L., Nguyen, H. T., Rainer, Q., Guiard, B. P., et al. (2011). Characterization of 5-HT(1A/1B)$^{-/-}$ mice: an animal model sensitive to anxiolytic treatments. *Neuropharmacology* 61, 478–488. doi: 10.1016/j.neuropharm.2011.02.009

Heisler, L. K., Chu, H. M., Brennan, T. J., Danao, J. A., Bajwa, P., Parsons, L. H., et al. (1998). Elevated anxiety and antidepressant-like responses in serotonin 5-HT1A receptor mutant mice. *Proc. Natl. Acad. Sci. U.S.A.* 95, 15049–15054. doi: 10.1073/pnas.95.25.15049

Hrdina, P. D., Foy, B., Hepner, A., and Summers, R. J. (1990). Antidepressant binding sites in brain: autoradiographic comparison of [3H]paroxetine and [3H]imipramine localization and relationship to serotonin transporter. *J. Pharmacol. Exp. Ther.* 252, 410–418.

Invernizzi, R. W. (2007). Role of TPH-2 in brain function: news from behavioral and pharmacologic studies. *J. Neurosci. Res.* 85, 3030–3035. doi: 10.1002/jnr.21330

Kuzelova, H., Ptacek, R., and Macek, M. (2010). The serotonin transporter gene (5-HTT) variant and psychiatric disorders: review of current literature. *Neuro Endocrinol. Lett.* 31, 4–10.

Lemonde, S., Turecki, G., Bakish, D., Du, L., Hrdina, P. D., Bown, C. D., et al. (2003). Impaired repression at a 5-hydroxytryptamine 1A receptor gene polymorphism associated with major depression and suicide. *J. Neurosci.* 23, 8788–8799.

Leonardo, E. D., and Hen, R. (2006). Genetics of affective and anxiety disorders. *Annu. Rev. Psychol.* 57, 117–137. doi: 10.1146/annurev.psych.57.102904.190118

Malagié, I., Trillat, A. C., Bourin, M., Jacquot, C., Hen, R., and Gardier, A. M. (2001). 5-HT1B Autoreceptors limit the effects of selective serotonin re-uptake inhibitors in mouse hippocampus and frontal cortex. *J. Neurochem.* 76, 865–871.

Malagié, I., Trillat, A. C., Douvier, E., Anmella, M. C., Dessalles, M. C., Jacquot, C., et al. (1996). Regional differences in the effect of the combined treatment of WAY 100635 and fluoxetine: an in vivo microdialysis study. *Naunyn Schmiedebergs Arch. Pharmacol.* 354, 785–790.

Malagié, I., Trillat, A. C., Jacquot, C., and Gardier, A. M. (1995). Effects of acute fluoxetine on extracellular serotonin levels in the raphe: an in vivo microdialysis study. *Eur. J. Pharmacol.* 286, 213–217. doi: 10.1016/0014-2999(95)00573-4

Malberg, J. E., Eisch, A. J., Nestler, E. J., and Duman, R. S. (2000). Chronic antidepressant treatment increases neurogenesis in adult rat hippocampus. *J. Neurosci.* 20, 9104–9110.

Maskos, U., Molles, B. E., Pons, S., Besson, M., Guiard, B. P., Guilloux, J. P., et al. (2005). Nicotine reinforcement and cognition restored by targeted expression of nicotinic receptors. *Nature* 436, 103–107. doi: 10.1038/nature03694

Nakahara, D., Hashiguti, H., Kaneda, N., Sasaoka, T., and Nagatsu, T. (1993). Normalization of tyrosine hydroxylase activity in vivo in the striatum of transgenic mice carrying human tyrosine hydroxylase gene: a microdialysis study. *Neurosci. Lett.* 158, 44–46. doi: 10.1016/0304-3940(93)90608-N

Nguyen, H. T., Guiard, B. P., Bacq, A., David, D. J., David, I., Quesseveur, G., et al. (2013). Blockade of the high-affinity norepinephrine transporter (NET) by the selective serotonin reuptake inhibitor escitalopram: an in vivo microdialysis study in mice. *Br. J. Pharmacol.* 168, 103–116. doi: 10.1111/j.1476-5381.2012.01850.x

Parks, C. L., Robinson, P. S., Sibille, E., Shenk, T., and Toth, M. (1998). Increased anxiety of mice lacking the serotonin1A receptor. *Proc. Natl. Acad. Sci. U.S.A.* 95, 10734–10739. doi: 10.1073/pnas.95.18.10734

Parrot, S., Lambás-Señas, L., Sentenac, S., Denoroy, L., and Renaud, B. (2007). Highly sensitive assay for the measurement of serotonin in microdialysates using capillary high-performance liquid chromatography with electrochemical detection. *J. Chromatogr. B Analyt. Technol. Biomed. Life Sci.* 850, 303–309.

Parsons, L. H., Smith, A. D., and Justice, J. B. Jr. (1991). Basal extracellular dopamine is decreased in the rat nucleus accumbens during abstinence from chronic cocaine. *Synapse* 9, 60–65. doi: 10.1002/syn.890090109

Paxinos, G., and Franklin, K. B. J. (2001). *The Mouse Brain in Stereotaxic Coordinates*, 2nd Edn. San Diego, CA: Academic Press.

Pineyro, G., Blier, P., Dennis, T., and de Montigny, C. (1994). Desensitization of the neuronal 5-HT carrier following its long-term blockade. *J. Neurosci.* 14, 3036–3047.

Pineyro, G., Castanon, N., Hen, R., and Blier, P. (1995). Regulation of [3H]5-HT release in raphe, frontal cortex and hippocampus of 5-HT1B knock-out mice. *Neuroreport* 7, 353–359.

Popa, D., Cerdan, J., Repérant, C., Guiard, B. P., Guilloux, J. P., David, D. J., et al. (2010). A longitudinal study of 5-HT outflow during chronic fluoxetine treatment using a new technique of chronic microdialysis in a highly emotional mouse strain. *Eur. J. Pharmacol.* 628, 83–90. doi: 10.1016/j.ejphar.2009.11.037

Porsolt, R. D., Le Pichon, M., and Jalfre, M. (1977). Depression: a new animal model sensitive to antidepressant treatments. *Nature* 266, 730–732. doi: 10.1038/266730a0

Portella, M. J., de Diego-Adeliño, J., Ballesteros, J., Puigdemont, D., Oller, S., Santosv, B., et al. (2011). Can we really accelerate and enhance the selective serotonin reuptake inhibitor antidepressant effect? A randomized clinical trial and a meta-analysis of pindolol in nonresistant depression. *J. Clin. Psychiatry* 72, 962–969. doi: 10.4088/JCP.09m05827blu

Ramboz, S., Oosting, R., Amara, D. A., Kung, H. F., Blier, P., Mendelsohn, M., et al. (1998). Serotonin receptor 1A knockout: an animal model of anxiety-related disorder. *Proc. Natl. Acad. Sci. U.S.A.* 95, 14476–14481. doi: 10.1073/pnas.95.24.14476

Reperant, C., Pons, S., Dufour, E., Rollema, H., Gardier, A. M., and Maskos, U. (2010). Effect of the alpha4beta2* nicotinic acetylcholine receptor partial agonist varenicline on dopamine release in beta2 knockout mice with selective re-expression of the beta2 subunit in the ventral tegmental area. *Neuropharmacology* 58, 346–350. doi: 10.1016/j.neuropharm.2009.10.007

Richardson-Jones, J. W., Craige, C. P., Guiard, B. P., Stephen, A., Metzger, K. L., Kung, H. F., et al. (2010). 5-HT1A autoreceptor levels determine vulnerability to stress and response to antidepressants. *Neuron* 65, 40–52. doi: 10.1016/j.neuron.2009.12.003

Richardson-Jones, J. W., Craige, C. P., Nguyen, T. H., Kung, H. F., Gardier, A. M., Dranovsky, A., et al. (2011). Serotonin-1A autoreceptors are necessary and sufficient for the normal formation of circuits underlying innate anxiety. *J. Neurosci.* 31, 6008–6018. doi: 10.1523/JNEUROSCI.5836-10.2011

Rocher, C., Bert, L., Robert, F., Renaud, B., Jacquot, C., and Gardier, A. M. (1996). Microdialysis monitoring of variations in extracellular levels of serotonin, GABA and excitatory amino acids in the frontal cortex of awake rats in response to a single peripheral or central administration of dexfenfluramine. *Brain Res.* 737, 221–230. doi: 10.1016/0006-8993(96)00735-4

Romero, L., Hervas, I., and Artigas, F. (1996). The 5-HT1A antagonist WAY-100635 selectively potentiates the presynaptic effects of serotonergic antidepressants in rat brain. *Neurosci. Lett.* 219, 123–126. doi: 10.1016/S0304-3940(96)13199-2

Rutter, J. J., Gundlah, C., and Auerbach, S. B. (1995). Systemic uptake inhibition decreases serotonin release via somatodendritic autoreceptor activation. *Synapse* 20, 225–233. doi: 10.1002/syn.890200306

Santarelli, L., Saxe, M., Gross, C., Surget, A., Battaglia, F., Dulawa, S., et al. (2003). Requirement of hippocampal neurogenesis for the behavioral effects of antidepressants. *Science* 301, 805–809. doi: 10.1126/science.1083328

Saudou, F., Amara, D. A., Dierich, A., LeMeur, M., Ramboz, S., Segu, L., et al. (1994). Enhanced aggressive behavior in mice lacking 5-HT1B receptor. *Science* 265, 1875–1878. doi: 10.1126/science.8091214

Silva, A. J., Paylor, R., Wehner, J. M., and Tonegawa, S. (1992). Impaired spatial learning in alpha-calcium-calmodulin kinase II mutant mice. *Science* 257, 206–211. doi: 10.1126/science.1321493

Solich, J., Faron-Gorecka, A., Kusmider, M., Palach, P., Gaska, M., and Dziedzicka-Wasylewska, M. (2011). Norepinephrine transporter (NET) knock-out upregulates dopamine and serotonin transporters in the mouse brain. *Neurochem. Int.* 59, 185–191. doi: 10.1016/j.neuint.2011.04.012

Sotnikova, T. D., and Gainetdinov, R. R. (2007). "Microdialysis in genetically altered animals," in *Handbook of Microdialysis: Methods, Applications and Clinical Aspects*, Vol. 16, eds B. H. C. Westerink and T. F. H. Cremers (Amsterdam: Academic Press), 399–417.

Steru, L., Chermat, R., Thierry, B., and Simon, P. (1985). The tail suspension test: a new method for screening antidepressants in mice. *Psychopharmacology (Berl.)* 85, 367–370. doi: 10.1007/BF00428203

Szapacs, M. E., Mathews, T. A., Tessarollo, L., Ernest Lyons, W., Mamounas, L. A., and Andrews, A. M. (2004). Exploring the relationship between serotonin and brain-derived neurotrophic factor: analysis of BDNF protein and extraneuronal 5-HT in mice with reduced serotonin transporter or BDNF expression. *J. Neurosci. Methods* 140, 81–92. doi: 10.1016/j.jneumeth.2004.03.026

Trillat, A. C., Malagié, I., Scearce, K., Pons, D., Jacquot, C., Hen, R., et al. (1997). Regulation of serotonin release in the frontal cortex and ventral hippocampus of homozygous mice lacking 5-HT1B receptors: in vivo microdialysis studies. *J. Neurochem.* 69, 2019–2025.

Weisstaub, N. V., Zhou, M., Lira, A., Lambe, E., Gonzalez-Maeso, J., Hornung, J. P., et al. (2006). Cortical 5-HT2A receptor signaling modulates anxiety-like behaviors in mice. *Science* 313, 536–540. doi: 10.1126/science.1123432

Wolf, W. A., Youdim, M. B., and Kuhn, D. M. (1985). Does brain 5-HIAA indicate serotonin release or monoamine oxidase activity? *Eur. J. Pharmacol.* 109, 381–387. doi: 10.1016/0014-2999(85)90399-1

Zetterström, T., Sharp, T., Marsden, C. A., and Ungerstedt, U. (1983). In vivo measurement of dopamine and its metabolites by intracerebral dialysis: changes after d-amphetamine. *J Neurochem.* 41, 1769–1773.

Zhou, F. C., Lesch, K. P., and Murphy, D. L. (2002). Serotonin uptake into dopamine neurons via dopamine transporters: a compensatory alternative. *Brain Res.* 942, 109–119. doi: 10.1016/S0006-8993(02)02709-9

Conflict of Interest Statement: H. Lundbeck A/S, supported the preclinical study with escitalopram.

2

Conservation of 5-HT_{1A} receptor-mediated autoinhibition of serotonin (5-HT) neurons in mice with altered 5-HT homeostasis

Naozumi Araragi[1]*[†], Boris Mlinar[2], Gilda Baccini[2], Lise Gutknecht[3], Klaus-Peter Lesch[1] and Renato Corradetti[2]

[1] Division of Molecular Psychiatry, Laboratory of Translational Neuroscience, Department of Psychiatry, Psychosomatics, and Psychotherapy, University of Wuerzburg, Wuerzburg, Germany
[2] Department of NEUROFARBA (Department of Neuroscience, Psychology, Drug Research and Child Health), University of Florence, Florence, Italy
[3] Department of Neurobiology, Institute of Functional Genomics, National Center for Scientific Research (UMR 5203), INSERM U661, University of Montpellier I and II, Montpellier, France

Edited by:
Laurence Lanfumey, Institut National de la Santé et de la Recherche Médicale, France

Reviewed by:
Heather Hain, PsychoGenics, Inc., USA
Laurence Lanfumey, Institut National de la Santé et de la Recherche Médicale, France

***Correspondence:**
Naozumi Araragi, Division of Molecular Psychiatry, Laboratory of Translational Neuroscience, Department of Psychiatry, Psychosomatics, and Psychotherapy, University of Wuerzburg, Fuechsleinstrasse 15, 97080 Wuerzburg, Germany
e-mail: naozumi.araragi@uni-wuerzburg.de

[†]Present address:
Naozumi Araragi, Experimental Neurosurgery, Department of Neurosurgery, University of Wuerzburg, Josef-Schneider-Strasse 11, 97080 Wuerzburg, Germany

Firing activity of serotonin (5-HT) neurons in the dorsal raphe nucleus (DRN) is controlled by inhibitory somatodendritic 5-HT_{1A} autoreceptors. This autoinhibitory mechanism is implicated in the etiology of disorders of emotion regulation, such as anxiety disorders and depression, as well as in the mechanism of antidepressant action. Here, we investigated how persistent alterations in brain 5-HT availability affect autoinhibition in two genetically modified mouse models lacking critical mediators of serotonergic transmission: 5-HT transporter knockout (*Sert−/−*) and tryptophan hydroxylase-2 knockout (*Tph2−/−*) mice. The degree of autoinhibition was assessed by loose-seal cell-attached recording in DRN slices. First, application of the 5-HT_{1A}-selective agonist R(+)-8-hydroxy-2-(di-n-propylamino)tetralin showed mild sensitization and marked desensitization of 5-HT_{1A} receptors in *Tph2−/−* mice and *Sert−/−* mice, respectively. While 5-HT neurons from *Tph2−/−* mice did not display autoinhibition in response to L-tryptophan, autoinhibition of these neurons was unaltered in *Sert−/−* mice despite marked desensitization of their 5-HT_{1A} autoreceptors. When the Tph2-dependent 5-HT synthesis step was bypassed by application of 5-hydroxy-L-tryptophan (5-HTP), neurons from both *Tph2−/−* and *Sert−/−* mice decreased their firing rates at significantly lower concentrations of 5-HTP compared to wildtype controls. Our findings demonstrate that, as opposed to the prevalent view, sensitivity of somatodendritic 5-HT_{1A} receptors does not predict the magnitude of 5-HT neuron autoinhibition. Changes in 5-HT_{1A} receptor sensitivity may rather be seen as an adaptive mechanism to keep autoinhibition functioning in response to extremely altered levels of extracellular 5-HT resulting from targeted inactivation of mediators of serotonergic signaling.

Keywords: serotonin transporter, tryptophan hydroxylase-2, knockout, dorsal raphe nucleus, autoinhibition, 5-HT_{1A} receptor

INTRODUCTION

The brain serotonin (5-HT) system has been implicated in emotion regulation and related psychopathological states, including anxiety, depression, impulsivity, and aggression (reviewed in Lesch et al., 2012). The 5-HT system originates from specified neurons located in distinct nuclei of the brainstem raphe complex. Among them, the dorsal raphe nucleus (DRN) contains the majority of 5-HT neurons and sends projections to various targets in the forebrain. 5-HT neurons in the DRN are known to exhibit spontaneous regular firing activities (Trulson and Jacobs, 1979; Vandermaelen and Aghajanian, 1983). The firing rate of 5-HT neurons is a determinant of 5-HT concentration and thus function in terminal regions, together with local mechanisms (Jacobs and Azmitia, 1992). In waking states, firing of 5-HT neurons is facilitated by noradrenergic input (Levine and Jacobs, 1992). Activity of 5-HT neurons is, in turn, limited by homeostatic negative feedback control exerted by extracellular 5-HT via somatodendritic inhibitory 5-HT_{1A} autoreceptors (Audero et al., 2008 and references therein). The role of 5-HT_{1A} receptors in suppression/regulation of 5-HT neuron firing activity is considered to be relevant to the pathophysiology of disorders of emotion regulation (Pineyro and Blier, 1999; Sharp et al., 2007). The importance of 5-HT_{1A} receptor function is further supported by the presumed mechanism of selective 5-HT reuptake inhibitor (SSRI) antidepressant action (Artigas et al., 1996; Pineyro and Blier, 1999). After acute administration of SSRI, extracellular 5-HT concentrations transiently increase and activate 5-HT_{1A} autoreceptors, inhibiting firing of 5-HT neurons. One criterion

Abbreviations: DRN, dorsal raphe nucleus; 5-HT, serotonin; 5-HTP, 5-hydroxy-L-tryptophan; R(+)-8-OH-DPAT, R(+)-8-hydroxy-2-(di-n-propylamino)tetralin; Sert, serotonin transporter; Tph2, tryptophan hydroxylase-2; Trp, L-tryptophan.

of antidepressants' therapeutic effects is desensitization of these $5\text{-}HT_{1A}$ receptors, leading to a net increase of 5-HT levels. In this context, dysfunction of autoinhibitory $5\text{-}HT_{1A}$ receptors has been proposed as a potential factor contributing to the pathogenesis of emotional disorders. However, studies on $5\text{-}HT_{1A}$ receptor expression in the raphe nuclei of patients with depression measured *in vivo* using positron emission tomography (PET) or in post-mortem brains have yielded contradictory findings: some investigators reported decreased expression (Drevets et al., 1999; Sargent et al., 2000; Arango et al., 2001; Meltzer et al., 2004), while others found enhanced expression (Stockmeier et al., 1998) or no difference compared to controls (Parsey et al., 2006). Moreover, PET imaging data revealed reduced $5\text{-}HT_{1A}$ binding in several brain regions including the raphe complex in panic disorder patients either with or without comorbid depression (Neumeister et al., 2004). To date, most studies concentrated on associations between expression levels of $5\text{-}HT_{1A}$ receptors with depressive disorders and there has been no direct evidence demonstrating how altered $5\text{-}HT_{1A}$ receptor availability translates into the extent of 5-HT neuron autoinhibition. The discrepancies among reports describing a relationship between $5\text{-}HT_{1A}$ receptor expression and depression indicate a need for better understanding of the precise mechanisms linking autoinhibition to $5\text{-}HT_{1A}$ receptor function.

Among various mediators of the brain 5-HT signaling, the 5-HT transporter (SERT, 5-HTT, SLC6A4) plays a central role because (i) it mediates the re-uptake of 5-HT from the extracellular space/synapse and thus terminates the 5-HT signaling and (ii) it is the target of numerous antidepressant drugs which inhibit its action. Carriers of the short variant (s-allele) of the transcriptional control region of the gene encoding SERT (5-HTT gene-linked polymorphic region, 5-HTTLPR), which leads to lower expression and thus a lower amount of SERT protein, are known to convey increased risk for emotional disorders in interaction with environmental factors (reviewed in Canli and Lesch, 2007). On the other hand, tryptophan hydroxylase (TPH) is the rate-limiting enzyme of 5-HT synthesis by converting the essential amino acid L-tryptophan (Trp) into 5-hydroxy-L-tryptophan (5-HTP). 5-HTP is then transformed into 5-HT by aromatic L-amino acid decarboxylase (AADC; Carlsson et al., 1972). While the first isoform TPH1 produces 5-HT in peripheral tissues and the pineal gland, the recently discovered TPH2 isoform is responsible for 5-HT synthesis in the brain (Gutknecht et al., 2009). Variation of the gene coding for TPH2 has been associated with personality traits related to emotional regulation (Gutknecht et al., 2007). Moreover, several polymorphisms in *TPH2*, which had previously been linked to mood disorders, were shown to lead to reduced expression of TPH2 (reviewed in Jacobsen et al., 2012a). Contribution of 5-HT to the regulation of emotion has been further verified by studies on mice with targeted inactivation of either *Sert* or *Tph2*. Indeed, *Sert* knockout (−/−) mice have been shown to display anxiety- and depression-like behaviors (reviewed in Murphy and Lesch, 2008). *Tph2*−/− mice have also been reported to have altered behaviors such as increased conditioned fear responses, aggression, depression-like behaviors, and impairment of maternal care (Savelieva et al., 2008; Alenina et al., 2009; Mosienko et al., 2012; for review, see Lesch et al., 2012).

Here, we investigated firing activity of DRN 5-HT neurons in brain slices obtained from *Sert*−/− mice and *Tph2*−/− mice using loose-seal cell-attached recording configuration. Compared to wildtype (*wt*) controls, *Sert*−/− mice were shown to have ~6- to 10-fold elevated extracellular 5-HT concentrations at baseline in several brain regions including the striatum and the frontal cortex, while heterozygous *Sert*+/− mice were shown to have milder increase, e.g., ~3-fold in the striatum (Fabre et al., 2000; Mathews et al., 2004; Shen et al., 2004). In contrast, *Tph2*−/− mice were reported to display an almost complete depletion of brain 5-HT, while *Tph2*+/− mice showed lower reduction in brain 5-HT, reaching 20–25% in the rostral raphe (Gutknecht et al., 2012). Both knockout mice therefore provide useful models to investigate potential modulation of autoinhibition of 5-HT neuron firing as a function of varying degrees of 5-HT availability in the cellular environment. Moreover, since both mouse lines have extensively been investigated as models for emotional disorders, investigating 5-HT neuron autoinhibitory functions in these mice will facilitate detection of potential alterations in autoinhibition related to disorders of emotion regulation.

In order to mimic *in vivo* 5-HT synthesis in *in vitro* experimental conditions, we applied 5-HT precursors through superfusion of brain slices under recording. Prior to this, we assessed the function of autoinhibitory $5\text{-}HT_{1A}$ receptors by applying their direct agonist. Feasibility of assessing autoinhibition in *in vitro* conditions had been established in previous studies (Liu et al., 2005; Mlinar et al., 2005; Evans et al., 2008; Gutknecht et al., 2012).

MATERIALS AND METHODS

ANIMALS

Animal handling followed the European Community guidelines for animal care (DL 116/92, application of the European Communities Council Directive 86/609/EEC) and approved by the local committees. The generation and genotyping procedure of *Tph2*−/− and *Sert*−/− animals were described previously (Bengel et al., 1998; Gutknecht et al., 2008). Animals were housed under a 12 h light/dark cycle (lights on: 08:00–20:00) at ambient temperature of 22 ± 1°C and a relative humidity of 40–50%. Data from *Tph2 wt* and *Sert wt* mice were treated together, since both mouse lines were backcrossed more than 10 generations into a C57BL/6J background and thus considered to have the same genetic background. Data from male and female mice were pooled.

DRUGS

SR-95531 (gabazine; $GABA_A$ receptor antagonist), D-AP5 (NMDA glutamate receptor antagonist), DNQX (AMPA/kainate receptor antagonist) were purchased from Ascent Scientific Ltd (Bristol, UK). *N*-[2-[4-(2-methoxyphenyl)-1-piperazinyl]ethyl]-*N*-2-pyridinylcyclohexanecarboxamide maleate (WAY-100635 maleate; selective $5\text{-}HT_{1A}$ receptor antagonist), CGP-55845 hydrochloride (selective $GABA_B$ receptor antagonist), and R(+)-8-hydroxy-2-(di-n-propylamino)tetralin (R(+)-8-OH-DPAT) were purchased from Tocris Bioscience (Bristol, UK). Strychnine (glycine receptor antagonist), Trp, 5-HTP, and L-phenylephrine were obtained from Sigma-Aldrich S.r.l. (Milan, Italy).

ELECTROPHYSIOLOGICAL RECORDING

Methods used follow those reported previously (Gutknecht et al., 2012). Mice (28–80 days old) were anesthetized with isoflurane and decapitated. The brain was immediately removed, dissected in ice-cold gassed (95% O_2,5% CO_2) artificial cerebrospinal fluid (ACSF) containing (in mM): 124 NaCl, 2.75 KCl, 1.25 NaH_2PO_4, 1.3 $MgCl_2$, 2 $CaCl_2$, 26 $NaHCO_3$, 11 D-glucose (pH 7.4), and the brainstem was sliced coronally into 200 μm thick slices with a vibratome (DSK-1000; Dosaka Co. Ltd, Kyoto, Japan) and transferred to a multi-well incubation chamber filled with bubbled ACSF at room temperature. After at least 90 min of recovery, the slices were individually transferred into the recording chamber and superfused continuously with gassed, warmed ACSF (34–35°C) at a rate of 2 ml min^{-1}. Superfusing ACSF was supplemented with 10 μM phenylephrine to facilitate firing (Vandermaelen and Aghajanian, 1983) and with a mixture of neurotransmitter blockers for glutamate, glycine, and GABA receptors (in μM: 10 DNQX; 20 D-AP5; 10 strychnine; 1 CGP-55845; 10 SR-95531) to functionally isolate the recorded neuron from synaptic input. Neurons were visualized by infrared differential interference contrast video microscopy with a Newicon C2400-07 camera (Hamamatsu, Hamamatsu City, Japan) mounted to an Axioskop microscope (Zeiss, Göttingen, Germany). Recordings were made using an EPC-10 amplifier (HEKA Elektronik, Lambrecht, Germany). Patch pipettes were prepared from thick-walled borosilicate glass on a P-97 Brown-Flaming electrode puller (Sutter Instruments, Novato, CA, USA) and had resistance of 3–6 MΩ when filled with solution containing (in mM): 125 NaCl, 10 HEPES, 2.75 KCl, 2 $CaCl_2$, 1.3 $MgCl_2$ (pH 7.4 with NaOH). Loose-seal cell-attached recordings (5–20 MΩ seal resistance) were acquired continuously in the voltage-clamp mode. Signals were filtered at 3 kHz and digitized at 10 kHz. Pipette potential was maintained at 0 mV. Recordings were aborted if firing rate was sensitive to changes in pipette holding potential or if shapes of action current changed. Data were analyzed using Clampfit 9.2 (Molecular Devices, Sunnyvale, CA, USA).

Neurons with likely serotonergic specification were first targeted according to morphological criteria (Brown et al., 2008): 5-HT neurons are clustered along the midline of the DRN and they have a larger soma (~20–25 μm long-axis diameter) than non-serotonergic neurons (~10–15 μm). Once loose-seal cell-attached recording configuration was established, 5-HT neurons were identified according to electrophysiological criteria (Vandermaelen and Aghajanian, 1983; Allers and Sharp, 2003). Neurons were considered serotonergic if, during at least 5 min-long baseline period at the beginning of the recording displayed slow and steady firing rate (<5 Hz); asymmetric action current with long upstroke to downstroke interval (proportional to action potential half-height width, >0.85 ms). According to these criteria, 250 out of 277 recorded neurons were identified as being serotonergic. Pharmacological experiments were done on 176 presumed serotonergic neurons, whose identity was pharmacologically confirmed based on 5-HT_{1A} receptor-mediated suppression of their firing rate. For all groups of neurons used in pharmacological experiments (**Figures 2–4**), the basal firing rate was matched and proved to be not different after *post hoc* statistical analysis (Kruskal–Wallis test, $p > 0.7$). Since experiments to assess autoinhibition depend on endogenous 5-HT, recordings were made from neurons located at least 50 μm below the slice surface (Mlinar et al., 2005). A single experiment was done in each slice.

For creating concentration–response curves for R(+)-8-OH-DPAT and 5-HTP application, drugs were applied for 10 min and mean firing rates were calculated from the last 1-min segment of each experimental epoch [e.g., baseline, R(+)-8-OH-DPAT 0.1 nM, 0.3 nM, etc.]. Trp was applied for 15 min and mean firing rates were obtained from the last 3-min segment of baseline and Trp application.

STATISTICAL ANALYSIS

All the statistical tests were performed by GraphPad Prism version 5.04 (GraphPad Software, San Diego, CA, USA). First, normality of data distribution was tested by D'Agostino–Pearson omnibus normality test. When the data were normally distributed, genotype effects were tested by one-way ANOVA [expressed as $F_{(df1,df2)}$ values] followed by Tukey's *post hoc* test. If not, data were analyzed by Kruskal–Wallis test [expressed as $H_{(df)}$ values] with Dunn's *post hoc* test. For testing effects of Trp in comparison to respective baseline, data (% change in firing rates) were analyzed by Wilcoxon signed rank test (two-tailed). In all cases, $p < 0.05$ was considered statistically significant.

RESULTS

COMPARISON OF BASAL FIRING RATES ACROSS GENOTYPES

In the absence of precursor supplementation (Trp or 5-HTP), and in the presence of receptor blockers for glutamate, GABA, and glycine receptors, the basal firing of 5-HT neurons in slices is relieved from the autoinhibitory control of endogenous 5-HT (Mlinar et al., 2005) and local action of major neurotransmitters. In these conditions of pharmacological isolation, the basal firing activity of 5-HT neurons reflects their *intrinsic* pacemaker activity, a characteristic that is difficult to study *in vivo*, where the firing activity is under control of both autoinhibition and synaptic input.

We compared the basal firing rates recorded before 5-HT precursor or 5-HT_{1A} receptor agonist application, across genotypes (**Figure 1**). Overall, 5-HT neurons showed typical regular pacemaker activity and firing rates similar to *wt* controls [in Hz: *Tph2−/−*, 1.61 ± 0.82 ($n = 54$); *Tph2+/−*, 1.90 ± 0.66 ($n = 45$); *wt*, 1.97 ± 0.69 ($n = 54$); *Sert+/−*, 1.85 ± 0.74 ($n = 47$); *Sert−/−*, 2.12 ± 0.75 ($n = 50$); mean ± SD; n = number of recorded neurons], except for *Tph2−/−* in which the firing rate was slightly, but significantly slower than in *wt* controls ($p < 0.05$, Kruskal–Wallis test followed by Dunn's multiple comparison test). These data show that basic electrophysiological properties underlying the typical pacemaker activity of 5-HT neurons are maintained regardless of genetic inactivation of *Tph2* or *Sert*.

COMPARISON OF 5-HT_{1A} RECEPTOR SENSITIVITY ACROSS GENOTYPES

Since 5-HT neuron autoinhibition is mediated by 5-HT_{1A} receptors, we investigated the functional response of 5-HT neurons to the 5-HT_{1A} receptor agonist R(+)-8-OH-DPAT in different genotypes. **Figure 2** illustrates typical experiments in which increasing

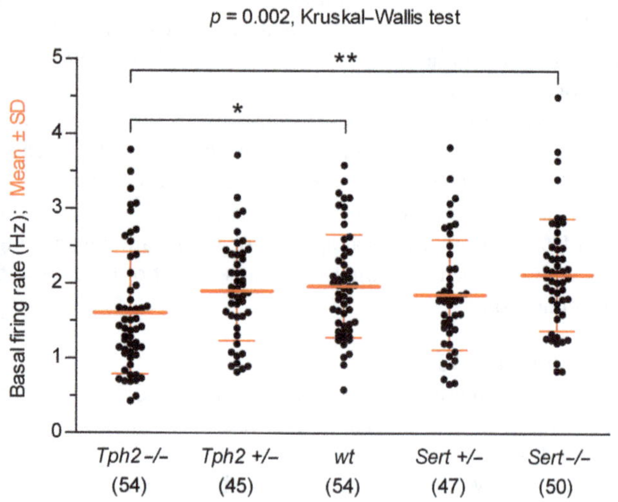

FIGURE 1 | Comparison of 5-HT neuron basal firing rates across genotypes. Data are shown as mean ± SD (number of cells shown in parentheses). Analysis of data using Kruskal–Wallis test revealed statistically significant differences among groups [$H_{(4)} = 16.67$, $p = 0.002$]. Dunn's multiple comparison *post hoc* test resulted in being significant for *Sert−/−* vs. *Tph2−/−* (**$p < 0.01$) and *wt* vs. *Tph2−/−* (*$p < 0.05$).

concentrations of R(+)-8-OH-DPAT were applied in slices from *wt* controls (**Figures 2A,B**), *Tph2−/−* (**Figures 2C,D**), and *Sert−/−* mice (**Figures 2E,F**). Application of R(+)-8-OH-DPAT reduced the firing rate of 5-HT neurons in a concentration-dependent manner, but with different effectiveness across genotypes, as shown by the comparison of log EC_{50} values obtained for each single neuron tested (log EC_{50} mean ± SD): *Tph2−/−*, −8.82 ± 0.29 ($n = 16$); *Tph2+/−*, −8.52 ± 0.19 ($n = 11$); *wt*, −8.52 ± 0.25 ($n = 12$); *Sert+/−*, −8.22 ± 0.27 ($n = 11$); *Sert−/−*, −7.17 ± 0.42 ($n = 8$; **Figure 2G**). Differences across genotypes were statistically significant [$F_{(4,53)} = 48.38$, $p < 0.0001$, one-way ANOVA]. Compared to *wt* controls, the response to application of R(+)-8-OH-DPAT resulted in slightly higher effectiveness of the agonist in *Tph2−/−* mice ($p < 0.05$) and very weak effectiveness in *Sert−/−* mice ($p < 0.001$). Although a small decrease in the sensitivity of 5-HT neurons was present also in *Sert+/−* mice, no statistically significant differences in log EC_{50} values were found for both *Tph2+/−* and *Sert+/−* vs. *wt* control mice, indicating that limited impairment of 5-HT synthesis and re-uptake did not result in relevant changes of 5-HT_{1A} autoreceptor sensitivity to R(+)-8-OH-DPAT. **Figure 2H** shows concentration–response curves fitted for each group on mean data obtained from the individual experiments shown in **Figure 2G**. It should be noted that in *Sert−/−* neurons, R(+)-8-OH-DPAT did not produce maximal inhibition of firing (see **Figure 2E**). Nevertheless, the average maximal inhibition was 60% compared to the other genotypes and the mean log value of concentrations producing an actual 50% decrease in firing of *Sert−/−* neurons was −6.91 ± 0.08 ($n = 8$), which did not affect the level of significance for decreased sensitivity of 5-HT_{1A} receptors shown in **Figure 2G**. Collectively, these data show that the sensitivity of 5-HT_{1A} receptors to agonist activation is markedly affected in *Sert−/−*.

ESTIMATION OF AUTOINHIBITION EXERTED BY ENDOGENOUS 5-HT ACROSS GENOTYPES

After assessing responsiveness to direct activation by the 5-HT_{1A} receptor agonist R(+)-8-OH-DPAT in the different genotypes, we investigated how specific genetic alterations translate into inhibition of 5-HT neuron activity by endogenous 5-HT. Once synthesis of 5-HT is restored in slices by supplementation of 5-HT precursors, the extent of autoinhibition in the different genotypes will depend on the balance between the level of extracellular 5-HT determined by the alteration of homeostatic mechanisms introduced by genetic manipulation and 5-HT_{1A} receptor sensitivity characteristic of each genotype.

Thus, we studied autoinhibition exerted by endogenous 5-HT, when *de novo* synthesis was restored in slices by supplementation of Trp or 5-HTP. Trp was used to estimate the extent of autoinhibition in respect to bioavailability of the natural precursor (Mlinar et al., 2005). 5-HTP was used to bypass the constraint in 5-HT synthesis produced by the rate-limiting enzyme Tph2. This allows reaching extracellular 5-HT concentrations greater than with Trp and permits quantification of the overall capacity of 5-HT neuron autoinhibition in different genotypes, including *Tph2−/−* mice.

Figure 3A shows that supplementation of Trp (30 μM) produced a decrease in firing rates of *Sert−/−* 5-HT neurons, an effect fully antagonized by WAY-100635, a selective 5-HT_{1A} receptor neutral antagonist (Corradetti et al., 1998). This demonstrates that 5-HT_{1A} receptor-mediated autoinhibition is present in *Sert−/−* mice. As shown in **Figure 3B**, 30 μM Trp significantly decreased firing rates of 5-HT neurons to a similar extent in all the genotypes tested (in % ± SD): *Tph2+/−*, 25.62 ± 15.37 ($n = 10$); *wt*, 25.55 ± 19.87 ($n = 7$); *Sert+/−*, 17.51 ± 12.99 ($n = 11$); *Sert−/−*, 22.03 ± 17.00 ($n = 14$). In all cases, the decrease in firing rates was significantly different from zero ($p < 0.05$; Wilcoxon signed rank test). Furthermore, responses to application of Trp were not statistically different across four genotypes [$H_{(3)} = 3.336$, $p = 0.3427$; Kruskal–Wallis test]. These data show that autoinhibition of DRN 5-HT neurons by endogenous 5-HT is conserved in all the genotypes to a similar level, irrespective of the genetic alteration.

To quantify the extent to which each genotype conserved the capacity to (auto)inhibit 5-HT neuron firing in response to different extracellular concentrations of endogenous 5-HT, we investigated the functional response of 5-HT neurons to 5-HTP in different genotypes.

Figure 4 illustrates firing rate changes of 5-HT neurons in response to increasing concentrations of 5-HTP in brain slices obtained from *wt* controls (**Figures 4A,B**), *Tph2−/−* (**Figures 4C,D**), and *Sert−/−* mice (**Figures 4E–H**). Application of 5-HTP reduced the firing rate of 5-HT neurons in a concentration-dependent manner, but with different effectiveness across genotypes [one-way ANOVA, $F_{(4,58)} = 6.723$, $p = 0.0002$], as shown by the comparison of log EC_{50} values obtained for each single neuron tested (log EC_{50} mean ± SD): *Tph2−/−*, −5.51 ± 0.41 ($n = 15$); *Tph2+/−*, −5.29 ± 0.30 ($n = 10$); *wt*, −5.17 ± 0.20 ($n = 14$); *Sert+/−*, −5.48 ± 0.36 ($n = 13$); *Sert−/−*, −5.76 ± 0.12 ($n = 11$; **Figure 4I**). Interestingly, the sensitivity to the effects of endogenous 5-HT synthesized

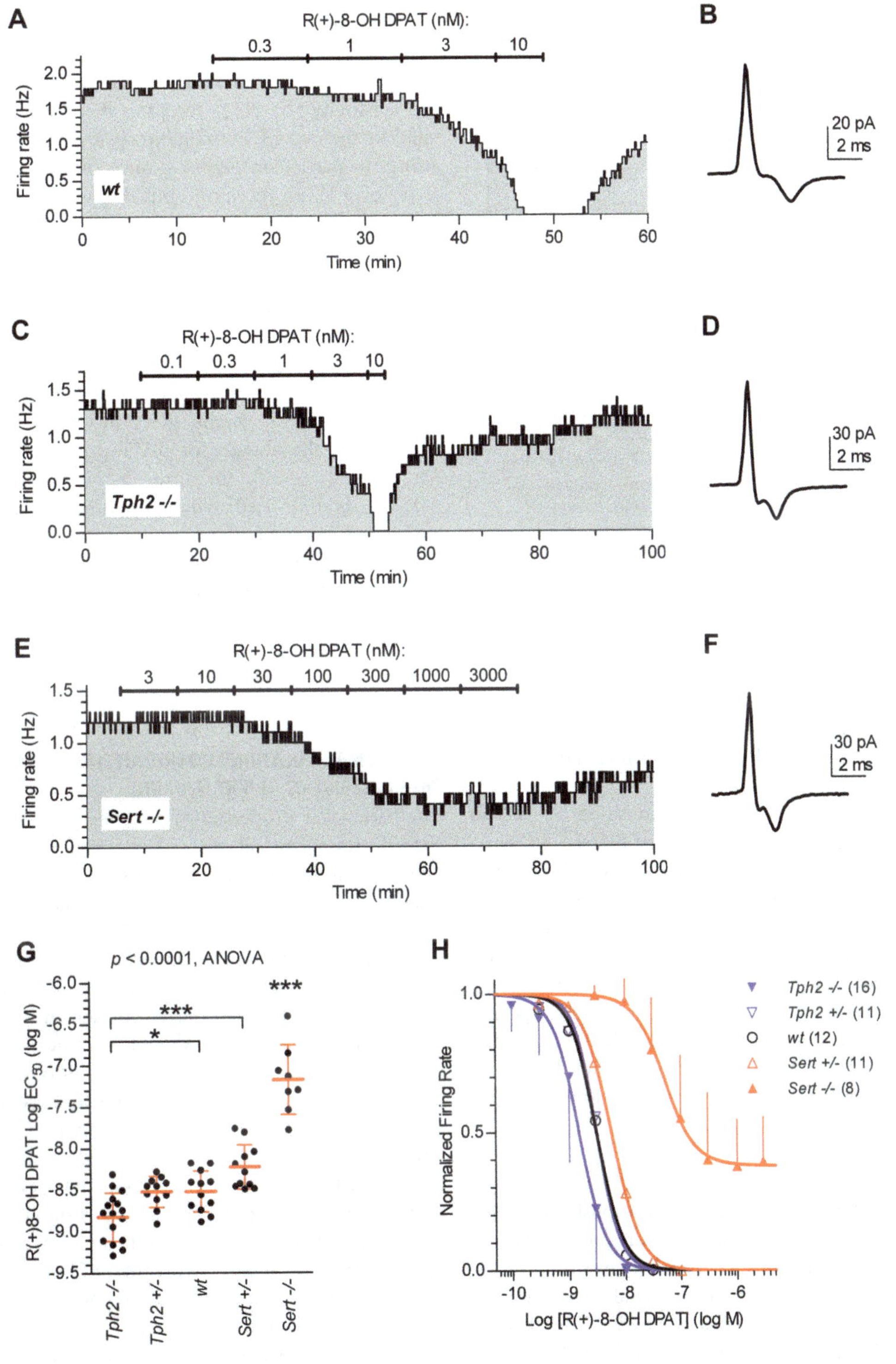

FIGURE 2 | Sensitivity of 5-HT neurons to R(+)-8-OH-DPAT differs across genotypes. Time courses of firing rate changes in response to increasing concentrations of R(+)-8-OH-DPAT of individual 5-HT neurons in brain slices obtained from *wt* **(A,B)**, *Tph2−/−* **(C,D)**, and *Sert−/−* mice **(E,F)**. Traces show action current of corresponding neurons recorded. **(G)** Dots represent log EC_{50} of concentration–responses from individual experiments. Red lines report mean ± SD of values. One-way ANOVA followed by Tukey's multiple comparison test showed statistically significant differences across genotypes [$F_{(4,53)} = 48.38$, $p < 0.0001$]. Asterisks indicate level of statistical significance between the indicated genotypes (for *Sert−/−*, vs. all the other four genotypes): $^{***}p < 0.001$, $^{*}p < 0.05$. **(H)** Average concentration–response curves obtained from all the experiments. Each data point corresponds to the mean from several neurons (numbers in parentheses). For the sake of clarity, error bars are shown only for *Sert−/−* mice and *Tph2−/−* mice in a single direction. Data are normalized on average baseline firing rates recorded before R(+)-8-OH-DPAT application. Note that, curves for *Sert−/−* mice did not achieve full inhibition of firing (see **E**).

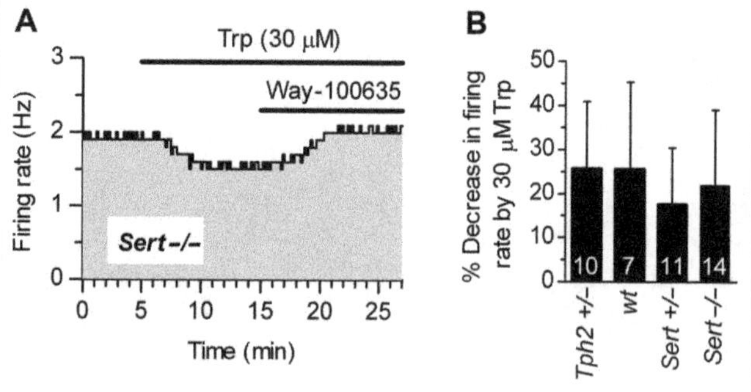

FIGURE 3 | Autoinhibition by endogenous 5-HT synthesized from Trp is conserved across genotypes. (A) Trp (30 μM) produced a 5-HT_{1A} receptor-mediated decrease in the firing rate of a 5-HT neuron from *Sert−/−* mice. Application of a selective 5-HT_{1A} receptor antagonist, WAY-100635 (50 nM; representative of three experiments) fully antagonized Trp effect, confirming that autoinhibition was mediated by 5-HT_{1A} autoreceptors. **(B)** Application of 30 μM Trp significantly suppressed firing activity of DRN serotonergic neurons in all the genotypes tested ($p < 0.05$; Wilcoxon signed rank test). Comparison of the effect of Trp among genotypes revealed no statistically significant differences among genotypes [$H_{(3)} = 3.336$, $p = 0.3427$; Kruskal–Wallis test]. Data are shown as mean ± SD. The number of neurons recorded for each genotype is shown at the bottom of the histograms.

from 5-HTP was increased both in *Tph2−/−* ($p < 0.05$) and *Sert−/−* ($p < 0.001$) mice compared to *wt* controls. **Figure 4J** shows concentration–response curves fitted for each group on mean data obtained from the individual experiments depicted in **Figure 4I**.

Whereas a stronger autoinhibitory response to 5-HTP in *Tph2−/−* mice is consistent with the observed increase in sensitivity of 5-HT_{1A} receptors to agonist activation, a similar increase in *Sert−/−* mice is unexpected in the presence of decreased sensitivity to R(+)-8-OH-DPAT. We suggest that, due to the absence of 5-HT re-uptake, in *Sert−/−* mice the extracellular 5-HT neosynthesized from 5-HTP attains higher levels than in *wt* control mice, leading to this apparent increase in response. Collectively, these results demonstrate that the changes in sensitivity to direct activation of 5-HT_{1A} receptors cannot directly be translated into the expected changes in autoinhibition exerted by endogenous 5-HT.

DISCUSSION

In the present study, we have investigated the relationship between the sensitivity of 5-HT_{1A} receptors and the concomitant degree of autoinhibition of 5-HT neurons in a panel of genetically modified mice characterized by impairment of cellular mechanisms crucial for homeostatic control of extracellular 5-HT levels (i.e., 5-HT synthesis and 5-HT re-uptake). *In vivo*, these genetic manipulations are likely to produce lifelong persistent modifications of 5-HT levels ranging from the absence of 5-HT in *Tph2−/−* mice (Savelieva et al., 2008; Alenina et al., 2009; Gutknecht et al., 2012) to a substantial increase in extracellular 5-HT levels in *Sert−/−* mice (Fabre et al., 2000; Mathews et al., 2004; Shen et al., 2004). The consequences of genetic alterations are maintained *in vitro*. This provides a set of conditions in which the relationship between the sensitivity of 5-HT_{1A} receptors and the autoinhibitory response of 5-HT neurons exerted by endogenous 5-HT could be quantitatively compared.

The major finding of the present study is that substantial and persistent alterations in 5-HT homeostasis produced changes in the sensitivity of 5-HT_{1A} receptors that did not translate in measurable changes of autoinhibitory regulation of 5-HT neuron firing. In particular, *Sert−/−* mice showed a marked subsensitivity of 5-HT_{1A} receptors, but displayed a normal capacity of autoinhibition. Interestingly, the sensitivity of 5-HT_{1A} receptors of both *Sert+/−* and *Tph2+/−* mice proved to be similar to that of *wt* control mice, showing that mild change in extracellular 5-HT levels is neither a strong stimulus for 5-HT_{1A} receptor adaptive changes in sensitivity, nor does it detectably affect autoinhibition.

In previous studies under similar recording conditions as used in this work, raphe slices showed substantial depletion of 5-HT in the absence of 5-HT precursors (Liu et al., 2005; Mlinar et al., 2005). *In vitro*, 5-HT content, together with 5-HT_{1A} receptor-mediated autoinhibition, can be restored by supplementation of Trp (Liu et al., 2005; Mlinar et al., 2005; Evans et al., 2008; Gutknecht et al., 2012). This allowed electrophysiological, quantitative, assessment of the modifications in sensitivity of 5-HT_{1A} receptors produced by altered 5-HT homeostasis *in vivo* and estimation of the functional state of autoinhibition when *de novo* synthesis of 5-HT was restored in slices.

GENETIC MANIPULATIONS DO NOT AFFECT PACEMAKER CHARACTERISTICS OF 5-HT NEURONS

The pacemaker properties of serotonergic neurons measured in slices in the virtual absence of endogenous 5-HT neosynthesis, hence of autoinhibition, were not substantially altered by genetic manipulation itself, as we observed similar baseline firing rates among genotypes, except for *Tph2−/−* mice, which had slightly lower baseline firing rates compared to the other genotypes. This shows that the basic characteristics of intrinsic pacemaker firing activity of 5-HT neurons are preserved independently from genetic manipulations that altered 5-HT homeostatic regulation. The small decrease in baseline firing rates observed in *Tph2−/−* mice may indicate that, in the chronic absence of 5-HT, neurons adapt their membrane properties, e.g., conductance, to compensate for absent autoinhibition and homeostatically keep pacemaker firing activity constant. The mechanism(s) underlying this adaptation is currently under investigation. It should be noted that the basal firing rate recorded under our experimental conditions, i.e., *in vitro*, results from the interplay of ion conductances responsible for pacemaking activity and likely do not correspond to the "basal" firing rate recorded *in vivo* (e.g., Gobbi et al., 2001; Bouali et al., 2003; see below) which is under the control of 5-HT_{1A} receptor-mediated autoinhibition in all genotypes (see **Figure 3**), except in *Tph2−/−* mice (Gutknecht et al., 2012).

LIFELONG EXPOSURE OF 5-HT NEURONS TO VARYING 5-HT LEVELS RESULTS IN CHANGES IN THE SENSITIVITY OF SOMATODENDRITIC 5-HT_{1A} RECEPTORS

Previous studies showed adaptive decrease in sensitivity of 5-HT_{1A} receptors in *Sert−/−* mice (Lanfumey et al., 2000; Mannoury

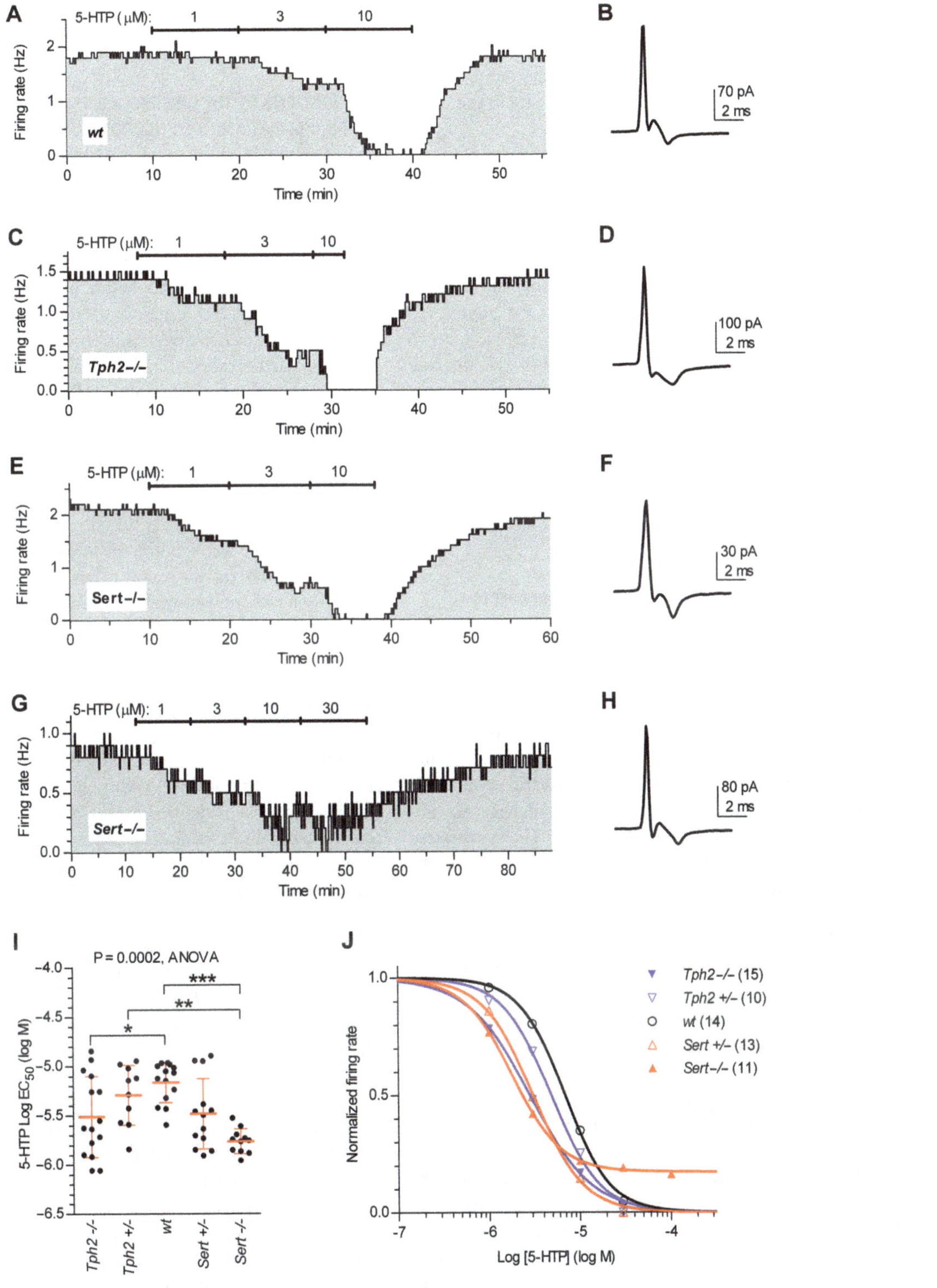

FIGURE 4 | Quantification of autoinhibition capacity of 5-HT neurons across genotypes by concentration–response curves for 5-HTP. Time courses of 5-HT neuron firing rate changes in response to increasing concentrations of 5-HTP in brain slices obtained from *wt* controls **(A,B)**, *Tph2–/–* **(C,D)**, and *Sert–/–* mice **(E–H)**. Traces show action current of corresponding neurons recorded. **(I)** Dots represent log EC_{50} of concentration–responses from individual experiments. Red lines report mean ± SD of values. One-way ANOVA followed by Tukey's multiple comparison test showed statistically significant differences [$F_{(4,58)} = 6.723$, $p = 0.0002$] Asterisks indicate level of statistical significance between the indicated genotypes: $***p < 0.001$, $**p < 0.01$, $*p < 0.05$. **(J)** Average concentration–response curves obtained from all the experiments. Each data point corresponds to the mean from several neurons (numbers shown in parentheses). For the sake of clarity, error bars are omitted. Data are normalized on average baseline firing rates recorded before 5-HTP application.

la Cour et al., 2001; Bouali et al., 2003). Our study extends the investigation to the opposite extreme, i.e., *Tph2−/−* mice, which are devoid of 5-HT and show a small, but significant increase in 5-HT_{1A} receptor sensitivity. This is consistent with neurochemical data showing an increase in 5-HT_{1A} receptor density in the raphe (Gutknecht et al., 2012).

In *Sert−/−* mice, we found a decrease in the maximal response to R(+)-8-OH-DPAT (~40%) and a similar reduction of autoinhibitory capacity as revealed by concentration–response curves with 5-HTP. This may reflect a downregulation of 5-HT_{1A} receptors due to lifelong exposure to increased stimulation by 5-HT or the emergence of a still-unknown adaptive mechanism directed to counteract increased autoinhibition exerted by high levels of extracellular 5-HT *in vivo*. In spite of the decrease, however, the remaining autoinhibition capacity of 5-HT neurons largely exceeded the magnitude of physiological autoinhibition produced by 5-HT when its synthesis was restored by Trp (see below).

Taken together, our data indicate that the level of 5-HT_{1A} receptor sensitivity of 5-HT neurons is inversely correlated with extracellular levels of 5-HT *in vivo*, at least in extreme conditions as represented by *Tph2−/−* and *Sert−/−* mice.

AUTOINHIBITION OF 5-HT NEURONS BY ENDOGENOUS 5-HT IS CONSERVED IN THE PHYSIOLOGICAL RANGE, REGARDLESS OF THE SENSITIVITY OF 5-HT_{1A} RECEPTORS

When the level of autoinhibition restored by Trp supplementation in slices from all the genotypes (except *Tph2−/−*) was measured, this resulted in being similar, irrespective of the sensitivity of 5-HT_{1A} receptors measured in each genotype. Notably, *Sert−/−* showed greatly decreased sensitivity to the agonist but normal autoinhibition, as estimated by Trp challenge. Accordingly, the autoinhibitory effect of endogenous 5-HT synthesized *de novo* from 5-HTP proved to be not decreased in all the mutants compared with *wt* controls, including *Tph2−/−* in which the absence of Tph2 was bypassed by 5-HTP. It should be noted that in *Sert−/−* mice the maximal inhibitory response was slightly decreased (~20%) in agreement with the reduced maximal response to the agonist, but the substantial residual inhibition capacity is apparently sufficient to produce a physiological level of autoinhibition as shown by Trp experiments. In conclusion, these data indicate that the marked subsensitivity of 5-HT_{1A} receptors observed in *Sert−/−* does not translate in the loss of normal autoinhibition capacity of 5-HT neurons.

Although counterintuitive, this notion is consistent with the observation that, *in vivo*, the firing rate of 5-HT neurons is not increased in *Sert−/−*, but similar to or even lower (Gobbi et al., 2001; Bouali et al., 2003) than that of *wt* controls, thus indicating that *in vivo* subsensitivity of 5-HT_{1A} receptors in *Sert−/−* mice does not relieve 5-HT neurons from autoinhibition. Furthermore, Fox et al. (2010) reported that in these mice antagonism of 5-HT_{1A} receptors by WAY-100635 resulted in the appearance of greater frequency of 5-HT_{2A} receptor-mediated head twitches than in *wt* controls. This suggests that the relief from autoinhibition, hence the increase in 5-HT neuron firing, produces an increase in 5-HT release sufficient to produce this 5-HT_{2A}-mediated behavioral effect (Willins and Meltzer, 1997), even in the presence of partial desensitization of 5-HT_{2A} receptors (Rioux et al., 1999; Li et al., 2003; Qu et al., 2005).

IMPLICATIONS OF THE DIVERGENCE BETWEEN SENSITIVITY TO R(+)-8-OH-DPAT AND 5-HT NEURON AUTOINHIBITION

The crucial role of somatodendritic 5-HT_{1A} receptors in regulating the firing rate of 5-HT neurons, hence the functional state of 5-HT system, has attracted interest in the attempt to infer the degree of activity of these neurons in pathological conditions of humans and in behavioral experiments of rodents. The present work may help to better understand the limits in the interpretation of the functional state of 5-HT system based on measurements of density/sensitivity of 5-HT_{1A} receptors of 5-HT neurons. Furthermore, since the knockout mice used in this investigation may model different risk factors (i.e., *TPH2* and *SERT* polymorphisms) for anxiety disorders and depression, our data showing that autoinhibition is not impaired in these mutants may provide a reference background for the interpretation of behavioral responses in these mice in the context of human psychopathology. For instance, functional autoinhibition in patients with depression were indirectly inferred from 5-HT_{1A} receptor imaging studies in the raphe (Drevets et al., 2007; Savitz et al., 2009). Overall, however, these studies failed to clarify whether the depression-related changes in 5-HT_{1A} receptor binding are genetically or environmentally driven during development, thus causative of the disorder, or whether they are simply an adaptation to acutely increased or decreased serotonergic transmission (Savitz et al., 2009).

Contradicting results were also gathered in the attempt to associate *SERT* polymorphisms with changes in the level of 5-HT_{1A} receptor expression/density. David et al. (2005) reported that carriers of the 5-HTTLPR s-allele had lower 5-HT_{1A} receptor binding potential in all the brain regions investigated compared to individuals homozygous for the l-allele. On the contrary, Lee et al. (2005) found that s-carriers had higher 5-HT_{1A} binding than ll-individuals in pregenual and subgenual cingulate cortex regions while in other regions, including the DRN, no difference was detected. More recently, Borg et al. (2009) could not reveal any differences in 5-HT_{1A} receptor density between carriers and non-carriers of the 5-HTTLPR s-allele and concluded that functional consequences of 5-HTTLPR are not likely to be mediated by differences in 5-HT_{1A} expression. Our results showing that 5-HT system autoinhibition is not reduced in mice with impaired Sert function even in the presence of altered 5-HT_{1A} receptor sensitivity would support this conclusion.

A second implication of our results involves the possibility to infer the degree of 5-HT system autoinhibition from functional assays using activation of 5-HT_{1A} receptors with direct agonists, in patients or in animal models. For example, one of the most consistent findings among depressed patients is their blunted hypothermia in response to 5-HT_{1A} receptor direct agonists (Lesch et al., 1990; Lesch, 1991; Jacobsen et al., 2012b and references therein). Such responses are usually ascribed to desensitization of somatodendritic 5-HT_{1A} receptors (reviewed in Jacobsen et al., 2012a). Our data suggest that, whereas blunted hypothermic response to direct agonists is likely to reflect subsensitivity of

5-HT_{1A} receptors in these patients, this decrease in response cannot directly be correlated to functional consequences that entail reduced autoinhibition and increase in the basal firing rate of 5-HT neurons.

On the other hand, the finding that 5-HT neurons in Tph2- and Sert-deficient mice display normal responsiveness to Trp and/or 5-HTP regarding autoinhibition of 5-HT neuron firing would support the use of Trp (or 5-HTP) as an appropriate challenge to test the functional state of 5-HT system in clinical settings and to reveal the involvement of altered autoinhibition in human psychopathology. Indeed, 5-HTP challenge has been successfully applied to reveal functional consequences dependent on 5-HTTLPR variation in humans (Maron et al., 2004).

Finally, the striking divergence between sensitivity to R(+)-8-OH-DPAT and 5-HT neuron autoinhibition in *Sert−/−* suggests the possibility that sustained increase in 5-HT levels by stressors or pharmacological treatments (e.g., SSRIs) may result in 5-HT_{1A} receptor subsensitivity, not accompanied by functional impairment of 5-HT neuron firing autoregulation. For instance, the rapid decrease in 5-HT_{1A} receptor sensitivity found in DRN 5-HT neurons following chronic ultramild stress and stressful uncontrolled environmental conditions is apparently not correlated with an increase in 5-HT system activity and has been suggested to be an adaptive mechanism to compensate for 5-HT fluctuations produced by stressful events (Laaris et al., 1999; Lanfumey et al., 1999). Interestingly, *in vivo* recording after chronic unpredictable stress in rats showed that the reduced ability of 8-OH-DPAT to inhibit 5-HT neuron firing was accompanied by a decrease in firing rate of DRN 5-HT neurons (Bambico et al., 2009), indicating that functional autoinhibition may be preserved in spite of 5-HT_{1A} receptor desensitization. Furthermore, desensitization of autoinhibitory 5-HT_{1A} receptors occurring with chronic SSRI administration (Le Poul et al., 2000; Hensler, 2002; Castro et al., 2003) has been proposed as a mechanism for 5-HT neurons to escape the sustained autoinhibition produced by the increase in 5-HT in raphe nuclei by blockade of Sert and to represent an important step to achieve enhanced therapeutic effects of SSRIs (Artigas et al., 1996). On the other hand, Richardson-Jones et al. (2010) showed that desensitization of 5-HT_{1A} autoreceptors is not sufficient for antidepressants to convey their efficacy, indicating dissociation between desensitization of 5-HT_{1A} autoreceptors and behavioral effects of chronic SSRI treatment. Thus, desensitization of 5-HT_{1A} autoreceptors appears rather to be an adaptive mechanism to neutralize elevated extracellular 5-HT levels, and not a primary factor leading to behavioral alteration.

Under a functional perspective, however, dynamic changes in the sensitivity/expression of 5-HT_{1A} receptors appear to be crucial to fulfill the requirements for physiological homeostasis of 5-HT system functioning. Thus, any impairment of adaptive mechanisms of 5-HT_{1A} receptors in response to sustained changes in 5-HT levels, or constitutive alteration of their expression even in the absence of altered 5-HT levels *in vivo*, becomes a potential source of pathological consequences. In fact, genetically induced overexpression of somatodendritic 5-HT_{1A} receptors in mice has been shown to produce autonomic dysregulation (Audero et al., 2008), behavioral alterations, and decreased response to antidepressant drugs (Richardson-Jones et al., 2010). In humans, the C(-1019)G 5-HT_{1A} promoter polymorphism leading to 5-HT_{1A} receptor overexpression is proposed to represent a risk factor for depression (Lemonde et al., 2003; Strobel et al., 2003; Rothe et al., 2004; reviewed in Albert and Francois, 2010) and response to antidepressant drugs (reviewed in Albert, 2012).

In conclusion, our data reveal that 5-HT neuron autoinhibition is similar in all *Tph2* and *Sert* genotypes studied, regardless of the different sensitivity of their somatodendritic 5-HT_{1A} receptors to R(+)-8-OH-DPAT. This suggests that adaptive changes in receptor sensitivity occur to compensate for variable extracellular 5-HT levels in different genotypes to homeostatically conserve autoinhibition in a physiological range. Thus, it appears that response to 5-HT_{1A} agonists *per se* is not always sufficient for evaluating the functional state of the 5-HT system, for which Trp and/or 5-HTP challenges may provide more informative data, both in clinical and animal experimental settings.

ACKNOWLEDGMENTS

Supported by the DFG (KFO 125, SFB TRR 58/A1 and A5), BMBF (IZKF Wuerzburg, 01KS9603), Compagnia di San Paolo (Programma Neuroscienze-2008.2265), and the EC (NEWMOOD LSHM-CT-2004-503474). Naozumi Araragi was supported by a grant of the German Excellence Initiative to the Graduate School of Life Sciences (GSLS), University of Wuerzburg. The article publishing fee was funded by the DFG and the University of Wuerzburg in the funding program Open Access Publishing.

REFERENCES

Albert, P. R. (2012). Transcriptional regulation of the 5-HT1A receptor: implications for mental illness. *Philos. Trans. R. Soc. Lond. B Biol. Sci.* 367, 2402–2415. doi: 10.1098/rstb.2011.0376

Albert, P. R., and Francois, B. L. (2010). Modifying 5-HT1A receptor gene expression as a new target for antidepressant therapy. *Front. Neurosci.* 4:35. doi: 10.3389/fnins.2010.00035

Alenina, N., Kikic, D., Todiras, M., Mosienko, V., Qadri, F., Plehm, R., et al. (2009). Growth retardation and altered autonomic control in mice lacking brain serotonin. *Proc. Natl. Acad. Sci. U.S.A.* 106, 10332–10337. doi: 10.1073/pnas.0810793106

Allers, K. A., and Sharp, T. (2003). Neurochemical and anatomical identification of fast- and slow-firing neurones in the rat dorsal raphe nucleus using juxtacellular labelling methods in vivo. *Neuroscience* 122, 193–204. doi: 10.1016/S0306-4522(03)00518-9

Arango, V., Underwood, M. D., Boldrini, M., Tamir, H., Kassir, S. A., Hsiung, S., et al. (2001). Serotonin 1A receptors, serotonin transporter binding and serotonin transporter mRNA expression in the brainstem of depressed suicide victims. *Neuropsychopharmacology* 25, 892–903. doi: 10.1016/S0893-133X(01)00310-4

Artigas, F., Romero, L., De Montigny, C., and Blier, P. (1996). Acceleration of the effect of selected antidepressant drugs in major depression by 5-HT1A antagonists. *Trends Neurosci.* 19, 378–383. doi: 10.1016/S0166-2236(96)10037-0

Audero, E., Coppi, E., Mlinar, B., Rossetti, T., Caprioli, A., Banchaabouchi, M. A., et al. (2008). Sporadic autonomic dysregulation and death associated with excessive serotonin autoinhibition. *Science* 321, 130–133. doi: 10.1126/science.1157871

Bambico, F. R., Nguyen, N. T., and Gobbi, G. (2009). Decline in serotonergic firing activity and desensitization of 5-HT1A autoreceptors after chronic unpredictable stress. *Eur. Neuropsychopharmacol.* 19, 215–228. doi: 10.1016/j.euroneuro.2008.11.005

Bengel, D., Murphy, D. L., Andrews, A. M., Wichems, C. H., Feltner, D., Heils, A., et al. (1998). Altered brain serotonin homeostasis and locomotor insensitivity to 3, 4-methylenedioxymethamphetamine ("Ecstasy") in serotonin transporter-deficient mice. *Mol. Pharmacol.* 53, 649–655.

Borg, J., Henningsson, S., Saijo, T., Inoue, M., Bah, J., Westberg, L., et al. (2009). Serotonin transporter genotype is associated with cognitive performance but not regional 5-HT1A receptor binding in humans. *Int. J. Neuropsychopharmacol.* 12, 783–792. doi: 10.1017/S1461145708009759

Bouali, S., Evrard, A., Chastanet, M., Lesch, K. P., Hamon, M., and Adrien, J. (2003). Sex hormone-dependent desensitization of 5-HT1A autoreceptors in knockout mice deficient in the 5-HT transporter. *Eur. J. Neurosci.* 18, 2203–2212. doi: 10.1046/j.1460-9568.2003.02960.x

Brown, R. E., Mckenna, J. T., Winston, S., Basheer, R., Yanagawa, Y., Thakkar, M. M., et al. (2008). Characterization of GABAergic neurons in rapid-eye-movement sleep controlling regions of the brainstem reticular formation in GAD67-green fluorescent protein knock-in mice. *Eur. J. Neurosci.* 27, 352–363. doi: 10.1111/j.1460-9568.2008.06024.x

Canli, T., and Lesch, K. P. (2007). Long story short: the serotonin transporter in emotion regulation and social cognition. *Nat. Neurosci.* 10, 1103–1109. doi: 10.1038/nn1964

Carlsson, A., Davis, J. N., Kehr, W., Lindqvist, M., and Atack, C. V. (1972). Simultaneous measurement of tyrosine and tryptophan hydroxylase activities in brain in vivo using an inhibitor of the aromatic amino acid decarboxylase. *Naunyn Schmiedebergs Arch. Pharmacol.* 275, 153–168. doi: 10.1007/BF00508904

Castro, M., Diaz, A., Del Olmo, E., and Pazos, A. (2003). Chronic fluoxetine induces opposite changes in G protein coupling at pre and postsynaptic 5-HT1A receptors in rat brain. *Neuropharmacology* 44, 93–101. doi: 10.1016/S0028-3908(02)00340-4

Corradetti, R., Laaris, N., Hanoun, N., Laporte, A. M., Le Poul, E., Hamon, M., et al. (1998). Antagonist properties of (−)-pindolol and WAY 100635 at somatodendritic and postsynaptic 5-HT1A receptors in the rat brain. *Br. J. Pharmacol.* 123, 449–462. doi: 10.1038/sj.bjp.0701632

David, S. P., Murthy, N. V., Rabiner, E. A., Munafo, M. R., Johnstone, E. C., Jacob, R., et al. (2005). A functional genetic variation of the serotonin (5-HT) transporter affects 5-HT1A receptor binding in humans. *J. Neurosci.* 25, 2586–2590. doi: 10.1523/JNEUROSCI.3769-04.2005

Drevets, W. C., Frank, E., Price, J. C., Kupfer, D. J., Holt, D., Greer, P. J., et al. (1999). PET imaging of serotonin 1A receptor binding in depression. *Biol. Psychiatry* 46, 1375–1387. doi: 10.1016/S0006-3223(99)00189-4

Drevets, W. C., Thase, M. E., Moses-Kolko, E. L., Price, J., Frank, E., Kupfer, D. J., et al. (2007). Serotonin-1A receptor imaging in recurrent depression: replication and literature review. *Nucl. Med. Biol.* 34, 865–877. doi: 10.1016/j.nucmedbio.2007.06.008

Evans, A. K., Reinders, N., Ashford, K. A., Christie, I. N., Wakerley, J. B., and Lowry, C. A. (2008). Evidence for serotonin synthesis-dependent regulation of in vitro neuronal firing rates in the midbrain raphe complex. *Eur. J. Pharmacol.* 590, 136–149. doi: 10.1016/j.ejphar.2008.06.014

Fabre, V., Beaufour, C., Evrard, A., Rioux, A., Hanoun, N., Lesch, K. P., et al. (2000). Altered expression and functions of serotonin 5-HT1A and 5-HT1B receptors in knock-out mice lacking the 5-HT transporter. *Eur. J. Neurosci.* 12, 2299–2310. doi: 10.1046/j.1460-9568.2000.00126.x

Fox, M. A., Stein, A. R., French, H. T., and Murphy, D. L. (2010). Functional interactions between 5-HT2A and presynaptic 5-HT1A receptor-based responses in mice genetically deficient in the serotonin 5-HT transporter (SERT). *Br. J. Pharmacol.* 159, 879–887. doi: 10.1111/j.1476-5381.2009.00578.x

Gobbi, G., Murphy, D. L., Lesch, K., and Blier, P. (2001). Modifications of the serotonergic system in mice lacking serotonin transporters: an in vivo electrophysiological study. *J. Pharmacol. Exp. Ther.* 296, 987–995.

Gutknecht, L., Araragi, N., Merker, S., Waider, J., Sommerlandt, F. M., Mlinar, B., et al. (2012). Impacts of brain serotonin deficiency following Tph2 inactivation on development and raphe neuron serotonergic specification. *PLoS ONE* 7:e43157. doi: 10.1371/journal.pone.0043157

Gutknecht, L., Jacob, C., Strobel, A., Kriegebaum, C., Muller, J., Zeng, Y., et al. (2007). Tryptophan hydroxylase-2 gene variation influences personality traits and disorders related to emotional dysregulation. *Int. J. Neuropsychopharmacol.* 10, 309–320. doi: 10.1017/S1461145706007437

Gutknecht, L., Kriegebaum, C., Waider, J., Schmitt, A., and Lesch, K. P. (2009). Spatio-temporal expression of tryptophan hydroxylase isoforms in murine and human brain: convergent data from Tph2 knockout mice. *Eur. Neuropsychopharmacol.* 19, 266–282. doi: 10.1016/j.euroneuro.2008.12.005

Gutknecht, L., Waider, J., Kraft, S., Kriegebaum, C., Holtmann, B., Reif, A., et al. (2008). Deficiency of brain 5-HT synthesis but serotonergic neuron formation in Tph2 knockout mice. *J. Neural. Transm.* 115, 1127–1132. doi: 10.1007/s00702-008-0096-6

Hensler, J. G. (2002). Differential regulation of 5-HT1A receptor-G protein interactions in brain following chronic antidepressant administration. *Neuropsychopharmacology* 26, 565–573. doi: 10.1016/S0893-133X(01)00395-5

Jacobs, B. L., and Azmitia, E. C. (1992). Structure and function of the brain serotonin system. *Physiol. Rev.* 72, 165–229.

Jacobsen, J. P., Medvedev, I. O., and Caron, M. G. (2012a). The 5-HT deficiency theory of depression: perspectives from a naturalistic 5-HT deficiency model, the tryptophan hydroxylase 2Arg439His knock in mouse. *Philos. Trans. R. Soc. Lond. B Biol. Sci.* 367, 2444–2459. doi: 10.1098/rstb.2012.0109

Jacobsen, J. P., Siesser, W. B., Sachs, B. D., Peterson, S., Cools, M. J., Setola, V., et al. (2012b). Deficient serotonin neurotransmission and depression-like serotonin biomarker alterations in tryptophan hydroxylase 2 (Tph2) loss-of-function mice. *Mol. Psychiatry* 17, 694–704. doi: 10.1038/mp.2011.50

Laaris, N., Le Poul, E., Laporte, A. M., Hamon, M., and Lanfumey, L. (1999). Differential effects of stress on presynaptic and postsynaptic 5-hydroxytryptamine-1A receptors in the rat brain: an in vitro electrophysiological study. *Neuroscience* 91, 947–958. doi: 10.1016/S0306-4522(98)00674-5

Lanfumey, L., Mannoury La Cour, C., Froger, N., and Hamon, M. (2000). 5-HT-HPA interactions in two models of transgenic mice relevant to major depression. *Neurochem. Res.* 25, 1199–1206. doi: 10.1023/A:1007683810230

Lanfumey, L., Pardon, M. C., Laaris, N., Joubert, C., Hanoun, N., Hamon, M., et al. (1999). 5-HT1A autoreceptor desensitization by chronic ultramild stress in mice. *Neuroreport* 10, 3369–3374. doi: 10.1097/00001756-199911080-00021

Lee, M., Bailer, U. F., Frank, G. K., Henry, S. E., Meltzer, C. C., Price, J. C., et al. (2005). Relationship of a 5-HT transporter functional polymorphism to 5-HT1A receptor binding in healthy women. *Mol. Psychiatry* 10, 715–716. doi: 10.1038/sj.mp.4001680

Lemonde, S., Turecki, G., Bakish, D., Du, L., Hrdina, P. D., Bown, C. D., et al. (2003). Impaired repression at a 5-hydroxytryptamine 1A receptor gene polymorphism associated with major depression and suicide. *J. Neurosci.* 23, 8788–8799.

Le Poul, E., Boni, C., Hanoun, N., Laporte, A. M., Laaris, N., Chauveau, J., et al. (2000). Differential adaptation of brain 5-HT1A and 5-HT1B receptors and 5-HT transporter in rats treated chronically with fluoxetine. *Neuropharmacology* 39, 110–122. doi: 10.1016/S0028-3908(99)00088-X

Lesch, K. P. (1991). 5-HT1A receptor responsivity in anxiety disorders and depression. *Prog. Neuropsychopharmacol. Biol. Psychiatry* 15, 723–733. doi: 10.1016/0278-5846(91)90001-H

Lesch, K. P., Araragi, N., Waider, J., Van Den Hove, D., and Gutknecht, L. (2012). Targeting brain serotonin synthesis: insights into neurodevelopmental disorders with long-term outcomes related to negative emotionality, aggression and antisocial behaviour. *Philos. Trans. R. Soc. Lond. B Biol. Sci.* 367, 2426–2443. doi: 10.1098/rstb.2012.0039

Lesch, K. P., Mayer, S., Disselkamp-Tietze, J., Hoh, A., Schoellnhammer, G., and Schulte, H. M. (1990). Subsensitivity of the 5-hydroxytryptamine1A (5-HT1A) receptor-mediated hypothermic response to ipsapirone in unipolar depression. *Life Sci.* 46, 1271–1277. doi: 10.1016/0024-3205(90)90359-Y

Levine, E. S., and Jacobs, B. L. (1992). Neurochemical afferents controlling the activity of serotonergic neurons in the dorsal raphe nucleus: microiontophoretic studies in the awake cat. *J. Neurosci.* 12, 4037–4044.

Li, Q., Wichems, C. H., Ma, L., Van De Kar, L. D., Garcia, F., and Murphy, D. L. (2003). Brain region-specific alterations of 5-HT2A and 5-HT2C receptors in serotonin transporter knockout mice. *J. Neurochem.* 84, 1256–1265. doi: 10.1046/j.1471-4159.2003.01607.x

Liu, R. J., Lambe, E. K., and Aghajanian, G. K. (2005). Somatodendritic autoreceptor regulation of serotonergic neurons: dependence on L-tryptophan and tryptophan hydroxylase-activating kinases. *Eur. J. Neurosci.* 21, 945–958. doi: 10.1111/j.1460-9568.2005.03930.x

Mannoury la Cour, C., Boni, C., Hanoun, N., Lesch, K. P., Hamon, M., and Lanfumey, L. (2001). Functional consequences of 5-HT transporter gene disruption on 5-HT(1a) receptor-mediated regulation of dorsal raphe and hippocampal cell activity. *J. Neurosci.* 21, 2178–2185.

Maron, E., Tasa, G., Toru, I., Lang, A., Vasar, V., and Shlik, J. (2004). Association between serotonin-related genetic polymorphisms and CCK-4-induced panic attacks with or without 5-hydroxytryptophan pretreatment in healthy volunteers. *World J. Biol. Psychiatry* 5, 149–154. doi: 10.1080/15622970410029927

Mathews, T. A., Fedele, D. E., Coppelli, F. M., Avila, A. M., Murphy, D. L., and Andrews, A. M. (2004). Gene dose-dependent alterations in extraneuronal serotonin but not dopamine in mice with reduced serotonin transporter expression. *J. Neurosci. Methods* 140, 169–181. doi: 10.1016/j.jneumeth.2004.05.017

Meltzer, C. C., Price, J. C., Mathis, C. A., Butters, M. A., Ziolko, S. K., Moses-Kolko, E., et al. (2004). Serotonin 1A receptor binding and treatment response in late-life depression. *Neuropsychopharmacology* 29, 2258–2265. doi: 10.1038/sj.npp.1300556

Mlinar, B., Tatini, F., Ballini, C., Nencioni, S., Della Corte, L., and Corradetti, R. (2005). Differential autoinhibition of 5-hydroxytryptamine neurons by 5-hydroxytryptamine in the dorsal raphe nucleus. *Neuroreport* 16, 1351–1355. doi: 10.1097/01.wnr.0000175249.25535.bf

Mosienko, V., Bert, B., Beis, D., Matthes, S., Fink, H., Bader, M., et al. (2012). Exaggerated aggression and decreased anxiety in mice deficient in brain serotonin. *Transl. Psychiatry* 2, e122. doi: 10.1038/tp.2012.44

Murphy, D. L., and Lesch, K. P. (2008). Targeting the murine serotonin transporter: insights into human neurobiology. *Nat. Rev. Neurosci.* 9, 85–96. doi: 10.1038/nrn2284

Neumeister, A., Bain, E., Nugent, A. C., Carson, R. E., Bonne, O., Luckenbaugh, D. A., et al. (2004). Reduced serotonin type 1A receptor binding in panic disorder. *J. Neurosci.* 24, 589–591. doi: 10.1523/JNEUROSCI.4921-03.2004

Parsey, R. V., Oquendo, M. A., Ogden, R. T., Olvet, D. M., Simpson, N., Huang, Y. Y., et al. (2006). Altered serotonin 1A binding in major depression: a [carbonyl-C-11]WAY100635 positron emission tomography study. *Biol. Psychiatry* 59, 106–113. doi: 10.1016/j.biopsych.2005.06.016

Pineyro, G., and Blier, P. (1999). Autoregulation of serotonin neurons: role in antidepressant drug action. *Pharmacol. Rev.* 51, 533–591.

Qu, Y., Villacreses, N., Murphy, D. L., and Rapoport, S. I. (2005). 5-HT2A/2C receptor signaling via phospholipase A2 and arachidonic acid is attenuated in mice lacking the serotonin reuptake transporter. *Psychopharmacology (Berl.)* 180, 12–20. doi: 10.1007/s00213-005-2231-5

Richardson-Jones, J. W., Craige, C. P., Guiard, B. P., Stephen, A., Metzger, K. L., Kung, H. F., et al. (2010). 5-HT1A autoreceptor levels determine vulnerability to stress and response to antidepressants. *Neuron* 65, 40–52. doi: 10.1016/j.neuron.2009.12.003

Rioux, A., Fabre, V., Lesch, K. P., Moessner, R., Murphy, D. L., Lanfumey, L., et al. (1999). Adaptive changes of serotonin 5-HT2A receptors in mice lacking the serotonin transporter. *Neurosci. Lett.* 262, 113–116. doi: 10.1016/S0304-3940(99)00049-X

Rothe, C., Gutknecht, L., Freitag, C., Tauber, R., Mossner, R., Franke, P., et al. (2004). Association of a functional 1019C > G 5-HT1A receptor gene polymorphism with panic disorder with agoraphobia. *Int. J. Neuropsychopharmacol.* 7, 189–192. doi: 10.1017/S1461145703004061

Sargent, P. A., Kjaer, K. H., Bench, C. J., Rabiner, E. A., Messa, C., Meyer, J., et al. (2000). Brain serotonin1A receptor binding measured by positron emission tomography with [11C]WAY-100635: effects of depression and antidepressant treatment. *Arch. Gen. Psychiatry* 57, 174–180. doi: 10.1001/archpsyc.57.2.174

Savelieva, K. V., Zhao, S., Pogorelov, V. M., Rajan, I., Yang, Q., Cullinan, E., et al. (2008). Genetic disruption of both tryptophan hydroxylase genes dramatically reduces serotonin and affects behavior in models sensitive to antidepressants. *PLoS ONE* 3:e3301. doi: 10.1371/journal.pone.0003301

Savitz, J., Lucki, I., and Drevets, W. C. (2009). 5-HT(1A) receptor function in major depressive disorder. *Prog. Neurobiol.* 88, 17–31. doi: 10.1016/j.pneurobio.2009.01.009

Sharp, T., Boothman, L., Raley, J., and Queree, P. (2007). Important messages in the 'post': recent discoveries in 5-HT neurone feedback control. *Trends Pharmacol. Sci.* 28, 629–636. doi: 10.1016/j.tips.2007.10.009

Shen, H. W., Hagino, Y., Kobayashi, H., Shinohara-Tanaka, K., Ikeda, K., Yamamoto, H., et al. (2004). Regional differences in extracellular dopamine and serotonin assessed by in vivo microdialysis in mice lacking dopamine and/or serotonin transporters. *Neuropsychopharmacology* 29, 1790–1799. doi: 10.1038/sj.npp.1300476

Stockmeier, C. A., Shapiro, L. A., Dilley, G. E., Kolli, T. N., Friedman, L., and Rajkowska, G. (1998). Increase in serotonin-1A autoreceptors in the midbrain of suicide victims with major depression-postmortem evidence for decreased serotonin activity. *J. Neurosci.* 18, 7394–7401.

Strobel, A., Gutknecht, L., Rothe, C., Reif, A., Mossner, R., Zeng, Y., et al. (2003). Allelic variation in 5-HT1A receptor expression is associated with anxiety- and depression-related personality traits. *J. Neural. Transm.* 110, 1445–1453. doi: 10.1007/s00702-003-0072-0

Trulson, M. E., and Jacobs, B. L. (1979). Raphe unit activity in freely moving cats: correlation with level of behavioral arousal. *Brain Res.* 163, 135–150. doi: 10.1016/0006-8993(79)90157-4

Vandermaelen, C. P., and Aghajanian, G. K. (1983). Electrophysiological and pharmacological characterization of serotonergic dorsal raphe neurons recorded extracellularly and intracellularly in rat brain slices. *Brain Res.* 289, 109–119. doi: 10.1016/0006-8993(83)90011-2

Willins, D. L., and Meltzer, H. Y. (1997). Direct injection of 5-HT2A receptor agonists into the medial prefrontal cortex produces a head-twitch response in rats. *J. Pharmacol. Exp. Ther.* 282, 699–706.

Conflict of Interest Statement: The authors declare that the research was conducted in the absence of any commercial or financial relationships that could be construed as a potential conflict of interest.

3

A method for biomarker measurements in peripheral blood mononuclear cells isolated from anxious and depressed mice: β-arrestin 1 protein levels in depression and treatment

***Indira Mendez-David*[1]*, Zeina El-Ali*[2]*, René Hen*[3,4]*, Bruno Falissard*[5]*, Emmanuelle Corruble*[5]*, Alain M. Gardier*[1]*, Saadia Kerdine-Römer*[2]† *and Denis J. David*[1]*†**

[1] *EA3544, Faculté de Pharmacie, Université Paris-Sud, Châtenay-Malabry, France*
[2] *INSERM UMR 996, Faculté de Pharmacie, Université Paris-Sud, Châtenay-Malabry, France*
[3] *Department of Neuroscience, Columbia University, New York, NY, USA*
[4] *Department of Psychiatry, Columbia University, New York, NY, USA*
[5] *INSERM U669, Département de Psychiatrie, Hôpital Bicêtre, Assistance Publique Hôpitaux de Paris, Université Paris-Sud, Le Kremlin-Bicêtre, France*

Edited by:
Thibault Renoir, Florey Institute of Neuroscience and Mental Health, Australia

Reviewed by:
Ciaran J. Faherty, Cadence Pharmaceuticals, USA
El Chérif Ibrahim, Aix-Marseille UNiversité - Centre National de la Recherche Scientifique, France

Correspondence:
Denis J. David, EA3544, Faculté de Pharmacie, Université Paris-Sud, 5, rue J-B Clement, Tour D1, 2e etage, F-92296 Châtenay-Malabry Cedex, France
e-mail: denis.david@u-psud.fr

†Saadia Kerdine-Römer and Denis J. David are joint last authors.

A limited number of biomarkers in the central and peripheral systems which are known may be useful for diagnosing major depressive disorders and predicting the effectiveness of antidepressant (AD) treatments. Since 60% of depressed patients do not respond adequately to medication or are resistant to ADs, it is imperative to delineate more accurate biomarkers. Recent clinical studies suggest that β-arrestin 1 levels in human mononuclear leukocytes may be an efficient biomarker. If potential biomarkers such as β-arrestin 1 could be assessed from a source such as peripheral blood cells, then they could be easily monitored and used to predict therapeutic responses. However, no previous studies have measured β-arrestin 1 levels in peripheral blood mononuclear cells (PBMCs) in anxious/depressive rodents. This study aimed to develop a method to detect β-arrestin protein levels through immunoblot analyses of mouse PBMCs isolated from whole blood. In order to validate the approach, β-arrestin levels were then compared in naïve, anxious/depressed mice, and anxious/depressed mice treated with a selective serotonin reuptake inhibitor (fluoxetine, 18 mg/kg/day in the drinking water). The results demonstrated that mouse whole blood collected by submandibular bleeding permitted isolation of enough PBMCs to assess circulating proteins such as β-arrestin 1. β-Arrestin 1 levels were successfully measured in healthy human subject and naïve mouse PBMCs. Interestingly, PBMCs from anxious/depressed mice showed significantly reduced β-arrestin 1 levels. These decreased β-arrestin 1 expression levels were restored to normal levels with chronic fluoxetine treatment. The results suggest that isolation of PBMCs from mice by submandibular bleeding is a useful technique to screen putative biomarkers of the pathophysiology of mood disorders and the response to ADs. In addition, these results confirm that β-arrestin 1 is a potential biomarker for depression.

Keywords: peripheral blood mononuclear cells, β-arrestin 1, anxiety, depression, mouse models, fluoxetine, biomarkers

INTRODUCTION

Elucidation of the neurobiological bases of depression and anxiety are significant challenges for today's society. Mood disorders impact 7% of the world's population and rank among the top 10 causes of disability (Kessler et al., 2005). Selective serotonin reuptake inhibitors (SSRIs) and serotonin and noradrenaline reuptake inhibitors (SNRIs) are the most commonly prescribed antidepressant (AD) drugs for major depressive disorders (MDD; Samuels et al., 2011). However, key questions about the molecular and cellular mechanisms underlying the effects of ADs remain unanswered. Approximately 60% of depression patients do not respond adequately or are resistant to these drugs (Samuels et al., 2011). Therefore, there are clear benefits of having valid, reliable, selective, and feasible biomarkers for MDD. Several studies have reported genome-wide expression changes associated with AD responses in MDD (Iga et al., 2007a,b; Belzeaux et al., 2010; Lakhan et al., 2010; Mamdani et al., 2011). However, candidate biomarkers that can accurately predict AD responses must be identified. While there are currently no specific markers that are considered "gold standards," a few candidates have emerged. Peripheral/serum brain-derived neurotrophic factor (BDNF), insulin-like growth factor 1 (IGF-1), and cytokines may serve as biomarkers of MDD and treatment response (for review, see Schmidt et al., 2011).

Recently, a substantial body of evidence indicates that β-arrestins (β-arrestin 1 and 2), proteins that regulate G protein receptor coupling, play major roles in the pathophysiology of mood disorders and in the mechanisms underlying AD actions (Avissar et al., 2004; Schreiber and Avissar, 2004; Matuzany-Ruban et al., 2005; Beaulieu et al., 2008; David et al., 2009; Schreiber et al., 2009; Golan et al., 2010). The β-arrestin-signaling cascade has recently gained attention as a potential pre-clinical/clinical bridging biomarker for depressive states and treatment effects. In naïve rats, SSRI, SNRI, and non-selective reuptake inhibitor ADs significantly elevate β-arrestin 1 levels in the cortex and the hippocampus (Avissar et al., 2004; Beaulieu and Caron, 2008; Beaulieu et al., 2008; David et al., 2009). Similarly, β-arrestin 1 expression is decreased in the hypothalamus and hippocampus in anxious/depressed mice exposed to glucocorticoid elevation, and is restored by chronic fluoxetine treatment (David et al., 2009). Moreover, β-arrestin 1 and 2 signaling is involved in mediating the response to fluoxetine and lithium (Beaulieu et al., 2008; David et al., 2009).

Clinical data from Avissar et al. (2004) suggest that β-arrestin 1 mRNA and protein levels are highest in peripheral blood leukocytes of MDD patients. Therefore, β-arrestin 1 may be a putative candidate biochemical marker in clinical practice for depressive pathophysiology and the response to ADs (for review, see Schreiber et al., 2009). β-Arrestin mRNA levels and β-arrestin 1 protein levels in mononuclear leukocytes of untreated patients with MDD are lower than the levels found in healthy subjects. Furthermore, reduced levels of β-arrestin 1 protein and mRNA are significantly correlated with the severity of depressive symptoms (Avissar et al., 2004; Schreiber et al., 2009). However, the low β-arrestin 1 protein and mRNA levels are alleviated by AD treatment. Therefore, these low levels can predict clinical improvement (Avissar et al., 2004; Golan et al., 2010).

These clinical data suggest that assessment of β-arrestin 1 levels may prove useful for diagnosing depression with high sensitivity and specificity (Golan et al., 2013). This hypothesis must first be validated in animal models of anxiety–depression. Most of the current understandings of mood disorders and AD activities are based on studies performed on animal models of anxiety–depression (Belzung and Lemoine, 2011). No animal studies have investigated whether β-arrestin 1 protein levels in peripheral blood mononuclear cells (PBMCs) area marker of the pathophysiology of depression and the AD response. However, if PBMCs can be successfully used to define biomarkers, they provide a system of circulating cells that can be easily collected from patients and monitored to predict therapeutic responses.

In this study, we developed a method to measure and assess circulating proteins (such as β-arrestin 1 in PBMCs) that are collected through submandibular bleeding from unanesthetized animals. Furthermore, we examined whether changes in β-arrestin 1 levels in mouse PBMCs were observed in a model of anxiety/depression (David et al., 2009; Guilloux et al., 2011; Rainer et al., 2012b), and whether these levels could be corrected by chronic treatment with the SSRI fluoxetine.

EXPERIMENTAL PROCEDURES

SUBJECTS

Adult male C57BL/6Ntac mice were purchased from Taconic Farms (Lille Skensved, Denmark). All mice were 7–8 weeks old, weighed 23–25 g at the beginning of the treatment and were maintained on a 12L:12D schedule (lights on at 0600 hours). The mice were group-housed with each cage containing five animals. Food and water were provided *ad libitum*. All testing were conducted in compliance with the laboratory animal care guidelines and with protocols approved by the Institutional Animal Care and Use Committee (Council directive # 87-848, October 19, 1987, Ministère de l'Agriculture et de la Forêt, Service Vétérinaire de la Santé et de la Protection Animale, permissions # 92-256B to Denis J. David).

DRUGS

Corticosterone (4-pregnen-11b-DIOL-3 20-DIONE 21-hemisuccinate from Sigma (Sigma-Aldrich, Saint-Quentin-Fallavier, France) was dissolved in 0.45% hydroxypropyl-β-cyclodextrin (Sigma-Aldrich, Saint-Quentin-Fallavier, France). Fluoxetine hydrochloride (18 mg/kg/day in the drinking water) was purchased from Anawa Trading (Zurich, Switzerland).

ISOLATION OF HUMAN AND MOUSE PERIPHERAL BLOOD MONONUCLEAR CELLS

Collection of human blood and isolation of peripheral blood mononuclear cells

Peripheral blood mononuclear cells were purified from 7.5 ml of human whole circulating blood obtained from Etablissement Français du Sang (Ivry-Sur-Seine, France) through density centrifugation (850 *g* at 20°C for 20 min) using a Ficoll gradient (PAA Laboratories GmbH, Pashing, Austria; **Figure 1A**). This centrifugation separated lymphocytes, monocytes, and plasma. The PBMC layers were carefully removed from the tube and transferred to a new 50 ml conical tube. The PBMCs were then washed twice (1 min each) with 1× phosphate-buffered saline (PBS)/fetal calf serum (FCS, 2%). After centrifugations (150 *g* at 20°C for 7 min), the cells were resuspended in the appropriate volume of 1× PBS. The human PBMCs were then recovered with a final centrifugation (1,000 *g* at 4°C for 5 min) and were stored at −80°C.

Collection of mouse blood and isolation of peripheral blood mononuclear cells

Blood was collected from unanesthetized mice as previously described (Golde et al., 2005; Joslin, 2009). In compliance with the laboratory animal care guidelines, approximately 0.4 ml of blood per mouse was collected in K_3EDTA tubes with a submandibular bleeding procedure. Five millimeters point size sterile lancets (MediPoint, Mineola, NY, USA; **Figure 1B**) were used to puncture the location where the orbital vein and the submandibular vein join to form the jugular vein (Joslin, 2009). A light pressure with dry gauze was applied to the punctured area for hemostasis. Separation and extraction of PBMCs were performed using an iodixanol mixer technique (Ford and Rickwood, 1990). Mouse PBMCs were purified from whole blood by density centrifugation (300 *g* at 20°C for 30 min) using solution B (see **Table 1** for preparation) of the OptiPrep^{TM} gradient solution (Sigma-Aldrich, Saint-Quentin-Fallavier, France). Specifically, the OptiPrep^{TM} gradient solution was used to separate blood into PBMC and plasma layers with centrifugation. The PBMC layers were then carefully removed from the tube and transferred to a new 50 ml conical tube. The PBMCs were then washed twice with solution B (1 min each). After another centrifugation (150 *g* at 20°C for 7 min) and two washing steps (1 min each), mouse

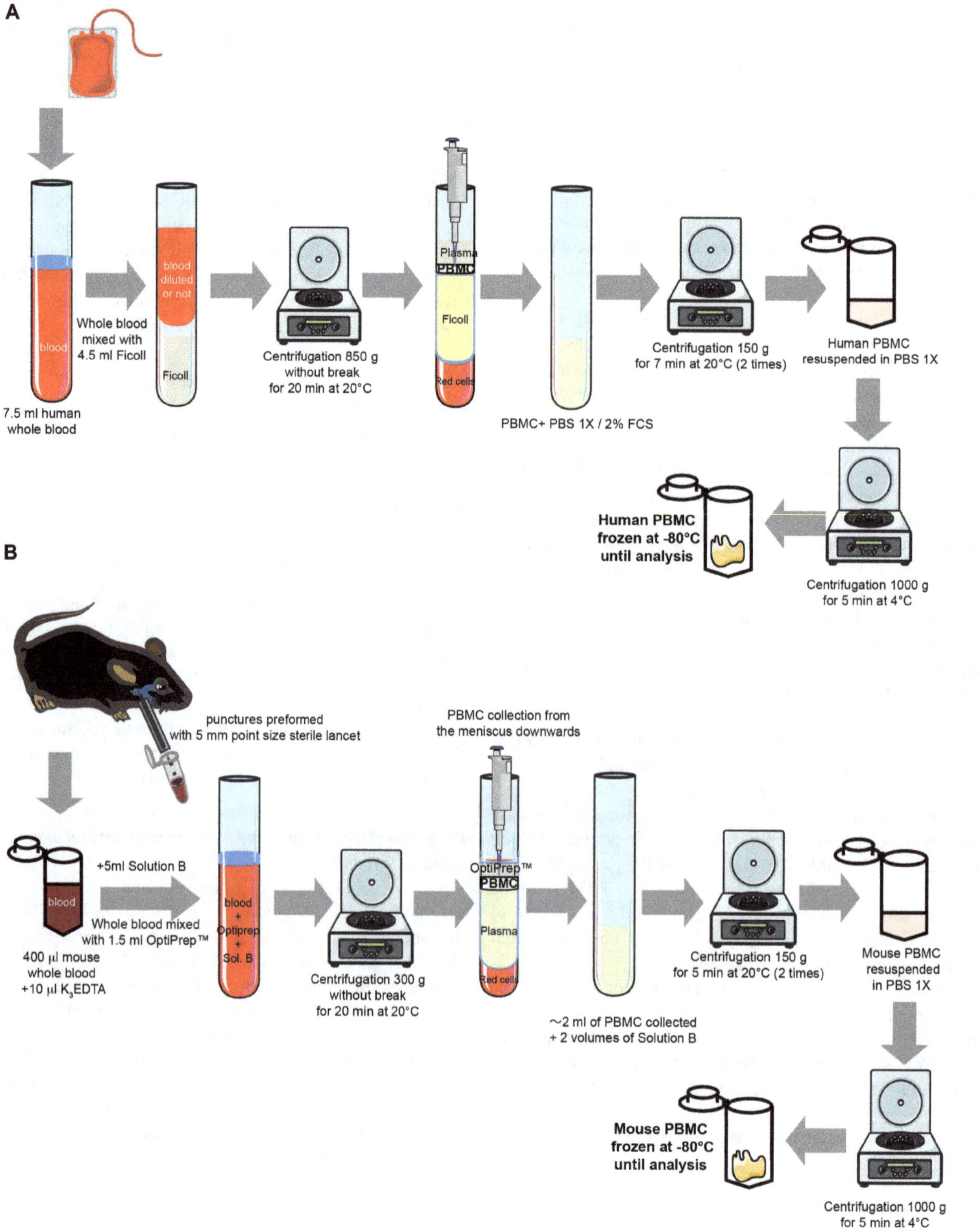

FIGURE 1 | Experimental protocol for isolating human and mouse peripheral blood mononuclear cells from whole blood. (A) Cartoon representing the different steps for isolating human PBMC from whole circulating blood (for full details of the method, see *Blood collection and Peripheral blood mononuclear cells Isolation in human* from the Section "Experimental Procedures"). Some elements of this figure were produced using Servier Medical Art image bank (www.servier.com). **(B)** Cartoon representing the different steps for isolating mouse PBMC from whole circulating blood (for full details of the method, see *Blood collection and Peripheral blood mononuclear cells Isolation in mouse* from the Section "Experimental Procedures"). Some elements of this figure were produced using Servier Medical Art image bank (www.servier.com).

Table 1 | Solution used to prepare peripheral blood mononuclear cells from mouse whole blood.

	OptiPrep™ density gradient medium	Tricine-buffered saline (TBS)	Solution B
Solutions	D1556-250ML (Sigma-Aldrich, France)	0.85% NaCl, 10 mM; Tricine-NaOH, pH 7.4 *(Tricine as 100 mM stock solution at 4°C; 1.79 g/100 ml water)*	Dissolve 0.85 g NaCl in 50 ml water; add 10 ml of Tricine stock; adjust to pH 7.4 with 1 M NaOH and make up to 100 ml

PBMCs were recovered with a final centrifugation (1,000 *g* at 4°C for 5 min) and were stored at −80°C.

β-ARRESTIN 1 LEVELS IN HUMAN AND MOUSE PERIPHERAL BLOOD MONONUCLEAR CELLS

Protein extraction from peripheral blood mononuclear cells and immunoblots

Peripheral blood mononuclear cells were thawed and homogenized with cell lysis buffer containing [20 mM Tris pH 7.4, 137 mM NaCl, 2 mM ethylenediaminetetraacetic acid (EDTA) pH 7.4, 1% Triton X-100, 25 mM β-glycerophosphate, 1 mM phenylmethylsulfonyl fluoride (PMSF), 10 μg/ml aprotinin, 10 μg/ml leupeptin, and 10 μg/ml pepstatin and 100 mM orthovanadate], were incubated on ice for 20 min, were then subjected to centrifugation at 21,130 *g* at 4°C for 20 min. Protein concentrations were quantified using a BCA Protein Assay Kit (Pierce Biotechnology).

β-Arrestin 1 level measurements with immunoblot analyses

Equal amounts of proteins were separated by 10% sodium dodecyl sulfate-polyacrylamide gel electrophoresis (SDS-PAGE) and transferred to polyvinylidene difluoride (PVDF) membranes (Amersham Biosciences, Les Ulis, France). The membranes were then incubated overnight with a primary mouse monoclonal anti-β-arrestin 1 antibody (#610551, BD Biosciences Pharmingen, France; 1:100). In order to ensure that equal amounts of total protein (30 μg) were loaded in each lane, β-actin protein levels were also assessed [β-actin (C4) horseradish peroxidase (HRP), Santa Cruz Biotechnology, Germany, 1:10,000]. Immune complexes were detected using appropriate peroxide-conjugated secondary antibodies and a chemiluminescent reagent kit (Pierce Biotechnology). Immunoblot quantifications were performed by densitometric scanning with Image Lab Software (Bio-Rad). Signals were in the linear range. The densitometry values were normalized against the β-actin values (**Figures 2** and **3**).

CORTICOSTERONE MODEL AND TREATMENT

The dose and duration of corticosterone treatment (CORT model) were selected based on previous studies (David et al., 2009; Guilloux et al., 2011; Hache et al., 2012; Rainer et al., 2012a,b). Exposure to chronic corticosterone results in a phenotype that is similar to a chronic stress phenotype, including a deterioration of the coat state and anxiety/depression-related behaviors. At the end, a higher emotionality score is observed (Guilloux et al., 2011). Corticosterone (35 μg/ml/day, equivalent to about 5 mg/kg/day) or vehicle (0.45% β-cyclodextrin, β-CD) were available to mice *ad libitum* in the drinking water in opaque bottles. Corticosterone-treated water was changed every 3 days to prevent degradation. Group-housed mice were also treated with the SSRI fluoxetine (18 mg/kg/day) for the last 4 weeks of the experiment (see the experimental protocol on **Figure 3A**).

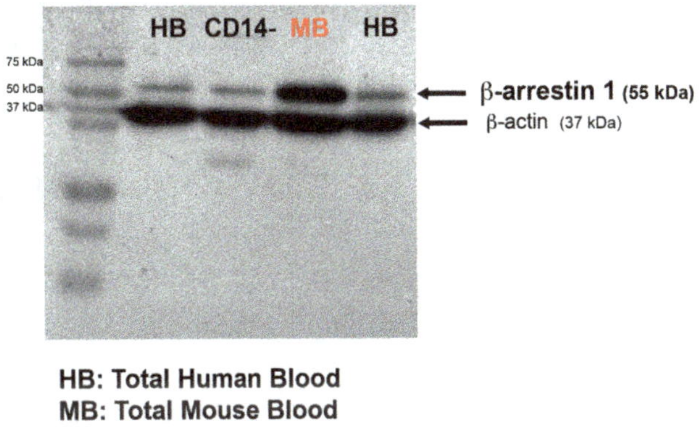

FIGURE 2 | β-Arrestin 1 is measurable in both human and mouse peripheral blood mononuclear cells obtained from a low collection volume of fresh blood. Representative western blot of β-arrestin 1 levels in PBMCs isolated either from CD14⁻ human cells, human or naïve mouse whole blood. In each blot, 30 μg of total protein were run. β-Actin was used as a control.

STATISTICAL ANALYSIS

β-Arrestin 1 levels were quantified and then expressed with a scatterplot or as mean ± SEM normalized to vehicle levels. Data were analyzed using Prism 6.0 software (GraphPad, La Jolla, USA). One-way ANOVAs were used to evaluate data when appropriate. Significant main effects were further analyzed by Fisher's *post hoc* test. Statistical significance was set at $p < 0.05$.

RESULTS

β-ARRESTIN 1 IS DETECTED IN HUMAN AND MOUSE PBMC

We first collected blood in order to assess whether β-arrestin 1 could be detected. Single-use lancets were used for submandibular bleeding and permitted drawing of ~0.4 ml of blood without the use of anesthesia (Golde et al., 2005). The mouse PBMCs were lysed and subjected to immunoblotting. A ~55 kDa band that corresponded to the molecular weight of β-arrestin 1 protein was detected with a monoclonal antibody against mouse anti-β-arrestin 1 that is known to detect human β-arrestin 1 (Avissar et al., 2004; Matuzany-Ruban et al., 2005; Golan et al., 2013; **Figure 2**). Therefore, this method of PBMC isolation from fresh mouse

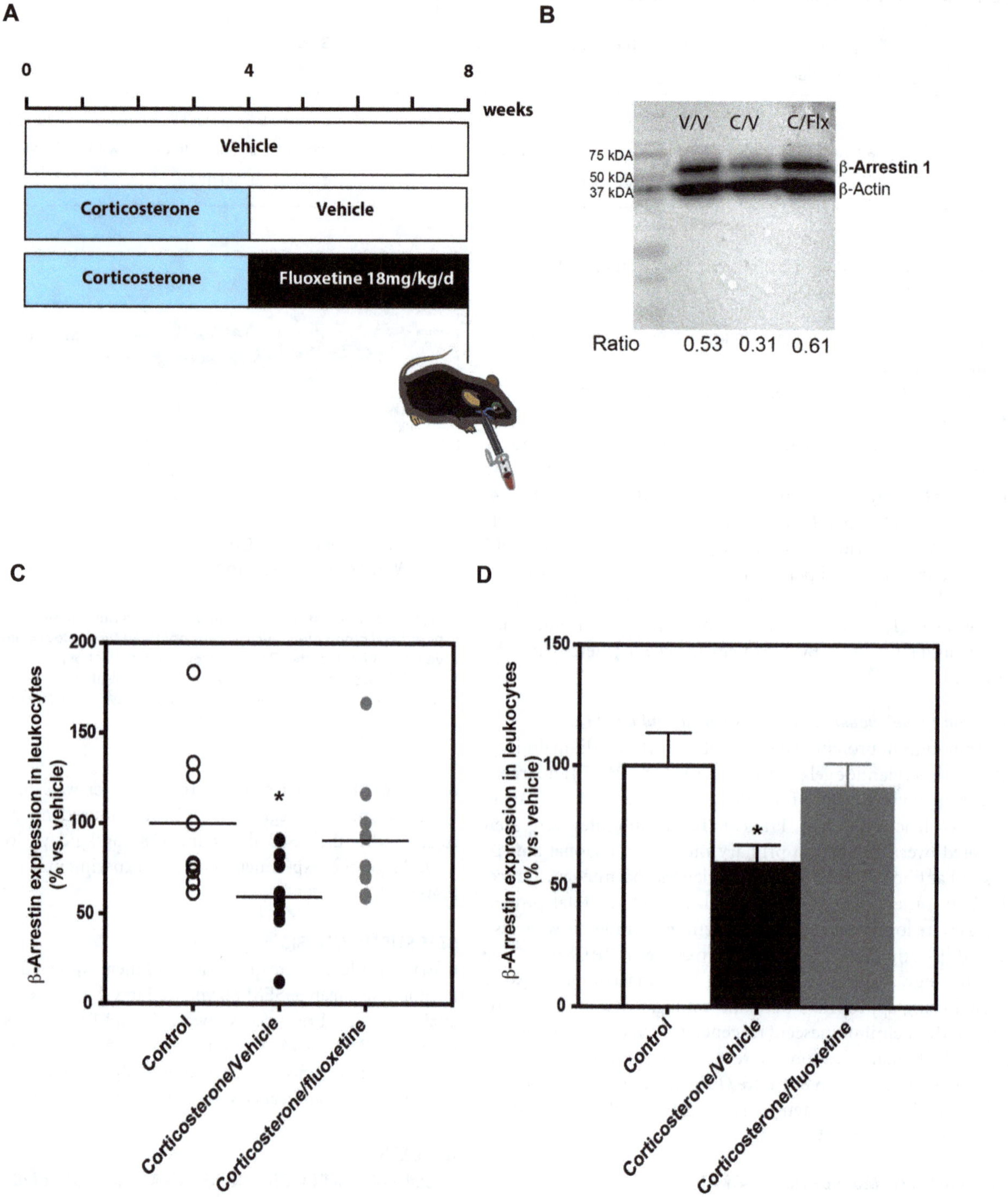

FIGURE 3 | Chronic fluoxetine treatment (18 mg/kg/day for 28 days) restored β-arrestin 1 levels in the peripheral blood mononuclear cells from anxio/depressive mice treated with chronic corticosterone treatment. **(A)** Experimental timeline used to measure β-arrestin 1 levels in peripheral blood mononuclear cells from naïve or anxio-depressive mouse submandibular bleeding chronically treated or not with fluoxetine during 28 days (18 mg/kg/day in the drinking water). **(B)** Representative western blot of β-arrestin 1 levels in peripheral blood mononuclear cells isolated from naïve (vehicle/vehicle, V/V), corticosterone (35 μg/ml/day; corticosterone/vehicle, C/V) or corticosterone/fluoxetine (18 mg/kg/day; corticosterone/fluoxetine, C/F) mouse whole blood. In each blot, 30 μg of protein from mouse PBMC were run. The densitometry values for each band allowed the calculation of a ratio: optical density for β-arrestin 1/optical density β-actin value. **(C,D)** Scatterplot of the individual effects **(C)** or bar charts of mean ± SEM of the effects **(D)** of a chronic administration (28 days) treatment with fluoxetine on β-arrestin 1 levels in the peripheral blood mononuclear cells from mice treated with chronic corticosterone in comparison to untreated animals. Data are expressed in percentage normalized to vehicle/vehicle expression; $n = 9–10$). $^{*}p < 0.05$, *versus* control vehicle/vehicle group.

blood successfully permitted measurements of β-arrestin 1 levels. This method can potentially be used to investigate levels of other proteins as well. Lysates of human total PBMCs and CD14 negative PBMC fraction cells ($CD14^-$) were used as positive controls. In addition, we were also able to detect β-arrestin 1 in human PBMCs isolated from low fresh circulating blood volume (7.5 ml) of healthy adult donors obtained from Etablissement Français du Sang (**Figure 2**). To our knowledge, this is the first study to detect β-arrestin 1 in this fashion.

Next, we decided to quantify β-arrestin 1 levels in PBMCs isolated from C57BL/6Ntac mice exposed to chronic corticosterone (David et al., 2009; Rainer et al., 2012b) that was given either alone or in combination with the SSRI fluoxetine (18 mg/kg/day; **Figure 3A**).

CHRONIC FLUOXETINE TREATMENT NORMALIZES β-ARRESTIN 1 EXPRESSION IN PBMC ISOLATED FROM ANXIOUS/DEPRESSIVE-LIKE MICE

In mouse PBMCs isolated from blood of mice treated chronically with corticosterone (35 μg/ml/day), we found that β-arrestin 1 levels were significantly lower (−41%; 59% of expression compared to 100% in the control group) than the levels in naïve animals [one-way ANOVA, $F(2,25) = 3.81$; $^*p < 0.05$; **Figures 3C,D**]. Interestingly, a 4-week treatment with the SSRI fluoxetine normalized these β-arrestin 1 expression levels so that they were not significantly different than the levels observed in naïve animals (**Figures 3C,D**).

DISCUSSION

We developed a new method to assess circulating proteins such as β-arrestin 1 through immunoblot analyses of mouse PBMCs isolated from whole blood. We showed significantly reduced β-arrestin 1 levels in PBMCs from anxious/depressed mice. These decreased β-arrestin 1 expression levels were restored to normal levels with chronic fluoxetine treatment.

PBMCs WERE ISOLATED FROM UNANESTHETIZED MICE

A recent review from Duman's group highlighted the need to develop a biomarker panel for depression. This biomarker panel should profile diverse peripheral factors that together will provide a biological signature of MDD subtypes and predict treatment response (Schmidt et al., 2011). Assessing peripheral protein levels in PBMCs is an attractive method because PBMCs are circulating cells that can be easily collected and monitored. Previous studies demonstrated that PBMCs can be isolated from mouse blood to assess immunological responses (Fuss et al., 2009). However, to our knowledge this is the first study to collect PBMCs from circulating blood of unanesthetized animals. Single-use lancets were used for submandibular bleeding. This method permitted PBMCs to be collected from peripheral blood circulation in living and unanesthetized mice. Thus, submandibular bleeding is a useful method to screen putative biomarkers of the pathophysiology of mood disorders and the response to ADs. This technique can be easily performed multiple times in the same animals and can be used with other rodent species such as rats.

β-ARRESTIN 1 PROTEIN LEVELS CAN BE MEASURED IN MOUSE AND HUMAN PBMCs

We measured β-arrestin 1 protein levels to determine whether mouse PBMCs are useful biological materials to screen biomarkers for MDD pathophysiology and the AD response. Over the last decade, several G protein receptor-related genes such as β-arrestins were found to be involved in the pathophysiology of mood disorders (Schreiber and Avissar, 2004; Beaulieu et al., 2008; David et al., 2009). Numerous data from clinical studies support the importance of measuring β-arrestin 1 levels as a peripheral biomarker of the pathophysiology of mood disorders and predicting the AD response (Avissar et al., 2004; Schreiber et al., 2009; Golan et al., 2013). However, no previous study demonstrated *ex vivo* measurements of β-arrestin 1 levels in leukocytes isolated from whole blood to compare levels between naïve and anxious/depressed rodents. In addition, this is the first study to assess β-arrestin 1 by immunoblot in human and in mouse leukocytes simultaneously by using the same monoclonal antibody.

In the human experiments, we were able to recover PBMCs from 7.5 ml of whole circulating blood from healthy volunteers. Previous studies showed that larger amounts of blood were needed for the detection of β-arrestin 1 in human leucocytes (Avissar et al., 2004; Matuzany-Ruban et al., 2005; Golan et al., 2013). Here, 7.5 ml was sufficient to acquire 30 μg of PBMC lysate for immunoblotting (**Figure 2**).

Avissar et al. (2004) demonstrated that β-arrestin 1 levels were elevated by chronic ADs in rat cortex and hippocampus. However, by contrast with their human study, they did not provide data showing that β-arrestin 1 levels in rat PBMCs are affected by chronic AD treatment (Avissar et al., 2004). Therefore, we also compared β-arrestin 1 levels in PBMCs of anxious/depressed mice before and after chronic AD treatment (**Figure 3**).

β-ARRESTIN 1 IS A PREDICTIVE MARKER OF THE PATHOPHYSIOLOGY OF DEPRESSION AND THE ANTIDEPRESSANT RESPONSE

To induce an anxious/depression-related phenotype, we utilized a chronic corticosterone treatment that results in hallmark characteristics of anxiety and depression (for review, see David et al., 2009; Mendez-David et al., 2013). In order to delineate a panel of biomarkers of the pathophysiology and the treatment of depression, it is first essential to screen putative candidates in a model of anxiety/depression. β-Arrestin 1 protein levels in leukocytes were reduced when mice were exposed to chronic corticosterone. As found in previous human studies (Matuzany-Ruban et al., 2005; Golan et al., 2013), these reduced β-arrestin 1 levels were alleviated by AD treatment.

LIMITATIONS OF THE STUDY

Measuring protein levels in mouse PBMCs at several time points is a powerful technique that can be used to reveal potential biomarkers for the pathophysiology of depression and the AD response. However, this study has some limitations that must be considered when interpreting the current findings. For example, it is important to distinguish diagnostic biomarkers from treatment biomarkers (Schmidt et al., 2011). This study does not address this difference. Further studies are required to assess whether β-arrestin 1 is a reasonable biomarker for diagnostic and/or drug treatments. A study that compares peripheral levels of β-arrestin 1 in stressed animals before and after AD treatment could definitively address this question. It also may be interesting to study whether there is a correlation between β-arrestin 1 levels and the severity of the anxio/depressive state (Guilloux et al., 2011). Moreover, disease conditions are most often signified by the dysregulation of complex biological pathways involving multiple key factors (Dudley and Butte, 2009). Thus, it is unlikely that β-arrestin 1 alone will be a sufficient diagnostic and treatment biomarker. However, mouse PBMCs might provide useful material to screen a panel of biomarkers and to provide biological signatures of MDD and AD treatments. Finally, in our study, β-arrestin 1 levels were measured using western blots, which is a semi-quantitative method of evaluating protein levels. The development of an enzyme-linked immunosorbent assay (ELISA) to assess β-arrestin 1 levels would provide a more quantitative method.

CONCLUSION

In this study, we demonstrated that PBMCs isolated from a small volume of whole blood in unanesthetized mice using a submandibular bleeding method may provide a useful biological tool to assess circulating proteins. This method will permit future studies to screen potential biomarkers for the pathophysiology of depression and AD responses. We also confirmed that measurements of β-arrestin 1 levels in PBMCs may serve as a biochemical marker of depression in humans (Avissar et al., 2004). Overall, we developed a powerful tool for translational studies that can easily be used to assess proteins measurements and to provide a biological signature of treatment response. Identification of a biological signature could predict the effectiveness of ADs (Fuss et al., 2009).

ACKNOWLEDGMENTS

We thank Valérie Domergue-Dupont and her staff in the animal care facility of the Institut Paris-Sud d'Innovation Therapeutique. We also thank Sylvain David (sylvain.david09@gmail.com) for designing the mouse submandibular bleeding method (**Figures 1B** and **3A**). This work was supported by grants from Agence Nationale pour la Recherche SAMENTA (ANR-12-SAMA-0007, to Alain M. Gardier) and by a NARSAD young investigator award (to Denis J. David). Finally, we are grateful to Dr. Benjamin A. Samuels (Columbia University, USA) for helpful discussions and critical reading of the manuscript.

AUTHOR CONTRIBUTIONS

Indira Mendez-David, Alain M. Gardier, René Hen, Saadia Kerdine-Römer, and Denis J. David designed research; Indira Mendez-David and Zeina El-Ali performed research and draw **Figure 2**; Indira Mendez-David analyzed data; Indira Mendez-David, Saadia Kerdine-Römer, and Denis J. David wrote the manuscript. Indira Mendez-David, Zeina El-Ali, René Hen, Emmanuelle Corruble, Bruno Falissard, Alain M. Gardier, Saadia Kerdine-Römer, and Denis J. David contributed to the preparation of the manuscript.

REFERENCES

Avissar, S., Matuzany-Ruban, A., Tzukert, K., and Schreiber, G. (2004). Beta-arrestin-1 levels: reduced in leukocytes of patients with depression and elevated by antidepressants in rat brain. *Am. J. Psychiatry* 161, 2066–2072. doi: 10.1176/appi.ajp.161.11.2066

Beaulieu, J. M., and Caron, M. G. (2008). Looking at lithium: molecular moods and complex behaviour. *Mol. Interv.* 8, 230–241. doi: 10.1124/mi.8.5.8

Beaulieu, J. M., Marion, S., Rodriguiz, R. M., Medvedev, I. O., Sotnikova, T. D., Ghisi, V., et al. (2008). A beta-arrestin 2 signaling complex mediates lithium action on behavior. *Cell* 132, 125–136. doi: 10.1016/j.cell.2007.11.041

Belzeaux, R., Formisano-Treziny, C., Loundou, A., Boyer, L., Gabert, J., Samuelian, J. C., et al. (2010). Clinical variations modulate patterns of gene expression and define blood biomarkers in major depression. *J. Psychiatr. Res.* 44, 1205–1213. doi: 10.1016/j.jpsychires.2010.04.011

Belzung, C., and Lemoine, M. (2011). Criteria of validity for animal models of psychiatric disorders: focus on anxiety disorders and depression. *Biol. Mood Anxiety Disord.* 1, 9. doi: 10.1186/2045-5380-1-9

David, D. J., Samuels, B. A., Rainer, Q., Wang, J. W., Marsteller, D., Mendez, I., et al. (2009). Neurogenesis-dependent and -independent effects of fluoxetine in an animal model of anxiety/depression. *Neuron* 62, 479–493. doi: 10.1016/j.neuron.2009.04.017

Dudley, J. T., and Butte, A. J. (2009). Identification of discriminating biomarkers for human disease using integrative network biology. *Pac. Symp. Biocomput.* 2009, 27–38.

Ford, T. C., and Rickwood, D. (1990). A new one-step method for the isolation of human mononuclear cells. *J. Immunol. Methods* 134, 237–241. doi: 10.1016/0022-1759(90)90385-9

Fuss, I. J., Kanof, M. E., Smith, P. D., and Zola, H. (2009). Isolation of whole mononuclear cells from peripheral blood and cord blood. *Curr. Protoc. Immunol.* Chapter 7, Unit 7.1. doi: 10.1002/0471142735.im0701s19

Golan, M., Schreiber, G., and Avissar, S. (2010). Antidepressants increase beta-arrestin 2 ubiquitinylation and degradation by the proteasomal pathway in C6 rat glioma cells. *J. Pharmacol. Exp. Ther.* 332, 970–976. doi: 10.1124/jpet.109.160218

Golan, M., Schreiber, G., and Avissar, S. (2013). Antidepressant-induced differential ubiquitination of beta-arrestins 1 and 2 in mononuclear leucocytes of patients with depression. *Int. J. Neuropsychopharmacol.* 16, 1745–1754. doi: 10.1017/S1461145713000291

Golde, W. T., Gollobin, P., and Rodriguez, L. L. (2005). A rapid, simple, and humane method for submandibular bleeding of mice using a lancet. *Lab Anim. (NY)* 34, 39–43. doi: 10.1038/laban1005-39

Guilloux, J. P., Seney, M., Edgar, N., and Sibille, E. (2011). Integrated behavioral *z*-scoring increases the sensitivity and reliability of behavioral phenotyping in mice: relevance to emotionality and sex. *J. Neurosci. Methods* 197, 21–31. doi: 10.1016/j.jneumeth.2011.01.019

Hache, G., Guiard, B. P., Le Dantec, Y., Orvoen, S., David, D. J., Gardier, A. M., et al. (2012). Antinociceptive effects of fluoxetine in a mouse model of anxiety/depression. *Neuroreport* 23, 525–529. doi: 10.1097/WNR.0b013e328353d70a

Iga, J., Ueno, S., Yamauchi, K., Numata, S., Kinouchi, S., Tayoshi-Shibuya, S., et al. (2007a). Altered HDAC5 and CREB mRNA expressions in the peripheral leukocytes of major depression. *Prog. Neuropsychopharmacol. Biol. Psychiatry* 31, 628–632. doi: 10.1016/j.pnpbp.2006.12.014

Iga, J., Ueno, S., Yamauchi, K., Numata, S., Tayoshi-Shibuya, S., Kinouchi, S., et al. (2007b). Gene expression and association analysis of vascular endothelial growth factor in major depressive disorder. *Prog. Neuropsychopharmacol. Biol. Psychiatry* 31, 658–663. doi: 10.1016/j.pnpbp.2006.12.011

Joslin, J. O. (2009). Blood collection techniques in exotic small mammals. *J. Exotic Pet Med.* 18, 117–139. doi: 10.1053/j.jepm.2009.04.002

Kessler, R. C., Chiu, W. T., Demler, O., Merikangas, K. R., and Walters, E. E. (2005). Prevalence, severity, and comorbidity of 12-month DSM-IV disorders in the National Comorbidity Survey Replication. *Arch. Gen. Psychiatry* 62, 617–627. doi: 10.1001/archpsyc.62.6.617

Lakhan, S. E., Vieira, K., and Hamlat, E. (2010). Biomarkers in psychiatry: drawbacks and potential for misuse. *Int. Arch Med.* 3, 1. doi: 10.1186/1755-7682-3-1

Mamdani, F., Berlim, M. T., Beaulieu, M. M., Labbe, A., Merette, C., and Turecki, G. (2011). Gene expression biomarkers of response to citalopram treatment in major depressive disorder. *Transl. Psychiatry* 1, e13. doi: 10.1038/tp.2011.12

Matuzany-Ruban, A., Avissar, S., and Schreiber, G. (2005). Dynamics of beta-arrestin1 protein and mRNA levels elevation by antidepressants in mononuclear leukocytes of patients with depression. *J. Affect. Disord.* 88, 307–312. doi: 10.1016/j.jad.2005.08.007

Mendez-David, I., Hen, R., Gardier, A. M., and David, D. J. (2013). Adult hippocampal neurogenesis: an actor in the antidepressant-like action. *Ann. Pharm. Fr.* 71, 143–149. doi: 10.1016/j.pharma.2013.02.006

Rainer, Q., Nguyen, H. T., Quesseveur, G., Gardier, A. M., David, D. J., and Guiard, B. P. (2012a). Functional status of somatodendritic serotonin 1A autoreceptor after long-term treatment with fluoxetine in a mouse model of anxiety/depression based on repeated corticosterone administration. *Mol. Pharmacol.* 81, 106–112. doi: 10.1124/mol.111.075796

Rainer, Q., Xia, L., Guilloux, J. P., Gabriel, C., Mocaer, E., Hen, R., et al. (2012b). Beneficial behavioural and neurogenic effects of agomelatine in a model of depression/anxiety. *Int. J. Neuropsychopharmacol.* 15, 321–335.

Samuels, B. A., Leonardo, E. D., Gadient, R., Williams, A., Zhou, J., David, D. J., et al. (2011). Modeling treatment-resistant depression. *Neuropharmacology* 61, 408–413. doi: 10.1016/j.neuropharm.2011.02.017

Schmidt, H. D., Shelton, R. C., and Duman, R. S. (2011). Functional biomarkers of depression: diagnosis, treatment, and pathophysiology. *Neuropsychopharmacology* 36, 2375–2394. doi: 10.1038/npp.2011.151

Schreiber, G., and Avissar, S. (2004). Editorial: complexity and future of biochemical differential diagnosis in psychiatry. *Isr. J. Psychiatry Relat. Sci.* 41, 79–81.

Schreiber, G., Golan, M., and Avissar, S. (2009). Beta-arrestin signaling complex as a target for antidepressants and as a depression marker. *Drug News Perspect.* 22, 467–480.

Conflict of Interest Statement: The authors declare that the research was conducted in the absence of any commercial or financial relationships that could be construed as a potential conflict of interest.

4

The role of the serotonergic and GABA system in translational approaches in drug discovery for anxiety disorders

Jocelien D. A. Olivier*[1,2], *Christiaan H. Vinkers*[3,4] and *Berend Olivier*[3,5]

[1] *Department of Women's and Children's Health, Uppsala University, Uppsala, Sweden*
[2] *Center for Gender Medicine, Karolinska Institutet, Stockholm, Sweden*
[3] *Division of Pharmacology, Utrecht Institute for Pharmaceutical Sciences and Rudolf Magnus Institute of Neuroscience, Utrecht University, Utrecht, Netherlands*
[4] *Department of Psychiatry, Rudolf Magnus Institute of Neuroscience, Utrecht Medical Center, Utrecht, Netherlands*
[5] *Department of Psychiatry, Yale University School of Medicine, New Haven, CT, USA*

Edited by:
Thibault Renoir, Florey Institute of Neuroscience and Mental Health, Australia

Reviewed by:
Alfredo Meneses, Center for Research and Advanced Studies, Mexico
Bruno Pierre Guiard, University of Paris XI, France

****Correspondence:***
Berend Olivier, Department of Psychiatry, Yale University School of Medicine, 333 Cedar Street, New Haven, CT 06510, USA
e-mail: b.olivier@uu.nl

There is ample evidence that genetic factors play an important role in anxiety disorders. In support, human genome-wide association studies have implicated several novel candidate genes. However, illumination of such genetic factors involved in anxiety disorders has not resulted in novel drugs over the past decades. A complicating factor is the heterogeneous classification of anxiety disorders in the Diagnostic and Statistical Manual of Mental Disorders (DSM-IV-TR) and diverging operationalization of anxiety used in preclinical and clinical studies. Currently, there is an increasing focus on the gene × environment (G × E) interaction in anxiety as genes do not operate in isolation and environmental factors have been found to significantly contribute to the development of anxiety disorders in at-risk individuals. Nevertheless, extensive research on G × E mechanisms in anxiety has not resulted in major breakthroughs in drug discovery. Modification of individual genes in rodent models has enabled the specific study of anxiety in preclinical studies. In this context, two extensively studied neurotransmitters involved in anxiety are the gamma-aminobutyric acid (GABA) and 5-HT (5-hydroxytryptamine) system. In this review, we illustrate the complex interplay between genes and environment in anxiety processes by reviewing preclinical and clinical studies on the serotonin transporter (5-HTT), 5-HT_{1A} receptor, 5-HT_2 receptor, and $GABA_A$ receptor. Even though targets from the serotonin and GABA system have yielded drugs with known anxiolytic efficacy, the relation between the genetic background of these targets and anxiety symptoms and development of anxiety disorders is largely unknown. The aim of this review is to show the vast complexity of genetic and environmental factors in anxiety disorders. In light of the difficulty with which common genetic variants are identified in anxiety disorders, animal models with translational validity may aid in elucidating the neurobiological background of these genes and their possible role in anxiety. We argue that, in addition to human genetic studies, translational models are essential to map anxiety-related genes and to enhance our understanding of anxiety disorders in order to develop potentially novel treatment strategies.

Keywords: translational, animal model, $GABA_A$, 5-HT, 5-HT_{1A} receptor, 5-HT_2 receptor, 5-HTT, 5-HTTLPR

INTRODUCTION

Anxiety disorders constitute one of the most prevalent classes of psychiatric disorders. Anxiety disorders in the Diagnostic and Statistical Manual of Mental Disorders (DSM-IV) include panic disorder (PD), generalized anxiety disorder (GAD), phobias, social phobia, obsessive compulsive disorder (OCD), and post-traumatic stress disorder (PTSD) and were the most common mental disorders within Europe in 2010 with 14% prevalence (Wittchen, 2011). The heterogeneous classification system of individual anxiety disorders in the DSM-IV is based on symptomatology rather than etiology (Friedman et al., 2011). Anxiety disorders are often comorbid with other psychiatric disorders such as mood disorders and substance abuse disorders which make anxiety disorders in general a heterogeneous class of psychiatric disorders. Moreover, specific anxiety disorders are often incomparable to each other with regard to the symptomatology. Specifically, OCD and PTSD are quite different with regard to their symptomatology compared to GAD or social phobia. Application of the DSM-V has not resulted in major changes in the classification of anxiety disorders (Friedman et al., 2011). The complex and specific classification of anxiety disorders may eventually hinder drug development as one-to-one translation to preclinical models is not possible. A classification based on the neurobiological mechanisms underlying pathological anxiety (intermediate phenotypes) has been proposed as a novel strategy to discover novel targets to treat anxiety symptoms (Ressler and Mayberg, 2007). However, so far, progress in understanding the neurobiology of emotional (dys)regulation has not resulted in novel treatments. Another approach is based on the hypothesis of dysfunctional neurotransmitter systems, which assumes that anxiety disorders are associated with abnormal functionality of specific neurotransmitter systems. However, the definition of a "dysfunctional" neurotransmitter system is difficult and not without confounds, and even more, a direct and consistent relation between specific neurotransmitters systems and anxiety disorders has not been established. The difficulty of developing novel anxiolytic drugs is illustrated by the fact that existing anxiolytic drugs such as benzodiazepines (BZs) and selective serotonin (5-hydroxytryptamine, 5-HT) reuptake inhibitors (SSRIs) have been developed several decades ago. The development of BZs was the result of serendipity and SSRIs were primarily developed to treat major depressive disorder. Interestingly, when patients start using SSRIs they experience anxiogenic effects of the drug, while after administration of several weeks SSRIs work anxiolytically. This is probably due to activation of 5-HT_{2C} receptors as antagonists for these receptors are able to reverse the acute anxiogenic effect of SSRIs (Bagdy et al., 2001). Moreover, chronic exposure to SSRIs has been shown to downregulate 5-HT_{2C} receptors in the cortex (Attar-Levy et al., 1999). Although extensive search has occurred in the ensuing decades to find new targets for anxiolytics based on the known and anticipated neurochemical mechanisms underlying anxiety, no real breakthroughs have emerged. Currently, SSRIs remain the preferred drugs for the treatment of anxiety disorders (augmented with BZs for a limited time interval). Although efficacious, some patients are treatment resistant, and inherent disadvantages with regard to side effects are attached to the use of SSRIs and BZs. Therefore, preclinical and clinical studies over the last decades have focused on other mechanisms to target anxiety processes in order to ultimately treat anxiety disorders. Since then, evidence has emerged for several novel anxiety targets, including the corticotropin-releasing factor 1 (CRF_1) receptors, neurokinin 1 (NK-1) receptors, and glucocorticoid receptors (for review, see Cryan and Sweeney, 2011). Although the preclinical efficacy of drugs targeting these neurotransmitters was often encouraging during development, no superior therapeutic anxiolytic effects have been found in subsequent clinical trials. Thus, no novel anxiolytic drug targets have reached the market to replace the current treatment choices. Surprisingly, even though targets such as the serotonin 1A (5-HT_{1A}) receptor, serotonin 2 (5-HT_2) receptor, the serotonin transporter (5-HTT), and the gamma-aminobutyric acid-A ($GABA_A$) receptor have yielded drugs with known efficacy, the relation between the genetic background of these targets and anxiety symptoms and disorders is little understood. The complexity of anxiety disorders calls for a multidisciplinary approach of the phenomenon of anxiety. In this review, we argue that by using translational preclinical models, anxiety-related genes can be mapped and this information may subsequently be used to enhance our understanding of clinical studies in order to identify novel drug targets for anxiety. To this end, this review focuses on the convincing evidence stemming from preclinical and clinical studies that genes involved in the serotonin and GABA system play a pivotal role in the development of anxiety disorders. These 5-HTergic and GABAergic genes are highlighted throughout this review to illustrate the complexity of the genetic background of anxiety disorders.

HERITABILITY OF ANXIETY DISORDERS

From family studies, the risk to develop an anxiety disorder such as PD, phobias, OCD, or GAD is three- to sixfold higher in first-degree relatives of affected probands compared to unaffected individuals (Chantarujikapong et al., 2001; Hettema et al., 2001). Also, twin studies have aided in estimating the genetic and environmental components of the variance in PTSD (Seedat et al., 2001). Moreover, concordance rates in monozygotic twins have been found to be increased compared to dizygotic twins for anxiety disorders with an estimated heritability in the range of 20–40% (Hettema et al., 2005). Thus, it is clear that genetic variability contributes to a certain extent to the risk for anxiety disorders. Nevertheless, the rather limited heritability implies that anxiety disorders are not mere genetically defined disorders.

LINKAGE MAPPING

When a disease runs in the family, genetic markers in several generations can be studied, and such linkage mapping has been found to be critical for identifying genes that are causal for anxiety disorders. It is assumed that a gene contributing to a disease is located in the same area of the genome as the genetic marker. Significant linkage for anxiety and PD has been reported at chromosomes 9q31 (Thorgeirsson et al., 2003), 2q (Fyer et al., 2006), 7p (Knowles et al., 1998), 13q (Hamilton et al., 2003), 15q (Fyer et al., 2006), and 22q (Hamilton et al., 2003). Significant linkages were also found for a "PD syndrome" (13q; Weissman et al., 2000). Additionally, suggestive-linkage regions were reported for agoraphobia (1q; Gelernter et al., 2001), PD and agoraphobia (12q; Smoller et al., 2001a), social phobia (Gelernter et al., 2004), and markers for specific phobia on chromosome 14 (Gelernter et al., 2003). Finally, Kaabi et al. (2006) detected a strong linkage signal for anxiety and PD on chromosome 4 (4q31-q34) at marker *D4S413*. Linkage studies for OCD have only revealed single nucleotide polymorphisms (SNPs) in the glutamate transporter gene SLC1A1 on 9p24 (Walitza et al., 2010). Although linkage studies have implicated several chromosomal regions that may harbor susceptibility genes (Smoller et al., 2008a), no candidate genes have emerged that play a straightforward role in the expression for a vulnerability to anxiety or anxiety disorders (Smoller et al., 2009). This is probably due to the fact that several genetic risk factors only explain a limited amount of variance. Moreover, the strongest linkage signals seem to derive from recessive and highly penetrant diseases. Linkage studies are good to detect regions involved in these recessive diseases and can narrow down the search for causal variants to a few million base pairs.

ASSOCIATION MAPPING

Association studies compare allelic variation in a group of patients to a healthy control population. When a certain allele plays a role in the development or susceptibility of a disease or is correlated with a causal allele, the frequency of this allele will be increased in the case population compared to the control population. Usually, linkage studies result in a signal of candidate genes in a certain region and are followed by a genetic association study on alleles in that genetic region. In this way, a specific gene or even a specific allele can be identified to play a causal role in a certain disorder. Genetic association studies have become the predominant method for identifying susceptibility loci for complex traits (Smoller et al., 2008a). Several genes have been associated with PD (Hovatta and Barlow, 2008), such as, e.g., catechol-*o*-methyl transferase (COMT; Hamilton et al., 2002; Domschke et al., 2004; Woo et al., 2004; Rothe et al., 2006), adenosine A2A receptor (ADORA2A; Deckert et al., 1998; Hamilton et al., 2004), cholecystokinin (CCK; Wang et al., 1998; Hattori et al., 2001; Maron et al., 2005), CCK-B receptor (Kennedy et al., 1999), 5-HT_{1A} receptor (HTR1A; Maron et al., 2004; Rothe et al., 2004; Fakra et al., 2009; Choi et al., 2010), 5-HT_{2A} receptor (HTR2A; Inada et al., 2003; Maron et al., 2005), 5-HTT (SLC6A4; Lesch et al., 1996; McDougle et al., 1998; Bengel et al., 1999; Ohara et al., 1999; Lee et al., 2005; Munafo et al., 2005), monoamine oxidase A (MAO-A; Deckert et al., 1999; Inada et al., 2003; Maron et al., 2004; Samochowiec et al., 2004), and the regulator of G protein signaling 2 (Rgs2; Smoller et al., 2008b). Genetic association studies have also revealed several genes involved in PTSD, with most attention for genes involved in the hypothalamus–pituitary–adrenal (HPA) axis and the regulation of neurobiological pathways such as the SLC6A4, DAT1, DRD2, DRD4, FKBP5, and GCCR (systematically reviewed in Digangi et al., 2013). Although linkage studies only found SNPs in the SLC1A1 to be associated with OCD, association studies have found more genes such as SLC6A4, HTR1D, HTR2A, HTR2C, DRD4, DRD2, SLC1a1, GRIN2B, GABBR1, COMT, MAO-A, TPH1, TPH2, BDNF (brain-derived neurotrophic factor), NTRK2, OLIG2, and MOG (reviewed in Walitza et al., 2010). For GAD the Gad2, Rgs2, and Ppargc1a (in anxiety-spectrum disorders) were found to be associated (Sokolowska and Hovatta, 2013). Moreover in general CDH2, ALAD, PSAP, EPB41L4A, DYNLL2, and PTGDS that were associated with anxiety disorders (Sokolowska and Hovatta, 2013). Among all these genes, the SLC6A4 (5-HTT) is one of the most widely investigated genes in relation to anxiety-related personality traits (Munafo et al., 2003). Most association studies of anxiety disorder have focused on candidate genes, which are suspected to play a role in a particular anxiety disorder. This can be based on earlier biological evidence (biological candidate) or because these genes are located within loci previously implicated via linkage studies (positional candidates). However, most likely more than one gene variant is involved in the regulation of distinct emotional responses, which together with the environmental influence will determine who will become affected. Studies in animal models of anxiety have provided evidence for the involvement of certain genes. The most intensively studied candidate genes are related to neurotransmitter systems implicated in the regulation of anxiety, to various neuropeptides, and to stress-related genes, and for that reason have functioned as targets to develop anxiolytic drugs. These targets include 5-HT, noradrenalin (NE), glutamate, dopamine, GABA, RGS2, and neuropeptides (CRF, neuropeptide Y, BDNF). To address the complexity of psychiatric disorders, two strategies have evolved; (1) going "big" and (2) going "deep" (Smoller et al., 2009).

GENOME-WIDE ASSOCIATION STUDIES

First studies have looked for SNPs based on an unbiased survey of the entire genome (genome-wide association studies, GWAS). The main aim of this strategy is to increase the explained variance of genetic studies by increasing the number of genes and, subsequently, sample size. By selecting a reduced set of SNPs that adequately represents the genetic variation, the whole DNA can be investigated with DNA chips measuring up to millions of SNPs. Although statistically stringent demands are uphold, the GWAS approach has resulted in the elucidation of genes and genetic variants involved in complex diseases such as autism and bipolar disorder although at a disappointing level (Chen et al., 2010; Gershon et al., 2011). With regard to anxiety, several anxiety genes have been found (Hovatta and Barlow, 2008), yet replication studies are lacking. Currently, GWAS are still on-going to localize and identify putative risk genes for anxiety disorders. The reason why GWAS were relatively unsuccessful for anxiety disorders is not fully clear. Several causes have been proposed, to name a few: (1) small effect sizes (Manolio et al., 2009); (2) new analytical approaches are necessary to detect more locations in the genome (Lubke et al., 2012); (3) epistasis, only a few genes together could contribute to a genetic risk while a gene on its own will never be identified. Network- and pathway-based methods are necessary in identifying candidate genes and to provide functional links to connect genetic variants to phenotypes (reviewed in Sun, 2012); (4) copy number variations (CNVs) might be responsible for a non-trivial proportion of common risk disease. The majority of CNVs remain invisible to current GWAS technology and would require whole-genome sequencing instead; (5) epigenetic inheritance, all technologies that are used in GWAS are based on DNA sequence, however not all inherited information is carried in the DNA. Therefore, GWAS are not detecting epigenetic variations and epigenome-wide association studies should be performed to discover epigenetically inherited variations; (6) gene × environment (G × E) effects, as in many psychiatric disorders, the environment induces complex G × E interactions which are hard to pick up by GWAS technology.

ENDOPHENOTYPES

Instead of going big, another strategy that has been increasingly applied is going "deep," i.e., the use of endophenotypes or intermediate phenotypes. These familiar or heritable traits are assumed to underlie anxiety disorders and may result in more insight into neurobiological mechanisms compared to classically defined anxiety disorder. Endophenotypes are particularly relevant in anxiety disorders, as the neural circuitry and central pathways mediating anxiety are relatively well known, partly because of extensive animal models and knowledge derived from functional magnetic resonance imaging (fMRI) studies in humans. Those enable the study of the relationship between activities in particular brain areas and anxiety. The amygdala, a limbic area involved in emotional processing, shows enhanced activity in phobias and PTSD compared to healthy individuals (Etkin and Wager, 2007). Such (endo) phenotypes are important targets for genetic studies because the link between genetic variation and disorder risk is reflected more directly, as, e.g., became clear when specific candidate polymorphism were associated with such brain parameters.

A polymorphism in the promoter of the 5-HTT gene has been frequently associated with amygdala reactivity (Hariri et al., 2002; Hariri and Holmes, 2006) implicating the S-allele (low transcriptional activity of the 5-HTT) in the increased amygdala reactivity toward external stimuli (Hariri, 2009). Anxiety and related stress responses are conserved in mammals at different levels. Therefore, similar genes in humans and rodents may regulate critical aspects of anxiety. While in humans it is difficult to control the genetic heterogeneity and environmental influences, animal models provide the possibility to identify novel candidate genes under controlled circumstances. In the section "preclinical genetic approaches to anxiety", we describe some animal models of anxiety that made it possible to study *in vivo* genetic associations at a functional level.

CONCLUSION

In conclusion, genetic studies aiming to unravel the neurobiological background of anxiety disorders have proven to be challenging. This is likely due to a complex and polygenic genetic background of anxiety disorders in which many genes influence the risk to develop anxiety disorders, each of them with a small effect. Moreover, epistatic processes, having the ability to mask the phenotype derived from other genes, are also very likely to be involved whereas environmental factors induce complex G × E interactions. The fact that different susceptibility genes segregate in different families possibly plays a role, making it extremely difficult to detect relatively small and diverse effects. Reported genes that have been associated with anxiety disorders have often been followed by non-replications. The risk of false positives is considerable and meta-analysis studies are needed to hint at a putative susceptibility gene or definitively reject it. Even if replications have been found, the number of negative studies often exceeds the number of positive studies (Smoller et al., 2009). These challenges have led to a generally critical perspective in the search of mental illness genes (Muglia, 2011; Klein et al., 2012). Moreover, Crow (2011) critically questions why only 1–2% of the 80–90% heritability of major psychiatric diseases can be attributed to genes identified by linkage and association. This suggests that many loci with small effects are involved for the heritability of anxiety-related personality traits (Shifman et al., 2008).

PRECLINICAL GENETIC APPROACHES TO ANXIETY

Despite extensive research, human linkage and association studies have not led to major breakthroughs so far. Therefore, it is of great importance to use other approaches in studying the involvement of genes in anxiety disorders as well. Animal pathology resembles human pathology to a certain (but varying) degree (Fernando and Robbins, 2011) and has greatly enhanced our knowledge in the neurobiological mechanisms underlying anxiety. Animal models can be powerful in dissecting putative genes in anxiety and anxiety-associated traits (Flint and Shifman, 2008; Kas et al., 2011), which can be used in parallel to human genetic studies. Because genomic technology advances rapidly, linkage between targets and neuronal circuitry and genetic factors involved in anxiety disorders are becoming increasingly elucidated. Fundamental research aimed at these targets may contribute to unraveling novel insights in anxiety processes and consequently engender new opportunities for drug discovery. The future needs a strict translational approach; data found in human (anxiety) research including genetic and environmental factors, should be used to formulate scientific approaches in animals and vice versa. In animals, we have the opportunity to apply cell-specific inducible knock-outs or knock-ins. Moreover, new optogenetic technology enables selective manipulation of cellular mechanisms and circuit functions linked to the gene's suggested function (Tye and Deisseroth, 2012). The 5-HT_{1A} receptor, the 5-HT_2 receptor, the 5-HTT, and the $GABA_A$ receptor complex belong to the most known and discussed targets in the field and will therefore be discussed below. Human and animal research continues to find new mechanisms around these targets and involvement of these targets in neural networks involved in anxiety modulation, opening new possibilities to apply in animal models and human psychopathology.

ANIMAL MODELS OF ANXIETY

The development of predictive animal models and genetically modified rodents has aided to clarify the role of several pharmacological molecules in brain circuits relevant to anxiety processes, including normal and abnormal behavior. Many animal models for anxiety are based on the natural behavior patterns of rodents (Rodgers et al., 1997). These ethologically based behavioral models include "approach-avoidance" tasks (Cryan and Holmes, 2005) where animals are exposed to aversive environments such as an open field, elevated plus maze or light/dark box and avoid the aversive arena (center of open field, open arms of elevated plus maze, light arena in light/dark box). Besides these unconditioned procedures also conditioned procedures have been used to model anxiety disorders, including conflict procedures such as the Vogel water-lick conflict test (Vogel et al., 1971), defensive burying tests (de Boer and Koolhaas, 2003), the four-plate test (Boissier et al., 1968), and fear-potentiated startle (Brown et al., 1951). Next to these tests also other parameters have been developed to assess anxiety such as the use of radiotelemetry to assess physiological parameters (Bouwknecht et al., 2007), social interaction tests (File and Seth, 2003), predator stress (Blanchard and Blanchard, 1971), and stress-induced vocalizations (Sanchez, 2003). All these models assess behavior that is functionally related to human anxiety as they show good face and construct validity.

THE 5-HT_{1A} RECEPTOR

The 5-HT_{1A} receptor has been implied in anxiety because 5-HT_{1A} receptor agonists exert anxiolytic activity in rodent models of anxiety (Olivier et al., 1999). Although clinically, development of new 5-HT_{1A} receptor agonists for anxiety disorders (e.g., ipsapirone, gepirone, tandospirone, flesinoxan) failed, the 5-HT_{1A} receptor has received considerable interest as a critical target implied in anxiety (Olivier et al., 1999; Holmes, 2008; Lanfumey et al., 2008; Akimova et al., 2009; Savitz et al., 2009). 5-HT_{1A} receptors are G protein-coupled inhibitory receptors expressed in 5-HTergic neurons as autoreceptors and in non-5-HTergic neurons as heteroreceptors. The somatodendritic 5-HT_{1A} autoreceptor controls 5-HTergic tone via feedback inhibition, although recently it was shown that not all 5-HT neurons express the somatodendritic 5-HT_{1A} autoreceptor mRNA (Kiyasova et al., 2013). It has been hypothesized that desensitized 5-HT_{1A} autoreceptors delay the onset of action of SSRIs that act by enhancing brain 5-HT levels

(Gardier et al., 1996; Blier et al., 1998). 5-HT_{1A} receptors are quite abundantly, although restrictedly present in some brain areas. Autoreceptors are mainly, if not only, found in the dorsal and median raphé nuclei, whereas postsynaptic heteroreceptors are found in high densities in limbic regions (including hippocampus) and in the frontal medial prefrontal and entorhinal cortices.

Human data

Genetic and imaging studies in humans suggest that 5-HT_{1A} receptor density or regulation are associated with anxiety, but also with the response to antidepressants (Lesch and Gutknecht, 2004). An association was found between a C(-1019)G polymorphism (rs6295G/C) in the promoter region of the 5-HT_{1A} receptor gene (Htr1a) and mood-related variables, including amygdala reactivity (Fakra et al., 2009). The G-allele is associated with enhanced raphé (presynaptic) 5-HT_{1A} autoreceptor expression but reduced postsynaptic 5-HT_{1A} heteroreceptor expression (Le FranÇois et al., 2008). How such changes contribute to an anxious phenotype is not known yet. More polymorphisms in the Htr1a gene exist, but it is not clear whether they influence anxiety (Drago et al., 2008).

Preclinical data

5-HT_{1A} receptors were found to modulate anxiety. All generated 5-HT_{1A} receptor knock-out (5-$HT_{1A}{}^{-/-}$) mice in several strains displayed enhanced anxiety (Heisler et al., 1998; Parks et al., 1998; Ramboz et al., 1998), although the anxious phenotype was dependent on the paradigm used (Pattij et al., 2001). Interestingly, the Swiss-Webster 5-$HT_{1A}{}^{-/-}$ mouse displayed a reduced sensitivity to the anxiolytic and sedative effects of diazepam, a non-α-subunit selective $GABA_A$-positive allosteric modulator (Sibille et al., 2000; Olivier et al., 2001), indicating changes in some α-subunits of the $GABA_A$–BZ receptor complex. However, this BZ insensitivity did not occur in other strains (Olivier et al., 2001; Pattij et al., 2002). Apparently, dysfunction of the $GABA_A$–BZ system is not a prerequisite for the "anxiogenic" phenotype of the 5-$HT_{1A}{}^{-/-}$ mouse. The anxiogenic phenotype in the 5-$HT_{1A}{}^{-/-}$ mouse was not responding to SSRIs (Santarelli et al., 2003), although Guilloux et al. (2006) showed that 5-$HT_{1A}{}^{-/-}$ mice on a C57Bl/6 background did respond better to SSRIs compared to wildtypes. Moreover, it appeared that overexpression of the 5-HT_{1A} receptor reduced anxiety (Kusserow et al., 2004). Rescue experiments of forebrain 5-HT_{1A} receptors showed that postsynaptic 5-HT_{1A} receptors are critical in the development of the anxiogenic phenotype in the null mutations (Gross et al., 2002). In addition, transgenic developmental overexpression of 5-HT_{1A} receptors in the rostral brain was sufficient to restore normal anxiety levels. Pharmacological blockade of 5-HT_{1A} receptors in early development, but not in adulthood, appeared sufficient to enhance anxious behavior in wildtype mice (Lo Iacono and Gross, 2008; Vinkers et al., 2010a). Zanettini et al. (2010) found increased social anxiety in the 5-$HT_{1A}{}^{-/-}$ mice, however this was reversed by postnatal handling, indicating that neural circuits involved with social anxiety are susceptible to early-life experiences. The complex regulation of anxiety processes during development and adulthood illustrates the complexity of the neural substrate. Also the genetic regulation of anxiety and its pathology makes it clear that straightforward and simple relationships between the function of a certain receptor and anxiety are not very likely. Richardson-Jones et al. (2010) were able to manipulate the level of presynaptic 5-HT_{1A} autoreceptors during adulthood without a concomitant change in postsynaptic 5-HT_{1A} heteroreceptors. Mice with higher (1A-high) or lower (1A-low) autoreceptor levels were tested on their stress vulnerability and response to antidepressants. 1A-low mice showed enhanced 5-HT tone and still respond to an SSRI, whereas 1A-high mice had decreased 5-HT tone and were unresponsive to SSRIs. The authors suggest that 1A-lows reflect human C/C, whereas 1A-highs model G/G carriers of the Htr1a C(-1019)G polymorphism. Such genetic mouse models are extremely useful in studying the underlying processes emerging in anxiety disorders. In addition, Bortolozzi et al. (2012) showed that C-1A-siRNA can be used *in vivo* to selectively silence the 5-HT_{1A} autoreceptor resulting in reduced 5-HT_{1A}-autoreceptor expression, but no alterations in postsynaptic 5-HT_{1A} receptors. Interestingly C-1A-siRNA increased the SSRI-induce elevation of extracellular 5-HT. Effects were seen after i.c.v. and intranasal C-1A-siRNA infusion which opens up new possible therapeutic applications. In conclusion, by genetic manipulation it was possible to study the exact role of specific 5-HT_{1A} receptors (e.g., presynaptic autoreceptors and postsynaptic heteroreceptors) in anxious behavior. Rodents can be manipulated in one specific gene, or even in a specific area. By doing so, the involvement of different 5-HT_{1A} receptors within anxiety disorders can be unraveled, and anxiolytic drugs can be developed for more specific targets (e.g., targeting only postsynaptical 5-HT_{1A} receptors in the rostral brain). Moreover, changes in other mechanisms in the brain in the modified mutant mouse can direct us to putative other and relevant targets and mechanisms involved in the complex anxiety phenotypes emerging. For example Pet1, a transcriptional factor of the ETS (E-twenty six) family, is important for determining the identity of 5-HT neurons in the raphe. Kiyasova et al. (2011) investigated 5-HT neurons in the Pet 1 knock-out mice and discovered a subset of 5-HT neurons that were either Pet1-dependent or Pet1-resistant, which resulted in different morphological features. Moreover, Pet1 knock-out mice showed reduced anxiety-like behavior in conflict-tests, but increased fear in aversive conditioning paradigms. Thus, Pet1 plays an important role in the acquisition and maintenance of 5-HT identity (Gaspar and Lillesaar, 2012; Andrade and Haj-Dahmane, 2013). These findings suggest that the differentiation of subpopulations of 5-HT neurons could also be a factor contributing to the development of anxiety disorders.

5-HT_2 RECEPTORS

Clinical data

The 5-HT_2 receptor subtypes are implicated in anxiety and in the mechanisms of related treatments (Quesseveur et al., 2012). 5-HT_2 receptors couple to multiple cellular signaling pathways and are involved in several physiological brain functions (Leysen, 2004). For example, when SSRIs are combined with 5-HT_{2C} receptor antagonists this may result in greater efficacy in reducing anxiety symptoms and improving sleep (Garner et al., 2009). Agomelatine is a melatonergic receptor (M1 and M2) agonist, but also contains 5-HT_{2C} receptor antagonistic properties, and has anxiolytic properties in patients with GAD (Stein et al., 2008). However, the initial promise for 5-HT_{2C} antagonists such as deramciclane in GAD

(Naukkarinen et al., 2005) has still to be confirmed consistently within large randomized placebo controlled studies.

Preclinical data

As in patients with GAD, agomelatine has been shown to relieve anxiety-like behavior in animals (Millan et al., 2005). Moreover, the 5-HT_{2C} receptor antagonist SB242084 increased the response of SSRIs in animal models (Cremers et al., 2004). Interestingly, Gomes and Nunes-de-Souza (2009) showed that stimulation of 5-$HT_{2A/2C}$ receptors rather than stimulation of 5-HT_{1A} receptors in the periaqueductal gray matter (PAG) attenuate anxiety-like behaviors in mice previously exposed to the elevated plus maze. Moreover, in mice intra-PAG infusions of mCPP (meta-chlorophenylpiperazine), a 5-$HT_{2B/2C}$ receptor agonist, attenuated anxiety-like behavior in the elevated plus maze which was blocked by the 5-$HT_{2A/2C}$ receptor antagonist ketanserin (Nunes-de-Souza et al., 2008). Thus 5-$HT_{2A/2C}$ receptors within the PAG play a key role in the regulation of anxiety-like behavior in mice. With respect to interactions of the 5-HT_2 receptor it was shown that CRF sensitized the 5-HT_2 receptor-mediated signaling through the CRF_1 receptor. This resulted into increased anxiety-like behavior in mice (Magalhaes et al., 2010), indicating a functional interaction between CRF and 5-HT. Furthermore, etifoxine, a $GABA_A$ receptor potentiator, dose-dependently increased the number of punished crossing in a four-plate test in mice (decreased anxiety). Interestingly this anti-punishment effect was blocked when a 5-HT_{2A} antagonist was administered (Bourin and Hascoet, 2010). In addition co-administration of the 5-HT_{2A} receptor agonist DOI together with a subthreshold dose of etifoxine induced an anti-punishment effect as well. Together these data indicate that the effect of etifoxine was modulated by 5-HT_{2A} ligands and that GABA and 5-HT can be co-released and act as co-transmitters in some regions of the central nervous system (CNS; Bourin and Hascoet, 2010). Several studies have suggested that 5-HT_{2A} receptors modulate learning and memory (Meneses, 2007a,b). As such, Zhang et al. (2013) found that stimulation of 5-HT_{2A} receptors with the agonist TCB-2 enhanced the extinction of cued fear memory in mice after trace and delay fear conditioning paradigms, while blockage with MDL 11,939 showed the opposite effect. With respect to G × E interaction it was shown that maternal separation increased adult anxiety behavior (Huot et al., 2001; Kalinichev et al., 2002). Interestingly, Benekareddy et al. (2011) have shown that blockade of the 5-HT_2 receptor (ketanserin) during early postnatal life prevented the increased anxiety seen in animals exposed to maternal separation. Moreover, the enhanced 5-HT_{2A} receptor mRNA in the prefrontal cortex was also blocked by postnatal treatment of ketanserin, implicating that the 5-HT_2 receptors are involved in the adverse effects of maternal separation. In addition to the pharmacological stimulation and blockage of the 5-HT_2 receptor, disruption of the 5-HT_{2A} receptor in mice increased anxiety-like behavior in conflict anxiety paradigms as well (Weisstaub et al., 2006). Martin et al. (2013) created a mouse model expressing only the fully edited VGV isoform of the 5-HT_{2C} receptor and showed that these mice had increased anxiety-like behavior after stimulation with a 5-HT_{2C} receptor agonist in the social interaction test. Moreover, in response to an innately aversive ultrasonic stimulus these mice freezed significantly more and displayed decreased brain 5-HT turnover during stress. When these results were put in relation with the 5-HT_{2C} receptor mRNA splicing process it turned out that the truncated protein (5-HT_{2C} receptor-Tr) interacted with the full-length receptor (5-HT_{2C} receptor-Fl). The 5-HT_{2C} receptor-Tr was localized in the endoplasmic reticulum where it bound to the 5-HT_{2C} receptor-Fl. As a result, the 5-HT_{2C} receptor-Fl could not reach the plasma membrane (Martin et al., 2013). These results show that the 5-HT_{2C} receptor pre-mRNA editing and splicing altering 5-HT_{2C} receptor levels are involved in pathological conditions. Finally, the decreased sociability and sniffing induced by mCPP (5-$HT_{2B/2C}$ agonist) in 5-$HTT^{+/+}$ mice, was not seen in 5-$HTT^{-/-}$ mice (Moya et al., 2011) which is probably due to increases in RNA editing of the 5-HT_{2C} receptor in the amygdala of 5-$HTT^{-/-}$ mice that generates less active reporter isoforms. In conclusion, the 5-HT_2 receptors are involved in anxiety processes; however more research is needed to further dissect the physiological relevance in different brain regions.

THE SEROTONIN TRANSPORTER (5-HTT)

Human data

The 5-HTT has been implied in processes underlying mood, anxiety and associate disorders mainly because SSRI anxiolytics block 5-HT uptake into the neuron thereby increasing 5-HTergic output. Polymorphisms in the promoter of the 5-HTT gene (5-HTTPRL) and its associated transcriptional control region, influence the functioning of the 5-HTergic system (Lesch, 2001). Variable numbers of tandem repeat polymorphisms are known in intron 2 as well as several SNPs that influence the structure of the 5-HTT protein (Murphy and Lesch, 2008). This makes the modulation of 5-HTergic transmission via the 5-HTT mechanism highly complex and gives probably an important insight in the factors that play a role in the genetic complexity of any psychiatric disorder. Gene variations influence intermediate biological phenotypes in concert with other genes, epigenetic variation, environmental and developmental factors. All these complex interactions contribute to the risk or resilience to develop a psychiatric condition. One avenue to pursue would be to try to find associations between specific candidate genes and intermediate phenotypes mediating between a moderating allele and a more complex disease phenotype (Murrough and Charney, 2011).

The 5-HTTLPR allele variations are called the short "S" allele and the long "L" allele. The S-allele has 44 base pairs less and lower transcriptional activity of the 5-HTT gene than the L-form. The S-allele has been the focus of many association studies (Hamilton, 2009). Although negative studies and non-replications with anxiety phenotypes have been reported (e.g., Risch et al., 2009; Grabe et al., 2011), many reported associations with anxiety-related traits and anxiety disorders (Lesch et al., 1996; McDougle et al., 1998; Bengel et al., 1999; Ohara et al., 1999; van Gestel et al., 2002; Lee et al., 2005; Munafo et al., 2005). Considerable evidence showed that after stressful life-events the low expression S-allele is associated with *poorer* outcomes (Lesch et al., 1996; Caspi et al., 2003). A significant interaction between maternal anxiety during gestation and subsequent levels of infant negative emotionality at 6 months of age was modulated by the 5-HTTLPR of the child (Pluess et al., 2011). Moreover, SS-allele carriers appeared particularly sensitive toward unpredictability as seen by modulated attention to the stress (Drabant et al., 2012), suggesting that such a mechanism may underlie the risk for psychopathology. In addition, deductive reasoning appeared also dependent on 5-HTTPRL genotype. Differences in 5-HTT functioning renders some individuals more vulnerable to emotional factors, thereby generating a deleterious effect on rational reasoning (Stollstorff et al., 2013). A gene × gene interaction was found between the 5-HTTLPR (measure in LL-variants) and an oxytocin receptor variant (TT variant of the SNP rs2268498) on individual differences in negative emotionality (Montag et al., 2011). Such data indicate that 5-HTergic and oxytocinergic neurotransmission processes are somewhere entwined and seem to play a role in affective disorders. In general, S-alleles of the 5-HTTLPR are associated with increased risk for a variety of psychiatric disorders, including anxiety. Thus, the S-allele is considered a "risk" or "vulnerability" allele (Caspi et al., 2010) whereas the function of the L-allele is far less clear although this allele has been suggested as a potential risk factor for the development of psychopathic traits too (Glenn, 2011). Because every human has either L, S or both alleles and most people do not suffer from psychiatric abnormalities; it must be assumed that the genome includes several "protective" alleles that make many individuals resilient to stress and pathology. Such protective genes have been suggested, e.g., the CRF_1-receptor variants that have been associated with protection from the extreme stresses of maltreatment during childhood (Polanczyk et al., 2009) and protective, emotional-resilience enhancing effects of the L-allele in students (Stein et al., 2009). Belsky et al. (2009) suggested that S-allele carriers are more vulnerable in general, not only negatively, but also positively. Thus "vulnerability genes" or "risk alleles" seem to make individuals more susceptible to environmental influences, for better and for worse. Homberg and Lesch (2011) take the hypothesis that S-carriers perform better in cognitive tasks than L-carriers and argue for a switch from a deficit-orientated connotation of the 5-HTTLPR variants to a cognitive superiority of S-allele carriers (which have enhanced reactivity of corticolimbic neural circuitry). Environmental conditions will determine whether a positive (cognitive) or negative (emotional) response will happen. Also Hankin et al. (2011) showed that SS-allele children were more sensitive to the environment. Under unsupportive, non-positive parenting SS-allele children exhibit low levels of positive affect, but with supportive/positive parenting these children displayed higher levels of positive affect. In addition to this, Eley et al. (2012) showed an association between the 5-HTTLPR and response to psychological treatment. That is, SS-allele children with anxiety disorder respond up to 20% better to psychotherapy compared to L-allele (SL/LL) carriers. This environmental sensitivity of the 5-HTTLPR makes it even more difficult, and should be taken into account when treating anxiety disorders.

Preclinical data

Several animal models were created to study the role of the 5-HTT and altered 5-HT signaling in the *in vivo* actions of SSRIs. For instance, Thompson et al. (2011) created a knock-in mouse expressing 5-HTT M172, which did not affect the recognition of 5-HT, but affected the serotonergic system and emotional behavior. Also, mice overexpressing 5-HTT have been generated resulting in reduced anxiety levels and bodyweight (Jennings et al., 2006; Line et al., 2011) and enhanced $5\text{-HT}_{2A/C}$ receptor function (Dawson et al., 2011). This model, together with 5-HTT knock-out (5-$\text{HTT}^{-/-}$) models might eliminate the effects of lifelong 5-HTT disturbances with all the compensatory effects occurring over the life span. Both 5-$\text{HTT}^{-/-}$ mouse (Bengel et al., 1998) and rat (Smits et al., 2006) have been created. 5-$\text{HTT}^{-/-}$ rodents display increased extracellular 5-HT in several brain regions (Fabre et al., 2000; Mathews et al., 2004; Shen et al., 2004; Homberg et al., 2007a; Olivier et al., 2008). Due to these increased extracellular 5-HT levels alterations in neurodevelopment and 5-HT synthesis/metabolism are found (reviewed in Murphy and Lesch, 2008; Homberg et al., 2010). 5-$\text{HTT}^{-/-}$ rodents have been considered as an extreme model of the 5-HTTLPR polymorphisms in humans, as brain and behavioral phenotypes of 5-$\text{HTT}^{-/-}$ animals resemble the heterogeneity observed for the 5-HTTLPR (Hariri and Holmes, 2006; Wellman et al., 2007; Homberg et al., 2008b; Olivier et al., 2008).5-$\text{HTT}^{-/-}$ animals have an altered ability to cope with stress and display anxiogenic and depressogenic behavior (Holmes et al., 2002; Tjurmina et al., 2002; Adamec et al., 2006; Wellman et al., 2007; Olivier et al., 2008; Jansen et al., 2010; Kalueff et al., 2010). Interestingly, when the environment is rewarding, 5-$\text{HTT}^{-/-}$ rodents are more hypersensitive as shown by their increased sensitivity for psychostimulants (Sora et al., 1998, 2001; Homberg et al., 2008a; Nonkes et al., 2013) indicating that 5-$\text{HTT}^{-/-}$ rodents are more sensitive to the environment. As found in S-allele carriers (Roiser et al., 2006a,b, 2007; Finger et al., 2007), improved cognition has been observed in 5-$\text{HTT}^{-/-}$ rodents (Homberg et al., 2007b, 2008b; Brigman et al., 2010) together with improved behavioral flexibility, directing their behavior toward the most rewarding stimuli (Brigman et al., 2010; Nonkes et al., 2013). Reduced conditioned freezing to a predicted foot shock is found in 5-$\text{HTT}^{-/-}$ rodents when a positive stimulus was given (Nonkes et al., 2012). However, it appears that phenotypical plasticity is not only present in 5-$\text{HTT}^{-/-}$ animals early in life, but also later in life (Homberg and van den Hove, 2012). This also accounts for heterozygous (5-$\text{HTT}^{+/-}$) rodents, which might be considered as a more valuable model for the 5-HTTLPR model as they have reduced expression of the 5-HTT, comparable to the S-allele carriers. For instance, low maternal care increased anxiety-like behavior in adult 5-$\text{HTT}^{+/-}$ mice, but not in wild-type littermates (Carola et al., 2008). This increased emotionality was linked to increased BDNF mRNA levels in the hippocampus, suggesting a role for BDNF in programing the 5-$\text{HTT}^{+/-}$ brain to become more susceptible to the environment. Interestingly, only 5-$\text{HTT}^{+/-}$ mice that experienced high maternal care showed increased 5-HT and norepinephrine levels in the hippocampus, together with decreased 5-HT turnover (Carola et al., 2011). At baseline level, 5-$\text{HTT}^{+/-}$ mice display decreased emotional behavior, however, upon prenatal maternal restraint stress, 5-$\text{HTT}^{+/-}$ offspring displayed increased emotional behavior (Van den Hove et al., 2011), although also decreased anxiety levels and enhanced memory performance were found in these mice. This is an important finding as individuals with anxiety symptoms have a range of biases in emotion processing, such as a willingness to selectively attend to thread cues (Bar-Haim et al., 2007; Waters et al., 2008) and to interpret emotionally ambiguous stimuli in a negative manner (Mathews and MacLeod, 2005). When 5-HTT$^{-/-}$ and 5-HTT$^{+/-}$ mice underwent a loser experience in a social defeat test they displayed delayed fear extinction and decreased recall of extinction to a higher extent than wild-types (Narayanan et al., 2011). In addition, 5-HTT$^{-/-}$ losers displayed increased anxiety levels and reduced exploration (Jansen et al., 2010). Similarly, increased escape latencies were found in 5-HTT$^{-/-}$ and 5-HTT$^{+/-}$ mice after repeated inescapable foot-shock stress (Muller et al., 2011). Moreover, chronic psychosocial stress due to an intruder in the cage resulted into decreased locomotor activity and increased social avoidance (Bartolomucci et al., 2010). It is clear that both the immature developing brain as well as the mature brain is sensitive to changes in the environment.

The advantage of having animal models for human disorders is that underlying mechanisms in the brain can be more easily studied as environmental influences can be regulated. With use of for example fMRI or microPET (micro-positron emission tomography) scanning, brain areas can be studied in humans. By doing so, it was discovered that the amygdala and prefrontal cortex of S-allele carriers showed hyperactivity upon environmental stimuli (Hariri et al., 2002; Kalin et al., 2008). However, a molecular understanding of this phenomenon is lacking, while such understanding might be helpful in identifying new targets for the diagnoses and therapy of anxiety disorders. With use of animal models it is possible to study the gene, the environment and their interactions. For example, low maternal care caused deficient $GABA_A$ receptor binding in the amygdala during adulthood. In pups with low maternal care increased α-amino-3-hydroxy-5-methyl-4-isoxazolepropionic acid receptor binding was found in the hippocampus, which correlated with BDNF mRNA levels in the somatosensory cortex. These effects are independent of genotype, and are only environmental. However, lower maternal care in 5-HTT$^{-/-}$ mice elevated BDNF mRNA levels in the hippocampus. Moreover, it was shown that loser stress in a resident-intruder test increased pronounced neuroplastic changes of pyramidal neurons in the prelimbic cortex and amygdala (Nietzer et al., 2011). Also effects on the corticolimbic system were found (reviewed in Homberg and van den Hove, 2012). While we now only discussed the G × E interactions, epigenetics is probably also a key contributor for these interactions. The relationship between genetic and epigenetic variation at the 5-HTT gene has so far not been studied in 5-HTT-deficient animal models. But 5-HTT-deficient rodents may be particularly suitable to study these interactions.

$GABA_A$ RECEPTOR α SUBUNITS AND ANXIETY

In the 1950s, BZs were serendipitously found as having therapeutically interesting activity with anxiolysis, sedation, anticonvulsive activity, and muscle relaxation. The molecular target of BZs is the $GABA_A$ receptor (Möhler and Okada, 1977). BZs mediate their actions via a modulatory binding site that is present on most, but not all $GABA_A$ receptors. The binding site for BZs is formed by one of the α subunits (α1, α2, α3, or α5) and a γ subunit (almost exclusively the γ2 subunit) $GABA_A$ receptors are the main inhibitory neurons in the CNS and it is estimated that 20–30% of all neurons in the CNS are of the $GABA_A$ type. BZs do not open the Cl^- channel in the absence of GABA. Only if the GABA receptor site is activated, activation of the BZ site may modulate the opening of the channel. Ligands at the BZ binding site are allosteric modulators. They modify the efficacy and/or affinity of GABA in positive (positive allosteric modulation, PAM), negative (negative allosteric modulation, NAM), or have neutral effects by stabilizing different three-dimensional conformations of the complex. Selectivity of a ligand for a specific receptor subtype can be obtained by affinity and/or by efficacy changes that determine the potential potency of a ligand.

Human data

Even though specific SNPs of the GABAergic system have been found to play a role in anxiety disorders (Nemeroff, 2003; Kalueff and Nutt, 2007), GWAS on anxiety disorders are scarce and GABAergic candidate genes emerging from the existing studies have been equivocal (Logue et al., 2012; Otowa et al., 2012). A limited number of studies suggested some link between the GABRA2 gene and anxiety. Nelson et al. (2009) found that polymorphisms in the GABRA2 gene interact with early childhood trauma and increase the risk for PTSD. Pham et al. (2009) found, investigating 26 SNPs in four $GABA_A$ receptor genes (GABRA2,3,6 and GABRG2) that none of the allelic variation in these genes was involved in liability to anxiety-spectrum disorders. Besides the GABRA subunit genes, several other GABAergic systems have been implicated in the genetic load of GABA system pathways on the psychobiology of anxiety. Suggestive signals for an association with anxiety disorders and anxiety-related personality traits have been found for other genes, e.g., glutamic acid decarboxylase 1 (Hettema et al., 2006) and 2 (Smoller et al., 2001b), b3 subunits of the GABAA receptor (Feusner et al., 2001), the diazepam binding inhibitor (Thoeringer et al., 2007), and the GABA transporter 1 (Thoeringer et al., 2009). The latter authors suggest a multiple system hit-theory in the genetic basis of anxiety disorders; many loci at different genes of the GABA system, each with a small effect, contribute to an individual's risk on anxiety disorder. If several risk genes are present, anxiety might develop depending upon adverse environmental (stress) factors.

Preclinical data

By making the GABA α subunits insensitive to the diazepam binding [α1(H101R) mice] strong evidence was gathered that α1 subunits were involved in sedative and anterograde amnesia effects of diazepam. As such α2 point mutations [α2(H101R) mice] led to absence of the anxiolytic and diminished muscle relaxant action, but intact anxiolysis. Point mutations in α3 [α3(H126R) mice] and α5 [α5(105R) mice] did not diazepam-induced myorelaxation, whereas sedation and anxiolysis were intact. Such data strongly suggest a functional differentiation in the $GABA_A$ receptors depending on the α-subunit composition (for review, see Möhler, 2006; Rudolph and Knoflach, 2011). Classic BZs are still frequently prescribed, have therapeutic activity but, inherent to the activation of all relevant α-subunits, come with build-in side effects. If used as anxiolytic tool, sedation is one of the troubling side effects. Furthermore, upon chronic use, BZs can lead to dependency, tolerance and induce abuse liability limiting long-term use (Tan et al., 2011). Recent efforts have tried to synthesize new drugs that have selectivity and potency for specific α subunits (Rudolph and Knoflach, 2011) although relatively selective drugs for the α1 subunit are already in use for sedation/hypnotic purposes (zolpidem, zopiclone, (S)-zopiclone, and zaleplon). Compounds that selectively activate the α2 subunits and have no effects on any other α subunit might constitute an ideal, non-sedative anxiolytic, although activation of α3 subunits might contribute to an anxiolytic profile (Dias et al., 2005; Vinkers et al., 2009; Atack, 2010). L-838417, a partial PAM at α2, α3, and α5 containing $GABA_A$ receptors and an antagonist at α1 containing receptors has a non-sedating anxiolytic profile in mice (McKernan et al., 2000; van Bogaert et al., 2006) and primates (Rowlett et al., 2005). Development of this compound has been stopped due to an unfavorable pharmacokinetic profile (Scott-Stevens et al., 2005). TPA023, an α2/α3 PAM, has anxiolytic and no sedative effects in rodents (Atack et al., 2006). TPA023 was evaluated in three phase 2 studies in GAD and showed preliminary indications of anxiolytic activity without sedation (Atack, 2010). However, this compound had to be withdrawn due to severe preclinical toxicity. A comparable story holds for ocinaplon, having a non-sedative anxiolytic profile in humans but also had to be withdrawn due to hepatotoxicity (Lippa et al., 2005; Czobor et al., 2010). Several other ligands have been synthetized and tested, mostly restricted to preclinical phases. It appears possible to make compounds with some selectivity for specific α subunits but *in vivo* efficacy is extremely difficult to design: both positive and negative allosteric modulators have been found, sometimes even mixed PAM/NAM effects on different α subunits are present or no selectivity is present *in vitro* whereas *in vivo* some efficacy is found (e.g., ocinaplon). MRK-409, an extremely low partial agonist (PAM) at α1, α2, and α5 containing $GABA_A$ receptors but higher intrinsic activity at α3 subunit $GABA_A$ receptors, appeared to be anxioselective in animals but sedative in humans, already at low (<10%) receptor occupancy (Atack et al., 2011). One of the unresolved issues around subunit selective GABAergic compounds is the issue of tolerance and abuse potential. Does activation of all α subunit containing $GABA_A$ receptors lead to addiction or is that caused by specific α subunits? This is an important issue because the development of potentially abusive medications will meet severe constraints if not impossible. There is some evidence that activation of α1 subunits is essential in the addictive properties of BZs (Tan et al., 2010, 2011). However, the processes of tolerance development are complex and endpoint-dependent (Vinkers et al., 2012). If the therapeutic effects of activation of α1-containing $GABA_A$ receptors cannot be separated from potential addictive side effects, no further development of α1 subunit specific ligands can be expected. However, if addictive properties are not entwined in (chronic) activation of the other α(2,3,5) subunits, new developments in the field of anxiety (and others like cognition and analgesia) might be expected (Mirza and Munro, 2010; Vinkers et al., 2010a).

THE INTERACTION BETWEEN 5-HT AND GABA

The GABA and the serotonergic system may directly interact (Lista et al., 1989; Gao et al., 1993; Fernandez-Guasti and Lopez-Rubalcava, 1998). However, the evidence is equivocal (Shephard et al., 1982; Thiebot, 1986). A serotonergic component in the anxiolytic actions of GABAergic BZs has been suggested (Stein et al., 1977; Thiebot et al., 1984; Harandi et al., 1987). Moreover, studies have found that a decreased serotonin activity and turnover emerges after the administration of BZs (Chase et al., 1970; Stein et al., 1977; Pratt et al., 1979; Trulson et al., 1982; Wright et al., 1992), although others have not found such effects (Shephard and Broadhurst, 1982; Thiebot et al., 1984; Thiebot, 1986). Also, the vast majority of serotonergic neurons express $GABA_A$ receptor α_3-subunit immunoreactivity but not $GABA_A$ receptor α_1-subunit staining (Gao et al., 1993). This is remarkable as the α_1 subunit is highly prevalent in the CNS. Thus, BZs could at least partially produce their anxiolytic effects by activating α_3 subunits located on serotonergic neurons (Vinkers et al., 2010b). In support, serotonergic raphe nuclei receive a prominent GABAergic input via distant sources as well as interneurons (Harandi et al., 1987; Bagdy et al., 2000; Gervasoni et al., 2000; Varga et al., 2001; Vinkers et al., 2010b). Together, the interaction of the GABA and serotonin system in anxiety disorders could be valuable in the search for novel anxiolytic drugs. Nevertheless, the fact that BZs acutely reduce anxiety, whereas SSRIs take several weeks before anxiolytic activity becomes apparent suggests that the two drug classes exert their effects via different mechanisms.

TRANSLATIONAL STUDIES INTO ANXIETY

Can the data on the involvement of 5-HT in anxiety and anxiety disorders (here illustrated with the 5-HTT, the $5\text{-}HT_2$ receptor and the $5\text{-}HT_{1A}$ receptor) be used to design translational research that possibly will generate new hypotheses and targets for anxiolytic therapeutics? Recently, Jasinska et al. (2012) formulated a hypothesis around the involvement of the 5-HTT gene, stress and raphe–raphe interactions in order to try to explain the risk of depression as a result of G × E interactions between the 5-HTT gene and stress. Different populations of 5-HTergic neurons in the dorsal raphe (DR) nucleus exist that differentially contribute to the response to stress. As mentioned before differentiation of subpopulations of 5-HT neurons could also be a factor contributing to the development of anxiety disorders (Gaspar and Lillesaar, 2012; Andrade and Haj-Dahmane, 2013). Although Jasinska et al. (2012) hypothesize this mechanism mainly for depression, there is no a priory reason why anxiety disorders would not be mediated by this or a similar mechanism. The authors propose that the variability in the reuptake of 5-HT during stressor-induced raphe–raphe interactions alters the balance in amygdala–ventromedial prefrontal cortex–DR (VMPFC–DR) circuitry. This VMPFC-DR circuitry is important in the reactivity to stressors and the regulation of emotion. In LL-individuals with an efficient 5-HT transport the circuitry is able to normalize, but not so in SS-individuals, potentially leading to abnormal activity and pathology. Whether such a mechanism also acts in human pathology is as yet unresolved but could lead to specific searches for new mechanisms causing pathological anxiety. Next to different functional 5-HTergic populations in the DR, 5-HTTs appear very dynamically regulated (Steiner et al., 2008), undergo regulated membrane trafficking as well as transitions between low and high activity states, with many signaling pathways involved. Moreover, 5-HTT exhibits dynamic associations with cytoskeletal binding proteins; actually Chang et al. (2012) found two pools of 5-HTT proteins on the surface of 5-HTergic cells, one relatively with free diffusion, the other with restricted mobility due to binding to the cytoskeleton.

Whether the 5-HTergic system exerts this kind of extremely variability which might lead to new and better understanding of the role of the 5-HTT complex, including its genetic variability is still a matter of the future but it remains fully possible that new mechanisms involved in anxiety and its disorders might emerge.

CONCLUDING REMARKS

This review has illustrated the complexity of research on the genetic background of anxiety disorders. Although we discuss only the serotonergic and the GABA system, more systems/candidates are of potential interest including glutamate, NE, dopamine, and some peptides (reviewed in Christmas et al., 2008), as well as specific translocator protein which promote neurosteroidogenesis (Taliani et al., 2009; Nothdurfter et al., 2012) and agomelatine (Stein et al., 2008). However, in the present review, four targets have been presented to exemplify the complexity of anxiety: the 5-HT_{1A} receptor, 5-HT_2 receptor, 5-HTT, and $GABA_A$ receptor. This is important as two known class of drugs (SSRIs and BZs) are effective anxiolytics. Even though these anxiolytic drugs have been around for decades, no subsequent breakthrough has become available. The reasons for the relative lack of progress in the anxiety field are not completely clear but may be due to the heterogeneous classification of anxiety disorders, but also the complex regulatory and financial regulations in the finding of new "druggable" targets (beyond the scope of this review, see, e.g., Knutsen, 2011). Nevertheless, a recurring theme is the continued paucity of novel targets for anxiolytic drugs and our limited knowledge of the mechanisms underlying the various anxiety disorders. This includes the limited contribution of genetic studies to novel anxiolytic targets. In this review, we have argued that it is vital to invest in fundamental research in the mechanisms involved in anxiety processes in animals and unaffected individuals. Because a direct investigation of the human brain is often not possible, animal research may contribute considerably in finding neural substrates for anxiety and its pathology. However, it is not realistic to think that such knowledge is completely translatable to the clinical situation. Moreover, in animal models it is not always possible to model specific symptoms related to human pathology, which might cause limitations in the development of novel drug targets.

The initial hope was, after elucidation of the human genome, that the identification of causative genes would be a matter of time. Notwithstanding a certain degree of heritability of anxiety disorders, no single gene or set of genes has emerged from a large number of studies on large cohorts of patients thus far. It becomes increasingly evident that anxiety disorders, probably similar to the neurobiological mechanisms underlying anxiety processes, are the result of many hundreds of genes with small effects which display complex interactions with both environmental factors and other genes. Therefore, genetic approaches in studies on anxiety disorders may be enriched with preclinical studies to identify relevant drug targets. It is improbable that a single gene contributes significantly to anxiety processes to a large degree. It is striking that the functionality of GABA and 5-HT system in "normal" or "pathological" anxiety in healthy individuals is largely unknown, In case of 5-HT modulation (via 5-HT_{1A} receptor activation or blockade of the 5-HTT) an indirect effect is possibly the most logical explanation, because treatment of anxiety disorders with SSRIs or buspirone takes weeks or even months before anxiolytic activity is seen (acute effects seen after administration of these drugs are even anxiogenic). The delayed effect therefore points to induction of mechanisms that slowly change and need time to become effective (plasticity changes). Anxiolytic effects after activation of $GABA_A$ receptors seem acute and might point to a primary mechanism directly involved in anxiety regulating mechanisms. Close collaboration between fundamental research and clinical studies into the mechanisms underlying anxiety might lead to breakthroughs in the search for novel anxiolytic drugs and enhance the success of research and development efforts aimed at drug discovery for anxiety disorders. In conclusion, we argue that animal models should play an important role in the future anxiolytic drug development as a fundamental component of a broad multidisciplinary approach. To be successful, novel clinical insights into the etiology of anxiety disorders from preclinical studies must be integrated in the broader context of human genetic studies and novel biopathway analysis.

REFERENCES

Adamec, R., Burton, P., Blundell, J., Murphy, D. L., and Holmes, A. (2006). Vulnerability to mild predator stress in serotonin transporter knockout mice. *Behav. Brain Res.* 170, 126–140. doi: 10.1016/j.bbr.2006.02.012

Akimova, E., Lanzenberger, R., and Kasper, S. (2009). The serotonin-1A receptor in anxiety disorders. *Biol. Psychiatry* 66, 627–635. doi: 10.1016/j.biopsych.2009.03.012

Andrade, R., and Haj-Dahmane, S. (2013). Serotonin neuron diversity in the dorsal raphe. *ACS Chem. Neurosci.* 4, 22–25. doi: 10.1021/cn300224n

Atack, J. R. (2010). GABAA receptor alpha2/alpha3 subtype-selective modulators as potential nonsedating anxiolytics. *Curr. Top. Behav. Neurosci.* 2, 331–360. doi: 10.1007/7854_2009_30

Atack, J. R., Wafford, K. A., Street, L. J., Dawson, G. R., Tye, S., Van Laere, K., et al. (2011). MRK-409 (MK-0343), a GABAA receptor subtype-selective partial agonist, is a non-sedating anxiolytic in preclinical species but causes sedation in humans. *J. Psychopharmacol.* 25, 314–328. doi: 10.1177/0269881109354927

Atack, J. R., Wafford, K. A., Tye, S. J., Cook, S. M., Sohal, B., Pike, A., et al. (2006). TPA023 [7-(1,1-dimethylethyl)-6-(2-ethyl-2H-1,2,4-triazol-3-ylmethoxy)-3-(2-fluorophenyl)-1,2,4-triazolo[4,3-b]pyridazine], an agonist selective for alpha2- and alpha3-containing GABAA receptors, is a nonsedating anxiolytic in rodents and primates. *J. Pharmacol. Exp. Ther.* 316, 410–422. doi: 10.1124/jpet.105.089920

Attar-Levy, D., Martinot, J. L., Blin, J., Dao-Castellana, M. H., Crouzel, C., Mazoyer, B., et al. (1999). The cortical serotonin2 receptors studied with positron-emission tomography and [18F]-setoperone during depressive illness and antidepressant treatment with clomipramine. *Biol. Psychiatry* 45, 180–186. doi: 10.1016/S0006-3223(98)00007-9

Bagdy, E., Kiraly, I., and Harsing, L. G. Jr. (2000). Reciprocal innervation between serotonergic and GABAergic neurons in raphe nuclei of the rat. *Neurochem. Res.* 25, 1465–1473. doi: 10.1023/A:1007672008297

Bagdy, G., Graf, M., Anheuer, Z. E., Modos, E. A., and Kantor, S. (2001). Anxiety-like effects induced by acute fluoxetine, sertraline or m-CPP treatment are reversed by pretreatment with the 5-HT2C receptor antagonist SB-242084 but not the 5-HT1A receptor antagonist WAY-100635. *Int. J. Neuropsychopharmacol.* 4, 399–408. doi: 10.1017/S1461145701002632

Bar-Haim, Y., Lamy, D., Pergamin, L., Bakermans-Kranenburg, M. J., and van IJzendoorn, M. H. (2007). Threat-related attentional bias in anxious and nonanxious individuals: a meta-analytic study. *Psychol. Bull.* 133, 1–24. doi: 10.1037/0033-2909.133.1.1

Bartolomucci, A., Carola, V., Pascucci, T., Puglisi-Allegra, S., Cabib, S., Lesch, K. P., et al. (2010). Increased vulnerability to psychosocial stress in heterozygous serotonin transporter knockout mice. *Dis. Model. Mech.* 3, 459–470. doi: 10.1242/dmm.004614

Belsky, J., Jonassaint, C., Pluess, M., Stanton, M., Brummett, B., and Williams, R. (2009). Vulnerability genes or plasticity genes? *Mol. Psychiatry* 14, 746–754. doi: 10.1038/mp.2009.44

Benekareddy, M., Vadodaria, K. C., Nair, A. R., and Vaidya, V. A. (2011). Postnatal serotonin type 2 receptor blockade prevents the emergence of anxiety behavior, dysregulated stress-induced immediate early gene responses, and specific transcriptional changes that arise following early life stress. *Biol. Psychiatry* 70, 1024–1032. doi: 10.1016/j.biopsych.2011.08.005

Bengel, D., Greenberg, B. D., Cora-Locatelli, G., Altemus, M., Heils, A., Li, Q., et al. (1999). Association of the serotonin transporter promoter regulatory region polymorphism and obsessive-compulsive disorder. *Mol. Psychiatry* 4, 463–466. doi: 10.1038/sj.mp.4000550

Bengel, D., Murphy, D. L., Andrews, A. M., Wichems, C. H., Feltner, D., Heils, A., et al. (1998). Altered brain serotonin homeostasis and locomotor insensitivity to 3, 4-methylenedioxymethamphetamine ("Ecstasy") in serotonin transporter-deficient mice. *Mol. Pharmacol.* 53, 649–655.

Blanchard, R. J., and Blanchard, D. C. (1971). Defensive reactions in the albino rat. *Learn. Motiv.* 21, 351–362. doi: 10.1016/0023-9690(71)90016-6

Blier, P., Pineyro, G., El, M. M., Bergeron, R., and de Montigny, C. (1998). Role of somatodendritic 5-HT autoreceptors in modulating 5-HT neurotransmission. *Ann. N. Y. Acad. Sci.* 861, 204–216. doi: 10.1111/j.1749-6632.1998.tb10192.x

Boissier, J. R., Simon, P., and Aron, C. (1968). A new method for rapid screening of minor tranquillizers in mice. *Eur. J. Pharmacol.* 4, 145–151. doi: 10.1159/000135006

Bortolozzi, A., Castane, A., Semakova, J., Santana, N., Alvarado, G., Cortes, R., et al. (2012). Selective siRNA-mediated suppression of 5-HT1A autoreceptors evokes strong anti-depressant-like effects. *Mol. Psychiatry* 17, 612–623. doi: 10.1038/mp.2011.92

Bourin, M., and Hascoet, M. (2010). Implication of 5-HT2 receptor subtypes in the mechanism of action of the GABAergic compound etifoxine in the four-plate test in Swiss mice. *Behav. Brain Res.* 208, 352–358. doi: 10.1016/j.bbr.2009.11.046

Bouwknecht, J. A., Olivier, B., and Paylor, R. E. (2007). The stress-induced hyperthermia paradigm as a physiological animal model for anxiety: a review of pharmacological and genetic studies in the mouse. *Neurosci. Biobehav. Rev.* 31, 41–59. doi: 10.1016/j.neubiorev.2006.02.002

Brigman, J. L., Mathur, P., Harvey-White, J., Izquierdo, A., Saksida, L. M., Bussey, T. J., et al. (2010). Pharmacological or genetic inactivation of the serotonin transporter improves reversal learning in mice. *Cereb. Cortex* 20, 1955–1963. doi: 10.1093/cercor/bhp266

Brown, J. S., Kalish, H. I., and Farber, I. E. (1951). Conditioned fear as revealed by magnitude of startle response to an auditory stimulus. *J. Exp. Psychol.* 41, 317–328. doi: 10.1037/h0060166

Carola, V., Frazzetto, G., Pascucci, T., Audero, E., Puglisi-Allegra, S., Cabib, S., et al. (2008). Identifying molecular substrates in a mouse model of the serotonin transporter × environment risk factor for anxiety and depression. *Biol. Psychiatry* 63, 840–846. doi: 10.1016/j.biopsych.2007.08.013

Carola, V., Pascucci, T., Puglisi-Allegra, S., Cabib, S., and Gross, C. (2011). Effect of the interaction between the serotonin transporter gene and maternal environment on developing mouse brain. *Behav. Brain Res.* 217, 188–194. doi: 10.1016/j.bbr.2010.10.020

Caspi, A., Hariri, A. R., Holmes, A., Uher, R., and Moffitt, T. E. (2010). Genetic sensitivity to the environment: the case of the serotonin transporter gene and its implications for studying complex diseases and traits. *Am. J. Psychiatry* 167, 509–527. doi: 10.1176/appi.ajp.2010.09101452

Caspi, A., Sugden, K., Moffitt, T. E., Taylor, A., Craig, I. W., Harrington, H., et al. (2003). Influence of life stress on depression: moderation by a polymorphism in the 5-HTT gene. *Science* 301, 386–389. doi: 10.1126/science.1083968

Chang, J. C., Tomlinson, I. D., Warnement, M. R., Ustione, A., Carneiro, A. M., Piston, D. W., et al. (2012). Single molecule analysis of serotonin transporter regulation using antagonist-conjugated quantum dots reveals restricted, p38 MAPK-dependent mobilization underlying uptake activation. *J. Neurosci.* 32, 8919–8929. doi: 10.1523/JNEUROSCI.0048-12.2012

Chantarujikapong, S. I., Scherrer, J. F., Xian, H., Eisen, S. A., Lyons, M. J., Goldberg, J., et al. (2001). A twin study of generalized anxiety disorder symptoms, panic disorder symptoms and post-traumatic stress disorder in men. *Psychiatry Res.* 103, 133–145. doi: 10.1016/S0165-1781(01)00285-2

Chase, T. N., Katz, R. I., and Kopin, I. J. (1970). Effect of diazepam on fate of intracisternally injected serotonin-C14. *Neuropharmacology* 9, 103–108. doi: 10.1016/0028-3908(70)90053-5

Chen, G., Henter, I. D., and Manji, H. K. (2010). Translational research in bipolar disorder: emerging insights from genetically based models. *Mol. Psychiatry* 15, 883–895. doi: 10.1038/mp.2010.3

Choi, W. S., Lee, B. H., Yang, J. C., and Kim, Y. K. (2010). Association study between 5-HT1A receptor gene C(-1019)G polymorphism and panic disorder in a Korean population. *Psychiatry Investig.* 7, 141–146. doi: 10.4306/pi.2010.7.2.141

Christmas, D., Hood, S., and Nutt, D. (2008). Potential novel anxiolytic drugs. *Curr. Pharm. Des* 14, 3534–3546. doi: 10.2174/138161208786848775

Cremers, T. I., Giorgetti, M., Bosker, F. J., Hogg, S., Arnt, J., Mork, A., et al. (2004). Inactivation of 5-HT(2C) receptors potentiates consequences of serotonin reuptake blockade. *Neuropsychopharmacology* 29, 1782–1789. doi: 10.1038/sj.npp.1300474

Crow, T. J. (2011). The missing genes: what happened to the heritability of psychiatric disorders? *Mol. Psychiatry* 16, 362–364. doi: 10.1038/mp.2010.92

Cryan, J. F., and Holmes, A. (2005). The ascent of mouse: advances in modelling human depression and anxiety. *Nat. Rev. Drug Discov.* 4, 775–790. doi: 10.1038/nrd1825

Cryan, J. F., and Sweeney, F. F. (2011). The age of anxiety: role of animal models of anxiolytic action in drug discovery. *Br. J. Pharmacol.* 164, 1129–1161. doi: 10.1111/j.1476-5381.2011.01362.x

Czobor, P., Skolnick, P., Beer, B., and Lippa, A. (2010). A multicenter, placebo-controlled, double-blind, randomized study of efficacy and safety of ocinaplon (DOV 273,547) in generalized anxiety disorder. *CNS Neurosci. Ther.* 16, 63–75. doi: 10.1111/j.1755-5949.2009.00109.x

Dawson, N., Ferrington, L., Lesch, K. P., and Kelly, P. A. (2011). Cerebral metabolic responses to 5-HT2A/C receptor activation in mice with genetically modified serotonin transporter (SERT) expression. *Eur. Neuropsychopharmacol.* 21, 117–128. doi: 10.1016/j.euroneuro.2010.10.006

de Boer, S. F., and Koolhaas, J. M. (2003). Defensive burying in rodents: ethology, neurobiology and psychopharmacology. *Eur. J. Pharmacol.* 463, 145–161. doi: 10.1016/S0014-2999(03)01278-0

Deckert, J., Catalano, M., Syagailo, Y. V., Bosi, M., Okladnova, O., Di, B. D., et al. (1999). Excess of high activity monoamine oxidase A gene promoter alleles in female patients with panic disorder. *Hum. Mol. Genet.* 8, 621–624. doi: 10.1093/hmg/8.4.621

Deckert, J., Nothen, M. M., Franke, P., Delmo, C., Fritze, J., Knapp, M., et al. (1998). Systematic mutation screening and association study of the A1 and A2a adenosine receptor genes in panic disorder suggest a contribution of the A2a gene to the development of disease. *Mol. Psychiatry* 3, 81–85. doi: 10.1038/sj.mp.4000345

Dias, R., Sheppard, W. F., Fradley, R. L., Garrett, E. M., Stanley, J. L., Tye, S. J., et al. (2005). Evidence for a significant role of alpha 3-containing GABAA receptors in mediating the anxiolytic effects of benzodiazepines. *J. Neurosci.* 25, 10682–10688. doi: 10.1523/JNEUROSCI.1166-05.2005

Digangi, J., Guffanti, G., McLaughlin, K. A., and Koenen, K. C. (2013). Considering trauma exposure in the context of genetics studies of posttraumatic stress disorder: a systematic review. *Biol. Mood Anxiety Disord.* 3, 2. doi: 10.1186/2045-5380-3-2

Domschke, K., Freitag, C. M., Kuhlenbaumer, G., Schirmacher, A., Sand, P., Nyhuis, P., et al. (2004). Association of the functional V158M catechol-*O*-methyl-transferase polymorphism with panic disorder in women. *Int. J. Neuropsychopharmacol.* 7, 183–188. doi: 10.1017/S146114570400416X

Drabant, E. M., Ramel, W., Edge, M. D., Hyde, L. W., Kuo, J. R., Goldin, P. R., et al. (2012). Neural mechanisms underlying 5-HTTLPR-related sensitivity to acute stress. *Am. J. Psychiatry* 169, 397–405. doi: 10.1176/appi.ajp.2011.10111699

Drago, A., Ronchi, D. D., and Serretti, A. (2008). 5-HT1A gene variants and psychiatric disorders: a review of current literature and selection of SNPs for future studies. *Int. J. Neuropsychopharmacol.* 11, 701–721. doi: 10.1017/S1461145707008218

Eley, T. C., Hudson, J. L., Creswell, C., Tropeano, M., Lester, K. J., Cooper, P., et al. (2012). Therapygenetics: the 5HTTLPR and response to psychological therapy.

Mol. Psychiatry 17, 236–237. doi: 10.1038/mp.2011.132

Etkin, A., and Wager, T. D. (2007). Functional neuroimaging of anxiety: a meta-analysis of emotional processing in PTSD, social anxiety disorder, and specific phobia. *Am. J. Psychiatry* 164, 1476–1488. doi: 10.1176/appi.ajp.2007.07030504

Fabre, V., Beaufour, C., Evrard, A., Rioux, A., Hanoun, N., Lesch, K. P., et al. (2000). Altered expression and functions of serotonin 5-HT1A and 5-HT1B receptors in knock-out mice lacking the 5-HT transporter. *Eur. J. Neurosci.* 12, 2299–2310. doi: 10.1046/j.1460-9568.2000.00126.x

Fakra, E., Hyde, L. W., Gorka, A., Fisher, P. M., Munoz, K. E., Kimak, M., et al. (2009). Effects of HTR1A C(-1019)G on amygdala reactivity and trait anxiety. *Arch. Gen. Psychiatry* 66, 33–40. doi: 10.1001/archpsyc.66.1.33

Fernandez-Guasti, A., and Lopez-Rubalcava, C. (1998). Modification of the anxiolytic action of 5-HT1A compounds by GABA-benzodiazepine agents in rats. *Pharmacol. Biochem. Behav.* 60, 27–32. doi: 10.1016/S0091-3057(97)00482-6

Fernando, A. B., and Robbins, T. W. (2011). Animal models of neuropsychiatric disorders. *Annu. Rev. Clin. Psychol.* 7, 39–61. doi: 10.1146/annurev-clinpsy-032210-104454

Feusner, J., Ritchie, T., Lawford, B., Young, R. M., Kann, B., and Noble, E. P. (2001). GABA(A) receptor beta 3 subunit gene and psychiatric morbidity in a post-traumatic stress disorder population. *Psychiatry Res.* 104, 109–117. doi: 10.1016/S0165-1781(01)00296-7

File, S. E., and Seth, P. (2003). A review of 25 years of the social interaction test. *Eur. J. Pharmacol.* 463, 35–53. doi: 10.1016/S0014-2999(03)01273-1

Finger, E. C., Marsh, A. A., Buzas, B., Kamel, N., Rhodes, R., Vythilingham, M., et al. (2007). The impact of tryptophan depletion and 5-HTTLPR genotype on passive avoidance and response reversal instrumental learning tasks. *Neuropsychopharmacology* 32, 206–215. doi: 10.1038/sj.npp.1301182

Flint, J., and Shifman, S. (2008). Animal models of psychiatric disease. *Curr. Opin. Genet. Dev.* 18, 235–240. doi: 10.1016/j.gde.2008.07.002

Friedman, M. J., Resick, P. A., Bryant, R. A., Strain, J., Horowitz, M., and Spiegel, D. (2011). Classification of trauma and stressor-related disorders in DSM-5. *Depress. Anxiety* 28, 737–749. doi: 10.1002/da.20845

Fyer, A. J., Hamilton, S. P., Durner, M., Haghighi, F., Heiman, G. A., Costa, R., et al. (2006). A third-pass genome scan in panic disorder: evidence for multiple susceptibility loci. *Biol. Psychiatry* 60, 388–401. doi: 10.1016/j.biopsych.2006.04.018

Gao, B., Fritschy, J. M., Benke, D., and Mohler, H. (1993). Neuron-specific expression of GABAA-receptor subtypes: differential association of the alpha 1- and alpha 3-subunits with serotonergic and GABAergic neurons. *Neuroscience* 54, 881–892. doi: 10.1016/0306-4522(93)90582-Z

Gardier, A. M., Malagie, I., Trillat, A. C., Jacquot, C., and Artigas, F. (1996). Role of 5-HT1A autoreceptors in the mechanism of action of serotoninergic antidepressant drugs: recent findings from in vivo microdialysis studies. *Fundam. Clin. Pharmacol.* 10, 16–27. doi: 10.1111/j.1472-8206.1996.tb00145.x

Garner, M., Mohler, H., Stein, D. J., Mueggler, T., and Baldwin, D. S. (2009). Research in anxiety disorders: from the bench to the bedside. *Eur. Neuropsychopharmacol.* 19, 381–390. doi: 10.1016/j.euroneuro.2009.01.011

Gaspar, P., and Lillesaar, C. (2012). Probing the diversity of serotonin neurons. *Philos. Trans. R. Soc. Lond. B Biol. Sci.* 367, 2382–2394. doi: 10.1098/rstb.2011.0378

Gelernter, J., Bonvicini, K., Page, G., Woods, S. W., Goddard, A. W., Kruger, S., et al. (2001). Linkage genome scan for loci predisposing to panic disorder or agoraphobia. *Am. J. Med. Genet.* 105, 548–557. doi: 10.1002/ajmg.1496

Gelernter, J., Page, G. P., Bonvicini, K., Woods, S. W., Pauls, D. L., and Kruger, S. (2003). A chromosome 14 risk locus for simple phobia: results from a genomewide linkage scan. *Mol. Psychiatry* 8, 71–82. doi: 10.1038/sj.mp.4001224

Gelernter, J., Page, G. P., Stein, M. B., and Woods, S. W. (2004). Genome-wide linkage scan for loci predisposing to social phobia: evidence for a chromosome 16 risk locus. *Am. J. Psychiatry* 161, 59–66. doi: 10.1176/appi.ajp.161.1.59

Gershon, E. S., Alliey-Rodriguez, N., and Liu, C. (2011). After GWAS: searching for genetic risk for schizophrenia and bipolar disorder. *Am. J. Psychiatry* 168, 253–256. doi: 10.1176/appi.ajp.2010.10091340

Gervasoni, D., Peyron, C., Rampon, C., Barbagli, B., Chouvet, G., Urbain, N., et al. (2000). Role and origin of the GABAergic innervation of dorsal raphe serotonergic neurons. *J. Neurosci.* 20, 4217–4225.

Glenn, A. L. (2011). The other allele: exploring the long allele of the serotonin transporter gene as a potential risk factor for psychopathy: a review of the parallels in findings. *Neurosci. Biobehav. Rev.* 35, 612–620. doi: 10.1016/j.neubiorev.2010.07.005

Gomes, K. S., and Nunes-de-Souza, R. L. (2009). Implication of the 5-HT2A and 5-HT2C (but not 5HT1A) receptors located within the periaqueductal gray in the elevated plus-maze test-retest paradigm in mice. *Prog. Neuropsychopharmacol. Biol. Psychiatry* 33, 1261–1269. doi: 10.1016/j.pnpbp.2009.07.015

Grabe, H. J., Schwahn, C., Appel, K., Mahler, J., Schulz, A., Spitzer, C., et al. (2011). Update on the 2005 paper: moderation of mental and physical distress by polymorphisms in the 5-HT transporter gene by interacting with social stressors and chronic disease burden. *Mol. Psychiatry* 16, 354–356. doi: 10.1038/mp.2010.45

Gross, C., Zhuang, X., Stark, K., Ramboz, S., Oosting, R., Kirby, L., et al. (2002). Serotonin1A receptor acts during development to establish normal anxiety-like behaviour in the adult. *Nature* 416, 396–400. doi: 10.1038/416396a

Guilloux, J. P., David, D. J., Guiard, B. P., Chenu, F., Reperant, C., Toth, M., et al. (2006). Blockade of 5-HT1A receptors by (+/−)-pindolol potentiates cortical 5-HT outflow, but not antidepressant-like activity of paroxetine: microdialysis and behavioral approaches in 5-HT1A receptor knockout mice. *Neuropsychopharmacology* 31, 2162–2172.

Hamilton, S. P. (2009). Linkage and association studies of anxiety disorders. *Depress. Anxiety* 26, 976–983. doi: 10.1002/da.20615

Hamilton, S. P., Fyer, A. J., Durner, M., Heiman, G. A., Baisre de Leon, A., Hodge, S. E., et al. (2003). Further genetic evidence for a panic disorder syndrome mapping to chromosome 13q. *Proc. Natl. Acad. Sci. U.S.A.* 100, 2550–2555. doi: 10.1073/pnas.0335669100

Hamilton, S. P., Slager, S. L., de Leon, A. B., Heiman, G. A., Klein, D. F., Hodge, S. E., et al. (2004). Evidence for genetic linkage between a polymorphism in the adenosine 2A receptor and panic disorder. *Neuropsychopharmacology* 29, 558–565. doi: 10.1038/sj.npp.1300311

Hamilton, S. P., Slager, S. L., Heiman, G. A., Deng, Z., Haghighi, F., Klein, D. F., et al. (2002). Evidence for a susceptibility locus for panic disorder near the catechol-*O*-methyltransferase gene on chromosome 22. *Biol. Psychiatry* 51, 591–601. doi: 10.1016/S0006-3223(01)01322-1

Hankin, B. L., Nederhof, E., Oppenheimer, C. W., Jenness, J., Young, J. F., Abela, J. R., et al. (2011). Differential susceptibility in youth: evidence that 5-HTTLPR x positive parenting is associated with positive affect 'for better and worse'. *Transl. Psychiatry* 1, e44. doi: 10.1038/tp.2011.44

Harandi, M., Aguera, M., Gamrani, H., Didier, M., Maitre, M., Calas, A., et al. (1987). gamma-Aminobutyric acid and 5-hydroxytryptamine interrelationship in the rat nucleus raphe dorsalis: combination of radioautographic and immunocytochemical techniques at light and electron microscopy levels. *Neuroscience* 21, 237–251. doi: 10.1016/0306-4522(87)90336-8

Hariri, A. R. (2009). The neurobiology of individual differences in complex behavioral traits. *Annu. Rev. Neurosci.* 32, 225–247. doi: 10.1146/annurev.neuro.051508.135335

Hariri, A. R., and Holmes, A. (2006). Genetics of emotional regulation: the role of the serotonin transporter in neural function. *Trends Cogn. Sci.* 10, 182–191. doi: 10.1016/j.tics.2006.02.011

Hariri, A. R., Mattay, V. S., Tessitore, A., Kolachana, B., Fera, F., Goldman, D., et al. (2002). Serotonin transporter genetic variation and the response of the human amygdala. *Science* 297, 400–403. doi: 10.1126/science.1071829

Hattori, E., Ebihara, M., Yamada, K., Ohba, H., Shibuya, H., and Yoshikawa, T. (2001). Identification of a compound short tandem repeat stretch in the 5′-upstream region of the cholecystokinin gene, and its association with panic disorder but not with schizophrenia. *Mol. Psychiatry* 6, 465–470. doi: 10.1038/sj.mp.4000875

Heisler, L. K., Chu, H. M., Brennan, T. J., Danao, J. A., Bajwa, P., Parsons, L. H., et al. (1998). Elevated anxiety and antidepressant-like responses in serotonin 5-HT1A receptor mutant mice. *Proc. Natl. Acad. Sci. U.S.A.* 95, 15049–15054. doi: 10.1073/pnas.95.25.15049

Hettema, J. M., An, S. S., Neale, M. C., Bukszar, J., van den Oord, E. J., Kendler, K. S., et al. (2006). Association between glutamic acid decarboxylase genes and anxiety disorders, major depression, and neuroticism.

Mol. Psychiatry 11, 752–762. doi: 10.1038/sj.mp.4001845

Hettema, J. M., Neale, M. C., and Kendler, K. S. (2001). A review and meta-analysis of the genetic epidemiology of anxiety disorders. *Am. J. Psychiatry* 158, 1568–1578. doi: 10.1176/appi.ajp.158.10.1568

Hettema, J. M., Prescott, C. A., Myers, J. M., Neale, M. C., and Kendler, K. S. (2005). The structure of genetic and environmental risk factors for anxiety disorders in men and women. *Arch. Gen. Psychiatry* 62, 182–189. doi: 10.1001/archpsyc.62.2.182

Holmes, A. (2008). Genetic variation in cortico-amygdala serotonin function and risk for stress-related disease. *Neurosci. Biobehav. Rev.* 32, 1293–1314. doi: 10.1016/j.neubiorev.2008.03.006

Holmes, A., Yang, R. J., Murphy, D. L., and Crawley, J. N. (2002). Evaluation of antidepressant-related behavioral responses in mice lacking the serotonin transporter. *Neuropsychopharmacology* 27, 914–923. doi: 10.1016/S0893-133X(02)00374-3

Homberg, J. R., de Boer, S. F., Raaso, H. S., Olivier, J. D., Verheul, M., Ronken, E., et al. (2008a). Adaptations in pre- and postsynaptic 5-HT(1A) receptor function and cocaine supersensitivity in serotonin transporter knockout rats. *Psychopharmacology (Berl.)* 200, 367–380. doi: 10.1007/s00213-008-1212-x

Homberg, J. R., van den Bos, R., den Heijer, E., Suer, R., and Cuppen, E. (2008b). Serotonin transporter dosage modulates long-term decision-making in rat and human. *Neuropharmacology* 55, 80–84. doi: 10.1016/j.neuropharm.2008.04.016

Homberg, J. R., and Lesch, K. P. (2011). Looking on the bright side of serotonin transporter gene variation. *Biol. Psychiatry* 69, 513–519. doi: 10.1016/j.biopsych.2010.09.024

Homberg, J. R., Olivier, J. D., Smits, B. M., Mul, J. D., Mudde, J., Verheul, M., et al. (2007a). Characterization of the serotonin transporter knockout rat: a selective change in the functioning of the serotonergic system. *Neuroscience* 146, 1662–1676. doi: 10.1016/j.neuroscience.2007.03.030

Homberg, J. R., Pattij, T., Janssen, M. C., Ronken, E., de Boer, S. F., Schoffelmeer, A. N., et al. (2007b). Serotonin transporter deficiency in rats improves inhibitory control but not behavioural flexibility. *Eur. J. Neurosci.* 26, 2066–2073. doi: 10.1111/j.1460-9568.2007.05839.x

Homberg, J. R., Schubert, D., and Gaspar, P. (2010). New perspectives on the neurodevelopmental effects of SSRIs. *Trends Pharmacol. Sci.* 31, 60–65. doi: 10.1016/j.tips.2009.11.003

Homberg, J. R., and van den Hove, D. L. (2012). The serotonin transporter gene and functional and pathological adaptation to environmental variation across the life span. *Prog. Neurobiol.* 99, 117–127. doi: 10.1016/j.pneurobio.2012.08.003

Hovatta, I., and Barlow, C. (2008). Molecular genetics of anxiety in mice and men. *Ann. Med.* 40, 92–109. doi: 10.1080/07853890701747096

Huot, R. L., Thrivikraman, K. V., Meaney, M. J., and Plotsky, P. M. (2001). Development of adult ethanol preference and anxiety as a consequence of neonatal maternal separation in Long Evans rats and reversal with antidepressant treatment. *Psychopharmacology (Berl.)* 158, 366–373. doi: 10.1007/s002130100701

Inada, Y., Yoneda, H., Koh, J., Sakai, J., Himei, A., Kinoshita, Y., et al. (2003). Positive association between panic disorder and polymorphism of the serotonin 2A receptor gene. *Psychiatry Res.* 118, 25–31. doi: 10.1016/S0165-1781(03)00064-7

Jansen, F., Heiming, R. S., Lewejohann, L., Touma, C., Palme, R., Schmitt, A., et al. (2010). Modulation of behavioural profile and stress response by 5-HTT genotype and social experience in adulthood. *Behav. Brain Res.* 207, 21–29. doi: 10.1016/j.bbr.2009.09.033

Jasinska, A. J., Lowry, C. A., and Burmeister, M. (2012). Serotonin transporter gene, stress and raphe–raphe interactions: a molecular mechanism of depression. *Trends Neurosci.* 35, 395–402. doi: 10.1016/j.tins.2012.01.001

Jennings, K. A., Loder, M. K., Sheward, W. J., Pei, Q., Deacon, R. M., Benson, M. A., et al. (2006). Increased expression of the 5-HT transporter confers a low-anxiety phenotype linked to decreased 5-HT transmission. *J. Neurosci.* 26, 8955–8964. doi: 10.1523/JNEUROSCI.5356-05.2006

Kaabi, B., Gelenter, J., Woods, S. W., Goddard, A., Page, G. P., and Elston, R. C. (2006). Genome scan for loci predisposing to anxiety disorders using a novel multivariate approach: strong evidence for a chromosome 4 risk locus. *Am. J. Hum. Genet.* 78, 543–553.

Kalin, N. H., Shelton, S. E., Fox, A. S., Rogers, J., Oakes, T. R., and Davidson, R. J. (2008). The serotonin transporter genotype is associated with intermediate brain phenotypes that depend on the context of eliciting stressor. *Mol. Psychiatry* 13, 1021–1027. doi: 10.1038/mp.2008.37

Kalinichev, M., Easterling, K. W., Plotsky, P. M., and Holtzman, S. G. (2002). Long-lasting changes in stress-induced corticosterone response and anxiety-like behaviors as a consequence of neonatal maternal separation in Long–Evans rats. *Pharmacol. Biochem. Behav.* 73, 131–140. doi: 10.1016/S0091-3057(02)00781-5

Kalueff, A. V., and Nutt, D. J. (2007). Role of GABA in anxiety and depression. *Depress. Anxiety* 24, 495–517. doi: 10.1002/da.20262

Kalueff, A. V., Olivier, J. D., Nonkes, L. J., and Homberg, J. R. (2010). Conserved role for the serotonin transporter gene in rat and mouse neurobehavioral endophenotypes. *Neurosci. Biobehav. Rev.* 34, 373–386. doi: 10.1016/j.neubiorev.2009.08.003

Kas, M. J., Krishnan, V., Gould, T. D., Collier, D. A., Olivier, B., Lesch, K. P., et al. (2011). Advances in multidisciplinary and cross-species approaches to examine the neurobiology of psychiatric disorders. *Eur. Neuropsychopharmacol.* 21, 532–544. doi: 10.1016/j.euroneuro.2010.12.001

Kennedy, J. L., Bradwejn, J., Koszycki, D., King, N., Crowe, R., Vincent, J., et al. (1999). Investigation of cholecystokinin system genes in panic disorder. *Mol. Psychiatry* 4, 284–285. doi: 10.1038/sj.mp.4000507

Kiyasova, V., Bonnavion, P., Scotto-Lomassese, S., Fabre, V., Sahly, I., Tronche, F., et al. (2013). A subpopulation of serotonergic neurons that do not express the 5-HT1A autoreceptor. *ACS Chem. Neurosci.* 4, 89–95. doi: 10.1021/cn300157s

Kiyasova, V., Fernandez, S. P., Laine, J., Stankovski, L., Muzerelle, A., Doly, S., et al. (2011). A genetically defined morphologically and functionally unique subset of 5-HT neurons in the mouse raphe nuclei. *J. Neurosci.* 31, 2756–2768. doi: 10.1523/JNEUROSCI.4080-10.2011

Klein, C., Lohmann, K., and Ziegler, A. (2012). The promise and limitations of genome-wide association studies. *JAMA*. doi: 10.1001/2012.jama.10823 [Epub ahead of print].

Knowles, J. A., Fyer, A. J., Vieland, V. J., Weissman, M. M., Hodge, S. E., Heiman, G. A., et al. (1998). Results of a genome-wide genetic screen for panic disorder. *Am. J. Med. Genet.* 81, 139–147. doi: 10.1002/(SICI)1096-8628(19980328)81:2<139::AID-AJMG4>3.0.CO;2-R

Knutsen, L. J. (2011). Drug discovery management, small is still beautiful: why a number of companies get it wrong. *Drug Discov. Today* 16, 476–484. doi: 10.1016/j.drudis.2011.04.002

Kusserow, H., Davies, B., Hortnagl, H., Voigt, I., Stroh, T., Bert, B., et al. (2004). Reduced anxiety-related behaviour in transgenic mice overexpressing serotonin 1A receptors. *Brain Res. Mol. Brain Res.* 129, 104–116. doi: 10.1016/j.molbrainres.2004.06.028

Lanfumey, L., Mongeau, R., Cohen-Salmon, C., and Hamon, M. (2008). Corticosteroid-serotonin interactions in the neurobiological mechanisms of stress-related disorders. *Neurosci. Biobehav. Rev.* 32, 1174–1184. doi: 10.1016/j.neubiorev.2008.04.006

Lee, H. J., Lee, M. S., Kang, R. H., Kim, H., Kim, S. D., Kee, B. S., et al. (2005). Influence of the serotonin transporter promoter gene polymorphism on susceptibility to posttraumatic stress disorder. *Depress. Anxiety* 21, 135–139. doi: 10.1002/da.20064

Le FranÇois, B., Czesak, M., Steubl, D., and Albert, P. R. (2008). Transcriptional regulation at a HTR1A polymorphism associated with mental illness. *Neuropharmacology* 55, 977–985. doi: 10.1016/j.neuropharm.2008.06.046

Lesch, K. P. (2001). Molecular foundation of anxiety disorders. *J. Neural. Transm.* 108, 717–746. doi: 10.1007/s007020170048

Lesch, K. P., Bengel, D., Heils, A., Sabol, S. Z., Greenberg, B. D., Petri, S., et al. (1996). Association of anxiety-related traits with a polymorphism in the serotonin transporter gene regulatory region. *Science* 274, 1527–1531. doi: 10.1126/science.274.5292.1527

Lesch, K. P., and Gutknecht, L. (2004). Focus on The 5-HT1A receptor: emerging role of a gene regulatory variant in psychopathology and pharmacogenetics. *Int. J. Neuropsychopharmacol.* 7, 381–385. doi: 10.1017/S1461145704004845

Leysen, J. E. (2004). 5-HT2 receptors. *Curr. Drug Targets CNS Neurol. Disord.* 3, 11–26. doi: 10.2174/1568007043482598

Line, S. J., Barkus, C., Coyle, C., Jennings, K. A., Deacon, R. M., Lesch, K. P., et al. (2011). Opposing alterations in anxiety and species-typical behaviours in serotonin transporter overexpressor and knockout mice. *Eur. Neuropsychopharmacol.* 21, 108–116. doi: 10.1016/j.euroneuro.2010.08.005

Lippa, A., Czobor, P., Stark, J., Beer, B., Kostakis, E., Gravielle, M., et al. (2005). Selective anxiolysis produced by ocinaplon, a GABA(A) receptor modulator. *Proc. Natl. Acad. Sci. U.S.A.* 102, 7380–7385. doi: 10.1073/pnas.0502579102

Lista, A., Blier, P., and de Montigny, C. (1989). In vivo presynaptic modulation of serotonergic neurotransmission in the rat hippocampus by diazepam. *Eur. J. Pharmacol.* 171, 229–231. doi: 10.1016/0014-2999(89)90111-8

Logue, M. W., Baldwin, C., Guffanti, G., Melista, E., Wolf, E. J., Reardon, A. F., et al. (2012). A genome-wide association study of post-traumatic stress disorder identifies the retinoid-related orphan receptor alpha (RORA) gene as a significant risk locus. *Mol. Psychiatry.* doi: 10.1038/mp.2012.113 [Epub ahead of print].

Lo Iacono, L., and Gross, C. (2008). Alpha-Ca^{2+}/calmodulin-dependent protein kinase II contributes to the developmental programming of anxiety in serotonin receptor 1A knock-out mice. *J. Neurosci.* 28, 6250–6257. doi: 10.1523/JNEUROSCI.5219-07.2008

Lubke, G. H., Hottenga, J. J., Walters, R., Laurin, C., de Geus, E. J., Willemsen, G., et al. (2012). Estimating the genetic variance of major depressive disorder due to all single nucleotide polymorphisms. *Biol. Psychiatry* 72, 707–709. doi: 10.1016/j.biopsych.2012.03.011

Magalhaes, A. C., Holmes, K. D., Dale, L. B., Comps-Agrar, L., Lee, D., Yadav, P. N., et al. (2010). CRF receptor 1 regulates anxiety behavior via sensitization of 5-HT2 receptor signaling. *Nat. Neurosci.* 13, 622–629. doi: 10.1038/nn.2529

Manolio, T. A., Collins, F. S., Cox, N. J., Goldstein, D. B., Hindorff, L. A., Hunter, D. J., et al. (2009). Finding the missing heritability of complex diseases. *Nature* 461, 747–753. doi: 10.1038/nature08494

Maron, E., Nikopensius, T., Koks, S., Altmae, S., Heinaste, E., Vabrit, K., et al. (2005). Association study of 90 candidate gene polymorphisms in panic disorder. *Psychiatr. Genet.* 15, 17–24. doi: 10.1097/00041444-200503000-00004

Maron, E., Tasa, G., Toru, I., Lang, A., Vasar, V., and Shlik, J. (2004). Association between serotonin-related genetic polymorphisms and CCK-4-induced panic attacks with or without 5-hydroxytryptophan pretreatment in healthy volunteers. *World J. Biol. Psychiatry* 5, 149–154. doi: 10.1080/15622970410029927

Martin, C. B., Ramond, F., Farrington, D. T., Aguiar, A. S. Jr., Chevarin, C., Berthiau, A. S., et al. (2013). RNA splicing and editing modulation of 5-HT2C receptor function: relevance to anxiety and aggression in VGV mice. *Mol. Psychiatry* 18, 656–665. doi: 10.1038/mp.2012.171

Mathews, A., and MacLeod, C. (2005). Cognitive vulnerability to emotional disorders. *Annu. Rev. Clin. Psychol.* 1, 167–195. doi: 10.1146/annurev.clinpsy.1.102803.143916

Mathews, T. A., Fedele, D. E., Coppelli, F. M., Avila, A. M., Murphy, D. L., and Andrews, A. M. (2004). Gene dose-dependent alterations in extraneuronal serotonin but not dopamine in mice with reduced serotonin transporter expression. *J. Neurosci. Methods* 140, 169–181. doi: 10.1016/j.jneumeth.2004.05.017

McDougle, C. J., Epperson, C. N., Price, L. H., and Gelernter, J. (1998). Evidence for linkage disequilibrium between serotonin transporter protein gene (SLC6A4) and obsessive compulsive disorder. *Mol. Psychiatry* 3, 270–273. doi: 10.1038/sj.mp.4000391

McKernan, R. M., Rosahl, T. W., Reynolds, D. S., Sur, C., Wafford, K. A., Atack, J. R., et al. (2000). Sedative but not anxiolytic properties of benzodiazepines are mediated by the GABA(A) receptor alpha1 subtype. *Nat. Neurosci.* 3, 587–592. doi: 10.1038/75761

Meneses, A. (2007a). Do serotonin(1-7) receptors modulate short and long-term memory? *Neurobiol. Learn. Mem.* 87, 561–572. doi: 10.1016/j.nlm.2006.12.005

Meneses, A. (2007b). Stimulation of 5-HT1A, 5-HT1B, 5-HT2A/2C, 5-HT3 and 5-HT4 receptors or 5-HT uptake inhibition: short- and long-term memory. *Behav. Brain Res.* 184, 81–90. doi: 10.1016/j.bbr.2007.06.026

Millan, M. J., Brocco, M., Gobert, A., and Dekeyne, A. (2005). Anxiolytic properties of agomelatine, an antidepressant with melatoninergic and serotonergic properties: role of 5-HT2C receptor blockade. *Psychopharmacology (Berl.)* 177, 448–458. doi: 10.1007/s00213-004-1962-z

Mirza, N. R., and Munro, G. (2010). The role of GABA(A) receptor subtypes as analgesic targets. *Drug News Perspect.* 23, 351–360. doi: 10.1358/dnp.2010.23.6.1489909.

Möhler, H. (2006). GABAA receptors in central nervous system disease: anxiety, epilepsy, and insomnia. *J. Recept. Signal Transduct. Res.* 26, 731–740. doi: 10.1080/10799890600920035

Möhler, H., and Okada, T. (1977). Benzodiazepine receptor: demonstration in the central nervous system. *Science* 198, 849–851. doi: 10.1126/science.918669

Montag, C., Fiebach, C. J., Kirsch, P., and Reuter, M. (2011). Interaction of 5-HTTLPR and a variation on the oxytocin receptor gene influences negative emotionality. *Biol. Psychiatry* 69, 601–603. doi: 10.1016/j.biopsych.2010.10.026

Moya, P. R., Fox, M. A., Jensen, C. L., LaPorte, J. L., French, H. T., Wendland, J. R., et al. (2011). Altered 5-HT2C receptor agonist-induced responses and 5-HT2C receptor RNA editing in the amygdala of serotonin transporter knockout mice. *BMC Pharmacol.* 11:3. doi: 10.1186/1471-2210-11-3

Muglia, P. (2011). From genes to therapeutic targets for psychiatric disorders – what to expect? *Curr. Opin. Pharmacol.* 11, 563–571. doi: 10.1016/j.coph.2011.08.003

Muller, J. M., Morelli, E., Ansorge, M., and Gingrich, J. A. (2011). Serotonin transporter deficient mice are vulnerable to escape deficits following inescapable shocks. *Genes Brain Behav.* 10, 166–175. doi: 10.1111/j.1601-183X.2010.00652.x

Munafo, M. R., Clark, T., and Flint, J. (2005). Does measurement instrument moderate the association between the serotonin transporter gene and anxiety-related personality traits? A meta-analysis. *Mol. Psychiatry* 10, 415–419. doi: 10.1038/sj.mp.4001627

Munafo, M. R., Clark, T. G., Moore, L. R., Payne, E., Walton, R., and Flint, J. (2003). Genetic polymorphisms and personality in healthy adults: a systematic review and meta-analysis. *Mol. Psychiatry* 8, 471–484. doi: 10.1038/sj.mp.4001326

Murphy, D. L., and Lesch, K. P. (2008). Targeting the murine serotonin transporter: insights into human neurobiology. *Nat. Rev. Neurosci.* 9, 85–96. doi: 10.1038/nrn2284

Murrough, J. W., and Charney, D. S. (2011). The serotonin transporter and emotionality: risk, resilience, and new therapeutic opportunities. *Biol. Psychiatry* 69, 510–512. doi: 10.1016/j.biopsych.2011.01.019

Narayanan, V., Heiming, R. S., Jansen, F., Lesting, J., Sachser, N., Pape, H. C., et al. (2011). Social defeat: impact on fear extinction and amygdala-prefrontal cortical theta synchrony in 5-HTT deficient mice. *PLoS ONE* 6:e22600. doi: 10.1371/journal.pone.0022600

Naukkarinen, H., Raassina, R., Penttinen, J., Ahokas, A., Jokinen, R., Koponen, H., et al. (2005). Deramciclane in the treatment of generalized anxiety disorder: a placebo-controlled, double-blind, dose-finding study. *Eur. Neuropsychopharmacol.* 15, 617–623. doi: 10.1016/j.euroneuro.2005.03.002

Nelson, E. C., Agrawal, A., Pergadia, M. L., Lynskey, M. T., Todorov, A. A., Wang, J. C., et al. (2009). Association of childhood trauma exposure and GABRA2 polymorphisms with risk of posttraumatic stress disorder in adults. *Mol. Psychiatry* 14, 234–235. doi: 10.1038/mp.2008.81

Nemeroff, C. B. (2003). The role of GABA in the pathophysiology and treatment of anxiety disorders. *Psychopharmacol. Bull.* 37, 133–146.

Nietzer, S. L., Bonn, M., Jansen, F., Heiming, R. S., Lewejohann, L., Sachser, N., et al. (2011). Serotonin transporter knockout and repeated social defeat stress: impact on neuronal morphology and plasticity in limbic brain areas. *Behav. Brain Res.* 220, 42–54. doi: 10.1016/j.bbr.2011.01.011

Nonkes, L. J., de Pooter, M., and Homberg, J. R. (2012). Behavioural therapy based on distraction alleviates impaired fear extinction in male serotonin transporter knockout rats. *J. Psychiatry Neurosci.* 37, 224–230. doi: 10.1503/jpn.110116

Nonkes, L. J., Maes, J. H., and Homberg, J. R. (2013). Improved cognitive flexibility in serotonin transporter knockout rats is unchanged following chronic cocaine self-administration. *Addict. Biol.* 18, 434–440. doi: 10.1111/j.1369-1600.2011.00351.x

Nothdurfter, C., Baghai, T. C., Schule, C., and Rupprecht, R. (2012). Translocator protein (18 kDa) (TSPO) as a therapeutic target for anxiety and neurologic disorders. *Eur. Arch. Psychiatry Clin. Neurosci.* 262(Suppl. 2), S107–S112. doi: 10.1007/s00406-012-0352-5

Nunes-de-Souza, V., Nunes-de-Souza, R. L., Rodgers, R. J., and Canto-de-Souza, A. (2008). 5-HT2 receptor activation in the midbrain periaqueductal grey (PAG) reduces anxiety-like behaviour in mice. *Behav. Brain Res.* 187, 72–79. doi: 10.1016/j.bbr.2007.08.030

Ohara, K., Suzuki, Y., Ochiai, M., Tsukamoto, T., Tani, K., and Ohara, K. (1999). A variable-number-tandem-repeat of the serotonin transporter gene and anxiety disorders. *Prog. Neuropsychopharmacol. Biol. Psychiatry* 23, 55–65. doi: 10.1016/S0278-5846(98)00091-8

Olivier, B., Pattij, T., Wood, S. J., Oosting, R., Sarnyai, Z., and Toth, M. (2001). The 5-HT(1A) receptor knockout mouse and anxiety. *Behav. Pharmacol.* 12, 439–450. doi: 10.1097/00008877-200111000-00004

Olivier, B., Soudijn, W., and van Wijngaarden, I. (1999). The 5-HT1A receptor and its ligands: structure and function. *Prog. Drug Res.* 52, 103–165. doi: 10.1007/978-3-0348-8730-4_3

Olivier, J. D., Van Der Hart, M. G., Van Swelm, R. P., Dederen, P. J., Homberg, J. R., Cremers, T., et al. (2008). A study in male and female 5-HT transporter knockout rats: an animal model for anxiety and depression disorders. *Neuroscience* 152, 573–584. doi: 10.1016/j.neuroscience.2007.12.032

Otowa, T., Kawamura, Y., Nishida, N., Sugaya, N., Koike, A., Yoshida, E., et al. (2012). Meta-analysis of genome-wide association studies for panic disorder in the Japanese population. *Transl. Psychiatry* 2, e186. doi: 10.1038/tp.2012.89

Parks, C. L., Robinson, P. S., Sibille, E., Shenk, T., and Toth, M. (1998). Increased anxiety of mice lacking the serotonin1A receptor. *Proc. Natl. Acad. Sci. U.S.A.* 95, 10734–10739. doi: 10.1073/pnas.95.18.10734

Pattij, T., Groenink, L., Oosting, R. S., van der Gugten, J., Maes, R. A., and Olivier, B. (2002). GABA(A)-benzodiazepine receptor complex sensitivity in 5-HT(1A) receptor knockout mice on a 129/Sv background. *Eur. J. Pharmacol.* 447, 67–74. doi: 10.1016/S0014-2999(02)01893-9

Pattij, T., Hijzen, T. H., Groenink, L., Oosting, R. S., van der Gugten, J., Maes, R. A., et al. (2001). Stress-induced hyperthermia in the 5-HT(1A) receptor knockout mouse is normal. *Biol. Psychiatry* 49, 569–574. doi: 10.1016/S0006-3223(00)01022-2

Pham, X., Sun, C., Chen, X., van den Oord, E. J., Neale, M. C., Kendler, K. S., et al. (2009). Association study between GABA receptor genes and anxiety spectrum disorders. *Depress. Anxiety* 26, 998–1003. doi: 10.1002/da.20628

Pluess, M., Velders, F. P., Belsky, J., van IJzendoorn, M. H., Bakermans-Kranenburg, M. J., Jaddoe, V. W., et al. (2011). Serotonin transporter polymorphism moderates effects of prenatal maternal anxiety on infant negative emotionality. *Biol. Psychiatry* 69, 520–525. doi: 10.1016/j.biopsych.2010.10.006

Polanczyk, G., Caspi, A., Williams, B., Price, T. S., Danese, A., Sugden, K., et al. (2009). Protective effect of CRHR1 gene variants on the development of adult depression following childhood maltreatment: replication and extension. *Arch. Gen. Psychiatry* 66, 978–985. doi: 10.1001/archgenpsychiatry.2009.114

Pratt, J., Jenner, P., Reynolds, E. H., and Marsden, C. D. (1979). Clonazepam induces decreased serotoninergic activity in the mouse brain. *Neuropharmacology* 18, 791–799. doi: 10.1016/0028-3908(79)90024-8

Quesseveur, G., Nguyen, H. T., Gardier, A. M., and Guiard, B. P. (2012). 5-HT2 ligands in the treatment of anxiety and depression. *Expert Opin. Investig. Drugs* 21, 1701–1725. doi: 10.1517/13543784.2012.719872

Ramboz, S., Oosting, R., Amara, D. A., Kung, H. F., Blier, P., Mendelsohn, M., et al. (1998). Serotonin receptor 1A knockout: an animal model of anxiety-related disorder. *Proc. Natl. Acad. Sci. U.S.A.* 95, 14476–14481. doi: 10.1073/pnas.95.24.14476

Ressler, K. J., and Mayberg, H. S. (2007). Targeting abnormal neural circuits in mood and anxiety disorders: from the laboratory to the clinic. *Nat. Neurosci.* 10, 1116–1124. doi: 10.1038/nn1944

Richardson-Jones, J. W., Craige, C. P., Guiard, B. P., Stephen, A., Metzger, K. L., Kung, H. F., et al. (2010). 5-HT1A autoreceptor levels determine vulnerability to stress and response to antidepressants. *Neuron* 65, 40–52. doi: 10.1016/j.neuron.2009.12.003

Risch, N., Herrell, R., Lehner, T., Liang, K. Y., Eaves, L., Hoh, J., et al. (2009). Interaction between the serotonin transporter gene (5-HTTLPR), stressful life events, and risk of depression: a meta-analysis. *JAMA* 301, 2462–2471. doi: 10.1001/jama.2009.878

Rodgers, R. J., Cao, B. J., Dalvi, A., and Holmes, A. (1997). Animal models of anxiety: an ethological perspective. *Braz. J. Med. Biol. Res.* 30, 289–304. doi: 10.1590/S0100-879X1997000300002

Roiser, J. P., Blackwell, A. D., Cools, R., Clark, L., Rubinsztein, D. C., Robbins, T. W., et al. (2006a). Serotonin transporter polymorphism mediates vulnerability to loss of incentive motivation following acute tryptophan depletion. *Neuropsychopharmacology* 31, 2264–2272. doi: 10.1038/sj.npp.1301084

Roiser, J. P., Rogers, R. D., Cook, L. J., and Sahakian, B. J. (2006b). The effect of polymorphism at the serotonin transporter gene on decision-making, memory and executive function in ecstasy users and controls. *Psychopharmacology (Berl.)* 188, 213–227. doi: 10.1007/s00213-006-0495-z

Roiser, J. P., Muller, U., Clark, L., and Sahakian, B. J. (2007). The effects of acute tryptophan depletion and serotonin transporter polymorphism on emotional processing in memory and attention. *Int. J. Neuropsychopharmacol.* 10, 449–461. doi: 10.1017/S146114570600705X

Rothe, C., Gutknecht, L., Freitag, C., Tauber, R., Mossner, R., Franke, P., et al. (2004). Association of a functional 1019C > G 5-HT1A receptor gene polymorphism with panic disorder with agoraphobia. *Int. J. Neuropsychopharmacol.* 7, 189–192. doi: 10.1017/S1461145703004061

Rothe, C., Koszycki, D., Bradwejn, J., King, N., Deluca, V., Tharmalingam, S., et al. (2006). Association of the Val158Met catechol O-methyltransferase genetic polymorphism with panic disorder. *Neuropsychopharmacology* 31, 2237–2242.

Rowlett, J. K., Platt, D. M., Lelas, S., Atack, J. R., and Dawson, G. R. (2005). Different GABAA receptor subtypes mediate the anxiolytic, abuse-related, and motor effects of benzodiazepine-like drugs in primates. *Proc. Natl. Acad. Sci. U.S.A.* 102, 915–920. doi: 10.1073/pnas.0405621102

Rudolph, U., and Knoflach, F. (2011). Beyond classical benzodiazepines: novel therapeutic potential of GABA(A) receptor subtypes. *Nat. Rev. Drug Discov.* 10, 685–697. doi: 10.1038/nrd3502

Samochowiec, J., Hajduk, A., Samochowiec, A., Horodnicki, J., Stepien, G., Grzywacz, A., et al. (2004). Association studies of MAO-A, COMT, and 5-HTT genes polymorphisms in patients with anxiety disorders of the phobic spectrum. *Psychiatry Res.* 128, 21–26. doi: 10.1016/j.psychres.2004.05.012

Sanchez, C. (2003). Stress-induced vocalisation in adult animals. A valid model of anxiety? *Eur. J. Pharmacol.* 463, 133–143. doi: 10.1016/S0014-2999(03)01277-9

Santarelli, L., Saxe, M., Gross, C., Surget, A., Battaglia, F., Dulawa, S., et al. (2003). Requirement of hippocampal neurogenesis for the behavioral effects of antidepressants. *Science* 301, 805–809. doi: 10.1126/science.1083328

Savitz, J., Lucki, I., and Drevets, W. C. (2009). 5-HT(1A) receptor function in major depressive disorder. *Prog. Neurobiol.* 88, 17–31. doi: 10.1016/j.pneurobio.2009.01.009

Scott-Stevens, P., Atack, J. R., Sohal, B., and Worboys, P. (2005). Rodent pharmacokinetics and receptor occupancy of the GABAA receptor subtype selective benzodiazepine site ligand L-838417. *Biopharm. Drug Dispos.* 26, 13–20. doi: 10.1002/bdd.423

Seedat, S., Niehaus, D. J., and Stein, D. J. (2001). The role of genes and family in trauma exposure and posttraumatic stress disorder. *Mol. Psychiatry* 6, 360–362. doi: 10.1038/sj.mp.4000867

Shen, H. W., Hagino, Y., Kobayashi, H., Shinohara-Tanaka, K., Ikeda, K., Yamamoto, H., et al. (2004). Regional differences in extracellular dopamine and serotonin assessed by in vivo microdialysis in mice lacking dopamine and/or serotonin transporters. *Neuropsychopharmacology* 29, 1790–1799. doi: 10.1038/sj.npp.1300476

Shephard, R. A., and Broadhurst, P. L. (1982). Hyponeophagia and arousal in rats: effects of diazepam, 5-methoxy-N,N-dimethyltryptamine, d-amphetamine and food deprivation. *Psychopharmacology (Berl.)* 78, 368–372. doi: 10.1007/BF00433744

Shephard, R. A., Buxton, D. A., and Broadhurst, P. L. (1982). Drug interactions do not support reduction in serotonin turnover as the mechanism of action of benzodiazepines. *Neuropharmacology* 21, 1027–1032. doi: 10.1016/0028-3908(82)90117-4

Shifman, S., Bhomra, A., Smiley, S., Wray, N. R., James, M. R., Martin, N. G., et al. (2008). A whole genome association study of neuroticism using DNA pooling. *Mol. Psychiatry* 13, 302–312. doi: 10.1038/sj.mp.4002048

Sibille, E., Pavlides, C., Benke, D., and Toth, M. (2000). Genetic inactivation of the Serotonin(1A) receptor in mice results in downregulation of major GABA(A) receptor alpha subunits, reduction of GABA(A) receptor binding, and benzodiazepine-resistant anxiety. *J. Neurosci.* 20, 2758–2765.

Smits, B. M., Mudde, J. B., van de Belt, J., Verheul, M., Olivier, J., Homberg, J., et al. (2006). Generation of gene knockouts and mutant models in the laboratory rat by ENU-driven target-selected mutagenesis. *Pharmacogenet. Genomics* 16, 159–169.

Smoller, J. W., Acierno, J. S. Jr., Rosenbaum, J. F., Biederman, J., Pollack, M. H., Meminger, S., et al. (2001a).

Targeted genome screen of panic disorder and anxiety disorder proneness using homology to murine QTL regions. *Am. J. Med. Genet.* 105, 195–206. doi: 10.1002/ajmg.1209

Smoller, J. W., Rosenbaum, J. F., Biederman, J., Susswein, L. S., Kennedy, J., Kagan, J., et al. (2001b). Genetic association analysis of behavioral inhibition using candidate loci from mouse models. *Am. J. Med. Genet.* 105, 226–235. doi: 10.1002/ajmg.1328

Smoller, J. W., Block, S. R., and Young, M. M. (2009). Genetics of anxiety disorders: the complex road from DSM to DNA. *Depress. Anxiety* 26, 965–975. doi: 10.1002/da.20623

Smoller, J. W., Gardner-Schuster, E., and Covino, J. (2008a). The genetic basis of panic and phobic anxiety disorders. *Am. J. Med. Genet. C Semin. Med. Genet.* 148C, 118–126. doi: 10.1002/ajmg.c.30174

Smoller, J. W., Paulus, M. P., Fagerness, J. A., Purcell, S., Yamaki, L. H., Hirshfeld-Becker, D., et al. (2008b). Influence of RGS2 on anxiety-related temperament, personality, and brain function. *Arch. Gen. Psychiatry* 65, 298–308. doi: 10.1001/archgenpsychiatry.2007.48

Sokolowska, E., and Hovatta, E. (2013). Anxiety genetics: findings from cross-species genome-wide approaches. *Biol. Mood Anxiety Disord.* 3, 9. doi: 10.1186/2045-5380-3-9

Sora, I., Hall, F. S., Andrews, A. M., Itokawa, M., Li, X. F., Wei, H. B., et al. (2001). Molecular mechanisms of cocaine reward: combined dopamine and serotonin transporter knockouts eliminate cocaine place preference. *Proc. Natl. Acad. Sci. U.S.A.* 98, 5300–5305. doi: 10.1073/pnas.091039298

Sora, I., Wichems, C., Takahashi, N., Li, X. F., Zeng, Z., Revay, R., et al. (1998). Cocaine reward models: conditioned place preference can be established in dopamine- and in serotonin-transporter knockout mice. *Proc. Natl. Acad. Sci. U.S.A.* 95, 7699–7704. doi: 10.1073/pnas.95.13.7699

Stein, D. J., Ahokas, A. A., and de Bodinat, C. (2008). Efficacy of agomelatine in generalized anxiety disorder: a randomized, double-blind, placebo-controlled study. *J. Clin. Psychopharmacol.* 28, 561–566. doi: 10.1097/JCP.0b013e318184ff5b

Stein, L., Belluzzi, J. D., and Wise, C. D. (1977). Benzodiazepines: behavioral and neurochemical mechanisms. *Am. J. Psychiatry* 134, 665–669.

Stein, M. B., Campbell-Sills, L., and Gelernter, J. (2009). Genetic variation in 5HTTLPR is associated with emotional resilience. *Am. J. Med. Genet. B Neuropsychiatr. Genet.* 150B, 900–906. doi: 10.1002/ajmg.b.30916

Steiner, J. A., Carneiro, A. M., and Blakely, R. D. (2008). Going with the flow: trafficking-dependent and -independent regulation of serotonin transport. *Traffic* 9, 1393–1402. doi: 10.1111/j.1600-0854.2008.00757.x

Stollstorff, M., Bean, S. E., Anderson, L. M., Devaney, J. M., and Vaidya, C. J. (2013). Rationality and emotionality: serotonin transporter genotype influences reasoning bias. *Soc. Cogn. Affect. Neurosci.* 8, 404–409. doi: 10.1093/scan/nss011

Sun, Y. V. (2012). Integration of biological networks and pathways with genetic association studies. *Hum. Genet.* 131, 1677–1686. doi: 10.1007/s00439-012-1198-7

Taliani, S., Da Settimo, F., Da Pozzo, E., Chelli, B., and Martini, C. (2009). Translocator protein ligands as promising therapeutic tools for anxiety disorders. *Curr. Med. Chem.* 16, 3359–3380. doi: 10.2174/092986709789057653

Tan, K. R., Brown, M., Labouebe, G., Yvon, C., Creton, C., Fritschy, J. M., et al. (2010). Neural bases for addictive properties of benzodiazepines. *Nature* 463, 769–774. doi: 10.1038/nature08758

Tan, K. R., Rudolph, U., and Luscher, C. (2011). Hooked on benzodiazepines: GABAA receptor subtypes and addiction. *Trends Neurosci.* 34, 188–197. doi: 10.1016/j.tins.2011.01.004

Thiebot, M. H. (1986). Are serotonergic neurons involved in the control of anxiety and in the anxiolytic activity of benzodiazepines? *Pharmacol. Biochem. Behav.* 24, 1471–1477. doi: 10.1016/0091-3057(86)90214-5

Thiebot, M. H., Soubrie, P., Hamon, M., and Simon, P. (1984). Evidence against the involvement of serotonergic neurons in the anti-punishment activity of diazepam in the rat. *Psychopharmacology (Berl.)* 82, 355–359. doi: 10.1007/BF00427685

Thoeringer, C. K., Binder, E. B., Salyakina, D., Erhardt, A., Ising, M., Unschuld, P. G., et al. (2007). Association of a Met88Val diazepam binding inhibitor (DBI) gene polymorphism and anxiety disorders with panic attacks. *J. Psychiatr. Res.* 41, 579–584. doi: 10.1016/j.jpsychires.2006.06.001

Thoeringer, C. K., Ripke, S., Unschuld, P. G., Lucae, S., Ising, M., Bettecken, T., et al. (2009). The GABA transporter 1 (SLC6A1): a novel candidate gene for anxiety disorders. *J. Neural. Transm.* 116, 649–657. doi: 10.1007/s00702-008-0075-y

Thompson, B. J., Jessen, T., Henry, L. K., Field, J. R., Gamble, K. L., Gresch, P. J., et al. (2011). Transgenic elimination of high-affinity antidepressant and cocaine sensitivity in the presynaptic serotonin transporter. *Proc. Natl. Acad. Sci. U.S.A.* 108, 3785–3790. doi: 10.1073/pnas.1011920108

Thorgeirsson, T. E., Oskarsson, H., Desnica, N., Kostic, J. P., Steffansson, J. G., Kolbeinsson, H., et al. (2003). Anxiety with panic disorder linked to chromosome 9q in Iceland. *Am. J. Hum. Genet.* 72, 1221–1230.

Tjurmina, O. A., Armando, I., Saavedra, J. M., Goldstein, D. S., and Murphy, D. L. (2002). Exaggerated adrenomedullary response to immobilization in mice with targeted disruption of the serotonin transporter gene. *Endocrinology* 143, 4520–4526. doi: 10.1210/en.2002-220416

Trulson, M. E., Preussler, D. W., Howell, G. A., and Frederickson, C. J. (1982). Raphe unit activity in freely moving cats: effects of benzodiazepines. *Neuropharmacology* 21, 1045–1050. doi: 10.1016/0028-3908(82)90120-4

Tye, K. M., and Deisseroth, K. (2012). Optogenetic investigation of neural circuits underlying brain disease in animal models. *Nat. Rev. Neurosci.* 13, 251–266. doi: 10.1038/nrn3171

van Bogaert, M. J., Oosting, R., Toth, M., Groenink, L., van Oorschot, R., and Olivier, B. (2006). Effects of genetic background and null mutation of 5-HT1A receptors on basal and stress-induced body temperature: modulation by serotonergic and GABAA-ergic drugs. *Eur. J. Pharmacol.* 550, 84–90. doi: 10.1016/j.ejphar.2006.08.058

Van den Hove, D., Jakob, S. B., Schraut, K. G., Kenis, G., Schmitt, A., Kneitz, S., et al. (2011). Differential effects of prenatal stress in 5-Htt deficient mice: towards molecular mechanisms of gene × environment interactions. *PLoS ONE* 6:e22715. doi: 10.1371/journal.pone.0022715

van Gestel, S., Forsgren, T., Claes, S., Del-Favero, J., Van Duijn, C. M., Sluijs, S., et al. (2002). Epistatic effect of genes from the dopamine and serotonin systems on the temperament traits of novelty seeking and harm avoidance. *Mol. Psychiatry* 7, 448–450. doi: 10.1038/sj.mp.4001005

Varga, V., Szekely, A. D., Csillag, A., Sharp, T., and Hajos, M. (2001). Evidence for a role of GABA interneurones in the cortical modulation of midbrain 5-hydroxytryptamine neurones. *Neuroscience* 106, 783–792. doi: 10.1016/S0306-4522(01)00294-9

Vinkers, C. H., Klanker, M., Groenink, L., Korte, S. M., Cook, J. M., Van Linn, M. L., et al. (2009). Dissociating anxiolytic and sedative effects of GABAAergic drugs using temperature and locomotor responses to acute stress. *Psychopharmacology (Berl.)* 204, 299–311. doi: 10.1007/s00213-009-1460-4

Vinkers, C. H., Mirza, N. R., Olivier, B., and Kahn, R. S. (2010a). The inhibitory GABA system as a therapeutic target for cognitive symptoms in schizophrenia: investigational agents in the pipeline. *Expert Opin. Investig. Drugs* 19, 1217–1233. doi: 10.1517/13543784.2010.513382

Vinkers, C. H., van Oorschot, R., Korte, S. M., Olivier, B., and Groenink, L. (2010b). 5-HT1A receptor blockade reverses GABA(A) receptor alpha3 subunit-mediated anxiolytic effects on stress-induced hyperthermia. *Psychopharmacology (Berl.)* 211, 123–130. doi: 10.1007/s00213-010-1895-7

Vinkers, C. H., van Oorschot, R., Nielsen, E. O., Cook, J. H., Hansen, H. H., Groenink, L., et al. (2012). GABA(A) receptor α subunits differentially contribute to diazepam tolerance after chronic treatment. *PLoS ONE* 7:e43054. doi: 10.1371/journal.pone.0043054

Vogel, J. R., Beer, B., and Clody, D. E. (1971). A simple and reliable conflict procedure for testing anti-anxiety agents. *Psychopharmacologia* 21, 1–7. doi: 10.1007/BF00403989

Walitza, S., Wendland, J. R., Gruenblatt, E., Warnke, A., Sontag, T. A., Tucha, O., et al. (2010). Genetics of early-onset obsessive-compulsive disorder. *Eur. Child Adolesc. Psychiatry* 19, 227–235. doi: 10.1007/s00787-010-0087-7

Wang, Z., Valdes, J., Noyes, R., Zoega, T., and Crowe, R. R. (1998). Possible association of a cholecystokinin promotor polymorphism (CCK-36CT) with panic disorder. *Am. J. Med. Genet.* 81, 228–234. doi: 10.1002/(SICI)1096-8628(19980508)81:3<228::AID-AJMG5>3.0.CO;2-S

Waters, A. M., Mogg, K., Bradley, B. P., and Pine, D. S. (2008). Attentional bias for emotional faces in children with generalized anxiety disorder. *J. Am. Acad. Child Adolesc. Psychiatry* 47, 435–442. doi: 10.1097/CHI.0b013e3181642992

Weissman, M. M., Fyer, A. J., Haghighi, F., Heiman, G., Deng, Z., Hen, R., et al. (2000). Potential panic disorder syndrome: clinical and genetic linkage evidence. *Am. J. Med. Genet.* 96,

24–35. doi: 10.1002/(SICI)1096-8628(20000207)96:1<24::AID-AJMG7>3.0.CO;2-E

Weisstaub, N. V., Zhou, M., Lira, A., Lambe, E., Gonzalez-Maeso, J., Hornung, J. P., et al. (2006). Cortical 5-HT2A receptor signaling modulates anxiety-like behaviors in mice. *Science* 313, 536–540. doi: 10.1126/science.1123432

Wellman, C. L., Izquierdo, A., Garrett, J. E., Martin, K. P., Carroll, J., Millstein, R., et al. (2007). Impaired stress-coping and fear extinction and abnormal corticolimbic morphology in serotonin transporter knock-out mice. *J. Neurosci.* 27, 684–691. doi: 10.1523/JNEUROSCI.4595-06.2007

Wittchen, H. U. (2011). The size and burden of mental disorders and other disorders of the brain in Europe 2010. *Eur Neuropsychopharmacol.* 21, 655–679. doi: 10.1016/j.euroneuro.2011.07.018

Woo, J. M., Yoon, K. S., Choi, Y. H., Oh, K. S., Lee, Y. S., and Yu, B. H. (2004). The association between panic disorder and the L/L genotype of catechol-*O*-methyltransferase. *J. Psychiatr. Res.* 38, 365–370. doi: 10.1016/j.jpsychires.2004.01.001

Wright, I. K., Upton, N., and Marsden, C. A. (1992). Effect of established and putative anxiolytics on extracellular 5-HT and 5-HIAA in the ventral hippocampus of rats during behaviour on the elevated X-maze. *Psychopharmacology (Berl.)* 109, 338–346. doi: 10.1007/BF02245882

Zanettini, C., Carola, V., Lo Lacono, L., Moles. A., Gross, C., and D'Amato, F. R. (2010). Postnatal handling reverses social anxiety in serotonin receptor 1A knockout mice. *Genes Brain Behav.* 9, 26–32. doi: 10.1111/j.1601-183X.2009.00531.x

Zhang, G., Asgeirsdottir, H. N., Cohen, S. J., Munchow, A. H., Barrera, M. P., and Stackman, R. W. Jr. (2013). Stimulation of serotonin 2A receptors facilitates consolidation and extinction of fear memory in C57BL/6J mice. *Neuropharmacology* 64, 403–413. doi: 10.1016/j.neuropharm.2012.06.007

Conflict of Interest Statement: The authors declare that the research was conducted in the absence of any commercial or financial relationships that could be construed as a potential conflict of interest.

5

Reduced brain somatostatin in mood disorders: a common pathophysiological substrate and drug target

Li-Chun Lin and Etienne Sibille*

Department of Psychiatry, Center for Neuroscience, University of Pittsburgh, Pittsburgh, PA, USA

Edited by:
Thibault Renoir, Florey Institute of Neuroscience and Mental Health, Australia

Reviewed by:
Jean-Philippe Guilloux, Université Paris Sud, France
Jacques Epelbaum, Université Paris Descartes, France
Elif Engin, McLean Hospital/Harvard Medical School, USA

****Correspondence:***
Etienne Sibille, Department of Psychiatry, Center for Neuroscience, University of Pittsburgh, Bridgeside Point II, 450 Technology Drive, Suite 231, Pittsburgh, PA 15219, USA
e-mail: sibilleel@upmc.edu

Our knowledge of the pathophysiology of affect dysregulation has progressively increased, but the pharmacological treatments remain inadequate. Here, we summarize the current literature on deficits in somatostatin, an inhibitory modulatory neuropeptide, in major depression and other neurological disorders that also include mood disturbances. We focus on direct evidence in the human postmortem brain, and review rodent genetic and pharmacological studies probing the role of the somatostatin system in relation to mood. We also briefly go over pharmacological developments targeting the somatostatin system in peripheral organs and discuss the challenges of targeting the brain somatostatin system. Finally, the fact that somatostatin deficits are frequently observed across neurological disorders suggests a selective cellular vulnerability of somatostatin-expressing neurons. Potential cell intrinsic factors mediating those changes are discussed, including nitric oxide induced oxidative stress, mitochondrial dysfunction, high inflammatory response, high demand for neurotrophic environment, and overall aging processes. Together, based on the co-localization of somatostatin with gamma-aminobutyric acid (GABA), its presence in dendritic-targeting GABA neuron subtypes, and its temporal-specific function, we discuss the possibility that deficits in somatostatin play a central role in cortical local inhibitory circuit deficits leading to abnormal corticolimbic network activity and clinical mood symptoms across neurological disorders.

Keywords: somatostatin, somatostatin-expressing interneurons, SST, SOM, SRIF, depression, mood disorders, GABA inhibition

INTRODUCTION

Mood disturbances are commonly observed in many neurological disorders. The chronic, recurrent and long duration of mood disturbances not only place an enormous emotional and financial burden on patients, but also on their families and society. Nearly 10% of all primary care office visits are depression-related (Stafford et al., 2000), but only 30% of patients with mood disturbances achieve remission with initial treatment (Trivedi et al., 2006). Somatostatin is a peptide expressed in multiple organs. In the brain, somatostatin (also known as somatotrophin release inhibiting factor and often abbreviated as SST, SRIF, or SOM) acts as a modulatory and inhibitory neuropeptide that is co-localized with gamma-aminobutyric acid (GABA), and that is involved in regulating multiple aspects of physiological and behavioral stress responses, including inhibition of hypothalamic hormone release, amygdala central nucleus output, and cortical local circuit integration of sensory input. Research advances over the past three decades suggest a critical role for somatostatin in the pathophysiology of mood disorders, and potential new therapeutic strategies. Several recent reviews have summarized the role of the somatostatin system, including in receptor subtypes (Patel, 1999; Csaba and Dournaud, 2001), pharmacological developments (Neggers and van der Lely, 2009), and during normal and pathological aging (Patel, 1999; Viollet et al., 2008; Martel et al., 2012).

This article highlights current findings on the functional roles of somatostatin in local neuronal circuits, and reviews somatostatin deficits across neurological disorders, including neuropsychiatric disorders [e.g., major depressive disorder (MDD), bipolar disorder, schizophrenia], and neurodegenerative disorders (e.g., Parkinson's, Alzheimer's, and Huntington's diseases; **Table 1**). This raises interesting questions, including first; whether the somatostatin deficits observed in neurological disorders represent common, distinct, or partly overlapping mechanisms of symptoms across disorders and, second, what may be the causes and biological mechanisms underlying the selective neuronal vulnerability of somatostatin-expressing neurons. In addition, we review somatostatin findings associated with affect regulation at the genetic, cellular, and pharmacological levels in animal studies. So far, these findings suggest that somatostatin deficits across different brain systems and diseases may play a central role in the affective symptom dimension rather than non-specific signals in neurological disorders (**Figure 1**). As somatostatin itself is not an ideal drug target, including for antidepressant effect, we suggest that further studies characterizing the intrinsic properties and biological vulnerabilities of somatostatin-expressing neurons, may identify novel targets with implications for understanding the function of local cell circuits and brain regions underlying affective symptoms across several neurological disorders.

Table 1 | Low somatostatin in human neurological disorders.

Neurological disorders	Brain region	Pathological findings	Reference
Major depressive disorder	CSF	Decreased	Agren and Lundqvist (1984), Kling et al. (1993), Molchan et al. (1993)
	Dorsolateral prefrontal cortex	Decreased (RNA expression)	Sibille et al. (2011)
	Anterior cingulate cortex	Decreased (RNA expression)	Tripp et al. (2011), Tripp et al. (2012)
	Amygdala	Decreased (RNA and protein expression)	Guilloux et al. (2012)
Schizophrenia	CSF	Decreased	Bissette et al. (1986), Reinikainen et al. (1990)
	Dorsolateral prefrontal cortex	Decreased (RNA expression)	Morris et al. (2008), Guillozet-Bongaarts et al. (2013)
	Hippocampus	Decreased (neuron number and density)	Konradi et al. (2011a)
	Caudal entorhinal cortex	Decreased (neuron number and density)	Wang et al. (2011)
	Parasubiculum	Decreased (neuron number and density)	Wang et al. (2011)
Bipolar disorder	Caudal entorhinal cortex	Decreased (neuron density)	Wang et al. (2011)
	Parasubiculum	Decreased (neuron density)	Wang et al. (2011)
	Hippocampus	Decreased (neuron number and RNA expression)	Konradi et al. (2011b)
	Dorsolateral prefrontal cortex	Decreased (RNA expression; trend level)	Sibille et al. (2011)
Alzheimer's disease	CSF	Decreased	Bissette et al. (1986); Tamminga et al. (1987)
	Temporal cortex	Decreased (immune-reactivity)	Rossor et al. (1980); Candy et al. (1985)
	Frontal cortex	Decreased (immune-reactivity)	Davies and Terry (1981); Candy et al. (1985)
	Hippocampus	Decreased (gene expression per cell)	Dournaud et al. (1994)
	Parahippocampal cortex	Decreased (neuronal density)	Dournaud et al. (1994)
Parkinson's disease	CSF	Decreased	Dupont et al. (1982)
	Frontal cortex	Decreased (radioimmune-reactivity)	Epelbaum et al. (1988)
Others	Temporal cortex	Decreased (immune-reactivity)	Beal et al. (1986)

LOW SOMATOSTATIN IN NEUROPSYCHIATRIC AND NEURODEGENERATIVE DISORDERS

MAJOR DEPRESSIVE DISORDER

Patients with major depressive disorder (MDD) show decreased somatostatin levels in the cerebrospinal fluid (CSF; Agren and Lundqvist, 1984; Molchan et al., 1991; Kling et al., 1993), and transiently decreased CSF somatostatin which normalize with recovery in MDD (Rubinow et al., 1985; Post et al., 1988). Evidence for low levels of CSF somatostatin was found to correlate significantly with elevated urinary cortisol in MDD patients (Molchan et al., 1993). This is consistent with the altered hypothalamic-pituitary-adrenal (HPA) axis function described in some depressed patients (Holsboer, 2000). The route and characterization, however, from CSF somatostatin to MDD pathophysiology is not direct, potentially due to a paucity of information on factors regulating CSF somatostatin, and to inconclusive somatostatin/HPA axis studies in MDD patients. Hence, despite these early findings, interest in somatostatin in mood disorders has declined over time.

Human post-mortem studies from our group have described region-specific somatostatin deficits in MDD patients, including a down-regulation of *somatostatin* gene expression in the dorsolateral prefrontal cortex (dlPFC), subgenual anterior cingulate cortex (sgACC), and amygdala (Sibille et al., 2011; Tripp et al., 2011, 2012; Guilloux et al., 2012). In addition, two peptides co-localized with somatostatin, neuropeptide Y and cortistatin, are both significantly down-regulated in MDD patients (Tripp et al., 2011, 2012).These three neuropeptides (somatostatin, neuropeptide Y, and cortistatin) are markers of GABAergic neurons that specifically target the dendritic compartment of pyramidal cells (de Lecea et al., 1997; Viollet et al., 2008), and that are essential in gating incoming sensory information (**Figure 1**). Other types of GABAergic cell markers, such as parvalbumin and cholecystokinin, are mostly not affected by MDD (although see Tripp et al., 2012). Interestingly, these somatostatin deficits were systematically more robust in female subjects across cohorts and regions (Sibille et al., 2011; Tripp et al., 2011, 2012; Guilloux et al., 2012), consistent with the female heightened vulnerability to develop MDD, and suggesting that low somatostatin may represent a molecular correlate of sexual dimorphism in vulnerability to affect dysregulation. Notably, these findings are also consistent with earlier postmortem studies showing reduced calbindin-positive cell numbers in MDD (Rajkowska et al., 2007; Maciag et al.,

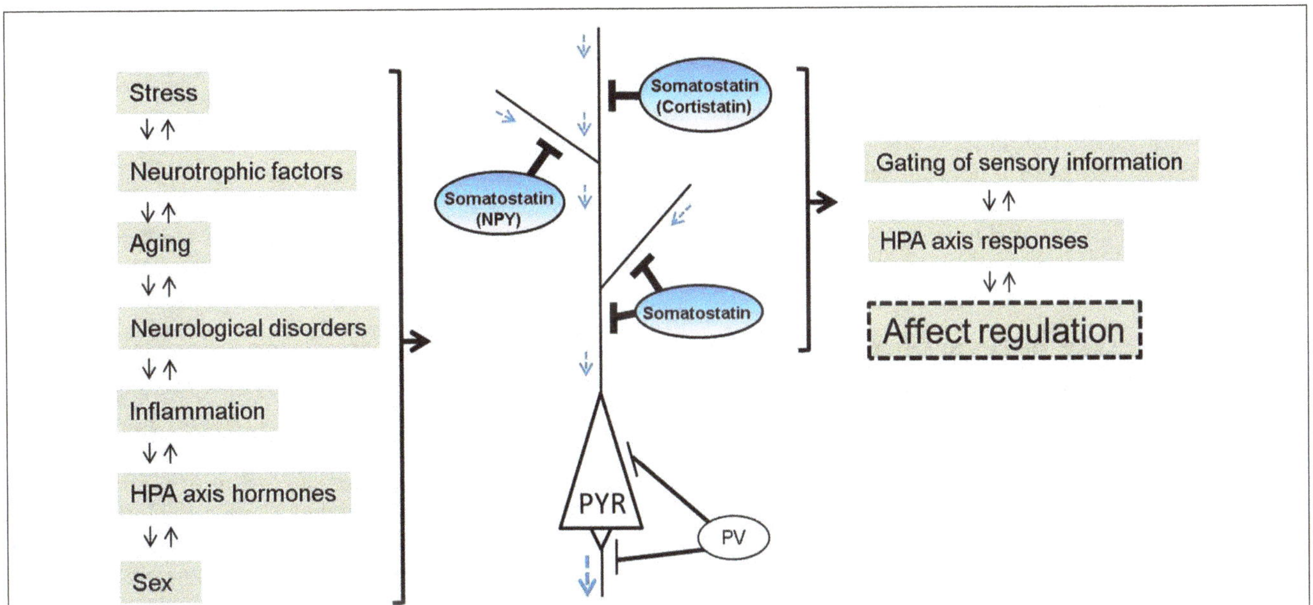

FIGURE 1 | Schematic of somatostatin signaling, pathological regulators and biological functions relevant to affect regulation. Somatostatin pathway activity is responsive to (left panel), and regulates (right panel), several biological events, and molecular and cellular properties that have been linked to mood disturbances. Somatostatin and somatostatin-expressing interneurons are key conduits for regulating incoming information and pyramidal cell function. In contrast, other GABA neurons subtypes targeting the perisomatic pyramidal cell compartment are mostly not affected in major depression. NPY, neuropeptide Y; PYR, pyramidal neuron; PV, parvalbumin.

2010), as somatostatin is mostly expressed in a subgroup of calbindin-positive cells (reviewed in Viollet et al., 2008). Converging evidence from down-regulation of *somatostatin* co-localized GABA markers in MDD across multiple human post-mortem studies suggests that this particular GABA subpopulation in the forebrain is selectively vulnerable, among other subtypes of GABA neurons. Furthermore, these local cell circuit-based findings introduce a new role for somatostatin in depression, which is distinct from its previously investigated role in the regulation of the HPA axis (Rubinow et al., 1983; Molchan et al., 1993; Weckbecker et al. 2003).

OTHER NEUROPSYCHIATRIC DISORDERS

Schizophrenia is a neuropsychiatric disorder characterized by positive (e.g., hallucination), negative symptoms (e.g., emotional blunting, apathy) and cognitive symptoms. Somatostatin deficits in schizophrenia are demonstrated by a reduction of CSF somatostatin (Bissette et al., 1986; Reinikainen et al., 1990), decreased *somatostatin* gene expression in the dlPFC (Morris et al., 2008; Guillozet-Bongaarts et al., 2013), and decreased number and density of somatostatin-expressing neurons in the hippocampus (Konradi et al., 2011a), caudal entorhinal cortex and parasubiculum (Wang et al., 2011). Changes in somatostatin are also identified in bipolar disorder, which is clinically characterized by fluctuating mood. Studies in subjects with bipolar disorder indicate decreases in somatostatin cellular density in the caudal entorhinal cortex and parasubiculum (Wang et al., 2011), number of somatostatin-expressing neurons in the hippocampus (Konradi et al., 2011b), *somatostatin* gene expression in the dlPFC (trend level; Sibille et al., 2011) and hippocampus (Konradi et al., 2011b). In addition, patients with bipolar disorder show elevated CSF somatostatin during manic states (Sharma et al., 1995).

NEURODEGENERATIVE DISORDERS

Alzheimer's disease is a neurodegenerative disease with neuropsychiatric symptoms (Bungener et al., 1996). Decreased CSF somatostatin (Bissette et al., 1986; Tamminga et al., 1987) and decreased somatostatin immune-reactivity across cortical and subcortical regions is reported in subjects with Alzheimer's disease, including temporal cortex, frontal cortex, and hippocampus (Davies et al., 1980; Rossor et al., 1980; Davies and Terry, 1981; Candy et al., 1985; Dournaud et al., 1994). Depression is a common comorbid symptom in Parkinson's disease and predicts greater disability at any assessment point (Aarsland et al., 1999). Decreased CSF somatostatin, decreased somatostatin immunoreactivity, and binding sites are also observed in the temporal cortex and frontal cortex of patients with Parkinson's disease (Beal et al., 1986; Epelbaum et al., 1988). Notably, reduced CSF somatostatin in Parkinson's disease appears to be irreversibly present at the onset of symptoms (Dupont et al., 1982).

REDUCED SOMATOSTATIN AND LOW MOOD?

The evidence outlined in this review provides only a glimpse of the potential full range of somatostatin deficits across neurological disorders, as multiple other brain regions and disease categories await further characterization (**Table 1**). Taken together, the cumulative evidence demonstrates that somatostatin deficits are common neurochemical and molecular features in individuals with neurological disorders, regardless of their categorical diagnosis. While somatostatin studies of cell number and gene expression in human postmortem brains suggest a specific alteration of somatostatin-positive neurons across neurological disorders, it is possible that changes and dys-synchronization of additional components of local neuronal circuits contribute to a common symptom dimension, which we speculate includes low affect and mood dysregulation. Hence, this review is not comprehensive, but rather, highlights the recent findings in brain somatostatin signaling and the potential role of somatostatin deficits in affect dysregulation for integrating categorical models of mood symptoms into a dimensional model across neurological disorders.

SOMATOSTATIN: GENES, NEURONS AND PHARMACOLOGY

SOMATOSTATIN SIGNALING

Somatostatin is a modulatory neuropeptide that synergizes with GABA-mediated inhibition, and that specifically targets the distal dendritic compartment of pyramidal neurons in cortical local circuits (Kawaguchi and Kubota, 1997; Gentet et al., 2012). Somatostatin inhibits release of numerous hormones from the hypothalamus, including corticotrophin releasing hormone (CRH; Wang et al., 1987; Patel, 1999). The somatostatin gene product is composed of 14 or 28 amino-acid residues. Both forms of somatostatin, somatostatin-14 and somatostatin-28, are generated by tissue-specific post-translational processing of the 116 amino-acid pre-pro-somatostatin peptide (Warren and Shields, 1984; Tostivint et al., 2008). Somatostatin-14 is predominantly produced in the central nervous system (CNS) but also in many peripheral organs (Epelbaum, 1986). Somatostatin-28 is mainly synthesized along the gastrointestinal tract (Fitz-Patrick and Patel, 1981). The 5′-upstream sequence of the *somatostatin* gene contains cyclic-AMP response element (CRE; Montminy et al., 1986), making its expression activity-dependent. Thus, *somatostatin* expression is preferentially altered by various stressors, such as seizures (Vezzani and Hoyer, 1999; Tallent and Qiu, 2008) and electrical foot shock (Ponomarev et al., 2010). Moreover, mice with conditional homozygous and constitutive heterozygous brain-derived neurotrophic factor (*Bdnf*) knockout or disruption of exon IV-expressing *Bdnf* transcripts show decreased *somatostatin* gene expression (Glorioso et al., 2006; Martinowich et al., 2011; Guilloux et al., 2012), demonstrating that *somatostatin* expression depends on *Bdnf* signaling. However, the molecular mechanisms by which this neurotrophic factor controls somatostatin and somatostatin-expressing neurons are still unknown.

Somatostatin, cortistatin and their receptors are closely intertwined systems (de Lecea et al., 1996, 1997; reviewed in Spier and de Lecea, 2000; de Lecea, 2008). Sharing high structural homology with somatostatin, cortistatin binds to all somatostatin receptor subtypes and is known to be regulated by exon IV-expressing *Bdnf* transcripts (Martinowich et al., 2011). However, distinct from somatostatin, cortistatin binds to additional receptors (e.g., growth hormone secretagogue receptor 1a and Mas-related gene X2 receptor) (Robas et al., 2003; Siehler et al., 2008) and has different physiological properties (e.g., activation of cation selective currents not responsive to somatostatin; Spier and de Lecea, 2000), suggesting that somatostatin and cortistatin may both contribute to affect regulation in an integrated, yet differential mode. The intracellular pathway of somatostatin signaling coupled to all five somatostatin receptors subtypes (Sst_{1-5}) is through the activation of inhibitory G protein (Gi) and the following inhibition of adenylyl cyclase, leading to reduction of cAMP levels, activation of phosphotyrosine phosphatases, and modulation of mitogen-activated protein kinases and phospholipase C (Koch and Schonbrunn, 1984; Koch et al., 1988).

Sst_{1-5} present different patterns of coexpression in the brain (Kluxen et al., 1992; Moller et al., 2003; reviewed in Martel et al., 2012). Sst1 is found in retina, basal ganglia and hypothalamus, Sst2 is highly abundant in several telencephalic structures (neocortex, hippocampus, and amygdala), Sst3 immunoreactivity has only been described in neuronal cilia (Schulz et al., 2000), Sst4 is expressed in olfactory bulb, cerebral cortex and CA1 region of the hippocampus (Schreff et al., 2000), and expression of Sst5 has been detected in cerebral cortex, hippocampus, amygdala, preoptic area, and hypothalamus (Stroh et al., 1999; Strowski et al., 2003; Olias et al., 2004). Interestingly, when co-expressed in the same cells, Sst5 influences Sst2 internalization and trafficking and modulates cellular desensitization to the effects of somatostatin-14 (Sharif et al., 2007), suggesting that the precise actions of somatostatin depend on the specific interaction of the Sst_{1-5} receptors expressed locally in each brain region.

GENETIC POLYMORPHISMS IN THE SOMATOSTATIN SYSTEM

The relatively high degree of amino acid conservation across species indicates that somatostatin-related genes have been highly constrained during evolution (Patel, 1999; Olias et al., 2004). Accordingly, there are currently very few reports linking *somatostatin* gene polymorphisms with neurological disorders. A primate-specific single nucleotide polymorphism (SNP) in the human *somatostatin* gene [C/T polymorphism (rs4988514)] is associated with increased risk in Alzheimer's disease progression and additive effect with the APOE epsilon4 allele (Vepsalainen et al., 2007; Xue et al., 2009), although this was not confirmed in larger genome-wide association studies (GWAS) (Hollingworth et al., 2011; Guerreiro et al., 2013). Leu48Met and Pro335Leu SNPs in the *SST5* gene are of potential significance to patients with bipolar disorder (Nyegaard et al., 2002), but no associations of SST5 SNPs are found in patients with autism (Lauritsen et al., 2003). The paucity of associations with somatostatin gene variants is surprising and may reflect either strong negative selection against genetic variations in this gene, or alternatively, dilution of signal due to heterogeneity of DSM-IV-based cohorts in genetic association studies. So, dimensional phenotypes, as defined by clusters of mood symptoms, which are closer to gene functions may have implications for future genetic studies of somatostatin and other genes.

SOMATOSTATIN-EXPRESSING NEURONS: DIVERSITY AND ROLES

Gamma-aminobutyric acid (GABA) neurons are a diverse group of inhibitory cells which co-release neuropeptides in order to support a fine-tuning of neuronal signaling and architecture. The local inhibitory circuits provide spatiotemporal control of information processing through at least 20 subtypes of cortical GABA neurons, which are based on their expression of different calcium binding proteins and neuropeptides, localization, targeting, and differential electrophysiological properties. Recent detailed reviews on GABA neuron subpopulations have been published (Csaba and

Dournaud, 2001; Di Cristo et al., 2004; Markram et al., 2004; Tan et al., 2008; Fishell and Rudy, 2011; Gentet et al., 2012; DeFelipe et al., 2013; Le Magueresse and Monyer, 2013). Approximately 20–30% of GABA neurons in the mouse somatosensory cortex express somatostatin (Lee et al., 2010; Rudy et al., 2011), and 40–50% of GABA neurons contain parvalbumin without overlapping with somatostatin in the frontal cortex, primary somatosensory cortex and visual cortex of mouse (Gonchar et al., 2007; Xu et al., 2010) and the visual cortex of rat (Gonchar and Burkhalter, 1997).

Recent reports focusing on the patterns of cortical neuronal connectivity show that somatostatin-expressing interneurons mediate the firing of pyramidal neurons with a fine level of specificity among cortical layers. Integrating optogenetic and electrophysiology approaches, mouse somatostatin-expressing interneurons in layer 2/3 of the somatosensory cortex provide a tonic inhibition to the distal dendrites of excitatory pyramidal neurons by sharpening selectivity during periods of quiet wakefulness, which may contribute to synchronized firing in cortical networks and sensorimotor integration (Gentet et al., 2012). Interestingly, in mouse somatosensory cortex, somatostatin-expressing interneurons show a spatially precise connectivity with pyramidal neurons through direct targeting in layers 2/3 or indirectly through inhibition of local parvalbumin interneurons in layer 4 (Xu et al., 2013). Moreover, in layers 2/3 of the mouse prefrontal cortex, somatostatin-expressing interneurons compartmentalizes inhibitions of calcium signaling to spine heads, not shafts, suggesting that dendrite-targeting inhibition through somatostatin-expressing interneurons may contribute to downstream cellular processes such as synaptic plasticity (Chiu et al., 2013). In mouse visual cortex, somatostatin-expressing interneurons are found to mediate response levels of specific subsets of pyramidal neurons whereas parvalbumin-expressing neurons alter response gain (Wilson et al., 2012). Parvalbumin-expressing neurons receive excitatory input from the thalamus and make strong synapses on the soma and axons of their target cells (Kawaguchi and Kubota, 1997) to control spike timing of the output neurons. In contrast, somatostatin-expressing neurons mostly do not receive input from thalamus (Beierlein et al., 2003; Cruikshank et al., 2010) and are instead activated through feed-forward mechanisms by activated pyramidal neurons. Somatostatin-expressing interneurons preferentially target distal dendrites of pyramidal neurons in layer 2/3 to modulate the processing of incoming sensory information before it is integrated at the soma level (Di Cristo et al., 2004; Markram et al., 2004; Tan et al., 2008; Murayama et al., 2009; Xu et al., 2013). Hence, the distinct GABAergic and prototypical inhibitory populations, expressing either parvalbumin or somatostatin, shape the spatiotemporal control of multiple post-synaptic potentials in cortical local circuits, and provide a framework to investigate the role of inhibitory circuits in physiology and pathology.

GENETIC APPROACHES TO INVESTIGATE THE SOMATOSTATIN SYSTEM

Mice mutant for somatostatin were created by deleting the coding region of the pre-pro-somatostatin (the last ten codons of the first exon; Zeyda et al., 2001). Somatostatin knockout (KO; Sst^{KO}) mice show intact motor coordination and motor learning, but have a significant impairment in motor learning as demands of motor coordination are increased. Overall, a detailed analysis demonstrated that Sst^{KO} mice are healthy, fertile, and show no overt behavioral phenotypes, including anxiety-like behavior in the open-field and fear conditioning tests. Notably, Sst^{KO} mice display high basal plasma levels of corticosterone and growth hormone (Zeyda et al., 2001), confirming a somatostatin-mediated inhibition of HPA axis function. Similarly, mice lacking individual Sst_{1-5} receptors have been tested in numerous biological fields. Of these, Sst_2 emerged as the primary receptor of interest (Zeyda and Hochgeschwender, 2008), and $Sst_2{}^{KO}$ mice display increased anxiety-like behavior in the elevated plus maze and open field, increased immobility in the forced swim test, decreased locomotion coupled with an increase of pituitary adrenocorticotropic hormone release instead of growth hormone (Viollet et al., 2000). In line with the observed changes in $Sst_2{}^{KO}$ mice, acute predator stress in rats led to up-regulated *Sst*$_2$ gene expression in the amygdala and cingulate cortex, shown correlated with Fos expression in the amygdala (Nanda et al., 2008). As the product of a different gene, cortistatin shares a high structural and functional similarity with somatostatin-14 (de Lecea et al., 1996, 1997). Notably, compared with the weak inhibitory effects of somatostatin on the basal release of CRH from rat hypothalamus and hippocampus, cortistatin exhibits strong inhibition of the expression and release of basal CRH (Tringali et al., 2012). These findings suggest that Sst2 may regulate affective phenotypes and HPA axis responses both through somatostatin and cortistatin. Given the limitations of human studies, Sst^{KO} mice provide an opportunity to explore the causal role of somatostatin in affect dysregulation and the underlying neural mechanisms. Such insights, however, will require systematic behavioral characterization with fine spatial and temporal resolution by including female cohorts and region-specific manipulation at different developmental stages. Based on the published studies to date, it is still unclear whether these mutants recapitulate behavioral features of mood disorders. Knowing the effects of somatostatin signaling on neuroendocrine regulation, future studies need to assess the molecular and cellular systems that somatostatin mutations converge upon, and where the exact neural circuits are affected. Moreover, combining genetic and environmental factors in animal models is critical to enhance the accuracy of disease modeling and translational efforts. For example, acute or chronic exposure to stress or to stress hormones may capture how such etiological factors determine the vulnerability to external insults, in contrast to baseline behavioral testing. In addition, mood disorder-related sex differences are observed in community-based epidemiological studies, where the factor of seeking treatment is removed (Kornstein et al., 2000; Festinger et al., 2008; Leach et al., 2008) and findings of low somatostatin in the amygdala appear more robust in postmortem studies of female MDD subjects (Tripp et al., 2012), suggesting that gender/sex may represent a biological predisposing factor, or at least a moderating factor, in the intrinsic vulnerability of the somatostatin system.

Although many mood disorders emerge during adolescence (Paus et al., 2008), behavioral abnormalities including affect dysregulation are often heritable and apparent before diagnostic criteria are met (McGuffin et al., 2003; Geller et al., 2006). It is unclear when somatostatin deficits occur and potentially begin to contribute to the formation of affective symptoms. Tracking somatostatin system using new anatomic techniques with refined cellular definition, from Brainbow (Livet et al., 2007) to CLARITY (Chung et al., 2013) and SeeDB (Ke et al., 2013), across different developmental stages may help identify age-dependent neural architecture and disease mechanisms related to somatostatin function.

SOMATOSTATIN ANALOG DEVELOPMENT AND PHARMACOLOGICAL STUDIES

As native somatostatin peptides have a very short half-life time (approximate 1–3 min; Sheppard et al., 1979), long-acting and highly potent somatostatin analogues are currently available for the treatment of acromegaly and neuroendocrine tumors, including octreotide (long-acting; LAR-OCT; Bauer et al., 1982) and Lanreotide (slow release or autogel; Bevan, 2005; Molitch, 2008). Compared to somatostatin, pharmacological tools of the five somatostatin receptor subtypes have lagged behind, partly due to the lack of high-affinity antagonists.

In addition, several novel somatostatin therapy models are available: (1) Universal somatostatin (Schmid and Schoeffter, 2004): a somatostatin molecular analog with high binding affinity to all or most human somatostatin receptors. An example is SOM230, which interacts with $Sst_{1,2,3,5}$ and particularly potent at Sst_5 compared with LAR-OCT; (2) Chimeric somatostatin/dopamine molecule (Saveanu et al., 2002; Pivonello et al., 2005): a somatostatin and dopamine hybrid agonist, based on reports that dopamine and somatostatin receptors can hetero-oligomerize to enhance functional responses (Rocheville et al., 2000). An example is BIM-23A760, which accelerates the suppression of growth hormone and adrenocorticotropic hormone by the interaction with Sst_2 and Drd2 simultaneously; (3) Chimeric-somatostatin vaccinations (Haffer, 2012): a fusion protein expressing chloramphenicol acetyl transferase protein and somatostatin. Two somatostatin vaccinations, JH17 and JH18, can effectively reduce weight gain and reduce final body weight percentage of normal, non-obese mice and mice with diet-induced obesity via the intra-peritoneal route; (4) Non-peptide antagonists, such as SRA880 (Sst_1 selective), ACQ090 (Sst_3 selective) and Sst_4 selective β peptide agonists (Rivier et al., 2003; Hoyer et al., 2004). Despite this extensive list, the practical use of somatostatin in the brain is hampered by the multiple effects of the peptide, by the need for small molecules targeting specific, high affinity receptors on the target cells in specific brain regions, and by the need for feasible routes of administration that lead to fast delivery into the brain.

The potential for using somatostatin analogues as treatment in the CNS is emerging for treatment of epilepsy (Vezzani and Hoyer, 1999; Tallent and Qiu, 2008), pain (Mollenholt et al., 1994; Taura et al., 1994) and headaches (Sicuteri et al., 1984; Kapicioglu et al., 1997); potential use for treatment of mood disorders is suggested by reversal of emotion-like behaviors in rodent models. Several pharmacological studies support a role of somatostatin in affect regulation. Intra-ventricular administration of somatostatin in rats produces anxiolytic- and antidepressant-like behaviors in the elevated plus-maze and forced swim tests, and a neurophysiological signature of anxiolytic drugs (e.g., reduction of theta frequency and theta frequency curve slope; Engin et al., 2008). Mice with intra-amygdalar and intra-septal microinfusions of somatostatin-14 and somatostatin-28 display reduced anxiety-like behavior in the elevated plus-maze and shock-probe tests (Yeung et al., 2011). Moreover, anxiolytic effects in the elevated plus-maze test are described after intra-cerebroventricular infusions of a selective Sst_2 receptor agonist, but not after infusions of the other four receptor agonists; antidepressant-like effects in the forced swim test are observed following infusions of either Sst_2 or Sst_3 agonists (Engin and Treit, 2009). Another agent to enhance somatostatin functioning, SRA880 (an antagonist of auto-receptor Sst_1), synergizes with imipramine in causing antidepressant-like effects in the tail suspension test and increases *Bdnf* mRNA expression in the mouse cerebral cortex (Nilsson et al., 2012).

EFFECTS OF ANTIDEPRESSANTS ON SOMATOSTATIN IN THE CNS

Significant efforts have been directed toward the characterization of the downstream targets of antidepressant treatment, with a focus on somatostatin. A recent study demonstrates that chronic imipramine treatment increases somatostatin expression in mouse hypothalamus (Nilsson et al., 2012). However, there is inconsistency regarding the effect of chronic citalopram treatment on somatostatin levels in rats (Kakigi et al., 1992; Prosperini et al., 1997; Pallis et al., 2006, 2009). Repeated administration of imipramine, maprotiline, mianserin, carbamazepine or zotepine has no effect on somatostatin levels in various brain regions of rats (Weiss et al., 1987; Kakigi et al., 1992). While some somatostatin receptors seem to exert anxiolytic or antidepressant-like effects, there is no direct evidence supporting somatostatin receptors as downstream targets of current antidepressants. Together, these findings suggest that somatostatin levels are mostly unchanged by antidepressants. It is unclear whether somatostatin, GABA, or GABA functioning in somatostatin-expressing interneurons may be the real mediators or antidepressant targets. Future studies are needed to determine the involvement of somatostatin receptors and associated intracellular signaling pathways in the therapeutic effects of antidepressants, or whether somatostatin effects are independent of current antidepressant modalities.

POTENTIAL MECHANISMS OF SELECTIVE VULNERABILITY OF SOMATOSTATIN-EXPRESSING INTERNEURONS

It is possible that low somatostatin in diseases acts as a biomarker for deregulated function of somatostatin-expressing neurons. As such, it is essential to identify upstream factors responsible for the dysfunction of somatostatin-expressing interneurons in neurological disorders. We speculate that intrinsic cellular properties in somatostatin-expressing neurons may determine their selective vulnerability to various insults. Pathways underlying this high vulnerability may include high intrinsic oxidative stress related to mitochondria, high sensitivity to inflammation, high dependence on neurotrophic environment, and cellular developmental and aging processes. These canonical pathways might provide novel cell-based perspectives in the treatment of affected somatostatin-expressing cells across neurological disorders.

OXIDATIVE STRESS AND MITOCHONDRIAL DYSFUNCTIONS

Oxidative stress produced by mitochondria during respiration is a common pathogenic mechanism implicated in neurological disorders (Sorce and Krause, 2009; Stefanescu and Ciobica, 2012). Depressed states in mood disorders are associated with decreased brain energy generation (Baxter et al., 1985, 1989). Mitochondrial dysfunction together with the oxidative stress accumulation has been proposed to synergistically contribute to the neuro-endangerment processes underlying depression (Gardner et al., 2003; Burnett et al., 2005) and neurodegenerative diseases (Lin and Beal, 2006; Mancuso et al., 2007; Petrozzi et al., 2007). Similarly, high baseline oxidative stress could be an intrinsic characteristic of vulnerable neuronal populations. Notably, neuronal nitric oxide synthase (nNOS) and NADPH diaphorase (NADPHd), two enzymes that produce reactive oxidative species, are extensively and almost exclusively co-localized with somatostatin and neuropeptide Y (Dun et al., 1994; Figueredo-Cardenas et al., 1996; Jaglin et al., 2012), hence providing a neurochemical basis for high susceptibility of somatostatin-expressing neurons to generate oxidative stress in response to pathophysiological insults.

HIGH DEPENDENCE ON NEUROTROPHIC ENVIRONMENT

Brain-derived neurotrophic factor (BDNF) and its receptor neurotrophic tyrosine kinase receptor type 2 (TrkB) have been implicated in mood disorders (Guilloux et al., 2012; Tripp et al., 2012). BDNF-TrkB signaling is one of the key mediators for maintaining normal *somatostatin* gene expression (Glorioso et al., 2006; Martinowich et al., 2011). Progressively impairing BDNF-TrkB signaling in patients with mood disturbances may directly impact the biology of somatostatin-expressing neurons, resulting in somatostatin deficits. In addition, Bdnf-TrkB signaling itself is vulnerable to increased inflammation (Goshen et al., 2008; Koo and Duman, 2008; Song and Wang, 2011) and high glucocorticoids insults (Hodes et al., 2012). Mild oxidative stress inhibits tyrosine phosphatases activity (Barrett et al., 2005), potentially leading to impaired TrkB downstream signaling. Cortistatin and neuropeptide Y expression partly overlaps with the somatostatin neuron population in rodents (Figueredo-Cardenas et al., 1996; de Lecea et al., 1997; Xu et al., 2010). Comparing the profile of gene changes between subjects with MDD and mice with genetically-altered Bdnf signaling suggest that the reduced *somatostatin*, *neuropeptide Y* and *cortistatin* are partly downstream from a combination of reduced constitutive and activity-dependent Bdnf signaling (Guilloux et al., 2012). In contrast, markers for other GABA neuron subtypes targeting the perisomatic area region cell body and axon initial segment of pyramidal neurons (i.e., cholecystokinin and calretinin), appear to be independent of BDNF signaling and unaffected in MDD patients (Guilloux et al., 2012; Tripp et al., 2012). Hence, it is possible that the somatostatin-specific cellular function and vulnerability are partly mediated by BDNF-TrkB signaling during both physiological and pathological processes of affect regulation.

INFLAMMATION AND CELLULAR AGING

Inflammation has been implicated as a contributing factor in the onset and progression of many neurological disorders (Di Filippo et al., 2008). Mood disturbances are associated with an activated inflammatory response system (Padmos et al., 2008; Miller et al., 2009), including increased levels of peripheral interleukins and tumor necrosis factor-alpha in MDD patients (Kaestner et al., 2005; Howren et al., 2009; Dowlati et al., 2010; Maes, 2011). Inflammatory illnesses are associated with more depressive episodes (Celik et al., 2010; Maes et al., 2012), suggesting that prior depression may sensitize inflammatory responses. Patients treated with inflammatory cytokines, such as interferon-α, are at greater risk of developing depressive episodes (Castera et al., 2006; Lotrich et al., 2007). Somatostatin released from sensory nerves and somatostatin receptors on peripheral blood mononuclear cells play a crucial role in anti-inflammation through inhibition of pro-inflammatory peptide release (Szolcsanyi et al., 1998; Kurnatowska and Pawlikowski, 2000; Helyes et al., 2004). Rats with chronic inflammation induced by lipopolysaccharide show decreased hippocampal *somatostatin* expression (Gavilan et al., 2007). It is possible that there is crosstalk among peripheral inflammation, somatostatin function, and central effects of somatostatin-expressing neurons. Hence, decreasing somatostatin expression due to cellular impairment in the progress of neurological diseases may further enhance inflammation in a vicious cycle, leading to exacerbated cellular vulnerability of somatostatin-expressing neurons.

Aging is associated with a considerable increase in an activated, pro-inflammatory state (Wei et al., 1992; Bruunsgaard and Pedersen, 2003), a decline in circulating levels of Bdnf (Erickson et al., 2010), and increased oxidative damage (Sohal and Weindruch, 1996). *Somatostatin* expression is significantly decreased with age in human cortical regions, but parvalbumin expression is not altered by age (Erraji-Benchekroun et al., 2005; Glorioso et al., 2011). Similarly, the number of hippocampal somatostatin-expressing interneurons decreases in aged rats, but the number of parvalbumin-expressing neurons remains the same (Vela et al., 2003). *Somatostatin* and *IL-1β* mRNA expression are negatively correlated in aged hippocampus of rats (Gavilan et al., 2007). Comparing the effects of aging on *somatostatin* expression in the sgACC, an accelerated reduction is found in patients with MDD compared to normal aging subjects (Tripp et al., 2012), suggesting a pattern resulting in an early aging phenomenon which we have speculated may be synergistically induced by normal age-related changes and depression-related pathological change (Douillard-Guilloux et al., 2013).

CONCLUSION

Here we have focused on somatostatin, a GABA marker, down-regulated in MDD, schizophrenia, bipolar disorder, and neurodegenerative diseases. Exploring cross-disease molecular (somatostatin) and cellular (somatostatin-expressing interneurons) pathological findings suggests a dimensional pathological phenotype that is specific to the somatostatin gene/cell biological entity rather than to categorical brain disorders. Based on these results we speculate that common risk factors affecting somatostatin and somatostatin-expressing neurons may impact information processing in the cortical local circuits (**Figure 1**). Clarifying the role of somatostatin and its regulation of GABA inhibition in affect regulation could provide new strategies for predicting, delaying, and treating neurological diseases with mood disturbances. A number of questions remain. For example, are the prevalent somatostatin deficits seen in multiple diseases reflected in a common symptom dimension, such as low mood, across neurological diseases? What are the critical events that determine the vulnerability of somatostatin-expressing neurons? And what are the pathogenic mechanisms that mediate the observed disease-related molecular and cellular phenotypes? One possibility is that inflammation, oxidative stress, aging, and reduced neurotrophic support may all converge to affect somatostatin-expressing neurons. Targeting these pathways may exert neuro-protective effects on somatostatin-expressing neurons, as a potential therapeutic approach with implications for several neuropsychiatric disorders and neurodegenerative diseases.

ACKNOWLEDGMENTS

This work was supported by National Institute of Mental Health (NIMH-MH093723, MH084060 and MH077159). We thank Beverly French for careful review of the manuscript.

REFERENCES

Aarsland, D., Larsen, J. P., Lim, N. G., Janvin, C., Karlsen, K., Tandberg, E., et al. (1999). Range of neuropsychiatric disturbances in patients with Parkinson's disease. *J. Neurol. Neurosurg. Psychiatry* 67, 492–496. doi: 10.1136/jnnp.67.4.492

Agren, H., and Lundqvist, G. (1984). Low levels of somatostatin in human CSF mark depressive episodes. *Psychoneuroendocrinology* 9, 233–248. doi: 10.1016/0306-4530(84)90003-9

Barrett, D. M., Black, S. M., Todor, H., Schmidt-Ullrich, R. K., Dawson, K. S., and Mikkelsen, R. B. (2005). Inhibition of protein-tyrosine phosphatases by mild oxidative stresses is dependent on *S*-nitrosylation. *J. Biol. Chem.* 280, 14453–14461. doi: 10.1074/jbc.M411523200

Bauer, W., Briner, U., Doepfner, W., Haller, R., Huguenin, R., Marbach. P., et al. (1982). SMS 201-995: a very potent and selective octapeptide analogue of somatostatin with prolonged action. *Life Sci.* 31, 1133–1140. doi: 10.1016/0024-3205(82)90087-X

Baxter, L. R. Jr., Phelps, M. E., Mazziotta, J. C., Schwartz, J. M., Gerner, R. H., Selin, C. E. et al. (1985). Cerebral metabolic rates for glucose in mood disorders. Studies with positron emission tomography and fluorodeoxyglucose F 18. *Arch. Gen. Psychiatry* 42, 441–447. doi: 10.1001/archpsyc.1985.01790280019002

Baxter, L. R. Jr., Schwartz, J. M., Phelps, M. E., Mazziotta, J. C., Guze, B. H., Selin, C. E. et al. (1989). Reduction of prefrontal cortex glucose metabolism common to three types of depression. *Arch. Gen. Psychiatry* 46, 243–250. doi: 10.1001/archpsyc.1989.01810030049007

Beal, M. F., Mazurek, M. F., and Martin, J. B. (1986). Somatostatin immunoreactivity is reduced in Parkinson's disease dementia with Alzheimer's changes. *Brain Res.* 397, 386–388. doi: 10.1016/0006-8993(86)90644-X

Beierlein, M., Gibson, J. R., and Connors, B. W. (2003). Two dynamically distinct inhibitory networks in layer 4 of the neocortex. *J. Neurophysiol.* 90, 2987–3000. doi: 10.1152/jn.00283.2003

Bevan, J. S. (2005). The antitumoral effects of somatostatin analog therapy in acromegaly. *J. Clin. Endocrinol. Metab.* 90, 1856–1863. doi: 10.1210/jc.2004-1093

Bissette, G., Widerlov, E., Walleus, H., Karlsson, I., Eklund, K., Forsman, A., et al. (1986). Alterations in cerebrospinal fluid concentrations of somatostatinlike immunoreactivity in neuropsychiatric disorders. *Arch. Gen. Psychiatry* 43, 1148–1151. doi: 10.1001/archpsyc.1986.01800120034008

Bruunsgaard, H., and Pedersen, B. K. (2003). Age-related inflammatory cytokines and disease. *Immunol. Allergy Clin. North Am.* 23, 15–39. doi: 10.1016/S0889-8561(02)00056-5

Bungener, C., Jouvent, R., and Derouesne, C. (1996). Affective disturbances in Alzheimer's disease. *J. Am. Geriatr. Soc.* 44, 1066–1071.

Burnett, B. B., Gardner, A., and Boles, R. G. (2005). Mitochondrial inheritance in depression, dysmotility and migraine? *J. Affect Disord.* 88, 109–116. doi: 10.1016/j.jad.2005.05.009

Candy, J. M., Gascoigne, A. D., Biggins, J. A., Smith, A. I., Perry, R. H., Perry, E. K., et al. (1985). Somatostatin immunoreactivity in cortical and some subcortical regions in Alzheimer's disease. *J. Neurol. Sci.* 71, 315–323. doi: 10.1016/0022-510X(85)90070-X

Castera, L., Constant, A., Henry, C., Champbenoit, P., Bernard, P. H., De Ledinghen, V., et al. (2006). Impact on adherence and sustained virological response of psychiatric side effects during peginterferon and ribavirin therapy for chronic hepatitis C. *Aliment. Pharmacol. Ther.* 24, 1223–1230. doi: 10.1111/j.1365-2036.2006.03107.x

Celik, C., Erdem, M., Cayci, T., Ozdemir, B., Ozgur Akgul, E., Kurt, Y. G., et al. (2010). The association between serum levels of neopterin and number of depressive episodes of major depression. *Prog. Neuropsychopharmacol. Biol. Psychiatry* 34, 372–375. doi: 10.1016/j.pnpbp.2010.01.002

Chiu, C. Q., Lur, G., Morse, T. M., Carnevale, N. T., Ellis-Davies, G. C., and Higley, M. J. (2013). Compartmentalization of GABAergic inhibition by dendritic spines. *Science* 340, 759–762. doi: 10.1126/science.1234274

Chung, K., Wallace, J., Kim, S. Y., Kalyanasundaram, S., Andalman, A. S., Davidson, T. J., et al. (2013). Structural and molecular interrogation of intact biological systems. *Nature* 497, 332–337. doi: 10.1038/nature12107

Cruikshank, S. J., Urabe, H., Nurmikko, A. V., and Connors, B. W. (2010). Pathway-specific feedforward circuits between thalamus and neocortex revealed by selective optical stimulation of axons. *Neuron* 65, 230–245. doi: 10.1016/j.neuron.2009.12.025

Csaba, Z., and Dournaud, P. (2001). Cellular biology of somatostatin receptors. *Neuropeptides* 35, 1–23. doi: 10.1054/npep.2001.0848

Davies, P., Katzman, R., and Terry, R. D. (1980). Reduced somatostatin-like immunoreactivity in cerebral cortex from cases of Alzheimer disease and Alzheimer senile dementa. *Nature* 288, 279–280. doi: 10.1038/288279a0

Davies, P., and Terry, R. D. (1981). Cortical somatostatin-like immunoreactivity in cases of Alzheimer's disease and senile dementia of the Alzheimer type. *Neurobiol. Aging* 2, 9–14. doi: 10.1016/0197-4580(81)90053-1

DeFelipe, J., Lopez-Cruz, P. L., Benavides-Piccione, R., Bielza, C., Larranaga, P., Anderson, S., et al. (2013). New insights into the classification and nomenclature of cortical GABAergic interneurons. *Nat. Rev. Neurosci.* 14, 202–216. doi: 10.1038/nrn3444

de Lecea, L. (2008). Cortistatin – functions in the central nervous system. *Mol. Cell. Endocrinol.* 286, 88–95. doi: 10.1016/j.mce.2007.12.014

de Lecea, L., Criado, J. R., Prospero-Garcia, O., Gautvik, K. M., Schweitzer, P., Danielson, P. E., et al. (1996). A cortical neuropeptide with neuronal depressant and sleep-modulating properties. *Nature* 381, 242–245. doi: 10.1038/381242a0

de Lecea, L., del Rio, J. A., Criado, J. R., Alcantara, S., Morales, M., Danielson, P. E., et al. (1997). Cortistatin is expressed in a distinct subset of cortical interneurons. *J. Neurosci.* 17, 5868–5880.

Di Cristo, G., Wu, C., Chattopadhyaya, B., Ango, F., Knott, G., Welker, E., et al. (2004). Subcellular domain-restricted GABAergic innervation in primary visual cortex in the absence of sensory and thalamic inputs. *Nat. Neurosci.* 7, 1184–1186. doi: 10.1038/nn1334

Di Filippo, M., Sarchielli, P., Picconi, B., and Calabresi, P. (2008). Neuroinflammation and synaptic plasticity: theoretical basis for a novel, immune-centred, therapeutic approach to neurological disorders. *Trends Pharmacol. Sci.* 29, 402–412. doi: 10.1016/j.tips.2008.06.005

Douillard-Guilloux, G., Guilloux, J. P., Lewis, D. A., and Sibille, E. (2013). Anticipated brain molecular aging in major depression. *Am. J. Geriatr. Psychiatry* 21, 450–460. doi: 10.1016/j.jagp.2013.01.040

Dournaud, P., Cervera-Pierot, P., Hirsch, E., Javoy-Agid, F., Kordon, C., Agid, Y., et al. (1994). Somatostatin messenger RNA-containing neurons in Alzheimer's disease: an in situ hybridization study in hippocampus, parahippocampal cortex and frontal cortex. *Neuroscience* 61, 755–764. doi: 10.1016/0306-4522(94)90399-9

Dowlati, Y., Herrmann, N., Swardfager, W., Liu, H., Sham, L., Reim, E. K., et al. (2010). A meta-analysis of cytokines in major depression. *Biol. Psychiatry* 67, 446–457. doi: 10.1016/j.biopsych.2009.09.033

Dun, N. J., Dun, S. L., Wong, R. K., and Forstermann, U. (1994). Colocalization of nitric oxide synthase and somatostatin immunoreactivity in rat dentate hilar neurons. *Proc. Natl. Acad. Sci. U.S.A.* 91, 2955–2959. doi: 10.1073/pnas.91.8.2955

Dupont, E., Christensen, S. E., Hansen, A. P., de Fine Olivarius, B., and Orskov, H. (1982). Low cerebrospinal fluid somatostatin in Parkinson disease: an irreversible abnormality. *Neurology* 32, 312–314. doi: 10.1212/WNL.32.3.312

Engin, E., Stellbrink, J., Treit, D., and Dickson, C. T. (2008). Anxiolytic and antidepressant effects of intracerebroventricularly administered somatostatin: behavioral and neurophysiological evidence. *Neuroscience* 157, 666–676. doi: 10.1016/j.neuroscience.2008.09.037

Engin, E., and Treit, D. (2009). Anxiolytic and antidepressant actions of somatostatin: the role of sst2 and sst3 receptors. *Psychopharmacology (Berl.)* 206, 281–289. doi: 10.1007/s00213-009-1605-5

Epelbaum, J. (1986). Somatostatin in the central nervous system: physiology and pathological modifications. *Prog. Neurobiol.* 27, 63–100. doi: 10.1016/0301-0082(86)90012-2

Epelbaum, J., Javoy-Agid, F., Enjalbert, A., Krantic, S., Kordon, C., and Agid, Y. (1988). Somatostatin concentrations and binding sites in human frontal cortex are differentially affected in Parkinson's disease associated dementia and in progressive supranuclear palsy. *J. Neurol. Sci.* 87, 167–174. doi: 10.1016/0022-510X(88)90242-0

Erickson, K. I., Prakash, R. S., Voss, M. W., Chaddock, L., Heo, S., McLaren, M., et al. (2010). Brain-derived neurotrophic factor is associated with age-related decline in hippocampal volume. *J. Neurosci.* 30, 5368–5375. doi: 10.1523/JNEUROSCI.6251-09.2010

Erraji-Benchekroun, L., Underwood, M. D., Arango, V., Galfalvy, H., Pavlidis, P., Smyrniotopoulos, P., et al. (2005). Molecular aging in human prefrontal cortex is selective and continuous throughout adult life. *Biol. Psychiatry* 57, 549–558. doi: 10.1016/j.biopsych.2004.10.034

Festinger, D. S., Marlowe, D. B., Dugosh, K. L., Croft, J. R., and Arabia, P. L. (2008). Higher magnitude cash payments improve research follow-up rates without increasing drug use or perceived coercion. *Drug Alcohol Depend.* 96, 128–135. doi: 10.1016/j.drugalcdep.2008.02.007

Figueredo-Cardenas, G., Morello, M., Sancesario, G., Bernardi, G., and Reiner, A. (1996). Colocalization of somatostatin, neuropeptide Y, neuronal nitric oxide synthase and NADPH-diaphorase in striatal interneurons in rats. *Brain Res.* 735, 317–324. doi: 10.1016/0006-8993(96)00801-3

Fishell, G., and Rudy, B. (2011). Mechanisms of inhibition within the telencephalon: "where the wild things are". *Annu. Rev. Neurosci.* 34, 535–567. doi: 10.1146/annurev-neuro-061010-113717

Fitz-Patrick, D., and Patel, Y. C. (1981). Evidence for somatostatin precursors in human stomach, placenta, and amniotic fluid. *J. Clin. Endocrinol. Metab.* 53, 372–376. doi: 10.1210/jcem-53-2-372

Gardner, A., Johansson, A., Wibom, R., Nennesmo, I., von Dobeln, U., Hagenfeldt, L., et al. (2003). Alterations of mitochondrial function and correlations with personality traits in selected major depressive disorder patients. *J. Affect. Disord.* 76, 55–68. doi: 10.1016/S0165-0327(02)00067-8

Gavilan, M. P., Revilla, E., Pintado, C., Castano, A., Vizuete, M. L., Moreno-González, I., et al. (2007). Molecular and cellular characterization of the age-related neuroinflammatory processes occurring in normal rat hippocampus: potential relation with the loss of somatostatin GABAergic neurons. *J. Neurochem.* 103, 984–996. doi: 10.1111/j.1471-4159.2007.04787.x

Geller, B., Tillman, R., Bolhofner, K., Zimerman, B., Strauss, N. A., and Kaufmann, P. (2006). Controlled, blindly rated, direct-interview family study of a prepubertal and early-adolescent bipolar I disorder phenotype: morbid risk, age at onset, and comorbidity. *Arch. Gen. Psychiatry* 63, 1130–1138. doi: 10.1001/archpsyc.63.10.1130

Gentet, L. J., Kremer, Y., Taniguchi, H., Huang, Z. J., Staiger, J. F., and Petersen, C. C. (2012). Unique functional properties of somatostatin-expressing GABAergic neurons in mouse barrel cortex. *Nat. Neurosci.* 15, 607–612. doi: 10.1038/nn.3051

Glorioso, C., Oh, S., Douillard, G. G., and Sibille, E. (2011). Brain molecular aging, promotion of neurological disease and modulation by sirtuin 5 longevity gene polymorphism. *Neurobiol. Dis.* 41, 279–290. doi: 10.1016/j.nbd.2010.09.016

Glorioso, C., Sabatini, M., Unger, T., Hashimoto, T., Monteggia, L. M., Lewis, D. A., et al. (2006). Specificity and timing of neocortical transcriptome changes in response to BDNF gene ablation during embryogenesis or adulthood. *Mol. Psychiatry* 11, 633–648. doi: 10.1038/sj.mp.4001835

Gonchar, Y., and Burkhalter, A. (1997). Three distinct families of GABAergic neurons in rat visual cortex. *Cereb. Cortex* 7, 347–358. doi: 10.1093/cercor/7.4.347

Gonchar, Y., Wang, Q., and Burkhalter, A. (2007). Multiple distinct subtypes of GABAergic neurons in mouse visual cortex identified by triple immunostaining. *Front. Neuroanat.* 1:3. doi: 10.3389/neuro.05.003.2007

Goshen, I., Kreisel, T., Ben-Menachem-Zidon, O., Licht, T., Weidenfeld, J., Ben-Hur, T., et al. (2008). Brain interleukin-1 mediates chronic stress-induced depression in mice via adrenocortical activation and hippocampal neurogenesis suppression. *Mol. Psychiatry* 13, 717–728. doi: 10.1038/sj.mp.4002055

Guerreiro, R., Wojtas, A., Bras, J., Carrasquillo, M., Rogaeva, E., Majounie, E., et al. (2013). TREM2 variants in Alzheimer's disease. *N. Engl. J. Med.* 368, 117–127. doi: 10.1056/NEJMoa1211851

Guilloux, J. P., Douillard-Guilloux, G., Kota, R., Wang, X., Gardier, A. M., Martinowich, K., et al. (2012). Molecular evidence for BDNF- and GABA-related dysfunctions in the amygdala of female subjects with major depression. *Mol. Psychiatry* 17, 1130–1142. doi: 10.1038/mp.2011.113

Guillozet-Bongaarts, A. L., Hyde, T. M., Dalley, R. A., Hawrylycz, M. J., Henry, A., Hof, P. R., et al. (2013). Altered gene expression in the dorsolateral prefrontal cortex of individuals with schizophrenia. *Mol. Psychiatry.* doi: 10.1038/mp.2013.30 [Epub ahead of print].

Haffer, K. N. (2012). Effects of novel vaccines on weight loss in diet-induced-obese (DIO) mice. *J. Anim. Sci. Biotechnol.* 3, 21. doi: 10.1186/2049-1891-3-21

Helyes, Z., Szabo, A., Nemeth, J., Jakab, B., Pinter, E., Banvolgyi, A., et al. (2004). Antiinflammatory and analgesic effects of somatostatin released from capsaicin-sensitive sensory nerve terminals in a Freund's adjuvant-induced chronic arthritis model in the rat. *Arthritis Rheum.* 50, 1677–1685. doi: 10.1002/art.20184

Hodes, G. E., Brookshire, B. R., Hill-Smith, T. E., Teegarden, S. L., Berton, O., and Lucki, I. (2012). Strain differences in the effects of chronic corticosterone exposure in the hippocampus. *Neuroscience* 222, 269–280. doi: 10.1016/j.neuroscience.2012.06.017

Hollingworth, P., Harold, D., Sims, R., Gerrish, A., Lambert, J. C., Carrasquillo, M. M., et al. (2011). Common variants at ABCA7, MS4A6A/MS4A4E, EPHA1, CD33 and CD2AP are associated with Alzheimer's disease. *Nat. Genet.* 43, 429–435. doi: 10.1038/ng.803

Holsboer, F. (2000). The corticosteroid receptor hypothesis of depression. *Neuropsychopharmacology* 23, 477–501. doi: 10.1016/S0893-133X(00)00159-7

Howren, M. B., Lamkin, D. M., and Suls, J. (2009). Associations of depression with C-reactive protein, IL-1, and IL-6: a meta-analysis. *Psychosom. Med.* 71, 171–186. doi: 10.1097/PSY.0b013e3181907c1b

Hoyer, D., Nunn, C., Hannon, J., Schoeffter, P., Feuerbach, D., Schuepbach, E., et al. (2004). SRA880, in vitro characterization of the first non-peptide somatostatin sst(1) receptor antagonist. *Neurosci. Lett.* 361, 132–135. doi: 10.1016/j.neulet.2004.02.017

Jaglin, X. H., Hjerling-Leffler, J., Fishell, G., and Batista-Brito, R. (2012). The origin of neocortical nitric oxide synthase-expressing inhibitory neurons. *Front. Neural Circuits* 6:44. doi: 10.3389/fncir.2012.00044

Kaestner, F., Hettich, M., Peters, M., Sibrowski, W., Hetzel, G., Ponath, G., et al. (2005). Different activation patterns of proinflammatory cytokines in melancholic and non-melancholic major depression are associated with HPA axis activity. *J. Affect. Disord.* 87, 305–311. doi: 10.1016/j.jad.2005.03.012

Kakigi, T., Maeda, K., Kaneda, H., and Chihara, K. (1992). Repeated administration of antidepressant drugs reduces regional somatostatin concentrations in rat brain. *J. Affect. Disord.* 25, 215–220. doi: 10.1016/0165-0327(92)90078-K

Kapicioglu, S., Gokce, E., Kapicioglu, Z., and Ovali, E. (1997). Treatment of migraine attacks with a long-acting somatostatin analogue (octreotide, SMS 201–995). *Cephalalgia* 17, 27–30. doi: 10.1046/j.1468-2982.1997.1701027.x

Kawaguchi, Y., and Kubota, Y. (1997). GABAergic cell subtypes and their synaptic connections in rat frontal cortex. *Cereb. Cortex* 7, 476–486. doi: 10.1093/cercor/7.6.476

Ke, M. T., Fujimoto, S., and Imai, T. (2013). SeeDB: a simple and morphology-preserving optical clearing agent for neuronal circuit reconstruction. *Nat. Neurosci.* 16, 1154–1161. doi: 10.1038/nn.3447

Kling, M. A., Rubinow, D. R., Doran, A. R., Roy, A., Davis, C. L., Calabrese, J. R., et al. (1993). Cerebrospinal fluid immunoreactive somatostatin concentrations in patients with Cushing's disease and major depression: relationship to indices of corticotropin-releasing hormone and cortisol secretion. *Neuroendocrinology* 57, 79–88. doi: 10.1159/000126345

Kluxen, F. W., Bruns, C., and Lubbert, H. (1992). Expression cloning of a rat brain somatostatin receptor cDNA. *Proc. Natl. Acad. Sci. U.S.A.* 89, 4618–4622. doi: 10.1073/pnas.89.10.4618

Koch, B. D., Blalock, J. B., and Schonbrunn, A. (1988). Characterization of the cyclic AMP-independent actions of somatostatin in GH cells. I. An increase in potassium conductance is responsible for both the hyperpolarization and the decrease in intracellular free calcium produced by somatostatin. *J. Biol. Chem.* 263, 216–225.

Koch, B. D., and Schonbrunn, A. (1984). The somatostatin receptor is directly coupled to adenylate cyclase in GH4C1 pituitary cell membranes. *Endocrinology* 114, 1784–1790. doi: 10.1210/endo-114-5-1784

Konradi, C., Yang, C. K., Zimmerman, E. I., Lohmann, K. M., Gresch, P., Pantazopoulos, H., et al. (2011a). Hippocampal interneurons are abnormal in schizophrenia. *Schizophr. Res.* 131, 165–173. doi: 10.1016/j.schres.2011.06.007

Konradi, C., Zimmerman, E. I., Yang, C. K., Lohmann, K. M., Gresch, P., Pantazopoulos, H., et al. (2011b). Hippocampal interneurons in bipolar disorder. *Arch. Gen. Psychiatry* 68, 340–350. doi: 10.1001/archgenpsychiatry.2010.175

Koo, J. W., and Duman, R. S. (2008). IL-1beta is an essential mediator of the antineurogenic and anhedonic effects of stress. *Proc. Natl. Acad. Sci. U.S.A.* 105, 751–756. doi: 10.1073/pnas.0708092105

Kornstein, S. G., Schatzberg, A. F., Thase, M. E., Yonkers, K. A., McCullough, J. P., Keitner, G. I., et al. (2000). Gender differences in chronic major and double depression. *J. Affect. Disord.* 60, 1–11. doi: 10.1016/S0165-0327(99)00158-5

Kurnatowska, I., and Pawlikowski, M. (2000). Effect of somatostatin analog-octreotide on the adjuvant arthritis in rat. *Neuro Endocrinol. Lett.* 21, 121–126.

Lauritsen, M. B., Nyegaard, M., Betancur, C., Colineaux, C., Josiassen, T. L., Kruse, T. A., et al. (2003). Analysis of transmission of novel polymorphisms in the somatostatin receptor 5 (SSTR5) gene in patients with autism. *Am. J. Med. Genet. B Neuropsychiatr. Genet.* 121B,100–104. doi: 10.1002/ajmg.b.20050

Leach, L. S., Christensen, H., Mackinnon, A. J., Windsor, T. D., and Butterworth, P. (2008). Gender differences in depression and anxiety across the adult lifespan: the role of psychosocial mediators. *Soc. Psychiatry Psychiatr. Epidemiol.* 43, 983–998. doi: 10.1007/s00127-008-0388-z

Lee, S., Hjerling-Leffler, J., Zagha, E., Fishell, G., and Rudy, B. (2010). The largest group of superficial neocortical GABAergic interneurons expresses ionotropic serotonin receptors. *J. Neurosci.* 30, 16796–16808. doi: 10.1523/JNEUROSCI.1869-10.2010

Le Magueresse, C., and Monyer, H. (2013). GABAergic interneurons shape the functional maturation of the cortex. *Neuron* 77, 388–405. doi: 10.1016/j.neuron.2013.01.011

Lin, M. T., and Beal, M. F. (2006). Mitochondrial dysfunction and oxidative stress in neurodegenerative diseases. *Nature* 443, 787–795. doi: 10.1038/nature05292

Livet, J., Weissman, T. A., Kang, H., Draft, R. W., Lu, J., Bennis, R. A., et al. (2007). Transgenic strategies for combinatorial expression of fluorescent proteins in the nervous system. *Nature* 450, 56–62. doi: 10.1038/nature06293

Lotrich, F. E., Rabinovitz, M., Gironda, P., and Pollock, B. G. (2007). Depression following pegylated interferon-alpha: characteristics and vulnerability. *J. Psychosom. Res.* 63, 131–135. doi: 10.1016/j.jpsychores.2007.05.013

Maciag, D., Hughes, J., O'Dwyer, G., Pride, Y., Stockmeier, C. A., Sanacora, G., et al. (2010). Reduced density of calbindin immunoreactive GABAergic neurons in the occipital cortex in major depression: relevance to neuroimaging studies. *Biol. Psychiatry* 67, 465–470. doi: 10.1016/j.biopsych.2009.10.027

Maes, M. (2011). Depression is an inflammatory disease, but cell-mediated immune activation is the key component of depression. *Prog. Neuropsychopharmacol. Biol. Psychiatry* 35, 664–675. doi: 10.1016/j.pnpbp.2010.06.014

Maes, M., Mihaylova, I., Kubera, M., and Ringel, K. (2012). Activation of cell-mediated immunity in depression: association with inflammation, melancholia, clinical staging and the fatigue and somatic symptom cluster of depression. *Prog. Neuropsychopharmacol. Biol. Psychiatry* 36, 169–175. doi: 10.1016/j.pnpbp.2011.09.006

Mancuso, C., Scapagini, G., Curro, D., Giuffrida Stella, A. M., De Marco, C., Butterfield, D. A., et al. (2007). Mitochondrial dysfunction, free radical generation and cellular stress response in neurodegenerative disorders. *Front. Biosci.* 12:1107–1123. doi: 10.2741/2130

Markram, H., Toledo-Rodriguez, M., Wang, Y., Gupta, A., Silberberg, G., and Wu, C. (2004). Interneurons of the neocortical inhibitory system. *Nat. Rev. Neurosci.* 5, 793–807. doi: 10.1038/nrn1519

Martel, G., Dutar, P., Epelbaum, J., and Viollet, C. (2012). Somatostatinergic systems: an update on brain functions in normal and pathological aging. *Front. Endocrinol. (Lausanne)* 3:154. doi: 10.3389/fendo.2012.00154

Martinowich, K., Schloesser, R. J., Jimenez, D. V., Weinberger, D. R., and Lu, B. (2011). Activity-dependent brain-derived neurotrophic factor expression regulates cortistatin-interneurons and sleep behavior. *Mol. Brain* 4, 11. doi: 10.1186/1756-6606-4-11

McGuffin, P., Rijsdijk, F., Andrew, M., Sham, P., Katz, R., and Cardno, A. (2003). The heritability of bipolar affective disorder and the genetic relationship to unipolar depression. *Arch. Gen. Psychiatry* 60, 497–502. doi: 10.1001/archpsyc.60.5.497

Miller, A. H., Maletic, V., and Raison, C. L. (2009). Inflammation and its discontents: the role of cytokines in the pathophysiology of major depression. *Biol. Psychiatry* 65, 732–741. doi: 10.1016/j.biopsych.2008.11.029

Molchan, S. E., Hill, J. L., Martinez, R. A., Lawlor, B. A., Mellow, A. M., Rubinow, D. R., et al. (1993). CSF somatostatin in Alzheimer's disease and major depression: relationship to hypothalamic-pituitary-adrenal axis and clinical measures. *Psychoneuroendocrinology* 18, 509–519. doi: 10.1016/0306-4530(93)90044-L

Molchan, S. E., Lawlor, B. A., Hill, J. L., Martinez, R. A., Davis, C. L., Mellow, A. M., et al. (1991). CSF monoamine metabolites and somatostatin in Alzheimer's disease and major depression. *Biol. Psychiatry* 29, 1110–1118. doi: 10.1016/0006-3223(91)90253-I

Molitch, M. E. (2008). Lanreotide Autogel in the management of acromegaly. *Drugs* 68, 724. doi: 10.2165/00003495-200868050-00014

Mollenholt, P., Rawal, N., Gordh, T. Jr., and Olsson, Y. (1994). Intrathecal and epidural somatostatin for patients with cancer. Analgesic effects and postmortem neuropathologic investigations of spinal cord and nerve roots. *Anesthesiology* 81, 534–542. doi: 10.1097/00000542-199409000-00004

Moller, L. N., Stidsen, C. E., Hartmann, B., and Holst, J. J. (2003). Somatostatin receptors. *Biochim. Biophys. Acta* 1616, 1–84. doi: 10.1016/S0005-2736(03)00235-9

Montminy, M. R., Sevarino, K. A., Wagner, J. A., Mandel, G., and Goodman, R. H. (1986). Identification of a cyclic-AMP-responsive element within the rat somatostatin gene. *Proc. Natl. Acad. Sci. U.S.A.* 83, 6682–6686. doi: 10.1073/pnas.83.18.6682

Morris, H. M., Hashimoto, T., and Lewis, D. A. (2008). Alterations in somatostatin mRNA expression in the dorsolateral prefrontal cortex of subjects with schizophrenia or schizoaffective disorder. *Cereb. Cortex* 18, 1575–1587. doi: 10.1093/cercor/bhm186

Murayama, M., Perez-Garci, E., Nevian, T., Bock, T., Senn, W., and Larkum, M. E. (2009). Dendritic encoding of sensory stimuli controlled by deep cortical interneurons. *Nature* 457, 1137–1141. doi: 10.1038/nature07663

Nanda, S. A., Qi, C., Roseboom, P. H., and Kalin, N. H. (2008). Predator stress induces behavioral inhibition and amygdala somatostatin receptor 2 gene expression. *Genes Brain Behav.* 7, 639–648. doi: 10.1111/j.1601-183X.2008.00401.x

Neggers, S. J., and van der Lely, A. J. (2009). Somatostatin analog and pegvisomant combination therapy for acromegaly. *Nat. Rev. Endocrinol.* 5, 546–552. doi: 10.1038/nrendo.2009.175

Nilsson, A., Stroth, N., Zhang, X., Qi, H., Falth, M., Skold, K., et al. (2012). Neuropeptidomics of mouse hypothalamus after imipramine treatment reveal somatostatin as a potential mediator of antidepressant effects. *Neuropharmacology* 62, 347–357. doi: 10.1016/j.neuropharm.2011.08.004

Nyegaard, M., Borglum, A. D., Bruun, T. G., Collier, D. A., Russ, C., Mors, O., et al. (2002). Novel polymorphisms in the somatostatin receptor 5 (SSTR5) gene associated with bipolar affective disorder. *Mol. Psychiatry* 7, 745–754. doi: 10.1038/sj.mp.4001049

Olias, G., Viollet, C., Kusserow, H., Epelbaum, J., and Meyerhof, W. (2004). Regulation and function of somatostatin receptors. *J. Neurochem.* 89, 1057–1091. doi: 10.1111/j.1471-4159.2004.02402.x

Padmos, R. C., Hillegers, M. H., Knijff, E. M., Vonk, R., Bouvy, A., Staal, F. J., et al. (2008). A discriminating messenger RNA signature for bipolar disorder formed by an aberrant expression of inflammatory genes in monocytes. *Arch. Gen. Psychiatry* 65, 395–407. doi: 10.1001/archpsyc.65.4.395

Pallis, E., Vasilaki, A., Fehlmann, D., Kastellakis, A., Hoyer, D., Spyraki, C., et al. (2009). Antidepressants influence somatostatin levels and receptor pharmacology in brain. *Neuropsychopharmacology* 34, 952–963. doi: 10.1038/npp.2008.133

Pallis, E. G., Spyraki, C., and Thermos, K. (2006). Chronic antidepressant treatment modulates the release of somatostatin in the rat nucleus accumbens. *Neurosci. Lett.* 395, 76–81. doi: 10.1016/j.neulet.2005.10.055

Patel, Y. C. (1999). Somatostatin and its receptor family. *Front. Neuroendocrinol.* 20:157–198. doi: 10.1006/frne.1999.0183

Paus, T., Keshavan, M., and Giedd, J. N. (2008). Why do many psychiatric disorders emerge during adolescence? *Nat. Rev. Neurosci.* 9, 947–957. doi: 10.1038/nrn2513

Petrozzi, L., Ricci, G., Giglioli, N. J., Siciliano, G., and Mancuso, M. (2007). Mitochondria and neurodegeneration. *Biosci. Rep.* 27, 87–104. doi: 10.1007/s10540-007-9038-z

Pivonello, R., Ferone, D., Lamberts, S. W., and Colao, A. (2005). Cabergoline plus lanreotide for ectopic Cushing's syndrome. *N. Engl. J. Med.* 352, 2457–2458. doi: 10.1056/NEJM200506093522322

Ponomarev, I., Rau, V., Eger, E. I., Harris, R. A., and Fanselow, M. S. (2010). Amygdala transcriptome and cellular mechanisms underlying stress-enhanced fear learning in a rat model of posttraumatic stress disorder. *Neuropsychopharmacology* 35, 1402–1411. doi: 10.1038/npp.2010.10

Post, R. M., Rubinow, D. R., Kling, M. A., Berrettini, W., and Gold, P. W. (1988). Neuroactive substances in cerebrospinal fluid. Normal and pathological regulatory mechanisms. *Ann. N. Y. Acad. Sci.* 531, 15–28. doi: 10.1111/j.1749-6632.1988.tb31808.x

Prosperini, E., Rizzi, M., Fumagalli, F., Tarizzo, G., Samanin, R., and Bendotti, C. (1997). Acute and chronic treatments with citalopram lower somatostatin levels in rat brain striatum through different mechanisms. *J. Neurochem.* 69, 206–213. doi: 10.1046/j.1471-4159.1997.69010206.x

Rajkowska, G., O'Dwyer, G., Teleki, Z., Stockmeier, C. A., and Miguel-Hidalgo, J. J. (2007). GABAergic neurons immunoreactive for calcium binding proteins are reduced in the prefrontal cortex in major depression. *Neuropsychopharmacology* 32, 471–482. doi: 10.1038/sj.npp.1301234

Reinikainen, K. J., Koponen, H., Jolkkonen, J., and Riekkinen, P. J. (1990). Decreased somatostatin-like immunoreactivity in the cerebrospinal fluid of chronic schizophrenic patients with cognitive impairment. *Psychiatry Res.* 33, 307–312. doi: 10.1016/0165-1781(90)90047-9

Rivier, J., Erchegyi, J., Hoeger, C., Miller, C., Low, W., Wenger, S., et al. (2003). Novel sst(4)-selective somatostatin (SRIF) agonists. 1. Lead identification using a betide scan. *J. Med. Chem.* 46, 5579–5586. doi: 10.1021/jm030243c

Robas, N., Mead, E., and Fidock, M. (2003). MrgX2 is a high potency cortistatin receptor expressed in dorsal root ganglion. *J. Biol. Chem.* 278, 44400–44404. doi: 10.1074/jbc.M302456200

Rocheville, M., Lange, D. C., Kumar, U., Patel, S. C., Patel, R. C., and Patel, Y. C. (2000). Receptors for dopamine and somatostatin: formation of hetero-oligomers with enhanced functional activity. *Science* 288, 154–157. doi: 10.1126/science.288.5463.154

Rossor, M. N., Emson, P. C., Mountjoy, C. Q., Roth, M., and Iversen, L. L. (1980). Reduced amounts of immunoreactive somatostatin in the temporal cortex in senile dementia of Alzheimer type. *Neurosci. Lett.* 20, 373–377. doi: 10.1016/0304-3940(80)90177-9

Rubinow, D. R., Gold, P. W., Post, R. M., and Ballenger, J. C. (1985). CSF somatostatin in affective illness and normal volunteers. *Prog. Neuropsychopharmacol. Biol. Psychiatry* 9, 393–400. doi: 10.1016/0278-5846(85)90192-7

Rubinow, D. R., Gold, P. W., Post, R. M., Ballenger, J. C., Cowdry, R., Bollinger, J., et al. (1983). CSF somatostatin in affective illness. *Arch. Gen. Psychiatry* 40, 409–412. doi: 10.1001/archpsyc.1983.01790040063009

Rudy, B., Fishell, G., Lee, S., and Hjerling-Leffler, J. (2011). Three groups of interneurons account for nearly 100% of neocortical GABAergic neurons. *Dev. Neurobiol.* 71, 45–61. doi: 10.1002/dneu.20853

Saveanu, A., Lavaque, E., Gunz, G., Barlier, A., Kim, S., Taylor, J. E., et al. (2002). Demonstration of enhanced potency of a chimeric somatostatin-dopamine molecule, BIM-23A387, in suppressing growth hormone and prolactin secretion from human pituitary somatotroph adenoma cells. *J. Clin. Endocrinol. Metab.* 87, 5545–5552. doi: 10.1210/jc.2002-020934

Schmid, H. A., and Schoeffter, P. (2004). Functional activity of the multiligand analog SOM230 at human recombinant somatostatin receptor subtypes supports its usefulness in neuroendocrine tumors. *Neuroendocrinology* 80(Suppl. 1), 47–50. doi: 10.1159/000080741

Schreff, M., Schulz, S., Handel, M., Keilhoff, G., Braun, H., Pereira, G., et al. (2000). Distribution, targeting, and internalization of the sst4 somatostatin receptor in rat brain. *J. Neurosci.* 20, 3785–3797.

Schulz, S., Handel, M., Schreff, M., Schmidt, H., and Hollt, V. (2000). Localization of five somatostatin receptors in the rat central nervous system using subtype-specific antibodies. *J. Physiol. Paris* 94, 259–264. doi: 10.1016/S0928-4257(00)00212-6

Sharif, N., Gendron, L., Wowchuk, J., Sarret, P., Mazella, J., Beaudet, A., et al. (2007). Coexpression of somatostatin receptor subtype 5 affects internalization and trafficking of somatostatin receptor subtype 2. *Endocrinology* 148, 2095–2105. doi: 10.1210/en.2006-1266

Sharma, R. P., Bissette, G., Janicak, P. G., Davis, J. M., and Nemeroff, C. B. (1995). Elevation of CSF somatostatin concentrations in mania. *Am. J. Psychiatry* 152, 1807–1809.

Sheppard, M., Shapiro, B., Pimstone, B., Kronheim, S., Berelowitz, M., and Gregory, M. (1979). Metabolic clearance and plasma half-disappearance time of exogenous somatostatin in man. *J. Clin. Endocrinol. Metab.* 48, 50–53. doi: 10.1210/jcem-48-1-50

Sibille, E., Morris, H. M., Kota, R. S., and Lewis, D. A. (2011). GABA-related transcripts in the dorsolateral prefrontal cortex in mood disorders. *Int. J. Neuropsychopharmacol.* 14, 721–734. doi: 10.1017/S1461145710001616

Sicuteri, F., Geppetti, P., Marabini, S., and Lembeck, F. (1984). Pain relief by somatostatin in attacks of cluster headache. *Pain* 18, 359–365. doi: 10.1016/0304-3959(84)90048-4

Siehler, S., Nunn, C., Hannon, J., Feuerbach, D., and Hoyer, D. (2008). Pharmacological profile of somatostatin and cortistatin receptors. *Mol. Cell. Endocrinol.* 286, 26–34. doi: 10.1016/j.mce.2007.12.007

Sohal, R. S., and Weindruch, R. (1996). Oxidative stress, caloric restriction, and aging. *Science* 273, 59–63. doi: 10.1126/science.273.5271.59

Song, C., and Wang, H. (2011). Cytokines mediated inflammation and decreased neurogenesis in animal models of depression. *Prog. Neuropsychopharmacol. Biol. Psychiatry* 35, 760–768. doi: 10.1016/j.pnpbp.2010.06.020

Sorce, S., and Krause, K. H. (2009). NOX enzymes in the central nervous system: from signaling to disease. *Antioxid. Redox. Signal.* 11, 2481–2504. doi: 10.1089/ars.2009.2578

Spier, A. D., and de Lecea, L. (2000). Cortistatin: a member of the somatostatin neuropeptide family with distinct physiological functions. *Brain Res. Brain Res. Rev.* 33, 228–241. doi: 10.1016/S0165-0173(00)00031-X

Stafford, R. S., Ausiello, J. C., Misra, B., and Saglam, D. (2000). National patterns of depression treatment in primary care. *Prim. Care Companion J. Clin. Psychiatry* 2, 211–216. doi: 10.4088/PCC.v02n0603

Stefanescu, C., and Ciobica, A. (2012). The relevance of oxidative stress status in first episode and recurrent depression. *J. Affect. Disord.* 143, 34–38. doi: 10.1016/j.jad.2012.05.022

Stroh, T., Kreienkamp, H. J., and Beaudet, A. (1999). Immunohistochemical distribution of the somatostatin receptor subtype 5 in the adult rat brain: predominant expression in the basal forebrain. *J. Comp. Neurol.* 412, 69–82. doi: 10.1002/(SICI)1096-9861(19990913)412:1<69::AID-CNE5>3.0.CO;2-V

Strowski, M. Z., Kohler, M., Chen, H. Y., Trumbauer, M. E., Li, Z., Szalkowski, D., et al. (2003). Somatostatin receptor subtype 5 regulates insulin secretion and glucose homeostasis. *Mol. Endocrinol.* 17, 93–106. doi: 10.1210/me.2001-0035

Szolcsanyi, J., Helyes, Z., Oroszi, G., Nemeth, J., and Pinter, E. (1998). Release of somatostatin and its role in the mediation of the anti-inflammatory effect induced by antidromic stimulation of sensory fibres of rat sciatic nerve. *Br. J. Pharmacol.* 123, 936–942. doi: 10.1038/sj.bjp.0701685

Tallent, M. K., and Qiu, C. (2008). Somatostatin: an endogenous antiepileptic. *Mol. Cell. Endocrinol.* 286, 96–103. doi: 10.1016/j.mce.2007.12.004

Tamminga, C. A., Foster, N. L., Fedio, P., Bird, E. D., and Chase, T. N. (1987). Alzheimer's disease: low cerebral somatostatin levels correlate with impaired cognitive function and cortical metabolism. *Neurology* 37, 161–165. doi: 10.1212/WNL.37.1.161

Tan, Z., Hu, H., Huang, Z. J., and Agmon, A. (2008). Robust but delayed thalamocortical activation of dendritic-targeting inhibitory interneurons. *Proc. Natl. Acad. Sci. U.S.A.* 105, 2187–2192. doi: 10.1073/pnas.0710628105

Taura, P., Planella, V., Balust, J., Beltran, J., Anglada, T., Carrero, E., et al. (1994). Epidural somatostatin as an analgesic in upper abdominal surgery: a double-blind study. *Pain* 59, 135–140. doi: 10.1016/0304-3959(94)90057-4

Tostivint, H., Lihrmann, I., and Vaudry, H. (2008). New insight into the molecular evolution of the somatostatin family. *Mol. Cell. Endocrinol.* 286, 5–17. doi: 10.1016/j.mce.2008.02.029

Tringali, G., Greco, M. C., Lisi, L., Pozzoli, G., and Navarra, P. (2012). Cortistatin modulates the expression and release of corticotrophin releasing hormone in rat brain. Comparison with somatostatin and octreotide. *Peptides* 34, 353–359. doi: 10.1016/j.peptides.2012.02.004

Tripp, A., Kota, R. S., Lewis, D. A., and Sibille, E. (2011). Reduced somatostatin in subgenual anterior cingulate cortex in major depression. *Neurobiol. Dis.* 42, 116–124. doi: 10.1016/j.nbd.2011.01.014

Tripp, A., Oh, H., Guilloux, J. P., Martinowich, K., Lewis, D. A., and Sibille, E. (2012). Brain-derived neurotrophic factor signaling and subgenual anterior cingulate cortex dysfunction in major depressive disorder. *Am. J. Psychiatry* 169, 1194–1202. doi: 10.1176/appi.ajp.2012.12020248

Trivedi, M. H., Rush, A. J., Wisniewski, S. R., Nierenberg, A. A., Warden, D., Ritz, L., et al. (2006). Evaluation of outcomes with citalopram for depression using measurement-based care in STAR*D: implications for clinical practice. *Am. J. Psychiatry* 163, 28–40. doi: 10.1176/appi.ajp.163.1.28

Vela, J., Gutierrez, A., Vitorica, J., and Ruano, D. (2003). Rat hippocampal GABAergic molecular markers are differentially affected by ageing. *J. Neurochem.* 85, 368–377. doi: 10.1046/j.1471-4159.2003.01681.x

Vepsalainen, S., Helisalmi, S., Koivisto, A. M., Tapaninen, T., Hiltunen, M., and Soininen, H. (2007). Somatostatin genetic variants modify the risk for Alzheimer's disease among Finnish patients. *J. Neurol.* 254, 1504–1508. doi: 10.1007/s00415-007-0539-2

Vezzani, A., and Hoyer, D. (1999). Brain somatostatin: a candidate inhibitory role in seizures and epileptogenesis. *Eur. J. Neurosci.* 11, 3767–3776. doi: 10.1046/j.1460-9568.1999.00838.x

Viollet, C., Lepousez, G., Loudes, C., Videau, C., Simon, A., and Epelbaum, J. (2008). Somatostatinergic systems in brain: networks and functions. *Mol. Cell. Endocrinol.* 286, 75–87. doi: 10.1016/j.mce.2007.09.007

Viollet, C., Vaillend, C., Videau, C., Bluet-Pajot, M. T., Ungerer, A., L'Héritier, A., et al. (2000). Involvement of sst2 somatostatin receptor in locomotor, exploratory activity and emotional reactivity in mice. *Eur. J. Neurosci.* 12, 3761–3770. doi: 10.1046/j.1460-9568.2000.00249.x

Wang, A. Y., Lohmann, K. M., Yang, C. K., Zimmerman, E. I., Pantazopoulos, H., Herring, N., et al. (2011). Bipolar disorder type 1 and schizophrenia are accompanied by decreased density of parvalbumin- and somatostatin-positive interneurons in the parahippocampal region. *Acta Neuropathol.* 122, 615–626. doi: 10.1007/s00401-011-0881-4

Wang, X. M., Tresham, J. J., Coghlan, J. P., and Scoggins, B. A. (1987). Intracerebroventricular infusion of a cyclic hexapeptide analogue of somatostatin inhibits hemorrhage-induced ACTH release. *Neuroendocrinology* 45, 325–327. doi: 10.1159/000124747

Warren, T. G., and Shields, D. (1984). Expression of preprosomatostatin in heterologous cells: biosynthesis, posttranslational processing, and secretion of mature somatostatin. *Cell* 39, 547–555. doi: 10.1016/0092-8674(84)90461-6

Weckbecker, G., Lewis, I., Albert, R., Schmid, H. A., Hoyer, D., and Bruns, C. (2003). Opportunities in somatostatin research: biological, chemical and therapeutic aspects. *Nat. Rev. Drug Discov.* 2, 999–1017. doi: 10.1038/nrd1255

Wei, J., Xu, H., Davies, J. L., and Hemmings, G. P. (1992). Increase of plasma IL-6 concentration with age in healthy subjects. *Life Sci.* 51, 1953–1956. doi: 10.1016/0024-3205(92)90112-3

Weiss, S. R., Nguyen, T., Rubinow, D. R., Helke, C. J., Narang, P. K., Post, R. M., et al. (1987). Lack of effect of chronic carbamazepine on brain somatostatin in the rat. *J. Neural. Transm.* 68, 325–333. doi: 10.1007/BF02098507

Wilson, N. R., Runyan, C. A., Wang, F. L., and Sur, M. (2012). Division and subtraction by distinct cortical inhibitory networks in vivo. *Nature* 488, 343–348. doi: 10.1038/nature11347

Xu, H., Jeong, H. Y., Tremblay, R., and Rudy, B. (2013). Neocortical somatostatin-expressing GABAergic interneurons disinhibit the thalamorecipient layer 4. *Neuron* 77, 155–167. doi: 10.1016/j.neuron.2012.11.004

Xu, X., Roby, K. D., and Callaway, E. M. (2010). Immunochemical characterization of inhibitory mouse cortical neurons: three chemically distinct classes of inhibitory cells. *J. Comp. Neurol.* 518, 389–404. doi: 10.1002/cne.22229

Xue, S., Jia, L., and Jia, J. (2009). Association between somatostatin gene polymorphisms and sporadic Alzheimer's disease in Chinese population. *Neurosci. Lett.* 465, 181–183. doi: 10.1016/j.neulet.2009.09.002

Yeung, M., Engin, E., and Treit, D. (2011). Anxiolytic-like effects of somatostatin isoforms SST 14 and SST 28 in two animal models (Rattus norvegicus) after intra-amygdalar and intra-septal microinfusions. *Psychopharmacology (Berl.)* 216, 557–567. doi: 10.1007/s00213-011-2248-x

Zeyda, T., Diehl, N., Paylor, R., Brennan, M. B., and Hochgeschwender, U. (2001). Impairment in motor learning of somatostatin null mutant mice. *Brain Res.* 906, 107–114. doi: 10.1016/S0006-8993(01)02563-X

Zeyda, T., and Hochgeschwender, U. (2008). Null mutant mouse models of somatostatin and cortistatin, and their receptors. *Mol. Cell. Endocrinol.* 286, 18–25. doi: 10.1016/j.mce.2007.11.029

Conflict of Interest Statement: The authors declare that the research was conducted in the absence of any commercial or financial relationships that could be construed as a potential conflict of interest.

6

Comorbid obsessive-compulsive symptoms in schizophrenia: contributions of pharmacological and genetic factors

Frederike Schirmbeck and Mathias Zink*

Central Institute of Mental Health, Department of Psychiatry and Psychotherapy, Faculty Medicine Mannheim, Heidelberg University, Mannheim, Germany

Edited by:
Maarten Van Den Buuse, Mental Health Research Institute, Australia

Reviewed by:
Bradley D. Pearce, Emory University, USA
Daniela Brunner, PsychoGenics, USA
Maarten Van Den Buuse, Mental Health Research Institute, Australia

****Correspondence:***
Mathias Zink, Central Institute of Mental Health, Department of Psychiatry and Psychotherapy, Medical Faculty Mannheim, Heidelberg University, PO Box 12 21 20, D-68072 Mannheim, Germany
e-mail: mathias.zink@zi-mannheim.de

A large subgroup of around 25% of schizophrenia patients suffers from obsessive-compulsive symptoms (OCS) and about 12% fulfill the diagnostic criteria of an obsessive-compulsive disorder (OCD). The additional occurrence of OCS is associated with high subjective burden of disease, additional neurocognitive impairment, poorer social and vocational functioning, greater service utilization and high levels of anxiety and depression. Comorbid patients can be assigned to heterogeneous subgroups. One hypothesis assumes that second generation antipsychotics (SGAs), most importantly clozapine, might aggravate or even induce second-onset OCS. Several arguments support this assumption, most importantly the observed chronological order of first psychotic manifestation, start of treatment with clozapine and onset of OCS. In addition, correlations between OCS-severity and dose and serum levels and duration of clozapine treatment hint toward a dose-dependent side effect. It has been hypothesized that genetic risk-factors dispose patients with schizophrenia to develop OCS. One study in a South Korean sample reported associations with polymorphisms in the gene *SLC1A1* (solute carrier family 1A1) and SGA-induced OCS. However, this finding could not be replicated in European patients. Preliminary results also suggest an involvement of polymorphisms in the *BDNF* gene (brain-derived neurotrophic factor) and an interaction between markers of *SLC1A1* and the gene *DLGAP3* (disc large associated protein 3) as well as GRIN2B (N-methyl-D-aspartate receptor subunit 2B). Further research of well-defined samples, in particular studies investigating possible interactions of genetic risk-constellations and pharmacodynamic properties, are needed to clarify the assumed development of SGA-induced OCS. Results might improve pathogenic concepts and facilitate the definition of at risk populations, early detection and monitoring of OCS as well as multimodal therapeutic interventions.

Keywords: antipsychotic agents, clozapine, comorbidity, compulsion, genetics, obsession, schizophrenia, SLC1A1

GENE AND ENVIRONMENT INTERACTIONS IN PSYCHIATRIC DISORDERS

Several frequent and disabling mental disorders manifest as a consequence of both genetic and environmental factors. Schizophrenia for instance is commonly perceived on the background of a gene-and-environment interaction (GxEI), where individual genetic properties dispose to a specific liability and sensitivity for specific stressors. These could include migration, other stressful life events, or effects of psychotropic substances (van Os and Kapur, 2009; van Os et al., 2008, 2010). Similar concepts were suggested regarding depression (Keers and Uher, 2012), anxiety disorders (Gregory et al., 2008; Nugent et al., 2011) and obsessive-compulsive disorder (OCD) (Nicolini et al., 2009; Pauls, 2010). Expanding the view to common comorbidities it is even more complex and demanding to investigate whether these might also be described on the basis of GxEI.

In this review we summarize evidence investigating possible pharmacological and genetic risk constellations underlying the co-occurrence of comorbid obsessive-compulsive symptoms (OCS) in schizophrenia.

EPIDEMIOLOGY OF OCS IN SCHIZOPHRENIA

Patients with schizophrenia have a high lifetime risk of about 25% for comorbid OCS and a recent meta-analysis reports that 12.1% also fulfill the criteria for an OCD (**Figure 1C**; Poyurovsky et al., 2004, 2012; Buckley et al., 2009; Lysaker and Whitney, 2009; Mukhopadhaya et al., 2009; Achim et al., 2011; Hadi et al., 2011). In contrast, prevalence rates of 1–2% for OCD in the general population are considerably lower (Murphy et al., 2010). Accordingly, primary OCD-patients carry a relatively low risk (1.7%) to develop comorbid psychotic symptoms (de Haan et al., 2009).

Abbreviations: AMS, amisulpride; APZ, aripiprazole; ARMS, at risk mental state; BDNF, brain derived neurotrophic factor; CBT, cognitive behavioral therapy; CLZ, clozapine; DLGAP3, disks large associated protein 3; GxEI: Gene and environment interaction; OCS, obsessive-compulsive symptoms; OCD, obsessive-compulsive disorder; OLZ, olanzapine; SGA, second generation antipsychotics; SLC1A1, solute carrier family gene 1A1; SNP, single nucleotide polymorphism; SSRI, selective serotonin reuptake inhibitor.

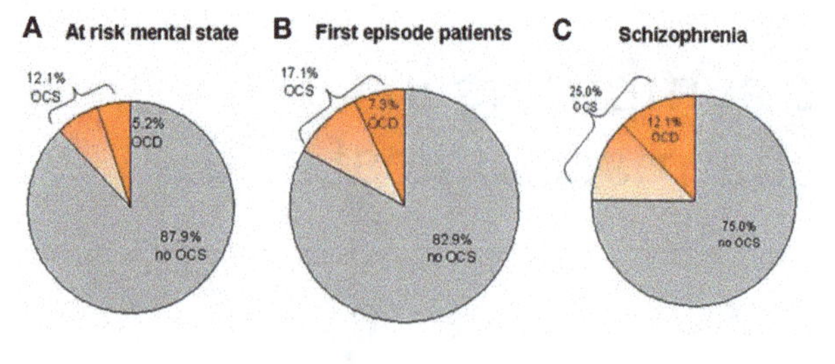

FIGURE 1 | Prevalence estimations of OCS and OCD within different samples of patients. (A) Mean prevalence rates in ARMS studies. **(B)** Mean prevalence rates in first-episode psychotic patients. **(C)** Mean prevalence rates in patients suffering from chronic schizophrenia.

Schizophrenia patients, who suffer from comorbid OCS often also display pronounced and sometimes treatment resistant positive and negative symptoms (Cunill et al., 2009; Sa et al., 2009). In addition, they present with specific neurocognitive deficits (Schirmbeck et al., 2012b), more often utilize health care services (Berman et al., 1995a), and show heightened levels of anxiety and depression (Lysaker and Whitney, 2009) when compared to schizophrenia patients without OCS. These pronounced impairments result in an additional burden of disease, in poorer social and vocational function (Fenton and McGlashan, 1986; Lysaker et al., 2004; Öngür and Goff, 2005; de Haan et al., 2013) and in a less favorable overall prognosis (Schirmbeck and Zink, 2013).

CLINICAL PRESENTATION AND EXPLANATORY CONCEPTS

Several heterogeneous subgroups of comorbid patients have been suggested depending on the diverse clinical course and phenotypic presentation. In order to unravel the specific interplay of genetic, psychosocial and pharmacological factors current research tries to focus on homogeneous subgroups. Subdivisions into such subgroups can for example be achieved according to the time point of first manifestation of comorbid OCS and the clinical course.

ONSET OF OCS

First onset of OCS has been described at different stages during the course of psychotic illness:

(1) Before psychosis as independent, co-existing symptoms or diagnosed OCD.
(2) Prior to psychotic manifestation as part of the at risk mental state (ARMS).
(3) Simultaneously with the first manifestation of psychosis.
(4) After the first psychotic episode during the course of chronic schizophrenia.
(5) As *de novo* OCS after initiation of antipsychotic treatment.

A remarkably large subgroup of patients already suffers from OCS during ARMS. Overall, sample-size weighted mean prevalence rates show that 12.1% (CI: 9.4–14.8%) of ARMS patients report OCS (Shioiri et al., 2007; Niendam et al., 2009; Bechdolf et al., 2011; Sterk et al., 2011; Hur et al., 2012), while 5.2% (CI: 4.1–6.3%) fulfill the criteria for OCD (Shioiri et al., 2007; Niendam et al., 2009; Rubino et al., 2009; Bechdolf et al., 2011; Fontenelle et al., 2011; DeVylder et al., 2012; Fusar-Poli et al., 2012; Sterk et al., 2011) (**Figure 1A**). Slightly higher averaged rates for OCS (17.1%, CI: 14.0–20.2) and OCD (7.3%, CI: 5.3–9.3%) can be found in first episode patients (**Figure 1B**; Poyurovsky et al., 1999a; de Haan et al., 2004; Sterk et al., 2011; de Haan et al., 2012; Zink et al., under review). Large variability of epidemiological data between studies can be explained by differences in the definition of ARMS criteria and differences in the psychometric assessment of OCS or OCD. Regarding the impact of OCS during the ARMS on other clinical variables, findings have been heterogeneous. Whereas higher impairment of psychosocial functioning (de Haan et al., 2012; DeVylder et al., 2012; Fusar-Poli et al., 2012; Hur et al., 2012) and more severe depressive symptoms (Niendam et al., 2009; DeVylder et al., 2012; Fontenelle et al., 2012; de Haan et al., 2013) have consistently been reported, findings regarding transition rates into psychosis (Niendam et al., 2009; Fontenelle et al., 2011, 2012; Fusar-Poli et al., 2012) and cognition (Van Dael et al., 2011){4854}(Hur et al., 2012) are contradicting.

Apart from OCS during the ARMS a growing body of evidence investigated the co-occurrence of OCS during manifest schizophrenia. A significant subgroup within these patients reports OCS development after treatment-start with second generation antipsychotic agents (SGA). The order of the three events "onset of psychosis," "start with SGA treatment" and subsequent "*de novo* development of OCS" hints toward the involvement of pharmacodynamic mechanisms (see **Figure 2E** and detailed description in section OCS induced by second-generation antipsychotics).

CLINICAL COURSE

In addition to varying time-points of first manifestation of OCS, the course of symptom severity over time also differs (**Figure 2**). OCS may appear as fluctuating symptoms, they may resolve, persist or even worsen over time. Within those patients who already reported manifest OCD prior to the psychotic illness, e.g., as adolescents, OCS will most likely persist or worsen independent of the course of schizophrenia (Hwang et al., 2009). Within those individuals who develop OCS sometime during the course of schizophrenia, only scarce longitudinal studies examined quantitative changes over time. One large investigation from the Netherlands followed participants over a period of 5 years and described a predominantly fluctuating course of OCS severity in over 70% of the comorbid sample: Some patients experienced the remission of OCS, others a fluctuating, more or less cyclic course, some reported first onset of OCS, whereas a forth group showed persisting symptom severity (Mahasuar et al., 2011). Another longitudinal study in a German sample investigated two pharmacological diverse groups and found persisting OCS severity over 12 months in the group treated with clozapine (CLZ) and olanzapine (OLZ) (Schirmbeck et al., 2012b, 2013). The diverse clinical course adds to the heterogeneous clinical presentation and suggests an involvement of different environmental factors and/or symptom interactions in the longitudinal development of comorbid OCS in schizophrenia (see section

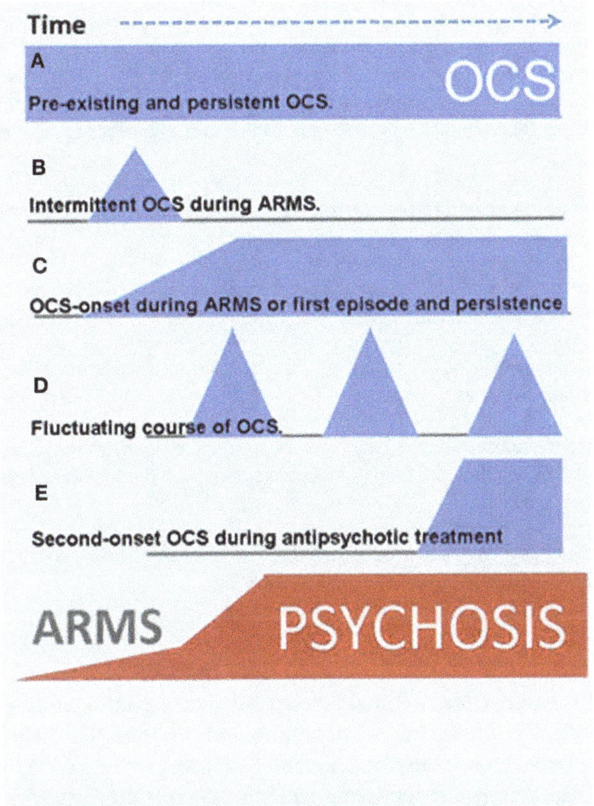

FIGURE 2 | OCS might manifest at different time points during the course of schizophrenia illness. In addition, the clinical course is highly variable. Blue symbols indicate the onset and severity of OCS, red ones are related to psychotic symptoms. **(A)** Pre-existing and persistent OCS. **(B)** Intermittent OCS during ARMS or later in the clinical course. **(C)** OCS-onset during ARMS and persistent course, strongly associated to the psychotic symptoms (schizo-obsessive concept). **(D)** Fluctuating course of OCS. **(E)** Second-onset OCS during antipsychotic treatment.

Underlying neurobiological mechanisms and environmental factors).

Furthermore, specific symptom dimensions of schizophrenia might overlap with the obsessive-compulsive phenotype (Fink and Taylor, 2001), making a careful differentiation and classification of presented symptoms necessary. Especially in cases of catatonic schizophrenia (Fink, 2013), a reliable assessment with established psychometric scales such as the catatonia rating scale (CRS) (Bräunig et al., 2000) and the Yale-Brown-Obsessive-Compulsive Scale (YBOCS) (Woody et al., 1995; de Haan et al., 2006) is often difficult. Historically, a more precise characterization was achieved by an undisguised view on the natural long-term course of schizophrenia, for instance published by Karl Leonhard (Beckmann et al., 2000). These descriptions allow clear discrimination between OCS and catatonic symptoms most importantly in patients with so-called "manneristic catatonia."

Clinical research and an improved pathogenic understanding of OCS in patients with schizophrenia is thus dependent on a careful exploration of symptoms. Several aspects help to discriminate delusions or hallucinations from typical OCS to ensure valid and reliable diagnosis (see **Table 1**).

PATHOGENIC CONCEPTS

In attempts to explain the co-occurrence of OCS in schizophrenia, heterogeneous, partly overlapping but also contradicting pathogenic concepts have been suggested.

The two rather common psychiatric syndromes could of course develop independently, representing a random association. Based on the above mentioned high prevalence rates and diverse clinical presentation this cannot be the only explanation for OCS in nearly every fourth patient with schizophrenia.

Early concepts assumed that patients with schizophrenia develop OCS as an attempt to reduce psychotic symptoms and thus, the presence of OCS was proposed to have protective effects regarding psychotic disintegration, based on single-case analyses or small case series (Stengel, 1945; Dowling et al., 1995). Similarly, Guillem et al. described negative correlations between specific OCS and the severity of psychotic disorganization in thinking and behavior, proposing compensating mechanisms (Guillem et al., 2009). However, in a broader perspective, subsequent research revealed higher severity of psychotic symptoms and more functional impairment if OCS were present (Cunill et al., 2009) (see above).

Approaching the co-occurrence from the OCD spectrum, the concept of "schizotypic OCD" has been described (Poyurovsky and Koran, 2005; Poyurovsky et al., 2008). This concept assumes that primary OCD-patients present beliefs, which can be classified on a spectrum between obsessions and delusions emphasizing the similarities as being irrational thoughts, the first with insight and the latter lacking insight. In line with this concept, the category of "obsessions without insight" was integrated into the fourth edition of the Diagnostic and Statistical Manual (DSM IV). OCD-patients without insight might therefore represent a subgroup with genetic, phenotypic and therapeutic vicinity to the schizophrenia-like spectrum (Tumkaya et al., 2009; Catapano et al., 2010).

Approaching the co-occurrence from the schizophrenia spectrum, a so-called "schizo-obsessive" subtype of psychosis has been proposed, based on cross-sectional evaluations (Poyurovsky, 2013). This subtype has been suggested to comprise OCS in addition to positive, negative and cognitive schizophrenia symptoms (Poyurovsky et al., 2012). Similar concepts have been proposed by Hwang et al. (2000), Bottas et al. (2005), and Reznik et al. (2001, 2005). Attempts to validate the "schizo-obsessive" subtype on a neurobiological level have been inconsistent. Some studies proposed specific neurological features (Sevincok et al., 2006; Poyurovsky et al., 2007b), cognitive deficits (Lysaker et al., 2002, 2009) and even structural abnormalities (Gross-Isseroff et al., 2003).

The mentioned high prevalence rates of OCS in the ARMS, led to the perception that specific OCS could be a part of the basic symptom cluster in the early course of schizophrenia (Sullwold and Huber, 1986; Ebel et al., 1989).

The summarized pathogenic concepts mirror the high degree of heterogeneity within the comorbid sample. They are currently discussed and the number of publications on this topic nearly doubles every year.

Table 1 | Identification of obsessive-compulsive symptoms in schizophrenia.

Insight-criterion	Patients suffering from OCD typically fulfill three symptom characteristics: they attribute the obsessions, impulsive symptoms and compulsions to their own thinking, declare with insight their unreasonableness and show some degree of resistance against them. In particular the first two properties allow a differentiation from hallucinations and delusions. Ruminations or stereotypic ego-dystonic cognitions with direct relation to the contents to psychotic thinking should not be diagnosed as obsessions.
OCS not solely related to the psychotic content	Cleaning or checking behavior should be diagnosed as compulsions only if it is accompanied by typical obsessions and not, if the patient currently suffers from delusions of contamination, intoxication or infection.
Re-evaluation of OCS after remission of psychotic symptoms	If first manifestation of OCS occurs simultaneously with the first psychotic exacerbation, the final decision on a valid comorbid condition should be postponed until the remission of psychotic symptoms.
Differentiation from catatonic symptoms	Repetitive behavior or stereotypic actions should carefully be discriminated from catatonic symptoms most importantly in patients with so-called "manieristic catatonia."
Obsessions presented as pseudohallucinations	A subgroups of OCS patients, who experience their obsessions as extremely aversive and burdening may try to distance themselves by using expressions such as "voices" or "foreign thought content", but in most cases these phenomena can be characterized as pseudohallucinations.
SGA-induced OCS	Patients without a previous history of OCS might develop these phenomena during antipsychotic treatment. This constellation hints toward the unfavorable effect of second-onset OCS induced by SGAs.

Clinical aspects that have to be considered when differentiating between psychotic symptoms (delusions, hallucinations) and OCS.

UNDERLYING NEUROBIOLOGICAL MECHANISMS AND ENVIRONMENTAL FACTORS

Neurobiology

While the described explanatory concepts mainly follow a clinical or psychopathological rationale, several investigations tried to improve the pathogenic understanding from a neurobiological perspective. So far, most emphasis has been given to a multimodal neurocognitive characterization. Preliminary investigations of neurological soft signs (Sevincok et al., 2006; Poyurovsky et al., 2007b) and neuroimaging techniques (Gross-Isseroff et al., 2003) need replication.

For primary OCD recent reviews of published literature reported specific cognitive deficits especially in the areas of cognitive shifting abilities, inhibitory control and the application of effective planning strategies (Kuelz et al., 2004). Based on these findings, the question arose whether OCS in schizophrenia might also be linked to additional cognitive impairment in these OCD-related domains (Lysaker and Whitney, 2009). Subsequently, several authors tried to differentiate schizophrenia samples with vs. without comorbid OCS on the basis of their neuropsychological performance. Findings have been contradicting. Whereas some investigations did not find any significant differences (Hermesh et al., 2003; Whitney et al., 2004; Öngür and Goff, 2005; Tumkaya et al., 2009; Tiryaki and Ozkorumak, 2010; Achim et al., 2011; Meijer et al., 2013), others even suggested that OCS may be associated with better cognitive abilities (Lee et al., 2009; Borkowska et al., 2013), especially in the prodromal states of schizophrenia (Van Dael et al., 2011; Fontenelle et al., 2012; Hur et al., 2012; Zink et al., under review). Most results, however, showed more pronounced deficits in the described domains of executive functioning (Hwang et al., 2000; Lysaker et al., 2002, 2009), cognitive flexibility (Kumbhani et al., 2010; Patel et al., 2010), and also delayed visual memory (Berman et al., 1998; Schirmbeck et al., 2011).

In a recent longitudinal assessment, Lysaker et al. prospectively analyzed executive functioning and reported that deficits were linked to greater concurrent and prospective self-report of OCS among schizophrenia patients (Lysaker et al., 2009). A comprehensive prospective investigation by Schirmbeck et al. explicitly included OCD-related cognitive domains in their analysis (Kuelz et al., 2004; Rajender et al., 2011). Over a period of 12 months schizophrenia patients with comorbid OCS showed significant pronounced deficits with increasing effect sizes regarding cognitive flexibility, visuo-spatial perception, and visual memory. Performance in these domains correlated with OCS severity (Schirmbeck et al., 2012b).

Based on these findings and with respect to possible causal pathways, it has been proposed that pronounced cognitive deficits reflect an underlying neurobiological risk factor for schizophrenia patients to develop OCS and mirror at least partially overlapping neurobiological mechanisms with OCD. In order to further substantiate this hypothesis neurobiological links that explain the pronounced deficits in the comorbid sample should be identified. Therefore, research should focus on candidate regions, which have been described in primary OCD, such as increased activation-levels in the orbitofrontal cortex (Whiteside et al., 2004; Friedlander and Desrocher, 2006)using fMRI approaches.

Regarding neurotransmission, current pathogenic theories of OCD assume a central serotonergic dysfunction in a network comprising cortical, striatal and thalamic centers (Pogarell et al., 2003). Corresponding evidence is provided by the therapeutic effects of selective serotonin reuptake inhibitors (SSRIs) and cognitive behavioral therapy (CBT) in OCD (Linden, 2006; Saxena et al., 2009). In addition, neuroimaging studies with structural and functional methods confirmed alterations in the suggested network (Friedlander and Desrocher, 2006; Menzies et al., 2008; Kwon et al., 2009a). Based on these findings it has been assumed that the strong serotonergic antagonism of CLZ

(Coward, 1992; Meltzer and Huang, 2008; Meltzer, 2012) and OLZ (Duggan et al., 2000) constitute a pathogenic mechanism in the development of second-onset OCS in schizophrenia (for more detail see section Epidemiological evidence and Pharmacological evidence). However, apart from serotonergic dysfunctions, alterations in dopaminergic activity (Van der Wee et al., 2004) and in glutamatergic neurotransmission, have also been related to OCD: Support for the involvement of glutamate in the development of OCD comes from animal models (Joel, 2006; Albelda et al., 2010; Yang and Lu, 2011), human MR spectroscopy (Whiteside et al., 2006; Starck et al., 2008), treatment approaches addressing the glutamatergic system (Coric et al., 2005; Poyurovsky et al., 2005, 2010; Lafleur et al., 2006; Pittenger et al., 2006) and the following results from genetic investigations.

Genetic disposition

Previous family and twin studies suggest a strong heritability of OCD (Nicolini et al., 2009; Pauls, 2010). In contrast, results from genetic association studies with a primary focus on candidate genes of serotonergic and dopaminergic neurotransmission were rather ambiguous. So far, only one linkage finding has consistently been replicated, which refers to single nucleotide polymorphisms (SNP) in the gene *SLC1A1* (solute carrier family) on chromosome 9p24, encoding the neuronal glutamate transporter EAAC1 (excitatory amino acid carrier 1) (Veenstra-VanderWeele et al., 2001; Arnold et al., 2006; Dickel et al., 2006; Stewart et al., 2007; Shugart et al., 2009; Wendland et al., 2009).

Possible neurogenetic disposition to develop OCS during the course of psychotic illness has just recently become a focus of interest. Research within this field is still scarce and needs further exploration. Progress has been achieved within a specific subgroup, suggesting a genetic disposition to develop OCS during SGA treatment (see section Genetic disposition).

Environmental factors

As briefly mentioned above, the majority of comorbid patients reports large fluctuation of OCS severity as either remitting, *de novo* development or intermittent OCS. However, the effect of environmental factors on onset or symptom severity as well as on interactions with other psychopathological processes has scarcely been investigated. Thus, the small number of longitudinal studies leaves important aspects unresolved. These include the following questions: (1) Do dynamic OCS and psychotic symptoms follow a parallel course? (2) Does a causal interaction of symptom variability exist? (3) Does experienced stress, life-events or antipsychotic medication influence the severity and course of OCS? Detailed follow-up analyses of the potential influence of environmental factors are therefore needed. Patients, who recently reported changes in their OCS should be investigated by means of an 'Experience Sampling Method' (ESM). This approach captures the reactivity to environmental factors and the course of symptoms in detail on a day to day basis, in real life situations, which allows to resolve symptom interactions and contextual triggers of variability. Results could provide the basis for individualized interventions, including adjusted modules of cognitive behavioral therapy (CBT).

Inconsistent results regarding associated neurobiological and environmental factors are most probably a consequence of the reported heterogeneity within the comorbid sample. Furthermore, methodological concerns such as the restriction to mainly cross-sectional evaluations and a lack of power due to small sample sizes add to inconclusive findings.

Thus, progress in pathogenic understanding seems most likely if future research focuses on the detailed characterization of homogeneous subsamples. One recent very promising approach has been achieved within the subgroup of patients who develop secondary OCS during SGA treatment. The following section summarizes evidence supporting the hypothesis of SGA-induced OCS and introduces possible genetic risk factors.

OCS INDUCED BY SECOND-GENERATION ANTIPSYCHOTICS

The subgroup of patients who report first onset or aggravation of OCS after psychotic manifestation and treatment initiation with SGAs has been briefly mentioned above. The simple assessment of the order of three important events (first psychotic manifestation, start of antipsychotic treatment and subsequent onset of OCS) helps to define this subgroup (Lykouras et al., 2003; Schirmbeck and Zink, 2012; Schirmbeck et al., 2013). The observation that schizophrenia patients develop OCS after psychotic manifestation and treatment initiation is mainly linked to SGAs and has rarely been reported under first generation antipsychotics. Several authors related this observation to the fact that SGAs carry the important pharmacodynamic feature of balanced antidopaminergic and antiserotonergic properties, which markedly exceed the low affinity of first generation antipsychotics to serotonergic receptors (Meltzer, 1995; Meltzer et al., 2003). In addition, differential effects on GABAergic and glutamatergic neurotransmission have to be considered (Lopez-Gil et al., 2010).

The hypothesis of SGA-induced OCS as a side-effect (Lykouras et al., 2003; Kwon et al., 2009b) first arose after the pioneer observations of Baker et al. (1992) and de Haan et al. (1999). Since then several studies show a clear association and possible causal interaction between SGA-treatment, most importantly CLZ (Schirmbeck and Zink, 2012), and the *de novo* occurrence of OCS (de Haan et al., 2004; Reznik et al., 2004; Kwon et al., 2009b; Schirmbeck et al., 2011).

Without a doubt, CLZ must be considered an indispensable part of the antipsychotic armament (Joober and Boksa, 2010; Kang and Simpson, 2010; Kane, 2011; Meltzer, 2012), especially in cases with otherwise treatment resistant psychoses (Kane et al., 1988). Several investigations (Asenjo Lobos et al., 2010) including the CATIE-study (McEvoy et al., 2006) have demonstrated its superior antipsychotic efficacy (Gupta and Daniel, 1995; Still et al., 1996; Kelly et al., 2003). Therefore, CLZ is considered the antipsychotic of first choice in treatment resistant schizophrenia. In addition, the substance demonstrates important anti-suicidal effects resulting in low mortality rates of CLZ-treated schizophrenia patients (Tiihonen et al., 2009). However, within a variety of other important side effects (Asenjo Lobos et al., 2010), the *de novo* occurrence or exacerbation of OCS under antipsychotic treatment has most often been observed with CLZ (Lykouras et al., 2003; Reznik et al., 2004; Schirmbeck and Zink, 2012). Due to a lack of controlled clinical trials, proposed causal interrelations cannot be confirmed, according to the general criteria suggested by Bradford Hill (2011). Nevertheless, several epidemiological (Epidemiological evidence) and pharmacological (Pharmacological evidence) arguments support this assumption (for summary see **Table 2**).

EPIDEMIOLOGICAL EVIDENCE

Increase of OCS prevalence after market approval of SGAs

Only few investigations reported comorbidity rates in samples treated with first generation antipsychotics (Fenton and McGlashan, 1986; Berman et al., 1995a,b; Nolfe et al., 2010). After market approval of SGAs, most importantly CLZ, in the 1970s in Europe and the late 1980s in the USA (Hippius, 1989; Kang and Simpson, 2010), prevalence estimations markedly rose. Although a potential publication bias and increased general awareness of this topic needs to be considered, these data provide a first indirect hint toward a possible interrelation.

Higher OCS prevalence during the chronic course of schizophrenia

As mentioned, prevalence estimations on OCS and OCD in ARMS and first episode samples clearly vary (see **Figure 1** and section Onset of OCS). However, when compared to established rates of 12% (OCD) and 25% (OCS) in chronic schizophrenia, they appear to be significantly smaller. The higher rates in the later stages of the disease might partly be attributed to antipsychotic treatment.

Onset of de novo OCS during antipsychotic treatment or marked aggravation

Several case reports and cases series, as well as systematic evaluations describe the *de novo* emergence of OCS during the treatment with atypical antipsychotics, most importantly CLZ (Schirmbeck and Zink, 2012). Poyurovski et al. estimated that up to 70% of schizophrenia patients treated with mainly antiserotonergic SGAs such as CLZ, OLZ or risperidone develop secondary OCS (Poyurovsky et al., 2004), while Lykouras et al. reviewed published data and even reported *de novo* OCS in 77% of CLZ treated patients (Lykouras et al., 2003). Independent studies reported high proportions of SGA-induced OCS within samples of comorbid patients: 25 of 28 (89%) (Schirmbeck et al., 2011), 29 of 39 (74%) (Lin et al., 2006) and 23 of 26 (88%) (Lim et al., 2007). Furthermore, retrospective assessments of the individual disease histories show that most patients experience the onset of OCS after first manifestation of psychosis and the start with SGA-treatment (Schirmbeck et al., 2012a) (**Figure 3**).

PHARMACOLOGICAL EVIDENCE

A variety of studies contribute to the assumption that antiserotonergic SGAs have pro-obsessive effects.

Higher prevalence of OCS in samples treated with CLZ

The risk for comorbid OCS markedly differs if patients are stratified according to their mode of antipsychotic treatment. As

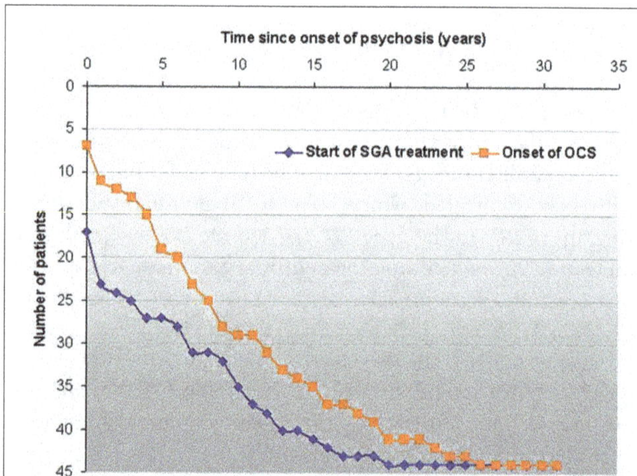

FIGURE 3 | In this sample of 44 comorbid patients the survival-curve shows the events "start of SGA treatment" and "first onset of OCS" on an individual basis related to the first manifestation of psychosis. The longitudinal course of OCS shows a high degree of variability and is not depicted here. The graphs shows that in all but 7 cases OCS developed subsequently to psychosis and the vast majority of patients reported OCS onset after treatment-start with SGAs (Schirmbeck et al., 2012a).

Table 2 | Arguments supporting SGA-induction of OCS.

Epidemiology	The prevalence rates of OCS in schizophrenia increased after market approval of clozapine (Schirmbeck and Zink, 2012). The comorbidity rates in later disease stages are higher than at first manifestation of schizophrenia (see **Figure 1**). Schizophrenia patients with comorbid OCS are most frequently found to be treated with clozapine. Vice versa high OCS prevalence in patients treated with clozapine (Poyurovsky et al., 2004; Lim et al., 2007; Poyurovsky et al., 2007a; Schirmbeck et al., 2011).
Pharmacology	The type of antipsychotic treatment is associated with the risk for OCS: Marked difference between samples treated with first generation antipsychotics or mainly dopaminergic SGAs (such as aripiprazole or amisulpride) compared to clozapine (Ertugrul et al., 2005; Sa et al., 2009; Schirmbeck et al., 2011). OCS manifest as a unfavorable drug effect *de novo* during treatment with potent antiserotonergic SGAs such as clozapine (see **Figure 3**) (Schirmbeck and Zink, 2012). The severity of OCS is positively correlated with duration, dosage and serum levels of clozapine treatment (Lin et al., 2006; Schirmbeck et al., 2011). The OCS severity is found stable over time in patients under stable clozapine treatment (Schirmbeck et al., 2013). The severity of OCS improves after reduction of clozapine dosage to minimally sufficient levels (due to augmentation or combination) (Rocha and Hara, 2006; Zink et al., 2006; Englisch et al., 2009).

Summary of epidemiological and pharmacological arguments supporting the assumption that OCS can be induced or at least markedly aggravated by SGA-treatment as an unfavorable side effect (Schirmbeck et al., 2012b).

reported, high prevalence rates in CLZ-treated patients (Ertugrul et al., 2005), contrast with low rates during treatment with first generation antipsychotics, for instance, haloperidol (Sa et al., 2009) or other SGAs. Differences in pharmacodynamic properties, in particular regarding inherent serotonergic blockade, monoaminergic reuptake inhibition or even partial serotonergic agonism might explain these diverging findings (Shapiro et al., 2003; Meltzer and Huang, 2008; Meltzer and Sumiyoshi, 2008; Remington, 2008; Lopez-Gil et al., 2010). Interestingly, Aripiprazole (APZ), a partial dopaminergic and serotonergic agonist, was associated with an inherent anti-obsessive effect in schizophrenia patients with OCS (Connor et al., 2005; Zink et al., 2006; Chang et al., 2008; Englisch and Zink, 2008; Englisch et al., 2009), quite similar to amisulpride (AMS), a dopamine D3/D2 receptor antagonist (Kim et al., 2008; Pani et al., 2008). A comparison of schizophrenia patients under antipsychotic monotherapy with either mainly antiserotonergic SGAs (CLZ or OLZ; group I) or mainly dopaminergic SGAs (AMS or APZ; group II) revealed that more than 70% of group-I-patients suffered from OCS while less than 10% of patients in group-II reported OCS (Schirmbeck et al., 2011). *Vice versa*, a stratification of schizophrenia patients according to presence or absence of comorbid OCS revealed that 77% of comorbid patients were treated with clozapine while only 36% of schizophrenia patients without OCS received this substance (Lim et al., 2007). These results clearly suggest an association between CLZ treatment and comorbid OCS. However, a possible confounding effect due to the selection of specific SGAs for specific subgroups of patients has to be considered.

Noteworthy, in some cases an alleviation of OCS severity after the addition of CLZ (Peters and de, 2009), an increase in CLZ dosage (Lykouras et al., 2003) or start with OLZ treatment (van Nimwegen et al., 2008; Poyurovsky, 2013) has been observed. Regarding these contradicting findings, some important aspects should be discussed. One explanation relates to the above mentioned diagnostic difficulties to differentiation between OCS and delusional or catatonic symptoms (**Table 1**). Patients with schizophrenia, who show obsessive ruminations or stereotypic thoughts during acute psychosis or repetitive ritualized behavior clearly related to the patient's primary psychotic condition might indeed benefit from treatment with CLZ. Thus, careful diagnostic evaluations are necessary. Furthermore, anti-obsessive effects of antipsychotics have also been reported in primary OCD, including OLZ, especially in cases with treatment-resistance to serotonergic antidepressants (Bloch et al., 2006; Bandelow et al., 2008; Dold et al., 2011; Muscatello et al., 2011). Nevertheless, even in treatment-resistant OCD current treatment guidelines do not recommend CLZ as an augmentation strategy.

Associations between the duration of treatment and OCS severity

Correlations between pharmacological variables and OCS provide further support for proposed causal interactions. Lin et al. (2006) compared CLZ-treated patients with and without comorbid OCS and found significantly longer CLZ treatment periods for the comorbid group, but no difference in duration of illness. Schirmbeck et al. reported a positive correlation between OCS severity and duration of CLZ-treatment (Schirmbeck et al., 2011). Accordingly, de Haan et al. reported this association for OLZ (de Haan et al., 2002).

ASSOCIATION BETWEEN DOSAGE AND BLOOD SERUM LEVELS AND OCS SEVERITY

Several authors demonstrated positive correlations between dose or serum levels of CLZ and severity of OCS (Lin et al., 2006; Reznik et al., 2004; Mukhopadhaya et al., 2009; Schirmbeck et al., 2011). Similarly, a reduction of daily CLZ-dosage, for instance through the combinations with another SGA, such as APZ, resulted in an alleviation of OCS severity (Rocha and Hara, 2006; Zink et al., 2006; Englisch et al., 2009). This observed effect might represent both a reduction of the suggested dose-related side effect of CLZ and/or a consequence of inherent anti-obsessive effects of APZ due to its partial dopaminergic and serotonergic agonism. The latter assumption was supported by a *placebo* controlled randomized trial, which showed reduced OCS severity after combination with APZ, but unchanged CLZ dose during the course of the study (Chang et al., 2008).

Differential effects of SGAs on the course of OCS

A recent longitudinal study revealed differential effects of antipsychotic agents on comorbid OCS. Within a 12 months observational period, changes in YBOCS scores significantly differed between two pharmacologically diverse groups (completer analysis: $p = 0.006$; full sample analysis: $p = 0.007$). Whereas the CLZ/OLZ group showed persistently high OCS severity over time, the AMS/APZ group reported further decrease of the initially low YBOCS-scores (Schirmbeck et al., 2013).

In conclusion, reported data show strong associations between comorbid OCS in schizophrenia and mainly antiserotonergic SGAs, most importantly CLZ. The published epidemiological and pharmacological evidence hint toward causal interactions, suggesting CLZ's strong inherent antiserotonergic properties (Steingard et al., 1993; Joober and Boksa, 2010; Kang and Simpson, 2010), most importantly the antagonism at 5-HT1C, 5-HT2A and 5HT2C receptors (Coward, 1992; Meltzer, 1994; Meltzer and Huang, 2008) as an relevant underlying mechanism. Low affinities to dopamine receptors result in a very small ratio of dopaminergic/serotonergic receptor blockade, which largely differs from SGAs such as AMS or APZ (Scatton et al., 1997; Shapiro et al., 2003; Correll, 2008). In addition, reciprocal interactions of dopaminergic and serotonergic neurotransmission with glutamatergic and GABAergic functions might play an important role (Lopez-Gil et al., 2010). Thus, pharmacotherapy constitutes a relevant environmental factor, which might exert pro-obsessive effects in schizophrenia patients. Within a broader perspective, additional questions arise concerning predisposing factors. These might comprise patient-inherent characteristics (neurocognitive profile, the subtype of psychosis, the stage of the illness, any kind of affective comorbidity or a family history for anxiety disorders) and the individual genetic disposition.

GENETIC DISPOSITION

Associations with the gene *SLC1A1* have consistently been replicated in primary OCD patients. Based on these findings a South Korean research group investigated the genetic risk to develop second-onset OCS during treatment with SGAs (Kwon et al., 2009b). Kwon et al evaluated associations between specific SNPs of the candidate gene *SLC1A1* and SGA-induced OCS and showed strong associations with the A/C/G dominant haplotype rs2228622 / rs3780413 / rs37801412. The odds ratio of 3.96 indicated an almost 4 times higher likelihood for patients, who carried this A/C/G haplotype to suffer from SGA-induced OCS. Neither the gene *SLC1A1* nor its chromosomal region has been associated with vulnerability to schizophrenia spectrum disorders (Deng et al., 2007). The same group further described a genetic interaction of the *SLC1A1* polymorphism with variants in the gene *DLGAP3* (disks large associated protein 3) and a link to SGA-induced OCS (Ryu et al., 2011). In addition, Cai et al reported on an interaction of SNPs in SLC1A1 and the type 2B subunit of the N-methyl-D-aspartate receptor gene (GRIN2B), as well as interactions with the YBOCS score in Chinese patients (Cai et al., 2013).

A replication approach of the results obtained by Kwon et al. (2009b) was conducted in 103 schizophrenia patients of European descent treated with SGAs. However, the described finding could not be reproduced, neither in single marker, nor in haplotype analyses. Because no genetic associations between *SLC1A1* polymorphisms and OCS were found within the power limits of this study, much larger samples seem necessary to untangle the interplay of pharmacological and genetic risk factors for OCS in schizophrenia (Schirmbeck et al., 2012a). The brain derived neurotrophic factor (*BDNF*) was recently proposed as a third candidate gene, because the Val66Met polymorphism was found to be associated with OCS in schizophrenia (Hashim et al., 2012). So far, independent replication approaches regarding *BDNF*, *DLGAP3* and GRIN2B have not been conducted.

RESEARCH PERSPECTIVES

GxEI ON A SECOND LEVEL OF COMPLEXITY

GxEIs are core elements within current theories of schizophrenia (van Os and Kapur, 2009; van Os et al., 2008, 2010), depression (Keers and Uher, 2012), anxiety disorders (Gregory et al., 2008; Nugent et al., 2011) and OCD (Nicolini et al., 2009; Pauls, 2010). High rates of bi-directional comorbidities lead to the obvious question, if these co-occurrences could also be explained by common GxEIs. One example of this experimental psychopathology has been illustrated by the described investigation of the risk to develop secondary OCS during treatment with SGAs. Here, the environmental factor is represented in the pharmacological treatment of schizophrenia with pro-obsessive SGAs.

As stated in chapter 4, SGAs increase the risk for secondary OCS via a pharmacodynamic mechanism. Independently, a set of SNPs within the gene *SLC1A1* seem to predispose to OCD. However, the initially reported high odds ratio by Kwon et al. (2009b) could not be replicated in a similar study performed with European patients (Schirmbeck et al., 2012a). Thus, the general genetic background of a patient (Asian or European) might be of importance when a specific SGA (balance between dopaminergic and serotonerigic blockade) is introduced as the treatment of choice. Furthermore, gene-x-gene interactions (SNPs in *SLC1A1*, *BDNF*, DLGAP3, and GRIN2B) have been suggested as further influencing factors (Ryu et al., 2011; Hashim et al., 2012) and should be considered in forthcoming studies. It is an important progress in recent neurobiological research to investigate how the interaction of these factors might influence the propensity of schizophrenia patients to suffer from comorbid OCS when being treated with SGAs.

Future progress might depend on two aspects: First, well defined homogeneous clinical cohorts should be defined to reduce the number of possible confounding causal factors to a minimum. Considering the order of symptom onset, the clinical course and the applied treatment for sample characterization might be helpful. Second, much larger cohorts have to be recruited in multicenter studies to investigate possible genetic risk constellations. If power analyses would be based on the much smaller genetic-risk estimations for the gene *SLC1A1* in the European sample (Schirmbeck et al., 2012a), group size calculations result in about five thousand participants, which would be necessary for replication.

Besides pharmacological treatment as a relevant factor, further non-pharmacological environmental factors could play an important role in the development of OCS in schizophrenia. Such factors might include, psychosocial stress induced by critical life events, interpersonal factors, changes of the vocational situation or the present state of general physical health. In addition, the reciprocal interaction and possible causal directions between OCS and psychotic positive, negative and cognitive symptoms of schizophrenia must be unraveled and considered. One important tool to unravel the interdependence of these variables are the above described experience sampling approaches. These allow to investigate the individual symptom variability in real life situations on a day to day basis.

Collected data will help to identify the time course of symptom-changes and its relation to important environmental factors. These studies are currently planned and will hopefully result in an improved understanding of etiological factors influencing the course of OCS in schizophrenia. Within this context it will also be desirable to collect DNA samples in order to analyse possible predisposing effects of the above mentioned polymorphisms to experience the development or aggravation of OCS after being exposed to stressful life events. Thus, combining experience sampling and genetic characterizations might markedly improve our insight into GxEI.

THERAPY

At present, pharmacological treatment interventions, most importantly combination as well as augmentation strategies, have been suggested to improve OCS in the highly impaired comorbid group (Schirmbeck et al., 2013). To address possible pro-obsessive effects of predominantly anti-serotonergic SGAs, the add-on of mainly dopaminergic SGAs such as AMS and APZ has been proposed (Connor et al., 2005; Zink et al., 2006; Englisch and Zink, 2008; Kim et al., 2008; Yang et al., 2008; Englisch et al., 2009; Muscatello et al., 2011). In addition, the augmentation with serotonergic antidepressants has been evaluated, for example with the tricyclic antidepressant clomipramine (Berman et al., 1995b) or with SSRIs, most often fluvoxamine (Poyurovsky et al., 1999b; Reznik and Sirota, 2000; Hwang et al., 2009). Results of these trials have been inconsistent with some studies failing to observe the

Table 3 | Therapeutic approaches.

Early recognition and monitoring	Definition of at-risk-constellations. Monitoring of subclinical levels of OCS or beginning cognitive impairment using sensitive sets of neurocognitive tests (Schirmbeck et al., 2011, 2012b).
Polypharmacy	Augmentation with antidepressants: Clomipramine, fluvoxamine and other SSRIs. [Level of evidence: RCTs, CS, CR] (Berman et al., 1995b; Poyurovsky et al., 1999b; Reznik and Sirota, 2000). Caveat: Additive (anticholinergic) side effects and pharmacokinetic interactions Augmentation with mood stabilizers (lamotrigine, valproic acid) aiming at a reduction of SGA-dosage to minimally sufficient levels [Level of evidence: CS, CR] (Zink et al., 2007; Poyurovsky et al., 2010; Rodriguez et al., 2010; Canas et al., 2012). Combination of pro-obsessive SGAs with neutral or anti-obsessive SGAs (amisulpride, aripiprazole) in order to reduce the clozapine-dosage to minimally sufficient levels [Level of evidence: RCT, CS, CR]. (Connor et al., 2005; Zink et al., 2006; Englisch and Zink, 2008; Kim et al., 2008; Yang et al., 2008; Englisch et al., 2009; Muscatello et al., 2011)
Psychotherapy	Cognitive behavioral therapy involving exposure and response prevention [Level of evidence: CS, CR] (Schirmbeck and Zink, 2012; Tundo et al., 2012).

Summary of therapeutic approaches for schizophrenia patients with comorbid OCS or OCD. The current level of empirical evidence is indicated in square brackets. Abbreviations: CR, case report; CS, case series; RCT, randomized controlled trial.

intended effects of OCS reduction. Furthermore, additive anticholinergic side effects and pharmacokinetic interactions have to be considered. Finally, first promising results were published reporting on the augmentation with mood stabilizers such as valproic acid (Zink et al., 2007; Canas et al., 2012) or lamotrigine (Poyurovsky et al., 2010; Rodriguez et al., 2010).

So far, very limited data exists on the efficacy and safety of cognitive behavioral therapy (CBT) for this group of patients. The small number of case reports and case series can hardly be reconciled with the fact, that CBT including exposure and response prevention is considered treatment of first choice for primary OCD with remarkably high effect sizes (Gava et al., 2007; Koran et al., 2007; Rosa-Alcazar et al., 2008; Kuelz and Voderholzer, 2011). With one exception, currently available CBT manuals for OCD do not provide guidelines for the treatment of OCS in schizophrenia (Emmelkamp and van Oppen, 2000; Lakatos and Reinecker, 2007; Oelkers et al., 2007; Foerstner et al., 2011). However, a summary of the published reports on 30 comorbid patients (Schirmbeck et al., 2013), who were treated with CBT including exposure elements or just exposure and response prevention alone showed favorable outcome measures with significant reduction of OCD severity in 24 patients. In the included case series by Tundo et al. (2012) 52% of investigated individuals were classified as "much or very much" improved, 33% as responders and 19% as remitters. The available evidence of CBT for OCS in schizophrenia is certainly limited by the small case numbers and further controlled clinical trials are needed. However, despite adverse clinical outcomes in 10%, and a total dropout rate of 20%, preliminary results suggest meaningful and marked reduction of OCS severity in 80% of participants (Schirmbeck et al., 2013). **Table 3** summarizes possible pharmacological and non-pharmacological approaches and current evidence of empirical support.

CONCLUSIONS

The summarized data substantiate the conclusions that OCS is a very frequent and relevant comorbid burden in schizophrenia. The clinical presentation of the co-occurrence is very diverse, suggesting different subgroups with heterogeneous pathogenic mechanisms. First insight into GxEI has been achieved for the subgroup of patients who experienced second-onset OCS during treatment with SGAs. In the future, a broader set of environmental variables, including non-pharmacological factors, and further genetic risk-constellations should be analysed, starting in the ARMS. In perspective, this will not only improve the risk prediction regarding comorbid OCS, but also early recognition and monitoring of emerging symptoms. Research within this field will further provide the individual framework of predisposing and disease-provoking factors with immediate impact for pharmacological and CBT approaches.

REFERENCES

Achim, A. M., Maziade, M., Raymond, E., Olivier, D., Merette, C., and Roy, M. A. (2011). How prevalent are anxiety disorders in schizophrenia? A meta-analysis and critical review on a significant association. *Schizophr. Bull.* 37, 811–821. doi: 10.1093/schbul/sbp148

Albelda, N., Bar-On, N., and Joel, D. (2010). The role of NMDA receptors in the signal attenuation rat model of obsessive-compulsive disorder. *Psychopharmacology* 210, 13–24. doi: 10.1007/s00213-010-1808-9

Arnold, P. D., Sicard, T., Burroughs, E., Richter, M. A., and Kennedy, J. L. (2006). Glutamate transporter gene SLC1A1 associated with obsessive-compulsive disorder. *Arch. Gen. Psychiatry* 63, 769–776. doi: 10.1001/archpsyc.63.7.769

Asenjo Lobos, C., Komossa, K., Rummel-Kluge, C., Hunger, H., Schmid, F., Schwarz, S., et al. (2010). Clozapine versus other atypical antipsychotics for schizophrenia. *Cochrane Database Syst. Rev.* 11:CD006633. doi: 10.1002/14651858.CD006633.pub2

Baker, R. W., Chengappa, K. N., Baird, J. W., Steingard, S., Christ, M. A., and Schooler, N. R. (1992). Emergence of obsessive compulsive symptoms during treatment with clozapine. *J. Clin. Psychiatry* 53, 439–442. doi: 10.1080/15622970802465807

Bandelow, B., Zohar, J., Hollander, E., Kasper, S., ller, H. J., WFSBP Task Force on Treatment Guidelines for Anxiety, O.-C. a. P.-T. S. D., et al. (2008). World Federation of Societies of Biological Psychiatry (WFSBP) guidelines for the pharmacological treatment of anxiety, obsessive-compulsive and post-traumatic stress disorders - first revision. *World J. Biol. Psychiatry* 9, 248–312. doi: 10.1080/15622970802465807

Bechdolf, A., Mueller, H., Stoetzer, H., Wagner, M., Maier, W., Lautenschlager, M., et al. (2011). Rationale and baseline characteristics of PREVENT: a second-generation intervention trial in subjects at-risk (Prodromal) of developing first-episode psychosis evaluating cognitive behavior therapy, aripiprazole, and placebo for the prevention of psychosis. *Schizophr. Bull.* 37, S111–S121. doi: 10.1093/schbul/sbr083

Beckmann, H., Bartsch, A. J., Neumärker, K.-J., Pfuhlmann, B., Verdaguer, M. F., and Franzek, E. (2000). Schizophrenias in the Wernicke-Kleist-Leonhard school. *Am. J. Psychiatry* 157, 1024–1025. doi: 10.1176/appi.ajp.157.6.1024-a

Berman, I., Kalinowski, A., Berman, S. M., Lengua, J., and Green, A. I. (1995a). Obsessive and compulsive symptoms in chronic schizophrenia. *Compr. Psychiatry* 36, 6–10. doi: 10.1016/0010-440X(95)90092-A

Berman, I., Sapers, B. L., Chang, H. H., Losonczy, M. F., Schmildler, J., and Green, A. I. (1995b). Treatment of obsessive-compulsive symptoms in schizophrenic patients with clomipramine. *J. Clin. Psychopharmacol.* 15, 206–210. doi: 10.1097/00004714-199506000-00009

Berman, I., Merson, A., Viegner, B., Losonczy, M. F., Pappas, D., and Green, A. I. (1998). Obsessions and compulsions as a distinct cluster of symptoms in schizophrenia: a neuropsychological study. *J. Nerv. Ment. Dis.* 186, 150–156. doi: 10.1097/00005053-199803000-00003

Bloch, M. H., Landeros-Weisenberger, A., Kelmendi, B., Coric, V., Bracken, M. B., and Leckman, J. F. (2006). A systematic review: antipsychotic augmentation with treatment refractory obsessive-compulsive disorder. *Mol. Psychiatry* 11, 622–632. doi: 10.1038/sj.mp.4001823

Borkowska, A., Pilaczynska, E., and Rybakowski, J. K. (2013). The frontal lobe neuropsychological tests in patients with schizophrenia and/or obsessive-compulsive disorder. *J. Neuropsychiatry Clin. Neurosci.* 15, 359–362. doi: 10.1176/appi.neuropsych.15.3.359

Bottas, A., Cooke, R. G., and Richter, M. A. (2005). Comorbidity and pathophysiology of obsessive-compulsive disorder in schizophrenia: is there evidence for a schizo-obsessive subtype of schizophrenia? *J. Psychiatry Neurosci.* 30, 187–193.

Bradford Hill, A. (2011). The environment and disease: association or causation? *Bull. World Health Organ.* 83, 295–300.

Bräunig, P., Krüger, S., Shugar, G., Höffler, J., and Börner, I. (2000). The catatonia rating scale I–development, reliability, and use. *Compr. Psychiatry* 41, 147–158. doi: 10.1016/S0010-440X(00)90148-2

Buckley, P. F., Miller, B. J., Lehrer, D. S., and Castle, D. J. (2009). Psychiatric comorbidities and schizophrenia. *Schizophr. Bull.* 35, 383–402. doi: 10.1093/schbul/sbn135

Cai, J., Zhang, W., Lu, W., Wu, Z., Chen, J., Yu, S., et al. (2013). Influence of polymorphisms in genes SLC1A1, GRIN2B, and GRIK2 on clozapine-induced obsessive-compulsive symptoms. *Psychopharmacology.* doi: 10.1007/s00213-013-3137-2. [Epub ahead of print].

Canas, F., Aydinoglu, U., and Sinani, G. (2012). Valproic acid augmentation in clozapine-associated hand-washing compulsion. *Psychiatry Clin. Neurosci.* 66, 463–464. doi: 10.111/j.14440-1819.2012.02361.x

Catapano, F., Perris, F., Fabrazzo, M., Cioffi, V., Giacco, D., De, S., et al. (2010). Obsessive-compulsive disorder with poor insight: a three-year prospective study. *Prog. Neuro-Psychopharmacol. Biol. Psychiatry* 34, 323–330. doi: 10.1016/j.pnpbp.2009.12.007

Chang, J. S., Ahn, Y.-M., Park, H. J., Lee, K. Y., Kim, S. H., Kang, U. G., et al. (2008). Aripiprazole augmentation in clozapine-treated patients with refractory schizophrenia: an 8-week, randomized, double-blind, placebo-controlled trial. *J. Clin. Psychiatry* 69, 720–731. doi: 10.4088/JCP.v69n0505

Connor, K. M., Payne, V. M., Gadde, K. M., Zhang, W., Davidson, J. R., Connor, K. M., et al. (2005). The use of aripiprazole in obsessive-compulsive disorder: preliminary observations in 8 patients. *J. Clin. Psychiatry* 66, 49–51. doi: 10.4088/JCP.v66n0107

Coric, V., Taskiran, S., Pittenger, C., Wasylink, S., Mathalon, D. H., Valentine, G., et al. (2005). Riluzole augmentation in treatment-resistant obsessive-compulsive disorder: an open-label trial. *Biol. Psychiatry* 58, 424–428. doi: 10.1016/j.biopsych.2005.04.043

Correll, C. U. (2008). Antipsychotic polypharmacy, part 2: why use 2 antipsychotics when 1 is not good enough? *J. Clin. Psychiatry* 69, 860–861. doi: 10.4088/JCP.v69n0521

Coward, D. M. (1992). General pharmacology of clozapine. *Br. J. Psychiatry Suppl.* 17, 5–11.

Cunill, R., Castells, X., and Simeon, D. (2009). Relationships between obsessive-compulsive symptomatology and severity of psychosis in schizophrenia: a systematic review and meta-analysis. *J. Clin. Psychiatry* 70, 70–82. doi: 10.4088/JCP.07r03618

de Haan, L., Beuk, N., Hoogenboom, B., Dingemans, P., and Linszen, D. (2002). Obsessive-compulsive symptoms during treatment with olanzapine and risperidone: a prospective study of 113 patients with recent-onset schizophrenia or related disorders. *J. Clin. Psychiatry* 63, 104–107. doi: 10.4088/JCP.v63n0203

de Haan, L., Dudek-Hodge, C., Verhoeven, Y., and Denys, D. (2009). Prevalence of psychotic disorders in patients with obsessive-compulsive disorder. *CNS Spectr.* 14, 415–417.

de Haan, L., Hoogeboom, B., Beuk, N., Wouters, L., Dingemans, P. M., and Linszen, D. H. (2006). Reliability and validity of the Yale-Brown Obsessive-Compulsive Scale in schizophrenia patients. *Psychopharmacol. Bull.* 39, 25–30.

de Haan, L., Linszen, D. H., and Gorsira, R. (1999). Clozapine and obsessions in patients with recent-onset schizophrenia and other psychotic disorders. *J. Clin. Psychiatry* 60, 364–365. doi: 10.4088/JCP.v60n0603

de Haan, L., Oekeneva, A., van, A. T., and Linszen, D. (2004). Obsessive-compulsive disorder and treatment with clozapine in 200 patients with recent-onset schizophrenia or related disorders. *Eur. Psychiatry* 19, 524. doi: 10.1016/j.eurpsy.2004.09.022

de Haan, L., Sterk, B., and van der Valk, R. (2012). Presence of obsessive compulsive symptoms in first-episode schizophrenia or related disorders is associated with subjective well-being and quality of life. *Early Interv. Psychiatry* 7, 285–290. doi: 10.1111/j.1751-7893.2012.00377.x

de Haan, L., Sterk, B., Wouters, L., and Linszen, D. H. (2013). The 5-year course of obsessive-compulsive symptoms and obsessive-compulsive disorder in first-episode schizophrenia and related disorders. *Schizophr. Bull.* 39, 151–160. doi: 10.1093/schbul/sbr077

Deng, X., Shibata, H., Takeuchi, N., Rachi, S., Sakai, M., Ninomiya, H., et al. (2007). Association study of polymorphisms in the glutamate transporter genes SLC1A1, SLC1A3, and SLC1A6 with schizophrenia. *Am. J. Med. Genet.* 144B, 271–278. doi: 10.1002/ajmg.b.30351

DeVylder, J. E., Oh, A. J., Ben-David, S., Azimov, N., Harkavy-Friedman, J. M., and Corcoran, C. M. (2012). Obsessive compulsive symptoms in individuals at clinical risk for psychosis: Association with depressive symptoms and suicidal ideation. *Schizophrenia Res.* 140, 110–113. doi: 10.1016/j.schres.2012.07.009

Dickel, D. E., Veenstra-VanderWeele, J., Cox, N. J., Wu, X., Fischer, D. J., Van Etten-Lee, M., et al. (2006). Association testing of the positional and functional candidate gene SLC1A1/EAAC1 in early-onset obsessive-compulsive disorder. *Arch. Gen. Psychiatry* 63, 778–785. doi: 10.1001/archpsyc.63.7.778

Dold, M., Aigner, M., Lanzenberger, R., and Kasper, S. (2011). Efficacy of antipsychotic augmentation therapy in treatment-resistant obsessive-compulsive disorder a meta-analysis of double-blind, randomised, placebo-controlled trials. *Fortschr. Neurol. Psychiatr.* 79, 453–466. doi: 10.1055/s-0031-1273397

Dowling, F. G., Pato, M. T., and Pato, C. N. (1995). Comorbidity of obsessive-compulsive and psychotic symptoms: a review. *Harv. Rev. Psychiatry* 3, 75–83. doi: 10.3109/10673229509017170

Duggan, L., Fenton, M., Dardennes, R. M., El-Dosoky, A., and Indran, S. (2000). Olanzapine for schizophrenia. *Cochrane Database Syst. Rev.* 2:CD001359. doi: 10.1002/14651858.CD001359

Ebel, H., Gross, G., Klosterkotter, J., Huber, G., Ebel, H., Gross, G., et al. (1989). Basic symptoms in schizophrenic and affective psychoses. *Psychopathology* 22, 224–232. doi: 10.1159/000284602

Emmelkamp, P. M. G., and van Oppen, P. (2000). *Zwangsstoerungen.* Göttingen: Hogrefe.

Englisch, S., Esslinger, C., Inta, D., Weinbrenner, A., Peus, V., Gutschalk, A., et al. (2009). Clozapine-induced obsessive compulsive syndromes improve in combination with aripiprazole. *Clin. Neuropharmacol.* 32, 227–229. doi: 10.1097/WNF.0b013e31819cc8e6

Englisch, S., and Zink, M. (2008). Combined antipsychotic treatment involving clozapine and aripiprazole. *Prog. Neuropsychopharmacol.*

Biol. Psychiatry 32, 1386–1392. doi: 10.1016/j.pnpbp.2008.02.010

Ertugrul, A., nil Yagcioglu, A. E., Eni, N., and Yazici, K. M. (2005). Obsessive-compulsive symptoms in clozapine-treated schizophrenic patients. *Psychiatry Clin. Neurosci.* 59, 219–222. doi: 10.1111/j.1440-1819.2005.01362.x

Fenton, W. S., and McGlashan, T. H. (1986). The prognostic significance of obsessive-compulsive symptoms in schizophrenia. *Am. J. Psychiatry* 143, 437–441.

Fink, M., and Taylor, M. A. (2001). The many varieties of catatonia. *Eur. Arch. Psychiatry Clin. Neurosci.* 251(Suppl. 1), I8–13. doi: 10.1007/PL00014200

Fink, M. (2013). Rediscovering catatonia: the biography of a treatable syndrome. *Acta Psychiatr. Scand. Suppl.* 127, 1–47. doi: 10.1111/acps.12038

Foerstner, U., Anne Marie, K., and Ulrich, V. (2011). *Störungsspezifische Behandlung der Zwangsstörungen: Ein Therapiemanual.* Stuttgart: Kohlhammer.

Fontenelle, L. F., Lin, A., Pantelis, C., Wood, S. J., Nelson, B., and Yung, A. R. (2012). Markers of vulnerability to obsessive-compulsive disorder in an ultra-high risk sample of patients who developed psychosis. *Early Interv. Psychiatry* 6, 201–206. doi: 10.1111/j.1751-7893.2012.00357.x

Fontenelle, L. F., Lin, A., Pantelis, C., Wood, S. J., Nelson, B., and Yung, A. R. (2011). A longitudinal study of obsessive-compulsive disorder in individuals at ultra-high risk for psychosis. *J. Psychiatr. Res.* 45, 1140–1145. doi: 10.1016/j.jpsychires.2011.03.005

Friedlander, L., and Desrocher, M. (2006). Neuroimaging studies of obsessive-compulsive disorder in adults and children. *Clin. Psychol. Rev.* 26, 32–49. doi: 10.1016/j.cpr.2005.06.010

Fusar-Poli, P., Nelson, B., Valmaggia, L., Yung, A. R., and McGuire, P. K. (2012). Comorbid depressive and anxiety disorders in 509 individuals with an at-risk mental state: impact on psychopathology and transition to psychosis. *Schizophr. Bull.* doi: 10.1093/schbul/sbs136. [Epub ahead of print].

Gava, I., Barbui, C., Aguglia, E., Carlino, D., Churchill, R., De, V. M., et al. (2007). Psychological treatments versus treatment as usual for obsessive compulsive disorder (OCD). *Cochrane Database Syst. Rev.* 2:CD005333. doi: 10.1002/14651858.CD005333.pub2

Gregory, A., Lau, J., and Eley, T. (2008). Finding gene-environment interactions for generalised anxiety disorder. *Eur. Arch. Psychiatry Clin. Neurosci.* 258, 69–75. doi: 10.1007/s00406-007-0785-4

Gross-Isseroff, R., Hermesh, H., Zohar, J., and Weizman, A. (2003). Neuroimaging communality between schizophrenia and obsessive compulsive disorder: a putative basis for schizo-obsessive disorder? *World J. Biol. Psychiatry* 4, 129–134. doi: 10.1080/15622970310029907

Guillem, F., Satterthwaite, J., Pampoulova, T., and Stip, E. (2009). Relationship between psychotic and obsessive compulsive symptoms in schizophrenia. *Schizophr. Res.* 115, 358–362. doi: 10.1016/j.schres.2009.06.004

Gupta, S., and Daniel, D. G. (1995). Cautions in the clozapine-to-risperidone switch. *Ann. Clin. Psychiatry* 7, 149. doi: 10.3109/10401239509149043

Hadi, E., Greenberg, Y., and Sirota, P. (2011). Obsessive-compulsive symptoms in schizophrenia: arevalence, clinical features and treatment. a literature review. *World J. Biol. Psychiatry* 13, 2–13. doi: 10.3109/15622975.2011.559271

Hashim, H. M., Fawzy, N., Fawzi, M. M., and Karam, R. A. (2012). Brain-derived neurotrophic factor Val66Met polymorphism and obsessive-compulsive symptoms in Egyptian schizophrenia patients. *J. Psychiatr. Res.* 46, 762–766. doi: 10.1016/j.jpsychires.2012.03.007

Hermesh, H., Weizman, A., Gur, S., Zalsman, G., Shiloh, R., Zohar, J., et al. (2003). Alternation learning in OCD/schizophrenia patients. *Eur. Neuropsychopharmacol.* 13, 87–91. doi: 10.1016/S0924-977X(02)00128-1

Hippius, H. (1989). The history of clozapine. *Psychopharmacology* 99(Suppl.), S3–S5. doi: 10.1007/BF00442551

Hur, J. W., Shin, N. Y., Jang, J. H., Shim, G., Park, H. Y., Hwang, J. Y., et al. (2012). Clinical and neurocognitive profiles of subjects at high risk for psychosis with and without obsessive-compulsive symptoms. *Aust. N.Z. J. Psychiatry* 46, 161–169. doi: 10.1177/0004867411432851

Hwang, M. Y., Kim, S. W., Yum, S. Y., and Opler, L. A. (2009). Management of schizophrenia with obsessive-compulsive features. *Psychiatr. Clin. North Am.* 32, 835–851. doi: 10.1016/j.psc.2009.08.002

Hwang, M. Y., Morgan, J. E., and Losconzcy, M. F. (2000). Clinical and neuropsychological profiles of obsessive-compulsive schizophrenia: a pilot study. *J. Neuropsychiatry Clin. Neurosci.* 12, 91–94.

Joel, D. (2006). Current animal models of obsessive compulsive disorder: a critical review. *Prog. Neuropsychopharmacol. Biol. Psychiatry* 30, 374–388. doi: 10.1016/j.pnpbp.2005.11.006

Joober, R., and Boksa, P. (2010). Clozapine: a distinct, poorly understood and under-used molecule. *J. Psychiatry Neurosci.* 35, 147–149. doi: 10.1503/jpn.100055

Kane, J., Honigfeld, G., Singer, J., and Meltzer, H. (1988). Clozapine for the treatment-resistant schizophrenic. a double-blind comparison with chlorpromazine. *Arch. Gen. Psychiatry* 45, 789–796. doi: 10.1001/archpsyc.1988.01800330013001

Kane, J. M. (2011). A user's guide to clozapine. *Acta Psychiatr. Scand.* 123, 407–408. doi: 10.1111/j.1600-0447.2011.01711.x

Kang, X., and Simpson, G. M. (2010). Clozapine: more side effects but still the best antipsychotic. *J. Clin. Psychiatry* 71, 982–983. doi: 10.4088/JCP.09com05497yel

Keers, R., and Uher, R. (2012). Gene-environment interaction in major depression and antidepressant treatment response. *Curr. Psychiatry Rep.* 14, 129–137. doi: 10.1007/s11920-011-0251-x

Kelly, D. L., Richardson, C. M., Tamminga, C. A., and Carpenter, W. T. (2003). The efficacy of high-dose olanzapine versus clozapine in treatment-resistant schizophrenia: a double-blind, crossover study. *J. Clin. Psychopharmacol.* 23, 668–670. doi: 10.1097/01.jcp.0000096246.29231.73

Kim, S. W., Shin, I. S., Kim, J. M., Yang, S. J., Hwang, M. Y., and Yoon, J. S. (2008). Amisulpride improves obsessive-compulsive symptoms in schizophrenia patients taking atypical antipsychotics: an open-label switch study. *J. Clin. Psychopharmacol.* 28, 349–352. doi: 10.1097/JCP.0b013e318172755a

Koran, L. M., Hanna, G. L., Hollander, E., Nestadt, G., Simpson, H. B., and American Psychiatric Association. (2007). Practice guideline for the treatment of patients with obsessive-compulsive disorder. *Am. J. Psychiatry* 164, 5–53.

Kuelz, A. K., Hohagen, F., and Voderholzer, U. (2004). Neuropsychological performance in obsessive-compulsive disorder: a critical review. *Biol. Psychol.* 65, 185–236. doi: 10.1016/j.biopsycho.2003.07.007

Kuelz, A. K., and Voderholzer, U. (2011). Psychotherapie der Zwangsstörung. *Der Nervenarzt* 82, 308–318. doi: 10.1007/s00115-010-2962-3

Kumbhani, S. R., Roth, R. M., Kruck, C. L., Flashman, L. A., and McAllister, T. W. (2010). Nonclinical obsessive-compulsive symptoms and executive functions in schizophrenia. *J. Neuropsychiatry Clin. Neurosci.* 22, 304–312. doi: 10.1176/appi.neuropsych.22.3.304

Kwon, J. S., Jang, J. H., Choi, J. S., and Kang, D. H. (2009a). Neuroimaging in obsessive-compulsive disorder. *Expert Rev. Neurother.* 9, 255–269. doi: 10.1586/14737175.9.2.255

Kwon, J. S., Joo, Y. H., Nam, H. J., Lim, M., Cho, E. Y., Jung, M. H., et al. (2009b). Association of the glutamate transporter gene SLC1A1 with atypical antipsychotics-induced obsessive-compulsive symptoms. *Arch. Gen. Psychiatry* 66, 1233–1241. doi: 10.1001/archgenpsychiatry.2009.155

Lafleur, D. L., Pittenger, C., Kelmendi, B., Gardner, T., Wasylink, S., Malison, R. T., et al. (2006). N-acetylcysteine augmentation in serotonin reuptake inhibitor refractory obsessive-compulsive disorder. *Psychopharmacology* 184, 254–256. doi: 10.1007/s00213-005-0246-6

Lakatos, A., and Reinecker, H. (2007). *Kognitive Verhaltenstherapie bei Zwangsstörungen: Ein Therapiemanual.* Göttingen: Hogrefe.

Lee, M.-J., Shin, Y.-B., Sunwoo, Y.-K., Jung, S.-H., Kim, W.-H., Kang, M.-H., et al. (2009). Comparative analysis of cognitive function in schizophrenia with and without obsessive compulsive disorder. *Psychiatry Invest.* 6, 286–293. doi: 10.4306/pi.2009.6.4.286

Lim, M., Park, D. Y., Kwon, J. S., Joo, Y. H., and Hong, K. S. (2007). Prevalence and clinical characteristics of obsessive-compulsive symptoms associated with atypical antipsychotics. *J. Clin. Psychopharmacol.* 27, 712–713. doi: 10.1097/JCP.0b013e31815a584c

Lin, S. K., Su, S. F., and Pan, C. H. (2006). Higher plasma drug concentration in clozapine-treated schizophrenic patients with side effects of obsessive/compulsive symptoms. *Ther. Drug Monit.* 28, 303–307. doi: 10.1097/01.ftd.0000211801.66569.80

Linden, D. E. (2006). How psychotherapy changes the brain - the contribution of functional neuroimaging. *Mol. Psychiatry* 11, 528–538. doi: 10.1038/sj.mp.4001816

Lopez-Gil, X., Artigas, F., and Adell, A. (2010). Unraveling monoamine receptors involved in the action of typical and atypical antipsychotics on glutamatergic and serotonergic transmission in prefrontal cortex. *Curr. Pharm. Des.* 16, 502–515. doi: 10.2174/138161210790361416

Lykouras, L., Alevizos, B., Michalopoulou, P., and Rabavilas, A. (2003). Obsessive-compulsive symptoms induced by atypical antipsychotics: a review of the reported cases. *Prog. Neuro-psychopharmacol. Biol. Psychiatry* 27, 333–346. doi: 10.1016/S0278-5846(03)00039-3

Lysaker, P. H., Lancaster, R. S., Nees, M. A., and Davis, L. W. (2004). Patterns of obsessive-compulsive symptoms and social function in schizophrenia. *Psychiatry Res.* 125, 139–146. doi: 10.1016/j.psychres.2003.12.007

Lysaker, P. H., and Whitney, K. A. (2009). Obsessive-compulsive symptoms in schizophrenia: prevalence, correlates and treatment. *Expert Rev. Neurother.* 9, 99–107. doi: 10.1586/14737175.9.1.99

Lysaker, P. H., Whitney, K. A., and Davis, L. W. (2009). Associations of executive function with concurrent and prospective reports of obsessive-compulsive symptoms in schizophrenia. *J. Neuropsychiatry Clin. Neurosci.* 21, 38–42. doi: 10.1176/appi.neuropsych.21.1.38

Lysaker, P. H., Bryson, G. J., Marks, K. A., Greig, T. C., and Bell, M. D. (2002). Association of obsessions and compulsions in schizophrenia with neurocognition and negative symptoms. *J. Neuropsychiatry Clin. Neurosci.* 14, 449–453. doi: 10.1176/appi.neuropsych.14.4.449

Mahasuar, R., Janardhan Reddy, Y. C., and Math, S. B. (2011). Obsessive-compulsive disorder with and without bipolar disorder. *Psychiatry Clin. Neurosci.* 65, 423–433. doi: 10.1111/j.1440-1819.2011.02247.x

McEvoy, J. P., Lieberman, J. A., Stroup, T. S., Davis, S. M., Meltzer, H. Y., Rosenheck, R. A., et al. (2006). Effectiveness of clozapine versus olanzapine, quetiapine, and risperidone in patients with chronic schizophrenia who did not respond to prior atypical antipsychotic treatment. *Am. J. Psychiatry* 163, 600–610. doi: 10.1176/appi.ajp.163.4.600

Meijer, J. H. M., Swets, M. M., Keeman, S. M., Nieman, D. H. P., Meijer, C. J. P., and GROUP, I. (2013). Is a schizo-obsessive subtype associated with cognitive impairment? Results from a large cross-sectional study in patients with psychosis and their unaffected relatives. *J. Nerv. Ment. Dis.* 201, 30–35. doi: 10.1097/NMD.0b013e31827ab2b2

Meltzer, H. Y. (1995). Role of serotonin in the action of atypical antipsychotic drugs. *Clin. Neurosci.* 3, 64–75.

Meltzer, H. Y. (1994). An overview of the mechanism of action of clozapine. *J. Clin. Psychiatry* 55, 47–52.

Meltzer, H. Y., and Huang, M. (2008). *In vivo* actions of atypical antipsychotic drug on serotonergic and dopaminergic systems. *Prog. Brain Res.* 172, 177–197. doi: 10.1016/S0079-6123(08)00909-6

Meltzer, H. Y., Li, Z., Kaneda, Y., and Ichikawa, J. (2003). Serotonin receptors: their key role in drugs to treat schizophrenia. *Prog. Neuropsychopharmacol. Biol. Psychiatry* 27, 1159–1172. doi: 10.1016/j.pnpbp.2003.09.010

Meltzer, H. Y., and Sumiyoshi, T. (2008). Does stimulation of 5-HT(1A) receptors improve cognition in schizophrenia? *Behav. Brain Res.* 195, 98–102. doi: 10.1016/j.bbr.2008.05.016

Meltzer, H. Y. (2012). Clozapine. *Clin. Schizophr. Relat. Psychoses* 6, 134–144. doi: 10.3371/CSRP.6.3.5

Menzies, L., Chamberlain, S. R., Laird, A. R., Thelen, S. M., Sahakian, B. J., and Bullmore, E. T. (2008). Integrating evidence from neuroimaging and neuropsychological studies of obsessive-compulsive disorder: the orbitofronto-striatal model revisited. *Neurosci. Biobehav. Rev.* 32, 525–549. doi: 10.1016/j.neubiorev.2007.09.005

Mukhopadhaya, K., Krishnaiah, R., Taye, T., Nigam, A., Bailey, A. J., Sivakumaran, T., et al. (2009). Obsessive-compulsive disorder in UK clozapine-treated schizophrenia and schizoaffective disorder: a cause for clinical concern. *J. Psychopharmacol.* 23, 6–13. doi: 10.1177/0269881108089582

Murphy, D. L., Timpano, K. R., Wheaton, M. G., Greenberg, B. D., and Miguel, E. C. (2010). Obsessive-compulsive disorder and its related disorders: a reappraisal of obsessive-compulsive spectrum concepts. *Dialogues Clin. Neurosci.* 12. 131–148.

Muscatello, M. R., Bruno, A., Pandolfo, G., Mico, U., Scimeca, G., Romeo, V. M., et al. (2011). Effect of aripiprazole augmentation of serotonin reuptake inhibitors or clomipramine in treatment-resistant obsessive-compulsive disorder: a double-blind, placebo-controlled study. *J. Clin. Psychopharmacol.* 31, 174–179. doi: 10.1097/JCP.0b013e31820e3db6

Nicolini, H., Arnold, P., Nestadt, G., Lanzagorta, N., and Kennedy, J. L. (2009). Overview of genetics and obsessive-compulsive disorder. *Psychiatry Res.* 170, 7–14. doi: 10.1016/j.psychres.2008.10.011

Niendam, T. A., Berzak, J., Cannon, T. D., and Bearden, C. E. (2009). Obsessive compulsive symptoms in the psychosis prodrome: correlates of clinical and functional outcome. *Schizophrenia Res.* 108, 170–175. doi: 10.1016/j.schres.2008.11.023

Nolfe, G., Milano, W., Zontini, G., Petrella, C., De, R. M., Rundle-Smith, S., et al. (2010). Obsessive-compulsive symptoms in schizophrenia: their relationship with clinical features and pharmacological treatment. *J. Psychiat. Pract.* 16, 235–242. doi: 10.1097/01.pra.0000386909.84289.ee

Nugent, N., Tyrka, A., Carpenter, L., and Price, L. (2011). Gene-environment interactions: early life stress and risk for depressive and anxiety disorders. *Psychopharmacology* 214, 175–196. doi: 10.1007/s00213-010-2151-x

Oelkers, C., Martin, H., and Miriam, B. (2007). *Zwangsst+Årungen: Ein kognitiv-verhaltensther apeutisches Behandlungsmanual.* Weinheim: Beltz Psychologie Verlags Union.

Öngür, D., and Goff, D. C. (2005). Obsessive-compulsive symptoms in schizophrenia: associated clinical features, cognitive function and medication status. *Schizophr. Res.* 75, 349–362. doi: 10.1016/j.schres.2004.08.012

Pani, L., Villagran, J. M., Kontaxakis, V. P., and Alptekin, K. (2008). Practical issues with amisulpride in the management of patients with schizophrenia. *Clin. Drug Invest.* 28, 465–477. doi: 10.2165/00044011-200828080-00001

Patel, D. D., Laws, K. R., Padhi, A., Farrow, J. M., Mukhopadhaya, K., Krishnaiah, R., et al. (2010). The neuropsychology of the schizo-obsessive subtype of schizophrenia: a new analysis. *Psychol. Med.* 40, 921–933. doi: 10.1017/S0033291709991255

Pauls, D. L. (2010). The genetics of obsessive-compulsive disorder: a review. *Dialogues Clin. Neurosci.* 12, 149–163.

Peters, B., and de, H. L. (2009). Remission of schizophrenia psychosis and strong reduction of obsessive-compulsive disorder after adding clozapine to aripiprazole. *Prog. Neuro-Psychopharmacol. Biol. Psychiatry* 33, 1576–1577. doi: 10.1016/j.pnpbp.2009.09.013

Pittenger, C., Krystal, J. H., and Coric, V. (2006). Glutamate-modulating drugs as novel pharmacotherapeutic agents in the treatment of obsessive-compulsive disorder. *NeuroRx* 3, 69–81. doi: 10.1016/j.nurx.2005.12.006

Pogarell, O., Hamann, C., Poepperl, G., Juckel, G., Chouker, M., Zaudig, M., et al. (2003). Elevated brain serotonin transporter availability in patients with obsessive-compulsive disorder. *Biol. Psychiatry* 54, 1406–1413. doi: 10.1016/S0006-3223(03)00183-5

Poyurovsky, M. (2013). *Schizoobsessive Disorder*, Vol. 1. Cambridge University Press, 1–245. ISBN: 1107 000122.

Poyurovsky, M., Faragian, S., Kleinman-Balush, V., Pashinian, A., Kurs, R., and Fuchs, C. (2007a). Awareness of illness and insight into obsessive-compulsive symptoms in schizophrenia patients with obsessive-compulsive disorder. *J. Nervous Mental Dis.* 195, 765–768. doi: 10.1097/NMD.0b013e318142ce67

Poyurovsky, M., Faragian, S., Pashinian, A., Levi, A., Viosbrod, A., Stryjer, R., et al. (2007b). Neurological soft signs in schizophrenia patients with obsessive-compulsive disorder. *J. Neuropsychiat. Clin. Neurosci.* 19, 145–150. doi: 10.1176/appi.neuropsych.19.2.145

Poyurovsky, M., Faragian, S., Pashinian, A., Heidrach, L., Fuchs, C., Weizman, R., et al. (2008). Clinical characteristics of schizotypal-related obsessive-compulsive disorder. *Psychiatry Res.* 159, 254–258. doi: 10.1016/j.psychres.2007.02.019

Poyurovsky, M., Fuchs, C., and Weizman, A. (1999a). Obsessive-compulsive disorder in patients with first-episode schizophrenia. *Am. J. Psychiatry* 156, 1998–2000.

Poyurovsky, M., Isakov, V., Hromnikov, S., Modai, I., Rauchberger, B., Schneidman, M., et al. (1999b). Fluvoxamine treatment of obsessivecompulsive symptoms in schizophrenic patients: an add-on open study. *Int. Clin. Psychopharmacol.* 14, 95–100. doi: 10.1097/00004850-199903000-00006

Poyurovsky, M., Glick, I., and Koran, L. M. (2010). Lamotrigine augmentation in schizophrenia and schizoaffective patients with obsessive-compulsive symptoms. *J. Psychopharmacol.* 24, 861–866. doi: 10.1177/0269881108099215

Poyurovsky, M., and Koran, L. M. (2005). Obsessive-compulsive disorder (OCD) with schizotypy vs. schizophrenia with OCD: diagnostic dilemmas and therapeutic implications. *J. Psychiatr. Res.* 39, 399–408. doi: 10.1016/j.jpsychires.2004.09.004

Poyurovsky, M., Weizman, A., and Weizman, R. (2004). Obsessive-compulsive disorder in schizophrenia: clinical characteristics and treatment. *CNS Drugs* 18, 989–1010. doi: 10.2165/00023210-200418140-00004

Poyurovsky, M., Weizman, R., Weizman, A., Koran, L., Poyurovsky, M., Weizman, R., et al. (2005). Memantine for treatment-resistant OCD. *Am. J. Psychiatry* 162, 2191–2192. doi: 10.1176/appi.ajp.162.11.2191-a

Poyurovsky, M., Zohar, J., Glick, I., Koran, L. M., Weizman, R., Tandon, R., et al. (2012). Obsessive-compulsive symptoms in schizophrenia: implications for future psychiatric classifications. *Comp. Psychiatry* 53, 480–483. doi: 10.1016/j.comppsych.2011.08.009

Rajender, G., Bhatia, M. S., Kanwal, K., Malhotra, S., Singh, T. B., and Chaudhary, D. (2011). Study of neurocognitive endophenotypes in drug-naive obsessive-compulsive disorder patients, their first-degree relatives and healthy controls. *Acta Psychiatr. Scand.* 124, 152–161. doi: 10.1111/j.1600-0447.2011.01733.x

Remington, G. (2008). Alterations of dopamine and serotonin transmission in schizophrenia. *Prog. Brain Res.* 172, 117–140. doi: 10.1016/S0079-6123(08)00906-0

Reznik, I., Kotler, M., and Weizman, A. (2005). Obsessive and compulsive symptoms in schizophrenia patients–from neuropsychology to clinical typology and classification. *J. Neuropsychiatry Clin. Neurosci.* 17, 254–255. doi: 10.1176/appi.neuropsych.17.2.254

Reznik, I., Mester, R., Kotler, M., and Weizman, A. (2001). Obsessive-compulsive schizophrenia: a new diagnostic entity? *J. Neuropsychiatry Clin. Neurosci.* 13, 115–116. doi: 10.1176/appi.neuropsych.13.1.115

Reznik, I., Yavin, I., Stryjer, R., Spivak, B., Gonen, N., Strous, R., et al. (2004). Clozapine in the treatment of obsessive-compulsive symptoms in schizophrenia patients: a case series study. *Pharmacopsychiatry* 37, 52–56. doi: 10.1055/s-2004-815525

Reznik, I. M., and Sirota, P. M. M. P. (2000). Obsessive and compulsive symptoms in schizophrenia: a randomized controlled trial with fluvoxamine and neuroleptics. *J. Clin. Psychopharmacol.* 20, 410–416. doi: 10.1097/00004714-200008000-00004

Rocha, F. L., and Hara, C. (2006). Benefits of combining aripiprazole to clozapine: three case reports. *Prog. Neuropsychopharmacol. Biol. Psychiatry* 30, 1167–1169. doi: 10.1016/j.pnpbp.2006.03.024

Rodriguez, C. I., Corcoran, C., and Simpson, H. B. (2010). Diagnosis and treatment of a patient with both psychotic and obsessive-compulsive symptoms. *Am. J. Psychiatry* 167, 754–761. doi: 10.1176/appi.ajp.2009.09070997

Rosa-Alcazar, A. I., Sanchez-Meca, J., Gomez-Conesa, A., and Marin-Martinez, F. (2008). Psychological treatment of obsessive-compulsive disorder: a meta-analysis. *Clin. Psychol. Rev.* 28, 1310–1325. doi: 10.1016/j.cpr.2008.07.001

Rubino, I. A., Frank, E., Croce, N. R., Pozzi, D., Lanza di, S. T., and Siracusano, A. (2009). A comparative study of axis I antecedents before age 18 of unipolar depression, bipolar disorder and schizophrenia. *Psychopathology* 42, 325–332. doi: 10.1159/000232975

Ryu, S., Oh, S., Cho, E. Y., Nam, H. J., Yoo, J. H., Park, T., et al. (2011). Interaction between genetic variants of DLGAP3 and SLC1A1 affecting the risk of atypical antipsychotics-induced obsessive-compulsive symptoms. *Am. J. Med. Genet.* 156, 949–959. doi: 10.1002/ajmg.b.31242

Sa, A. R., Hounie, A. G., Sampaio, A. S., Arrais, J., Miguel, E. C., and Elkis, H. (2009). Obsessive-compulsive symptoms and disorder in patients with schizophrenia treated with clozapine or haloperidol. *Compr. Psychiatry* 50, 437–442. doi: 10.1016/j.comppsych.2008.11.005

Saxena, S., Gorbis, E., O'Neill, J., Baker, S. K., Mandelkern, M. A., Maidment, K. M., et al. (2009). Rapid effects of brief intensive cognitive-behavioral therapy on brain glucose metabolism in obsessive-compulsive disorder. *Mol. Psychiatry* 14, 197. doi: 10.1038/sj.mp.4002134

Scatton, B., Claustre, Y., Cudennec, A., Oblin, A., Perrault, G., Sanger, D. J., et al. (1997). Amisulpride: from animal pharmacology to therapeutic action. *Int. Clin. Psychopharmacol.* 12, S29–S36. doi: 10.1097/00004850-199705002-00006

Schirmbeck, F., Esslinger, C., Rausch, F., Englisch, S., Meyer-Lindenberg, A., and Zink, M. (2011). Antiserotonergic antipsychotics are associated with obsessive-compulsive symptoms in schizophrenia. *Psychol. Med.* 41, 2361–2374. doi: 10.1017/S0033291711000419

Schirmbeck, F., Nieratschker, V., Frank, J., Englisch, S., Rausch, F., Meyer-Lindenberg, A., et al. (2012a). Polymorphisms in the glutamate transporter gene SLC1A1 and obsessive compulsive symptoms induced by second generation antipsychotic agents. *Psychiatr. Genet.* 22, 245–252. doi: 10.1097/YPG.0b013e328353fbee

Schirmbeck, F., Rausch, F., Englisch, S., Eifler, S., Esslinger, C., Meyer-Lindenberg, A., et al. (2012b). Stable cognitive deficits in schizophrenia patients with comorbid obsessive-compulsive symptoms: a 12 months longitudinal study. *Schizophr. Bull.* doi: 10.1093/schbul/sbs123. [Epub ahead of print].

Schirmbeck, F., and Zink, M. (2012). Clozapine-induced obsessive-compulsive symptoms in schizophrenia: a critical review. *Curr. Neuropharmacol.* 10, 88–95. doi: 10.2174/157015912799362724

Schirmbeck, F., Rausch, F., Englisch, S., Eifler, S., Esslinger, C., Meyer-Lindenberg, A., et al. (2013). Differential effects of antipsychotic agents on obsessive-compulsive symptoms in schizophrenia: a longitudinal study. *J. Psychopharmacol.* 27, 349–357. doi: 10.1177/0269881112463470

Schirmbeck, F., and Zink, M. (2013). "Obsessive-compulsive syndromes in schizophrenia: a case for polypharmacy?" in *Polypharmacy in Psychiatric Practice*, ed M. Ritsner (Dordrecht; Heidelberg; New York; London: Springer), 233–261.

Sevincok, L., Akoglu, A., and Arslantas, H. (2006). Schizo-obsessive and obsessive-compulsive disorder: comparison of clinical characteristics and neurological soft signs. *Psychiatry Res.* 145, 241–248. doi: 10.1016/j.psychres.2005.11.010

Shapiro, D. A., Renock, S., Arrington, E., Chiodo, L. A., Liu, L. X., Sibley, D. R., et al. (2003). Aripiprazole, a novel atypical antipsychotic drug with a unique and robust pharmacology. *Neuropsychopharmacology* 28, 1400–1411. doi: 10.1038/sj.npp.1300203

Shioiri, T., Shinada, K., Kuwabara, H., and, Someya, T. (2007). Early prodromal symptoms and diagnoses before first psychotic episode in 219 inpatients with schizophrenia. *Psychiatry Clin. Neurosci.* 61, 348–354. doi: 10.1111/j.1440-1819.2007.01685.x

Shugart, Y. Y., Wang, Y., Samuels, J. F., Grados, M. A., Greenberg, B. D., Knowles, J. A., et al. (2009). A family-based association study of the glutamate transporter gene SLC1A1 in obsessive-compulsive disorder in 378 families. *Am. J. Med. Genet. B Neuropsychiatr. Genet.* 150B, 886–892. doi: 10.1002/ajmg.b.30914

Starck, G., Ljungberg, M., Nilsson, M., Jonsson, L., Lundberg, S., Ivarsson, T., et al. (2008). A 1H magnetic resonance spectroscopy study in adults with obsessive compulsive disorder: relationship between metabolite concentrations and symptom severity. *J. Neural Trans.* 115, 1051–1062. doi: 10.1007/s00702-008-0045-4

Steingard, S., Chengappa, K. N. R., Baker, R., and, Schooler, N. R. (1993). Clozapine, obsessive symptoms, and serotonergic mechanisms. *Am. J. Psychiatry* 150, 1435.

Stengel, E. (1945). A study on some clinical aspects of the relationship between obsessional neurosis and psychotic reaction types. *J. Ment. Sci.* 91, 166–187.

Sterk, B., Lankreijer, K., Linszen, D. H., and de, Haan, L. (2011). Obsessive-compulsive symptoms in first episode psychosis and in subjects at ultra high risk for developing psychosis, onset and relationship to psychotic symptoms. *Aust. N.Z. J. Psychiatry* 45, 400–405. doi: 10.3109/00048674.2010.533363

Stewart, S. E., Fagerness, J. A., Platko, J., Smoller, J. W., Scharf, J. M., Illmann, C., et al. (2007). Association of the SLC1A1 glutamate transporter gene and obsessive-compulsive disorder. *Am. J. Med. Genet.* 144 B, 1027–1033. doi: 10.1002/ajmg.b.30533

Still, D. J., Dorson, P. G., Crismon, M. L., and, Pousson, C. (1996). Effects of switching inpatients with treatment-resistant schizophrenia from clozapine to risperidone. *Psychiatr. Serv.* 47, 1382–1384.

Sullwold, L., and Huber, G. (1986). Basic schizophrenic disorders. *Monogr. Gesamtgeb. Psychiatr. Psychiatry Ser.* 42, 1–177. doi: 10.1007/978-3-642-82842-3

Tiihonen, J., Lonnqvist, J., Wahlbeck, K., Klaukka, T., Niskanen, L., Tanskanen, A., et al. (2009). 11-year follow-up of mortality in patients with schizophrenia: a population-based cohort study (FIN11 study). *Lancet* 374, 620–627. doi: 10.1016/S0140-6736(09)60742-X

Tiryaki, A., and Ozkorumak, E. (2010). Do the obsessive-compulsive symptoms have an effect in schizophrenia? *Compr. Psychiatry* 51, 357–362. doi: 10.1016/j.comppsych.2009.10.007

Tumkaya, S., Karadag, F., Oguzhanoglu, N. K., Tekkanat, C., Varma, G., Ozdel, O., et al. (2009). Schizophrenia with obsessive-compulsive disorder and obsessive-compulsive disorder with poor insight: a neuropsychological comparison. *Psychiatry Res.* 165, 38–46. doi: 10.1016/j.psychres.2007.07.031

Tundo, A., Salvati, L., Di Spigno, D., Cieri, L., Parena, A., Necci, R., et al. (2012). Cognitive-behavioral therapy for obsessive-compulsive disorder as a comorbidity with schizophrenia or schizoaffective disorder. *Psychother. Psychosom.* 81, 58–60. doi: 10.1159/000329455

Van Dael, F., van, Os, J., de Graaf, R., ten Have, M., Krabbendam, L., and Myin-Germeys, I. (2011). Can obsessions drive you mad? Longitudinal evidence that obsessive-compulsive symptoms worsen the outcome of early psychotic experiences. *Acta Psychiatr. Scand.* 123, 136–146. doi: 10.1111/j.1600-0447.2010.01609.x

Van der Wee, N. J., Stevens, H., Hardeman, J. A., Mandl, R. C., Denys, D. A., van Megen, H. J., et al. (2004). Enhanced dopamine transporter density in psychotropic-naive patients with obsessive-compulsive disorder shown by $[^{123}I]\beta$-CIT SPECT. *Am. J. Psychiatry* 161, 2201–2206. doi: 10.1176/appi.ajp.161.12.2201

van Nimwegen, L., de Haan, L., van, B. N., Laan, W., van den, B. W., and Linszen, D. (2008). Obsessive-compulsive symptoms in a randomized, double-blind study with olanzapine or risperidone in young patients with early psychosis. *J. Clin. Psychopharmacol.* 28, 214–218. doi: 10.1097/JCP.0b013e318166f520

van Os, J., and Kapur, S. (2009). Schizophrenia. *Lancet* 374, 635–645. doi: 10.1016/S0140-6736(09)60995-8

van Os, J., Kenis, G., and Rutten, B. P. (2010). The environment and schizophrenia. *Nature* 468, 203–212. doi: 10.1038/nature09563

van Os, J., Rutten, B. P., and Poulton, R. (2008). Gene-environment interactions in schizophrenia: review of epidemiological findings and future directions. *Schizophr. Bull.* 34, 1066–1082. doi: 10.1093/schbul/sbn117

Veenstra-VanderWeele, J., Kim, S. J., Gonen, D., Hanna, G. L., Leventhal, B. L., and Cook, E. H. Jr. (2001). Genomic organization of the SLC1A1/EAAC1 gene and mutation screening in early-onset obsessive-compulsive disorder. *Mol. Psychiatry* 6, 160–167. doi: 10.1038/sj.mp.4000806

Wendland, J. R., Moya, P. R., Timpano, K. R., Anavitarte, A. P., Kruse, M. R., Wheaton, M. G., et al. (2009). A haplotype containing quantitative trait loci for, SLC1A1 gene expression and its association with obsessive-compulsive disorder. *Arch. Gen. Psychiatry* 66, 408–416. doi: 10.1001/archgenpsychiatry.2009.6

Whiteside, S. P., Port, J. D., and Abramowitz, J. S. (2004). A meta-analysis of functional neuroimaging in obsessive-compulsive disorder. *Psychiatry Res.* 132, 69–79. doi: 10.1016/j.pscychresns.2004.07.001

Whiteside, S. P., Port, J. D., Deacon, B. J., and Abramowitz, J. S. (2006). A magnetic resonance spectroscopy investigation of obsessive-compulsive disorder and anxiety. *Psychiatry Res.* 146, 137–147. doi: 10.1016/j.pscychresns.2005.12.006

Whitney, K. A., Fastenau, P. S., Evans, J. D., and Lysaker, P. H. (2004). Comparative neuropsychological function in obsessive-compulsive disorder and schizophrenia with and without obsessive-compulsive symptoms. *Schizophr. Res.* 69, 75–83. doi: 10.1016/j.schres.2003.08.013

Woody, S. R., Steketee, G., and Chambless, D. L. (1995). Reliability and validity of the Yale-Brown Obsessive-Compulsive Scale. *Behav. Res. Ther.* 33, 597–605. doi: 10.1016/0005-7967(94)00076-V

Yang, K. C., Su, T. P., and Chou, Y. H. (2008). Effectiveness of aripiprazole in treating obsessive compulsive symptoms. *Prog. Neuropsychopharmacol. Biol. Psychiatry* 32, 585–586. doi: 10.1016/j.pnpbp.2007.10.009

Yang, X. W., and Lu, X. H. (2011). Molecular and cellular basis of obsessive-compulsive disorder-like behaviors: emerging view from mouse models. *Curr. Opin. Neurol.* 24, 114–118. doi: 10.1097/WCO.0b013e32834451fb

Zink, M., Englisch, S., Knopf, U., Kuwilsky, A., and Dressing, H. (2007). Augmentation of clozapine with valproic acid for clozapine-induced obsessive compulsive symptoms. *Pharmacopsychiatry* 40, 202–203. doi: 10.1055/s-2007-985885

Zink, M., Knopf, U., and Kuwilsky, A. (2006). Management of clozapine-induced obsessive compulsive symptoms in a man with schizophrenia. *Aust. N.Z. J. Psychiatry* 41, 293–294. doi: 10.1080/00048670601172806

Conflict of Interest Statement: Frederike Schirmbeck was supported by an unrestricted scientific grant of Evangelisches Studienwerk. Mathias Zink received unrestricted scientific grants of the European Research Advisory Board (ERAB), German Research Foundation (DFG), Pfizer Pharma GmbH, Servier and Bristol Myers Squibb Pharmaceuticals; further speaker and travel grants were provided from Astra Zeneca, Lilly, Pfizer Pharma GmbH, Bristol Myers Squibb Pharmaceuticals, Servier, Otsuka, Roche and Janssen Cilag.

Antipsychotic treatments: focus on lurasidone

Tomiki Sumiyoshi*

Neurocognition and Pharmacology Laboratory, Department of Neuropsychiatry, University of Toyama Graduate School of Medicine and Pharmaceutical Sciences, Toyama, Japan

Edited by:
Maarten Van Den Buuse, Mental Health Research Institute, Australia

Reviewed by:
Jared W. Young, University of California, San Diego, USA
Anand Gururajan, The Florey Institute of Neuroscience and Mental Health, Australia

***Correspondence:**
Tomiki Sumiyoshi, Neurocognition and Pharmacology Laboratory, Department of Neuropsychiatry, University of Toyama Graduate School of Medicine and Pharmaceutical Sciences, 2630 Sugitani, Toyama 930-0194, Japan e-mail: tomikisumiyoshi840@hotmail.com

The introduction of atypical antipsychotic drugs (AAPDs), or second-generation antipsychotics, with clozapine as the prototype, has largely changed the clinicians' attitudes toward the treatment of mental illnesses including, but not limited to schizophrenia. Initially, there was optimism that AAPDs would be superior over typical antipsychotic drugs (TAPDs), or first-generation antipsychotic drugs, in terms of efficacy in various phenomenological aspects, including cognitive impairment, and less likelihood of causing adverse events. However, these views have been partly challenged by results from recent meta-analysis studies. Specifically, cardio-metabolic side effects of AAPDs, in spite of a relative paucity of extrapyramidal symptoms, may sometimes limit the use of these agents. Accordingly, attempts have been made to develop newer compounds, e.g., lurasidone, with the aim of increasing efficacy and tolerability. Further investigations are warranted to determine if a larger proportion of patients will be benefitted by treatment with AAPDs compared to TAPDs in terms of remission and recovery.

Keywords: antipsychotic drugs, second generation, schizophrenia, effectiveness, side effects, remission

INTRODUCTION

Antipsychotic drugs have been considered to represent a series of compounds to treat specific symptoms of schizophrenia, i.e., positive (delusions, hallucinations, disorganized thoughts, and etc.) and negative (blunt affect, avolition, social withdrawal, and etc.) symptoms. Conventional, or "typical," antipsychotic drugs (TAPDs) exert antipsychotic effects at doses that cause extrapyramidal motor side effects due to dopamine (DA)-D_2 receptor blocking properties. Selective actions on psychotic symptoms, with less chance to cause extrapyramidal side effects (EPS), have become possible with the advent of newer class agents, so-called "atypical antipsychotic drugs (AAPDs)" (Meltzer, 1991a). In addition to positive symptoms of schizophrenia, which antipsychotic drugs were initially expected to ameliorate, there is a recent trend to use AAPDs for other psychiatric diseases, e.g., mood disorders, as discussed below.

The development of antipsychotic drugs has been coupled with more intricate theories on the pathophysiology of schizophrenia (Meltzer, 1991b). For example, hyperactivity of DA neurons projecting to the limbic regions, e.g., nucleus accumbens and amygdala, has been shown to be associated with positive symptoms, while a decrease in DA activity in the prefrontal cortex has been considered to cause negative symptoms (Seeman et al., 2006). On the other hand, phencyclidine (PCP), an antagonist at the N-methyl-D-aspartate (NMDA) type glutamate receptor, has been found to produce schizophrenia-like symptoms. This observation led to the glutamate hypothesis of the disease, which is proposed to be linked to the DA hypothesis (Toru et al., 1994).

This article aims to provide theoretical issues on AAPDs in relation to efficacy for treating psychotic symptoms and cognition, as well as safety and tolerability. Specifically, cognitive benefits of lurasidone, a novel AAPD are a focus of this paper. Based on previous discussions (Oliveira et al., 2009; Melnik et al., 2010; Meltzer, 2013) and updated information on these issues, the author present a hypothesis for future directions of therapeutics of schizophrenia and related disorders.

HISTORY OF ANTIPSYCHOTIC DRUGS

The serendipitous discovery of the ability of chlorpromazine to treat psychomotor excitation of schizophrenia confirmed the concept that the illness is a medical entity related to brain chemistry (Delay and Deniker, 1955) (**Figure 1**). The subsequent development of haloperidol, also inhibiting psychomotor symptoms, provided a clue to the pharmacological target shared by most antipsychotic agents; the DA-D_2 receptor (Seeman et al., 2006). This property of TAPDs (**Figure 2**) is associated with the incidence of motor dysfunction, e.g., parkinsonisms, akashisia, dystonia and dyskinesia, as well as endocrinological derangements, e.g., hyperprolactinemia (Sumiyoshi, 2008).

The search for improved medications for schizophrenia led to the implementation of clozapine, the prototype of AAPDs (Kane et al., 1988; Meltzer, 1989). Clozapine shows strong blocking effects for serotonin (5-HT)-5-HT_{2A} and DA-D_4 receptors relative to D_2 receptors, which is thought to underlie the ability of this compound to ameliorate not only positive symptoms, but also negative symptoms to some extent, without causing EPS (Meltzer et al., 1989; Stockmeier et al., 1993; Sumiyoshi et al., 1995).

The experience with clozapine prompted the development of a series of AAPDs with relatively potent 5-HT_{2A} vs. D_2 receptor blocking effects, in an attempt to decrease the likelihood of EPS and elevation of plasma prolactin (pPRL) levels. Consequently, risperidone, olanzapine, quetiapine, aripiprazole, ziprasidone, have been developed (**Figure 3**). In addition, paliperidone, an active metabolite of risperidone, as well as lurasidone, asenapine

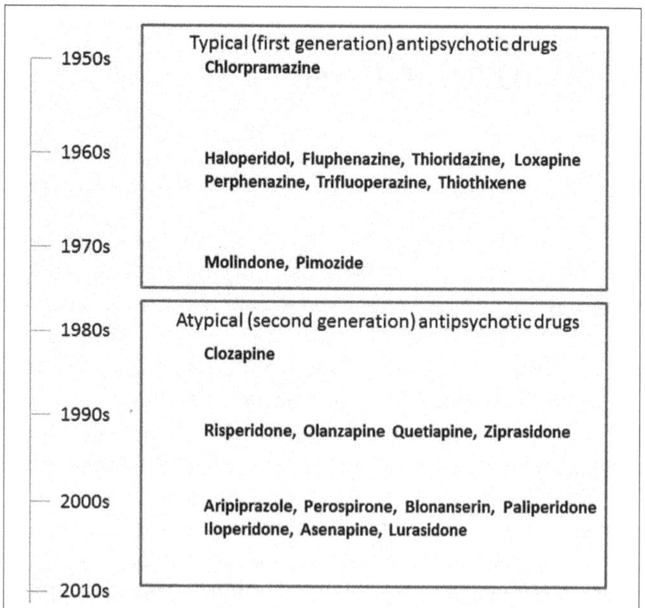

FIGURE 1 | Historical overview of the development of antipsychotic drugs.

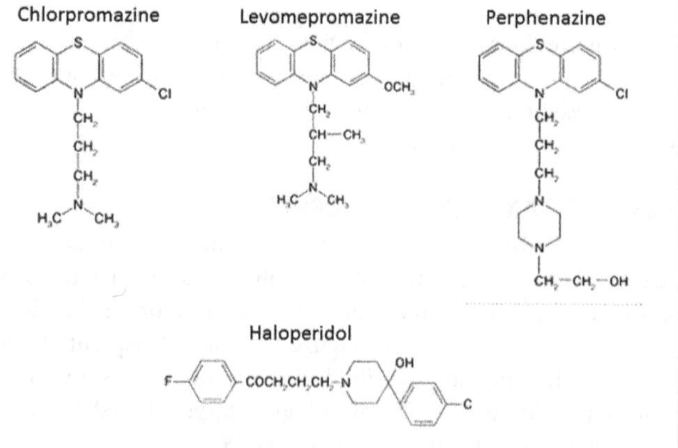

FIGURE 2 | Representative typical (first generation) antipsychotic drugs.

and iloperidone (in the USA), amisulpiride (in Europe), and perospirone and blonanserin (in Japan), have enriched the choice of AAPDs (**Figure 4**).

PHARMACOLOGY

The above AAPDs, except amisulpiride, a relatively selective D_2/D_3 ligand, share a property of relatively high 5-HT_{2A} vs. D_2 receptor affinity (Meltzer et al., 1989; Stockmeier et al., 1993; Sumiyoshi et al., 1995). Some of them, e.g., clozapine, olanzapine and quetiapine, also exhibit considerable affinities for D_1, histamine H_1, adrenalin-α_1, and muscarinic-M_1, receptors, and etc. (Meltzer et al., 2003; Newman-Tancredi and Kleven, 2011). Pharmacologic profiles for representative AAPDs can be summarized as eliciting relatively strong affinities for 5-HT_{1A}, 5-HT_{2C} and NA-α_1 receptors, in addition to 5-HT_{2A} and D_2 receptors, as indicated in **Figure 5** (Newman-Tancredi and Kleven, 2011).

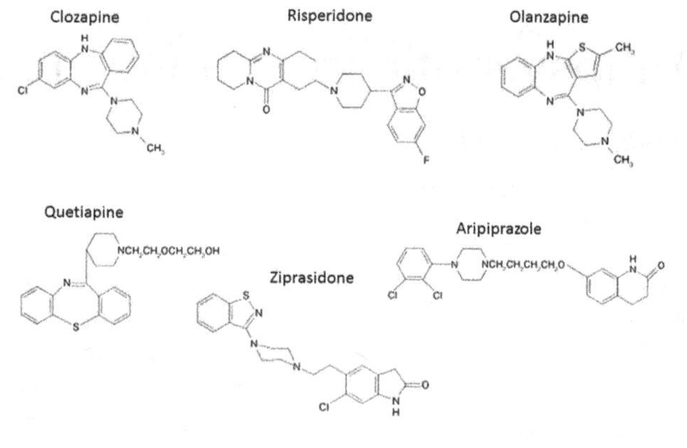

FIGURE 3 | Atypical (second generation) antipsychotic drugs widely used.

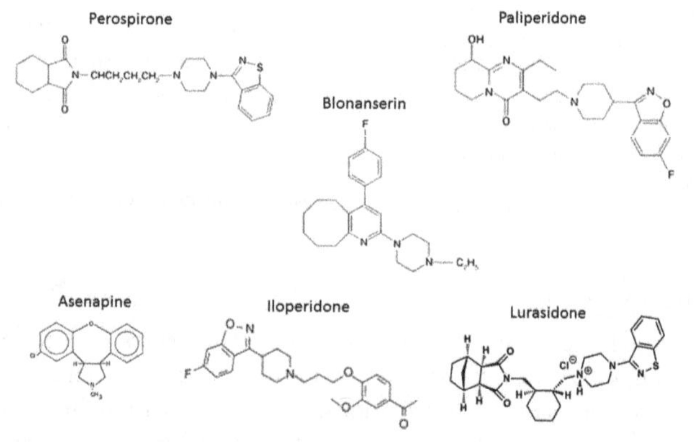

FIGURE 4 | Atypical (second generation) antipsychotic drugs recently developed.

Other common pharmacologic features of AAPDs include the ability to increase extracellular concentrations of DA and acetylcholine in the prefrontal cortex, as measured by *in vivo* microdialysis (Kuroki et al., 1998; Ichikawa et al., 2002). This property has been associated with beneficial effects of these compounds on negative symptoms and cognitive impairment (Kuroki et al., 1998; Ichikawa et al., 2002; Meltzer et al., 2003). It should be noted that the mechanisms of action of antipsychotic drugs were largely derived from studies using animal models of behavioral abnormalities, e.g., sensorimotor gating deficits (Swerdlow et al., 1994).

EFFICACY

GENERAL VIEWS

A recent meta-analysis comparing AAPDs and TAPDs in the treatment of chronic schizophrenia suggests the advantage of clozapine, risperidone, olanzapine, and amisulpiride over TAPDs (Leucht et al., 2009b) for overall efficacy. However, the effect sizes were small (Leucht et al., 2009b), and specific side effects of these agents, e.g., hyperprolactinemia for risperidone and weight

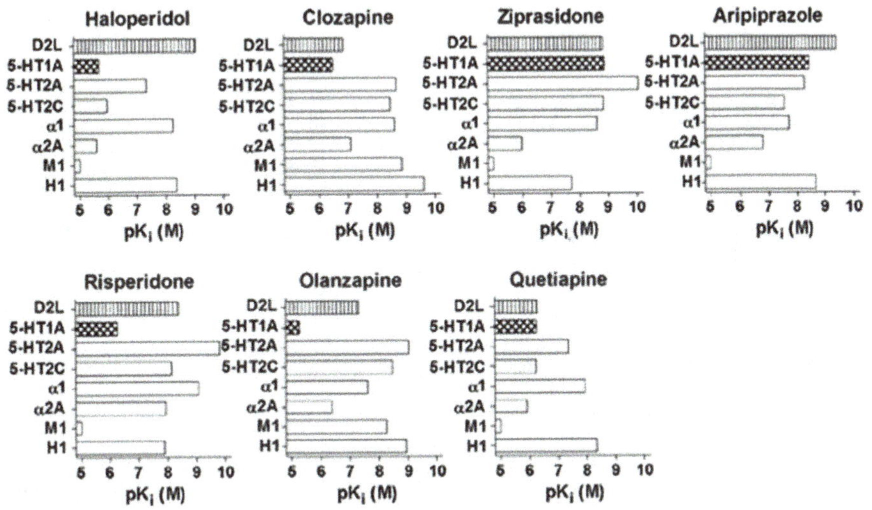

FIGURE 5 | Receptor binding profiles of antipsychotic drugs. A larger pKi value represents a stronger affinity for the particular receptor. [Data from Newman-Tancredi and Kleven (2011)].

gain/metabolic syndrome for olanzapine and clozapine, should be considered (Zhang et al., 2013).

For first-episode patients, Zhang et al. (2013) conducted a meta-analysis of acute, randomized trials with AAPDs vs. TAPDs comparison. The results indicate AAPDs as a whole showed superior efficacy for negative symptoms, and that olanzapine and amisulpiride specifically showed greater benefits than TAPDs (Zhang et al., 2013).

COGNITION

Patients with schizophrenia demonstrate a 1–2.5 standard deviation decline in performance on neuropsychological tests of a range of cognitive domains, e.g., several types of memory, executive function (planning, flexibility of thinking and etc.), attention/information processing, verbal fluency, and motor function (Harvey and Keefe, 1997; Keefe et al., 2004) (**Figure 6**). Cognitive impairment in schizophrenia has been suggested to largely determine the outcome for patients (Green, 1996; Addington and Addington, 2000; Green et al., 2000).

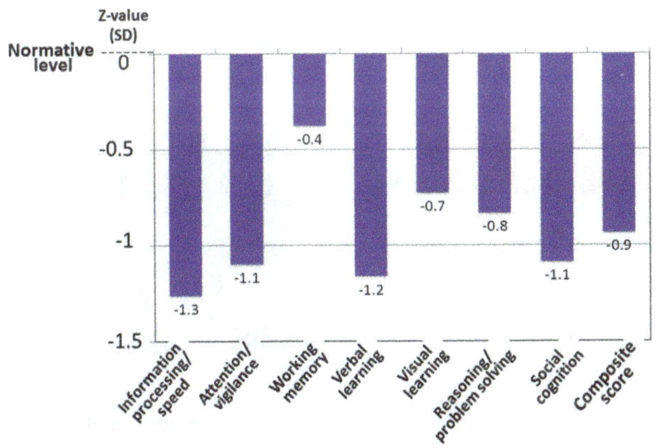

FIGURE 6 | Cognitive impairment of schizophrenia, as evaluated by the MATRICS Consensus Cognitive Battery–Japanese version. Patients with schizophrenia ($N = 30$) demonstrate about a one-standard deviation decline from the normative value in the performance on tests of several cognitive domains. Data were obtained from Outpatient Clinic of University of Toyama Hospital.

Although TAPDs, e.g., haloperidol, exert detrimental influence on cognition in healthy subjects (Saeedi et al., 2006; Veselinovic et al., 2013), there has been controversy about whether AAPDs are more advantageous over TAPDs for its enhancement in schizophrenia (Meltzer et al., 1999; Woodward et al., 2005; Goldberg et al., 2007). Results of the large scale trials, such as the Clinical Antipsychotic Trials of Intervention Effectiveness (CATIE) study, suggest AAPDs may not elicit superiority over TAPDs on cognition (Keefe et al., 2007). However, observations in the CATIE trial should be interpreted with caution, as it did not include a placebo arm, and the results were from chronic patients (Lieberman et al., 2005).

Besides a trial with chronic schizophrenia (Weickert et al., 2003), there has been little study on cognition in acute schizophrenia that includes a placebo arm. Accordingly, we recently reported a double-blind placebo-controlled trial to examine the effect of lurasidone, a novel AAPD (Meyer et al., 2009; Sumiyoshi et al., 2013), on cognitive performance in patients with acute psychosis, followed by a long-term extension study (Sumiyoshi et al., 2013) (**Figure 7**).

In the acute study patients were randomized to receive treatment with lurasidone 80 mg ($N = 125$), 160 mg ($N = 121$), quetiapine 600 mg ($N = 120$), or placebo ($N = 122$). Subjects who completed the 6-week treatment were eligible for the double-blind extension study to receive a once-daily flexible dose of lurasidone (40–160 mg/day; $N = 151$) or quetiapine (200–800 mg/day; $N = 85$). Subjects who received placebo in the acute study were administered lurasidone (40–160 mg/day; $N = 56$). Cognitive performance was examined with the computerized CogState battery (Pietrzak et al., 2009) at baseline

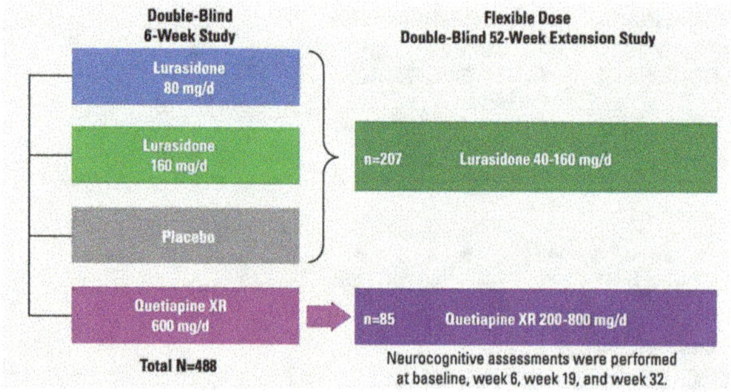

FIGURE 7 | Schema of the protocol for the double-blind study of the effect of lurasidone on cognitive function in patients with acute schizophrenia (Sumiyoshi et al., 2013; **3rd Asian Congress on Schizophrenia Research).**

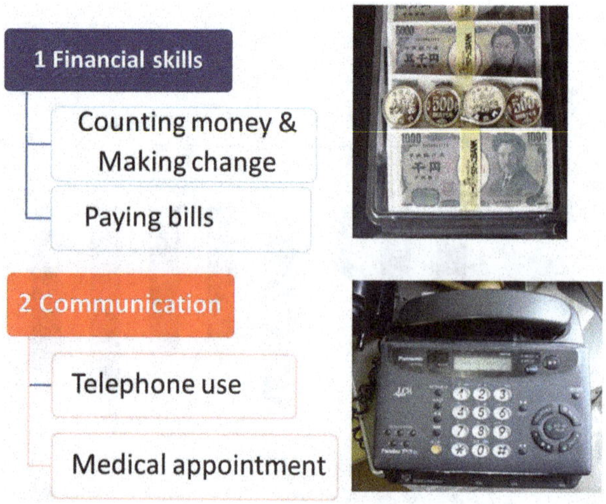

FIGURE 8 | UCSD Performance-based Skills Assessment—Brief version (UPSA-B).

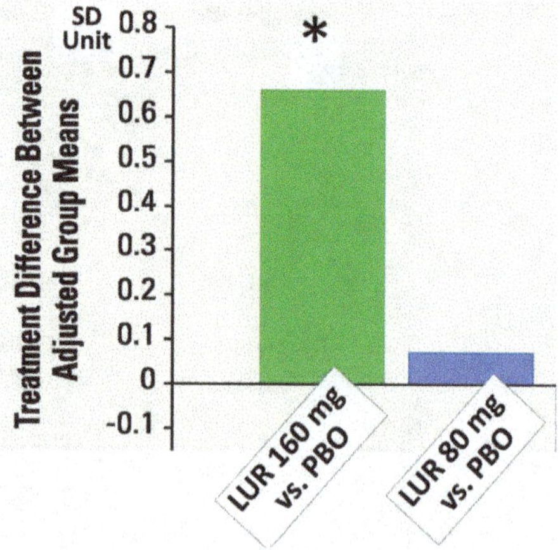

FIGURE 9 | Cognitive composite z-scores in double-blind 6-week acute phase study of lurasidone (LUR) relative to placebo (PBO). Data are based on LOCF analysis of CogState composite score (standardized z-score) at week 6 in the evaluable-test sample set ($N = 267$). $^*P < 0.05$, ANCOVA adjusted for baseline and pooled center.

of the acute phase, and after 6, 19, and 32 weeks of treatment. The battery consists of eight tasks that measure verbal learning, speed of processing, attention/vigilance, visual working memory, visual memory, spatial working memory, reasoning and problem solving, and social cognition (Pietrzak et al., 2009). The average of standardized Z-scores from each task was used as the valid neurocognitive composite Z-score. Functional capacity was evaluated with UCSD Performance-based Skills Assessment—Brief version (UPSA-B) (Mausbach et al., 2011) (**Figure 8**).

At 6 weeks, the change in the neurocognitive composite Z-score did not differ significantly among all groups in intent-to-treat population ($N = 488$). In the evaluable analysis sample ($N = 267$) according to pre-specific criteria, lurasidone, at 160 mg, was superior to both placebo ($p < 0.05$, $d = 0.367$) and quetiapine XR ($p < 0.05$, $d = 0.411$) (**Figure 9**). Patients with any of the active treatments elicited greater improvement in the UPSA-B score than did those given placebo. In the 6-month extension study, lurasidone, at flexible doses of 40–160 mg/day, showed a significantly greater cognitive benefit compared to quetiapine XR, at flexible doses of 200–800 mg/day, at week 32 ($p < 0.01$, $d = 0.57$). Mixed effects model analysis demonstrated significant cross-sectional and longitudinal relationship between the cognitive composite score and UPSA-B total score.

Data from the placebo-controlled acute phase study provide robust evidence for the ability of lurasidone to enhance cognitive function and functional capacity in patients with schizophrenia. The relatively high rate of subjects who did not provide evaluable data may be associated with awareness of illness, or insight, of study participants (Harvey et al., 2013).

In spite of some beneficial effects, discussed above, no treatments have been approved for treating cognitive or negative symptoms in schizophrenia. Therefore, further efforts are required in this area.

MOOD DISORDERS

Recently, AAPDs have been used for a variety of psychiatric conditions, in addition to schizophrenia, e.g., mood disorders, although the mechanisms underlying their therapeutic effects remain unknown. So far, the Food and Drug Administration in the US has approved indications for olanzapine, quetiapine, risperidone, aripiprazole, and asenapine to treat bipolar disorder, as shown in **Table 1** (Bobo, 2013; Spielmans et al., 2013). As for major depressive disorder, a recent meta-analysis (Spielmans et al., 2013) indicates adjunctive treatment with AAPDs, e.g., aripiprazole, olanzapine/fluoxetine, quetiapine, or risperidone, is effective in reducing depressive symptoms, with small-to-moderate effect sizes. Olanzapine, quetiapine, and aripiprazole are indicated to treat major depression (Spielmans et al., 2013), as shown in **Table 2**.

OTHER DISEASES

Some AAPDs have been suggested to ameliorate part of symptoms or caregiver's burden in other conditions, such as

Table 1 | Year of approval by FDA of AAPDs for bipolar disorder.

	Acute mania/ mixed episodes	Bipolar disorder maintenance Tx	Acute bipolar depression
Olanzapine	2000	2004	2003[a]
Quetiapine	2004	2004[b]	2008
Risperidone	2003	2009[c]	
Aripiprazole	2004	2004	
Asenapine	2007		
Lurasidone			2013[d]

[a] *Olanzapine/flluoxetine combination.*
[b] *In combination with valproate/lithium.*
[c] *Depot formulation.*
[d] *Both for monotherapy and in combination with valproate/lithium.*

Table 2 | Year of approval for major depression.

	Add-on to antidepressants	Monotherapy
Quetiapine	2009	Applying
Olanzapine	2009[a]	
Aripiprazole	2007	

[a] *Olanzapine/flluoxetine combination.*

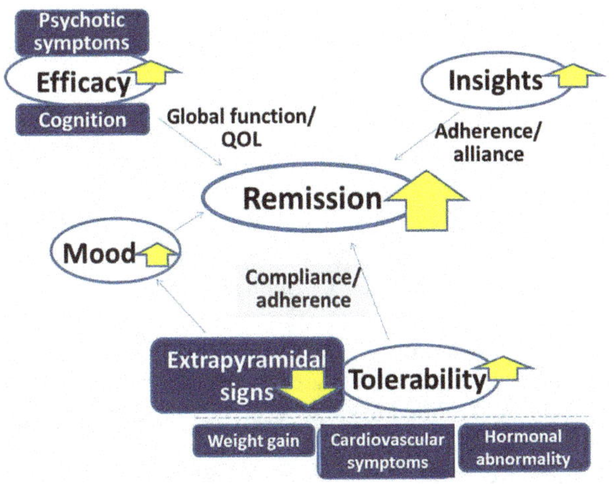

FIGURE 10 | Advantage of atypical antipsychotic drugs (AAPDs) for improving outcome in the treatment of psychotic disorders. Compared to typical antipsychotic drugs, AAPDs elicit fewer incidences of extrapyramidal signs, which enhance compliance and adherence. AAPDs may also demonstrate greater efficacy for mood symptoms. The superiority of AAPDs in terms of ameliorating psychotic symptoms and cognitive impairment is under debate. The development of newer antipsychotic drugs with minimal adverse events associated with some existing AAPDs, e.g., weight gain, cardiovascular symptoms, and hormonal abnormalities, may provide an effective strategy to attain greater remission rates.

Alzheimer's disease (Mohamed et al., 2012), Huntington disease (Adam and Jankovic, 2008), Parkinson's disease (Friedman, 2011), and Tourette's syndrome (Maher and Theodore, 2012). For example, AAPDs have been reported to reduce psychosis, agitation, and/or aggressive behavior in Alzheimer's disease and Huntington disease (Mohamed et al., 2012; Adam and Jankovic, 2008). Clozapine, as well as quetiapine to some extent, has been shown to be effective in controlling psychotic symptoms of Parkinson's disease (Friedman, 2011).

TOLERABILITY

Compared to TAPDs, AAPDs have been associated with reduced risk of EPS and tardive dyskinesia, although the latter compounds may more frequently induce weight gain and cardio-metabolic side effects in schizophrenia (De Hert et al., 2012a). Further, some large scale studies with chronic patients did not find noticeable differences in efficacy between the two antipsychotic classes (Lieberman et al., 2005; Jones et al., 2006; Leucht et al., 2009a), raising a question about the advantage of AAPDs. However, there is a suggestion that higher benefit/risk ratios for AAPDs would be expected in acute patients compared with chronic patients (Zhang et al., 2013). In fact, a recent meta-analysis (Zhang et al., 2013) indicates olanzapine, amisulpiride, risperidone and quetiapine, elicit superior efficacy, greater treatment persistence and less EPS than TAPDs. These authors also found greater weight increase and metabolic changes for some of these AAPDs, such as olanzapine (Zhang et al., 2013).

These lines of evidence prompted the development of newer antipsychotic drugs with minimal adverse events associated with the above AAPDs, e.g., weight gain, lipid metabolism, cardiovascular risk, and glucose intolerance. Accordingly, the FDA approved iloperidone and asenapine in 2009, followed by lurasidone in 2010, for the treatment of adults with acute schizophrenia. De Hert et al. (2012b) conducted a systematic review and exploratory meta-analysis of these new AAPDs together with paliperidone in the treatment of schizophrenia and bipolar disorder. The findings suggest a relatively greater tolerability for lurasidone in comparison with placebo, and indicate the need for further controlled studies comparing the newer agents with other antipsychotic drugs currently available (De Hert et al., 2012b).

PERSPECTIVES

In the pursuit of novel therapeutics, critical issues to be addressed, or "unmet needs," include (1) treatment-resistant patients, (2) prevention of psychosis, and (3) remission/recovery. There have been some suggestions for the former two, e.g., clozapine for treatment-resistant schizophrenia (Kane et al., 1988; Meltzer, 1989), and risperidone and olanzapine for prevention (McGorry et al., 2002; McGlashan et al., 2006). On the other hand, there seems to be a relative paucity of information on whether AAPDs increase remission in schizophrenia (Takeuchi et al., 2012), due, partly, to the limited number of valid assessment methods (Alaqeel and Margolese, 2012).

Such measures include the Remission in Schizophrenia Working Group (RSWG) criteria (Andreasen et al., 2005), which has been developed to operationally define symptomatic remission. Using the RSWG criteria, Alaqeel et al. (2013) recently conducted a meta-analysis to compare remission rates between AAPD and TAPD treatments. Results from four eligible studies, with 3433 schizophrenia patients, suggest AAPDs are associated with a 1.46 increased probability of attaining remission relative to TAPDs (Alaqeel et al., 2013). The lower dropout rate with AAPDs may explain the modest but significant increase in the rate of enduring symptomatic remission, which deserves further study.

CONCLUSIONS

Antipsychotic drugs play a major role in the treatment of schizophrenia and related disorders. However, there remain a number of issues to be solved to more effectively improve clinical practice, e.g., dealing with treatment-resistant patients. As discussed, some evidence suggests the superiority of AAPDs as a group over TAPDs in terms of compliance/adherence, although controversy exists. At least, it is legitimate to confirm that AAPDs elicit lower incidence of EPS compared to TAPDs. Accordingly, AAPDs may also demonstrate greater efficacy for mood symptoms, and less likelihood to cause secondary negative symptoms related to EPS (**Figure 10**).

Further investigations are warranted to determine if a larger proportion of patients can be benefitted by treatment with AAPDs compared with TAPDs in terms of remission and recovery. Specifically, efforts to develop newer antipsychotic compounds with minimal adverse events associated with some existing AAPDs, e.g., weight gain, cardiovascular symptoms, and hormonal abnormalities, will provide a promising strategy to attain this goal.

ACKNOWLEDGMENTS

This study was funded by grants-in-aid for Scientific Research from Japan Society for the Promotion of Science, Health and Labour Sciences Research Grants for Comprehensive Research on Disability, Health, and Welfare (H23-Seishin-Ippan-002; H24-Seishin-Ippan-002), and SENSHIN Medical Research Foundation.

The author acknowledges Drs. Herbert Y. Meltzer, Philip Harvey, Cynthia Siu, Adrian Newman-Tancredi, and Chika Sumiyoshi for discussions.

REFERENCES

Adam, O. R., and Jankovic, J. (2008). Symptomatic treatment of Huntington disease. *Neurotherapeutics* 5, 181–197. doi: 10.1016/j.nurt.2008.01.008

Addington, J., and Addington, D. (2000). Neurocognitive and social functioning in schizophrenia: a 2.5 year follow-up study. *Schizophr. Res.* 44, 47–56. doi: 10.1016/S0920-9964(99)00160-7

Alaqeel, B., and Margolese, H. C. (2012). Remission in schizophrenia: critical and systematic review. *Harv. Rev. Psychiatry* 20, 281–297. doi: 10.3109/10673229.2012.747804

Alaqeel, B., Rej, S., Annable, L., and Margolese, H. C. (2013). "Do second-generation antipsychotics increase remission in schizophrenia? A meta-analysis," in *14th International Congress of Schizophrenia Research* (Orlando, FL).

Andreasen, N. C., Carpenter, W. T. Jr., Kane, J. M., Lasser, R. A., Marder, S. R., et al. (2005). Remission in schizophrenia: proposed criteria and rationale for consensus. *Am. J. Psychiatry* 162, 441–449. doi: 10.1176/appi.ajp.162.3.441

Bobo, W. V. (2013). Asenapine, iloperidone and lurasidone: critical appraisal of the most recently approved pharmacotherapies for schizophrenia in adults. *Expert Rev. Clin. Pharmacol.* 6, 61–91. doi: 10.1586/ecp.12.70

De Hert, M., Detraux, J., Van Winkel, R., Yu, W., and Correll, C. U. (2012a). Metabolic and cardiovascular adverse effects associated with antipsychotic drugs. *Nat. Rev. Endocrinol.* 8, 114–126. doi: 10.1038/nrendo.2011.156

De Hert, M., Yu, W., Detraux, J., Sweers, K., Van Winkel, R., and Correll, C. U. (2012b). Body weight and metabolic adverse effects of asenapine, iloperidone, lurasidone and paliperidone in the treatment of schizophrenia and bipolar disorder: a systematic review and exploratory meta-analysis. *CNS Drugs* 26, 733–759. doi: 10.2165/11634500-000000000-00000

Delay, J., and Deniker, P. (1955). Neuroleptic effects of chlorpromazine in therapeutics of neuropsychiatry. *J. Clin. Exp. Psychopathol.* 16, 104–112.

Friedman, J. H. (2011). Atypical antipsychotic drugs in the treatment of Parkinson's disease. *J. Pharm. Pract.* 24, 534–540. doi: 10.1177/0897190011426556

Goldberg, T. E., Goldman, R. S., Burdick, K. E., Malhotra, A. K., Lencz, T., Patel, R. C., et al. (2007). Cognitive improvement after treatment with second-generation antipsychotic medications in first-episode schizophrenia: is it a practice effect? *Arch. Gen. Psychiatry* 64, 1115–1122. doi: 10.1001/archpsyc.64.10.1115

Green, M. F. (1996). What are the functional consequences of neurocognitive deficits in schizophrenia? [see comments]. *Am. J. Psychiatry* 153, 321–330.

Green, M. F., Kern, R. S., Braff, D. L., and Mintz, J. (2000). Neurocognitive deficits and functional outcome in schizophrenia: are we measuring the "right stuff"? *Schizophr. Bull.* 26, 119–136. doi: 10.1093/oxfordjournals.schbul.a033430

Harvey, P., Siu, C., Cucchiaro, J., Pikalov, A., and Loebel, A. (2013). "Awareness of illness as a predictor of cooperation with cognitive assessments and cognitive benefits of atypical antipsychotic medication," in *14th International Congress on Schizophrenia Research* (Orland, FL).

Harvey, P. D., and Keefe, R. S. (1997). Cognitive impairment in schizophrenia and implication of atypical neuroleptic treatment. *CNS Spectrums* 2, 41–55.

Ichikawa, J., Dai, J., O'laughlin, I. A., Fowler, W. L., and Meltzer, H. Y. (2002). Atypical, but not typical, antipsychotic drugs increase cortical acetylcholine release without an effect in the nucleus accumbens or striatum. *Neuropsychopharmacology* 26, 325–339. doi: 10.1016/S0893-133X(01)00312-8

Jones, P. B., Barnes, T. R., Davies, L., Dunn, G., Lloyd, H., Hayhurst, K. P., et al. (2006). Randomized controlled trial of the effect on quality of life of second- vs first-generation antipsychotic drugs in schizophrenia: cost utility of the latest antipsychotic drugs in schizophrenia study (CUtLASS 1). *Arch. Gen. Psychiatry* 63, 1079–1087. doi: 10.1001/archpsyc.63.10.1079

Kane, J., Honigfeld, G., Singer, J., Meltzer, H. Y., and Group, C. C. S. (1988). Clozapine for the treatment-resistant schizophrenic: a double-blind comparison with chlorpromazine. *Arch. Gen. Psychiatry* 45, 789–796. doi: 10.1001/archpsyc.1988.01800330013001

Keefe, R. S., Bilder, R. M., Davis, S. M., Harvey, P. D., Palmer, B. W., Gold, J. M., et al. (2007). Neurocognitive effects of antipsychotic medications in patients with chronic schizophrenia in the CATIE Trial. *Arch. Gen. Psychiatry* 64, 633–647. doi: 10.1001/archpsyc.64.6.633

Keefe, R. S., Goldberg, T. E., Harvey, P. D., Gold, J. M., Poe, M. P., and Coughenour, L. (2004). The brief assessment of cognition in Schizophrenia: reliability, sensitivity, and comparison with a standard neurocognitive battery. *Schizophr. Res.* 68, 283–297. doi: 10.1016/j.schres.2003.09.011

Kuroki, H., Meltzer, H. Y., and Ichikawa, J. (1998). Effect of antipsychotic drugs on extracellular dopamine levels in rat medial prefrontalcortex and nucleus accumbens. *J. Pharmacol. Exp. Ther.* 288, 774–781.

Leucht, S., Corves, C., Arbter, D., Engel, R. R., Li, C., and Davis, J. M. (2009a). Second-generation versus first-generation antipsychotic drugs for schizophrenia: a meta-analysis. *Lancet* 373, 31–41. doi: 10.1016/S0140-6736(08)61764-X

Leucht, S., Komossa, K., Rummel-Kluge, C., Corves, C., Hunger, H., Schmid, F., et al. (2009b). A meta-analysis of head-to-head comparisons of second-generation antipsychotics in the treatment of schizophrenia. *Am. J. Psychiatry* 166, 152–163. doi: 10.1176/appi.ajp.2008.08030368

Lieberman, J. A., Stroup, T. S., McEvoy, J. P., Swartz, M. S., Rosenheck, R. A., Perkins, D. O., et al. (2005). Effectiveness of antipsychotic drugs in patients with chronic schizophrenia. *N. Engl J. Med.* 353, 1209–1223. doi: 10.1056/NEJMoa051688

Maher, A. R., and Theodore, G. (2012). Summary of the comparative effectiveness review on off-label use of atypical antipsychotics. *J. Manag. Care Pharm.* 18, S1–S20.

Mausbach, B. T., Depp, C. A., Bowie, C. R., Harvey, P. D., McGrath, J. A., Thronquist, M. H., et al. (2011). Sensitivity and specificity of the UCSD Performance-based Skills Assessment (UPSA-B) for identifying functional milestones in schizophrenia. *Schizophr. Res.* 132, 165–170. doi: 10.1016/j.schres.2011.07.022

McGlashan, T. H., Zipursky, R. B., Perkins, D., Addington, J., Miller, T., Woods, S. W., et al. (2006). Randomized, double-blind trial of olanzapine versus placebo in patients prodromally symptomatic for psychosis. *Am. J. Psychiatry* 163, 790–799. doi: 10.1176/appi.ajp.163.5.790

McGorry, P. D., Yung, A. R., Phillips, L. J., Yuen, H. P., Francey, S., Cosgrave, E. M., et al. (2002). Randomized controlled trial of interventions designed to reduce the risk of progression to first-episode psychosis in a clinical sample with subthreshold symptoms. *Arch. Gen. Psychiatry* 59, 921–928. doi: 10.1001/archpsyc.59.10.921

Melnik, T., Soares, B. G., Puga, M. E., and Atallah, A. N. (2010). Efficacy and safety of atypical antipsychotic drugs (quetiapine, risperidone, aripiprazole and paliperidone) compared with placebo or typical antipsychotic drugs for treating refractory schizophrenia: overview of systematic reviews. *Sao Paulo Med. J.* 128, 141–166. doi: 10.1590/S1516-31802010000300007

Meltzer, H. Y. (1989). Clinical studies on the mechanism of action of clozapine: the dopamine- serotonin hypothesis of schizophrenia. *Psychopharmacology (Berl)* 99, S18–S27. doi: 10.1007/BF00442554

Meltzer, H. Y. (1991a). The mechanism of action of novel antipsychotic drugs. *Schizophr. Bull.* 17, 263–287. doi: 10.1093/schbul/17.2.263

Meltzer, H. Y. (1991b). The neurobiology of schizophrenia. *Curr. Opin. Psychiatry* 4, 90–95. doi: 10.1097/00001504-199102000-00021

Meltzer, H. Y. (2013). Update on typical and atypical antipsychotic drugs. *Annu. Rev. Med.* 64, 393–406. doi: 10.1146/annurev-med-050911-161504

Meltzer, H. Y., Li, Z., Kaneda, Y., and Ichikawa, J. (2003). Serotonin receptors: their key role in drugs to treat schizophrenia. *Prog. Neuropsychopharmacol. Biol. Psychiatry* 27, 1159–1172. doi: 10.1016/j.pnpbp.2003.09.010

Meltzer, H. Y., Matsubara, S., and Lee, J. C. (1989). Classification of typical and atypical antipsychotic drugs on the basis of dopamine D-1, D-2 and serotonin2 pKi values. *J. Pharmacol. Exp. Ther.* 251, 238–246.

Meltzer, H. Y., Park, S., and Kessler, R. (1999). Cognition, schizophrenia, and the atypical antipsychotic drugs. *Proc. Nat. Acad. Sci. U.S.A.* 96, 13591–13593. doi: 10.1073/pnas.96.24.13591

Meyer, J. M., Loebel, A. D., and Schweizer, E. (2009). Lurasidone: a new drug in development for schizophrenia. *Expert. Opin. Investig. Drugs* 18, 1715–1726. doi: 10.1517/13543780903286388

Mohamed, S., Rosenheck, R., Lyketsos, C. G., Kaczynski, R., Sultzer, D. L., and Schneider, L. S. (2012). Effect of second-generation antipsychotics on caregiver burden in Alzheimer's disease. *J. Clin. Psychiatry* 73, 121–128. doi: 10.4088/JCP.10m06574

Newman-Tancredi, A., and Kleven, M. S. (2011). Comparative pharmacology of antipsychotics possessing combined dopamine D2 and serotonin 5-HT1A receptor properties. *Psychopharmacology* 216, 451–473. doi: 10.1007/s00213-011-2247-y

Oliveira, I. R., Nunes, P. M., Coutinho, D. M., and Sena, E. P. (2009). Review of the efficacy of placebo in comparative clinical trials between typical and atypical antipsychotics. *Rev. Bras. Psiquiatr* 31, 52–56. doi: 10.1590/S1516-44462009000100013

Pietrzak, R. H., Olver, J., Norman, T., Piskulic, D., Maruff, P., and Snyder, P. J. (2009). A comparison of the CogState schizophrenia battery and the measurement and treatment research to improve cognition in schizophrenia (MATRICS) battery in assessing cognitive impairment in chronic schizophrenia. *J. Clin. Exp. Neuropsychol.* 31, 848–859. doi: 10.1080/13803390802592458

Saeedi, H., Remington, G., and Christensen, B. K. (2006). Impact of haloperidol, a dopamine D2 antagonist, on cognition and mood. *Schizophr. Res.* 85, 222–231. doi: 10.1016/j.schres.2006.03.033

Seeman, P., Schwarz, J., Chen, J. F., Szechtman, H., Perreault, M., McKnight, G. S., et al. (2006). Psychosis pathways converge via D2high dopamine receptors. *Synapse* 60, 319–346. doi: 10.1002/syn.20303

Spielmans, G. I., Berman, M. I., Linardatos, E., Rosenlicht, N. Z., Perry, A., and Tsai, A. C. (2013). Adjunctive atypical antipsychotic treatment for major depressive disorder: a meta-analysis of depression, quality of life, and safety outcomes. *PLoS Med.* 10:e1001403. doi: 10.1371/journal.pmed.1001403

Stockmeier, C. A., Dicarlo, J. J., Zhang, Y., Thompson, P., and Meltzer, H. Y. (1993). Characterization of typical and atypical antipsychotic drugs based on *in vivo* occupancy of $serotonin_2$ and $dopamine_2$ receptors. *J. Pharmacol. Exp. Ther.* 266, 1374–1384.

Sumiyoshi, T. (2008). A possible dose-side effect relationship of antipsychotic drugs: relevance to cognitive function in schizophrenia. *Expert Rev. Clin. Pharmacol.* 1, 791–802. doi: 10.1586/17512433.1.6.791

Sumiyoshi, T., Miyanishi, T., Harvey, P., Siu, C., Loebel, A., and Ogasa, M. (2013). "Cognitive performance in patients with schizophrenia treated with lurasidone: results from a placebo- and active-controlled acute phase study followed by a 6-month double-blind extension," in *3rd Asian Congress on Schizophrenia Research* (Bali).

Sumiyoshi, T., Suzuki, K., Sakamoto, H., Yamaguchi, N., Mori, H., Shiba, K., et al. (1995). Atypicality of several antipsychotics on the basis of *in vivo* dopamine- D_2 and serotonin-$5HT_2$ receptor occupancy. *Neuropsychopharmacology* 12, 57–64.

Swerdlow, N. R., Braff, D. L., Taaid, N., and Geyer, M. A. (1994). Assessing the validity of an animal model of deficient sensorimotor gating in schizophrenic patients. *Arch. Gen. Psychiatry* 51, 139–154. doi: 10.1001/archpsyc.1994.03950020063007

Takeuchi, H., Suzuki, T., Uchida, H., Watanabe, K., and Mimura, M. (2012). Antipsychotic treatment for schizophrenia in the maintenance phase: a systematic review of the guidelines and algorithms. *Schizophr. Res.* 134, 219–225. doi: 10.1016/j.schres.2011.11.021

Toru, M., Kurumaji, A., and Ishimaru, M. (1994). Excitatory amino acids: implications for psychiatric disorders research. *Life Sci.* 55, 1683–1699. doi: 10.1016/0024-3205(94)00337-8

Veselinovic, T., Schorn, H., Vernaleken, I. B., Hiemke, C., Zernig, G., Gur, R., and Grunder, G. (2013). Effects of antipsychotic treatment on cognition in healthy subjects. *J. Psychopharmacol.* 27, 374–385. doi: 10.1177/0269881112466183

Weickert, T. W., Goldberg, T. E., Marenco, S., Bigelow, L. B., Egan, M. F., and Weinberger, D. R. (2003). Comparison of cognitive performances during a placebo period and an atypical antipsychotic treatment period in schizophrenia: critical examination of confounds. *Neuropsychopharmacology* 28, 1491–1500. doi: 10.1038/sj.npp.1300216

Woodward, N. D., Purdon, S. E., Meltzer, H. Y., and Zald, D. H. (2005). A meta-analysis of neuropsychological change to clozapine, olanzapine, quetiapine, and risperidone in schizophrenia. *Int. J. Neuropsychopharmacol.* 8, 457–472. doi: 10.1017/S146114570500516X

Zhang, J. P., Gallego, J. A., Robinson, D. G., Malhotra, A. K., Kane, J. M., and Correll, C. U. (2013). Efficacy and safety of individual second-generation vs. first-generation antipsychotics in first-episode psychosis: a systematic review and meta-analysis. *Int. J. Neuropsychopharmacol.* 16, 1205–1218. doi: 10.1017/S1461145712001277

Conflict of Interest Statement: The author has received advisory board and/or speaker's honoraria from Dainippon-Sumitomo, Yoshitomi-yakuhin, Tanabe-Mitsubishi, Otsuka, Eli Lilly, and Takeda Pharmaceuticals.

8

Hippocampal serotonin depletion unmasks differences in the hyperlocomotor effects of phencyclidine and MK-801: quantitative versus qualitative analyses

Wendy K. Adams[1,2]†, Adam L. Halberstadt[3] and Maarten van den Buuse[1,4]*

[1] Behavioural Neuroscience Laboratory, Florey Institute for Neuroscience and Mental Health, University of Melbourne, Melbourne, VIC, Australia
[2] Centre for Neuroscience, University of Melbourne, Melbourne, VIC, Australia
[3] Department of Psychiatry, University of California San Diego, La Jolla, CA, USA
[4] Department of Pharmacology, University of Melbourne, Melbourne, VIC, Australia

Edited by:
Thibault Renoir, Florey Institute of Neuroscience and Mental Health, Australia

Reviewed by:
Charles H. Large, Autifony Therapeutics Limited, Italy
Enrico Sanna, University of Cagliari, Italy

***Correspondence:**
Maarten van den Buuse, Florey Institute for Neuroscience and Mental Health, University of Melbourne, Kenneth Myer Building, 30 Royal Parade, Parkville, VIC 3010, Australia
e-mail: mvdbuuse@unimelb.edu.au
†

Antagonism of *N*-methyl-D-aspartate (NMDA) receptors by phencyclidine (PCP) is thought to underlie its ability to induce a schizophrenia-like syndrome in humans, yet evidence indicates it has a broader pharmacological profile. Our previous lesion studies highlighted a role for serotonergic projections from the median, but not dorsal, raphe nucleus in mediating the hyperlocomotor effects of PCP, without changing the action of the more selective NMDA receptor antagonist, MK-801. Here we compared locomotor responses to PCP and MK-801 in rats that were administered 5,7-dihydroxytryptamine (5,7-DHT) into either the dorsal or ventral hippocampus, which are preferentially innervated by median and dorsal raphe, respectively. Dorsal hippocampus lesions potentiated PCP-induced hyperlocomotion (0.5, 2.5 mg/kg), but not the effect of MK-801 (0.1 mg/kg). Ventral hippocampus lesions did not alter the hyperlocomotion elicited by either compound. Given that PCP and MK-801 may induce different spatiotemporal patterns of locomotor behavior, together with the known role of the dorsal hippocampus in spatial processing, we also assessed whether the 5,7-DHT-lesions caused any qualitative differences in locomotor responses. Treatment with PCP or MK-801 increased the smoothness of the path traveled (reduced spatial d) and decreased the predictability of locomotor patterns within the chambers (increased entropy). 5,7-DHT-lesions of the dorsal hippocampus did not alter the effects of PCP on spatial d or entropy – despite potentiating total distance moved – but caused a slight reduction in levels of MK-801-induced entropy. Taken together, serotonergic lesions targeting the dorsal hippocampus unmask a functional differentiation of the hyperlocomotor effects of PCP and MK-801. These findings have implications for studies utilizing NMDA receptor antagonists in modeling glutamatergic dysfunction in schizophrenia.

Keywords: serotonin, hippocampus, phencyclidine, MK-801, 5,7-dihydroxytryptamine, locomotor hyperactivity, spatial d, entropy

INTRODUCTION

Phencyclidine (PCP) and MK-801 are often used interchangeably in the psychopharmacological literature as they are both non-competitive antagonists of the glutamatergic *N*-methyl-D-aspartate (NMDA) receptor. It is well-established, however, that MK-801 is more potent at this receptor site than PCP, and that both agents have direct, and dissimilar, effects on other neurotransmitter systems (Lodge and Johnson, 1990; Morris et al., 2005). For example, PCP is a more potent catecholaminergic reuptake inhibitor than MK-801 (Snell et al., 1988; Hiramatsu et al., 1989) and is reported to block reuptake at the serotonin transporter (Hiramatsu et al., 1989; Rothman, 1994; Millan et al., 1999). More recent *in vitro* binding studies distinguish PCP and MK-801 by their relative affinities to the dopamine D_2 receptor (Kapur and Seeman, 2002; Seeman et al., 2005), although negative findings have also been reported (Millan et al., 1999; Jordan et al., 2006). It is also suggested that PCP has moderate affinity for the serotonin 5-HT_{2A} receptor (Kapur and Seeman, 2002) but this has not been replicated by other studies (Millan et al., 1999; Rabin et al., 2000).

The functional mechanism of action of PCP and its analog, ketamine, is of great interest as they are able to evoke a syndrome in humans resembling the spectrum of symptoms in schizophrenia. These "dissociative anesthetics" are thus distinct from psychostimulants like amphetamine, as they can induce not only positive symptoms but also the negative symptoms and cognitive deficits characteristic of the illness (Luby et al., 1959; Krystal et al., 1994; Halberstadt, 1995; Jentsch and Roth, 1999; Morris et al., 2005). Moreover, while psychostimulants typically require chronic use to elicit psychotic states in healthy subjects, a single dose of a PCP or ketamine can induce schizophrenia-like behavioral disturbances (Abi-Saab et al., 1998; Moghaddam and Jackson, 2003; Stone and Pilowsky, 2006). Indeed, their pharmacological characterisation as NMDA receptor antagonists in the 1980s (Anis et al., 1983; Lodge and Johnson, 1990) led to the development of the "NMDA receptor hypofunction hypothesis of schizophrenia," which suggests that dopaminergic dysfunction may be secondary to a primary glutamatergic deficit (Jentsch and Roth, 1999; Olney et al., 1999; Svensson, 2000; Javitt, 2004; Coyle, 2006). The ubiquitous distribution of glutamatergic neurons in the brain, and their regulation by neuromodulatory transmitters, make them a likely candidate for dysfunction in schizophrenia. Interactions between the glutamate system and the dopamine or serotonin systems have been widely studied in this context (Aghajanian and Marek, 2000; Svensson, 2000; Coyle, 2006; Meltzer et al., 2011). However, while PCP may be an appropriate pharmacological tool used in modeling the disorder (Lipska and Weinberger, 2000; Morris et al., 2005), whether its schizophrenia-like effects are due entirely to NMDA receptor antagonism remains to be determined (Kapur and Seeman, 2002; Seeman et al., 2005; Seeman and Lasaga, 2005).

Previous studies have provided evidence of differential serotonergic involvement in the hyperlocomotor effects of PCP and MK-801. For example, PCP-induced locomotor behavior in rats is attenuated by the administration of 5-HT_{2A} receptor antagonists (Maurel-Remy et al., 1995; Krebs-Thomson et al., 1998; Millan et al., 1999). In contrast, 5-HT_{2A} receptor blockade has less consistent effects on MK-801-elicited hyperactivity (Maj et al., 1996; Higgins et al., 2003), suggesting subtle differences in the mechanism of action of these NMDA receptor antagonists. Indeed, when administered alone, locomotor behaviors such as forward ambulation and stereotypic movements induced by PCP and MK-801 are qualitatively different (Hiramatsu et al., 1989; Tricklebank et al., 1989; Lehmann-Masten and Geyer, 1991; Danysz et al., 1994; Ogren and Goldstein, 1994; Gilmour et al., 2009). Some suggest that this is mediated by the ability of PCP to increase serotonin turnover (Hiramatsu et al., 1989), yet others have reported that MK-801 alters serotonin turnover but not PCP (Martin et al., 1998b). Both PCP- and MK-801-induced locomotor hyperactivity, however, is enhanced by pre-treatment with a 5-HT_{2C} receptor antagonist (Hutson et al., 2000). In fact, the 5-HT_{2C} receptor is emerging as a key serotonin receptor subtype involved in the modulation of locomotor behaviors (Takahashi et al., 2001; Giorgetti and Tecott, 2004; Halberstadt et al., 2009). Serotonergic projections to the hippocampus, in particular, are implicated in the modulation of locomotion (Takahashi et al., 2000; Kusljic and van den Buuse, 2004; Dias Soares et al., 2007) and the 5-HT_2 receptor family seems especially involved in this region (Takahashi et al., 2001; Dave et al., 2004).

We have extensively studied the role of brain serotonin in models of schizophrenia in rats using the approach of selective lesions. Injection of the serotonergic neurotoxin, 5,7-dihydroxytryptamine (5,7-DHT), into the median, but not the dorsal, raphe nucleus (MnR, DR) was found to potentiate PCP-induced locomotor behaviors (Kusljic et al., 2003, 2005), but not the effect of MK-801 (Kusljic et al., 2005), providing evidence of a pharmacological distinction between these drugs at the level of serotonergic projections originating in the MnR. Local 5,7-DHT administration into MnR projection regions revealed that lesions of the dorsal, but not ventral, hippocampus enhanced both PCP- and ketamine-induced hyperlocomotion (Kusljic and van den Buuse, 2004; Adams et al., 2009). Taken together, these findings raised questions about both the selectivity and sensitivity of lesion effects. Specifically, we wanted to clarify: (1) whether 5,7-DHT-lesions of the dorsal hippocampus are sufficient to distinguish between the actions of PCP and MK-801, like MnR lesions; and (2) whether the lesions also enhance locomotor responses to PCP at a five-fold lower dose. To this end, our first experiment investigated both dorsal and ventral hippocampal lesion effects on locomotor hyperactivity induced by 0.5 and 2.5 mg/kg of PCP or 0.1 mg/kg of MK-801.

In addition, we wished to examine more qualitative aspects of locomotor behavior using a novel method of analyses. Previously, such high resolution approaches have shown that PCP and MK-801 induce different spatiotemporal patterns of locomotor behavior (Lehmann-Masten and Geyer, 1991), and that pre-treatment with serotonin receptor ligands modulates the type of patterns elicited by PCP, creating an entirely new behavioral profile (Krebs-Thomson et al., 1998). Therefore, we conducted a second experiment focusing on more qualitative aspects of locomotor responses to PCP (2.5 mg/kg) and MK-801 (0.1 mg/kg) in dorsal hippocampus lesioned rats, including the "smoothness" and "predictability" of locomotor paths. Given the prominent role of the dorsal hippocampus in spatial information processing, with visuospatial inputs directed mainly to the dorsal, but not ventral, domain (Moser and Moser, 1998; Small, 2002; Bast, 2007), we anticipated our lesions might modulate such spatial aspects of locomotor behavior, either at baseline or following drug treatment.

MATERIALS AND METHODS

ANIMALS

Sixty four male Sprague-Dawley rats (aged 4–5 weeks) were obtained from the Department of Pathology, University of Melbourne (Parkville, VIC, Australia), or Monash Animal Services (Clayton, VIC, Australia). Colony conditions were standardized, with a 12/12 h light/dark cycle (lights on 7:00–19:00) and the temperature maintained at approximately 22°C. All procedures were performed in the light phase. Rats were housed in groups of 2–3 in cages enriched with shredded paper and cardboard boxes, with standard food and tap water available *ad libitum*. All surgical and experimental protocols were approved by the Animal Experimentation Ethics Committee of the University of Melbourne or the Howard Florey Institute (Parkville, VIC, Australia), and adhered to the guidelines outlined in the Australian Code of Practise for the Care and Use of Animals for Scientific Purposes (National Health and Medical Research Council of Australia, 2004).

DRUGS AND SOLUTIONS

To prevent oxidation, 5,7-DHT (5,7-dihydroxytryptamine creatinine sulfate salt, Fluka BioChemika, Sigma-Aldrich, St. Louis, MO, USA) was dissolved in 0.9% saline containing 0.1% ascorbic acid. The selective noradrenaline reuptake inhibitor, desmethylimipramine hydrochloride (DMI; Sigma-Aldrich), was prepared in distilled water and dissolved by sonication. The non-steroidal anti-inflammatory agent, Carprofen (Rimadyl®, 50 mg/ml, Pfizer, West Ryde, NSW, Australia) was diluted in 0.9% saline. Consistent with previous work in our laboratory, PCP hydrochloride (Experiment 1: Sigma-Aldrich; Experiment 2: National

Measurement Institute, Pymble, NSW, Australia) and (+)-MK-801 hydrogen maleate (dizocilpine, Sigma-Aldrich) were dissolved in 0.9% saline and administered subcutaneous (s.c.). All doses were taken as the weight of the salt and injection volume was 1 mg/kg body weight.

STEREOTAXIC LESION SURGERY

Surgery was conducted when animals were 7–8 weeks old as described previously (Kusljic and van den Buuse, 2004; Adams et al., 2008, 2009; Adams and van den Buuse, 2011). In brief, rats were randomly allocated to one of four groups: dorsal hippocampus-injected (DHI), ventral hippocampus-injected (VHI) or their equivalent sham-operated controls. At the outset of surgery, 30 min prior to 5,7-DHT infusion, DMI (20 mg/kg, i.p.) was injected to prevent the destruction of noradrenergic neurons. Animals were then anesthetized using a 10% isoflurane/oxygen mixture and transferred to a stereotaxic apparatus affixed with a nose cone to maintain anesthesia. Carprofen (5 mg/kg, s.c.) was used to minimize post-operative discomfort. Holes were drilled in the skull above the dorsal or ventral hippocampus, using the following coordinates relative to bregma: posterior −3.6 mm, lateral ±1.5 and ±3.5 mm, and ventral −3.8 mm for the dorsal hippocampus; posterior −5.6 mm, lateral ±4.8 mm and ventral −8.0 mm for the ventral hippocampus (Paxinos and Watson, 1998). 5,7-DHT (1 μl, 5 μg/μl) was injected bilaterally into the dorsal or ventral hippocampus over 2 min; for the DHI infusions, two 0.5 μl injections were used. Sham-operated rats received equivalent volumes of vehicle solution. Rats were allowed two weeks to recover from surgery before behavioral experiments started.

LOCOMOTOR HYPERACTIVITY TESTING

Locomotor activity was measured in eight automated photocell cages (43 cm × 43 cm × 31 cm, l × w × h, ENV-520, Med Associates Inc., St. Albans, VT, USA). Each cage had 16 evenly-spaced infrared transmitters and receivers on each of its four sides, which detected a rat's position in three dimensions (*x*, *y* and *z*). Software (Activity Monitor 4.0, Med Associates Inc.) recorded the status of the infrared beams every 50 ms, effectively generating a spatio-temporal map of an animal's movement throughout a testing session. Every 5 min, the software calculated the total distance moved from these data, reflecting the gross distance traveled by an animal with small repetitive movements filtered out.

Each session included a random allocation of 5,7-DHT-lesioned rats and sham-operated controls. Baseline locomotor activity was initially recorded for 30 min, allowing the animals to habituate to the cages before receiving drug treatment. Post-injection locomotor activity was then recorded for further 90 min. Testing sessions were separated by 3–4 days to allow for drug clearance, and the order of treatment in each experiment was pseudo-randomized to offset potential interactions, such as sensitisation, that could occur between treatments. Baseline activity differences were assessed by averaging pre-injection distance moved across all testing sessions within each experiment. As baseline activity was unaffected by the serotonergic lesions in both experiments, these data were subsequently removed from analyses of drug effects.

ENZYME-LINKED IMMUNOSORBENT ASSAY (ELISA)

Lesions were confirmed by measuring serotonin levels in the dorsal and ventral hippocampus using Serotonin ELISA kits (Labor Diagnostika Nord GmbH & Co. KG, Nordhorn, Germany), with minor adjustments as described before (Adams et al., 2009; Adams and van den Buuse, 2011). Rats were decapitated at least three days after the end of locomotor testing, and the dorsal and ventral hippocampi dissected out, weighed, and stored at −80°C until ELISA. Serotonin levels were normalized for tissue wet weight. Analyses of ELISA data from DHI- and VHI-sham-operated rats in each experiment found no differences in hippocampal serotonin levels between the two types of controls; therefore, these groups were combined. In line with our previous work (Adams and van den Buuse, 2011), DHI or VHI rats were excluded if the percentage serotonin depletion was <20% in the relevant hippocampal domain compared to sham-operated animals; presently, only one VHI rat was excluded from Experiment 1.

DESIGN AND ANALYSES

Animals were used in two experimental cohorts. Experiment 1 contained DHI ($n = 16$), VHI ($n = 8$) and equivalent sham-operated controls ($n = 17$); all rats received saline, 0.5 and 2.5 mg/kg PCP, and 0.1 mg/kg MK-801 in locomotor activity tests. Experiment 2 contained only DHI ($n = 12$) and DHI-sham-operated ($n = 11$) rats; all animals received saline, 2.5 mg/kg PCP and 0.1 mg/kg MK-801 in locomotor activity tests; 0.02 mg/kg MK-801 was also tested in these animals yet these data are not presented as this dose had negligible effect on locomotor responses. Using a within-subjects design to assess drug responses was important for comparing the effects of PCP and MK-801 by minimizing the variation that is inherent in between-group comparisons; in addition, it greatly reduced the number of animals required.

In Experiment 1, distance moved data were calculated by the activity monitor software. In Experiment 2, raw *x*, *y*, *t* data were extracted from the software as ASCII text files and analyzed for qualitative aspects of locomotor activity. Analysis of the spatial structure of locomotor paths was performed by calculating the descriptive statistic, spatial d. As described by Paulus and Geyer (1991), spatial d is based conceptually on fractal geometry and calculated using scaling arguments. Changes in d reflect smoother (reduced d values) or rougher (increased d values) locomotor paths. Entropy was used to quantify the predictability of locomotor paths, specifically the predictability of sequences of transitions across different zones of the test chamber (Paulus and Geyer, 1993). For example, a rat repeatedly circling along the outer edges of the chamber would move through zones 1, 2, 3, 6, 9, 4, and back to 1; repetition of this sequence many times would result in a low entropy measure. By contrast, a rat that moves through different zones of the chamber via more diverse routes would result in higher entropy levels.

Analysis of variance (ANOVA) with repeated measures, as appropriate, was used to compare differences between and within groups using SYSTAT software (SYSTAT 9.0, SPSS Inc., Chicago, IL, USA). All data were analyzed separately, initially in an overall ANOVA with data from each group (Experiment 1: sham-operated, DHI, VHI; Experiment 2: sham-operated, DHI). When significant main effects of, or interactions with, group were found in the main analyses, planned (a priori) ANOVA comparisons ensued, with either DHI or VHI groups compared to controls, and drug effects compared to that of saline injection.

Distance moved data from Experiment 1 were analyzed in 5-min intervals to assess possible time-dependent drug effects, whereas distance moved, spatial d and entropy data from Experiment 2 were assessed in 30-min intervals. Post-injection spatial d and entropy data were analyzed for 60 min as low activity levels in the 60–90 min block following saline treatment rendered measurement of these variables unreliable. Thus, overall ANOVAs of all post-injection activity data contained the repeated measures variables, "drug" (Experiment 1: four saline/drug treatments; Experiment 2: three saline/drug treatments) and "time" (Experiment 1: 18 5-min intervals; Experiment 2: two or three 30-min intervals).

Enzyme-linked immunosorbent assay data were analyzed by comparing absolute serotonin levels in either the dorsal or ventral hippocampus. Data are presented as percentage depletion relative to sham-operated animals to control for inter-assay variability.

Differences were considered significant if $p < 0.05$.

RESULTS

SEROTONIN DEPLETION IN THE DORSAL AND VENTRAL HIPPOCAMPUS

In Experiment 1, DHI rats showed a comparable level of serotonin depletion in the ventral hippocampus as VHI rats, but a greater extent of depletion in the dorsal hippocampus (**Table 1**). VHI rats in this cohort also showed a slight, but significant, depletion of serotonin in the dorsal hippocampus. Like those in Experiment 1, DHI rats in Experiment 2 showed serotonin depletion in both the dorsal and ventral hippocampus compared to sham-operated controls (**Table 1**).

EXPERIMENT 1: LESION EFFECTS ON LOCOMOTOR HYPERACTIVITY INDUCED BY 0.5 AND 2.5 mg/kg PCP AND 0.1 mg/kg MK-801

Analysis of variance of average pre-injection distance moved found no group differences, indicating that 5,7-DHT administration into the dorsal or ventral hippocampus did not affect levels of baseline activity (**Figure 1**). Locomotor activity diminished over this

Table 1 | Serotonin depletion pattern in the dorsal and ventral hippocampus of 5,7-DHT-lesioned rats.

	Dorsal hippocampus		Ventral hippocampus	
	% Depletion	*F, p*	% Depletion	*F, p*
Experiment 1				
DHI	77 ± 4**	177.0, <0.001	54 ± 5**	34.3, <0.001
VHI	19 ± 8*	5.4, 0.029	45 ± 8*	14.0, 0.001
Experiment 2				
DHI	79 ± 5**	130.1, <0.001	82 ± 2**	138.1, <0.001

*Data are expressed as mean percentage depletion of serotonin ± SEM in each hippocampal domain relative to the sham-operated controls in each experiment. Statistical results in adjacent columns refer to the F- and p-values obtained in ANOVA comparison of absolute serotonin levels. *p < 0.05, **p < 0.001 compared to sham-operated controls.*

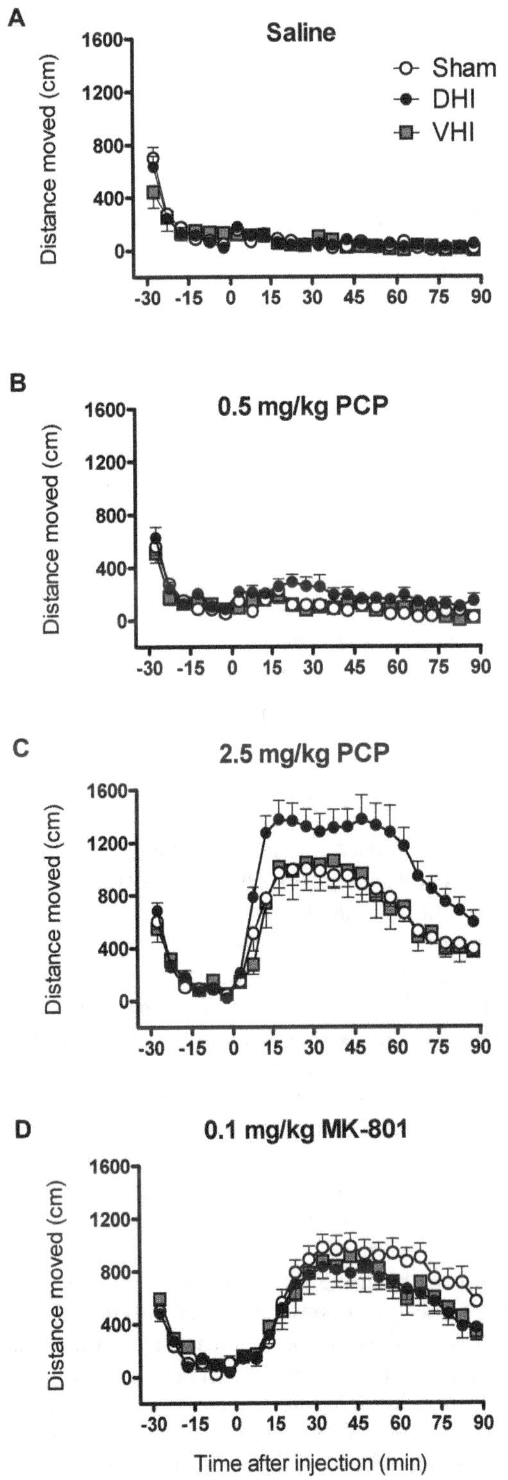

FIGURE 1 | Effect of 5,7-DHT-lesions targeting the dorsal or ventral hippocampus on locomotor hyperactivity induced by 0.5 and 2.5 mg/kg PCP and 0.1 mg/kg MK-801. Panels show mean distance moved (cm) in 5 min intervals ± SEM for DHI (n = 16), VHI (n = 8) and sham-operated rats (n = 17) treated with **(A)** saline **(B)** 0.5 and **(C)** 2.5 mg/kg PCP and **(D)** 0.1 mg/kg MK-801. Total distance moved following 0.5 and 2.5 mg/kg PCP injection was significantly higher in DHI rats compared to controls (see text for details).

30 min pre-injection habituation period similarly in all animals (main effect of time: $F_{5,190} = 163.5, p < 0.001$).

Analysis of all post-injection distance moved data revealed significant lesion effects (main effect of group: $F_{2,38} = 3.7, p=0.034$; drug by group interaction: $F_{6,114} = 3.7, p = 0.002$; **Figure 1**). Rats that were administered 5,7-DHT into the dorsal hippocampus showed enhanced locomotor hyperactivity following 0.5 mg/kg PCP treatment, with a 109 ± 37% increase in total post-injection distance moved compared to controls (main effect of group: $F_{1,31} = 7.2, p = 0.012$; drug by group interaction: $F_{1,31} = 6.0, p = 0.020$; **Figure 1B**). Confirming our previous findings (Kusljic and van den Buuse, 2004), DHI rats also showed potentiated hyperlocomotor effects of 2.5 mg/kg PCP treatment (51 ± 15% increase in total distance moved; main effect of group: $F_{1,31} = 10.6, p = 0.003$; drug by group interaction: $F_{1,31} = 9.3, p = 0.005$; **Figure 1C**). The enhancement of PCP-induced hyperlocomotion was uniform throughout the session for both doses (lack of significant interactions with time and group; **Figures 1B,C**). In contrast, VHI and sham-operated animals showed similar PCP-induced locomotor hyperactivity at both doses (main effects of drug: 0.5 mg/kg, $F_{1,23} = 13.4, p = 0.001$; 2.5 mg/kg, $F_{1,23} = 133.3, p < 0.001$; **Figures 1B,C**). Notably, treatment with MK-801 evoked locomotor hyperactivity to a similar extent and temporal magnitude in sham-operated, DHI and VHI rats (main effect of drug: $F_{1,38} = 127.3, p < 0.001$; drug by time interaction: $F_{17,646} = 42.3, p < 0.001$), indicating that the potentiated hyperlocomotor effect in DHI rats is unique to PCP (**Figure 1D**).

EXPERIMENT 2: FURTHER ANALYSIS OF DORSAL HIPPOCAMPUS LESION EFFECTS ON LOCOMOTOR HYPERACTIVITY INDUCED BY 2.5 mg/kg PCP AND 0.1 mg/kg MK-801

Distance moved

As observed in Experiment 1, average pre-injection distance moved did not differ between DHI and sham-operated rats in this experiment. Both groups habituated to the chambers with similar levels of activity (**Figure 2A**).

Analysis of variance of all post-injection distance moved data found that the effects of drug treatment were, again, dependent on lesion group (drug by group interaction: $F_{2,42} = 6.3, p = 0.004$; **Figure 2A**). As expected, total PCP-induced hyperactivity was greater in DHI rats than in sham-operated controls (51 ± 13% increase in total distance moved; main effect of group: $F_{1,21} = 8.5, p = 0.008$; drug by group interaction: $F_{1,21} = 11.3, p = 0.003$; **Figure 2A**, middle panel). In addition, MK-801 treatment caused a time-dependent increase in locomotor activity that was unaffected by dorsal hippocampus lesions (main effect of drug: $F_{1,21} = 125.1, p < 0.001$; drug by time interaction: $F_{2,42} = 52.1, p < 0.001$; **Figure 2A**, bottom panel). The lack of significant interactions between time and group in analyses of distance moved data for both compounds also corresponded with Experiment 1. Representative plots of post-injection activity are provided in **Figure 3**, in which enhanced PCP-induced hyperlocomotion in a DHI animal is clearly depicted (**Figure 3B**, bottom panel).

Spatial d

Assessment of average pre-injection spatial d revealed no difference in baseline levels between DHI and sham-operated rats (**Figure 2B**). After saline treatment, spatial d values increased over the course of the test sessions as the animals habituated to the chambers and made fewer smooth, linear exploratory movements (saline data only, comparison of all three time blocks: main effect of time, $F_{2,42} = 18.9, p < 0.001$; **Figure 2B**, top panel). Spatial d values exceeded baseline levels during the 30–60 min block ($F_{1,21} = 27.7, p < 0.001$) but not during the 0–30 min block.

Overall ANOVA of post-injection data found time-dependent, drug effects on spatial d that were unaffected by the lesions (main effect of drug: $F_{2,42} = 45.3, p < 0.001$; drug by time interaction: $F_{2,42} = 46.4, p < 0.001$). Compared to saline, both PCP and MK-801 treatments reduced spatial d in DHI and sham-operated rats (main effects of drug: PCP, $F_{1,21} = 67.7, p < 0.001$; MK-801, $F_{1,21} = 61.4, p < 0.001$), with more pronounced effects occurring in the 30–60 min time block (drug by time interactions: PCP, $F_{1,21} = 9.5, p = 0.006$; MK-801, $F_{1,21} = 82.6, p < 0.001$; **Figure 2B**). Further analyses for each time block revealed that PCP treatment reduced spatial d in both blocks (0-30 min, $F_{1,21} = 23.5, p < 0.001$; 30–60 min, $F_{1,21} = 75.3, p < 0.001$), whereas the effect of MK-801 treatment was significant in the 30–60 min interval only (0–30 min, $F_{1,21} = 3.6, p = 0.071$; 30–60 min, $F_{1,21} = 135.5, p < 0.001$). 5,7-DHT-lesions targeting the dorsal hippocampus, however, did not influence the changes in overall smoothness of the paths traveled following treatment with either compound.

Entropy

Analysis of mean pre-injection entropy data found no group differences, highlighting that the predictably of the paths traveled at baseline was unchanged by 5,7-DHT administration into the dorsal hippocampus (**Figure 2C**). In saline-treated animals, entropy values declined over the course of the session as the animals became habituated to the test chambers, indicating that the locomotor paths became progressively more repetitive (saline data only, comparison of all three time blocks: main effect of time, $F_{2,42} = 51.6, p < 0.001$; **Figure 2C**, top panel). Entropy levels were lower than baseline during both post-injection time blocks (0–30 min, $F_{1,21} = 11.0, p = 0.003$; 30–60 min, $F_{1,21} = 103.5, p < 0.001$).

Assessment of all post-injection data found an overall, time-dependent influence of drug treatment on entropy levels (main effect of drug: $F_{2,42} = 34.6, p < 0.001$; drug by time interaction: $F_{2,42} = 35.5, p < 0.001$; **Figure 2C**). Drug effects on entropy were further influenced by hippocampal 5,7-DHT lesions (drug by group interaction: $F_{2,42} = 3.7, p = 0.032$). PCP administration increased entropy compared to saline injection (main effect of drug: $F_{1,21} = 51.1, p < 0.001$), indicating that the animals traveled in less predictable manner around the chambers. While entropy levels following saline treatment decreased over time, after PCP injection entropy was elevated throughout the session (drug by time interaction: $F_{1,21} = 28.5, p < 0.001$; 0–30 min, $F_{1,21} = 8.4, p = 0.009$; 30–60 min, $F_{1,21} = 65.1, p < 0.001$). This effect was similar in sham-operated and DHI animals (**Figure 2C**, middle panel). Treatment with MK-801 also increased entropy compared to saline injection (main effect of drug: $F_{1,21} = 36.5, p < 0.001$) yet, similar to its effect on spatial d, this was significant only in the 30–60 min

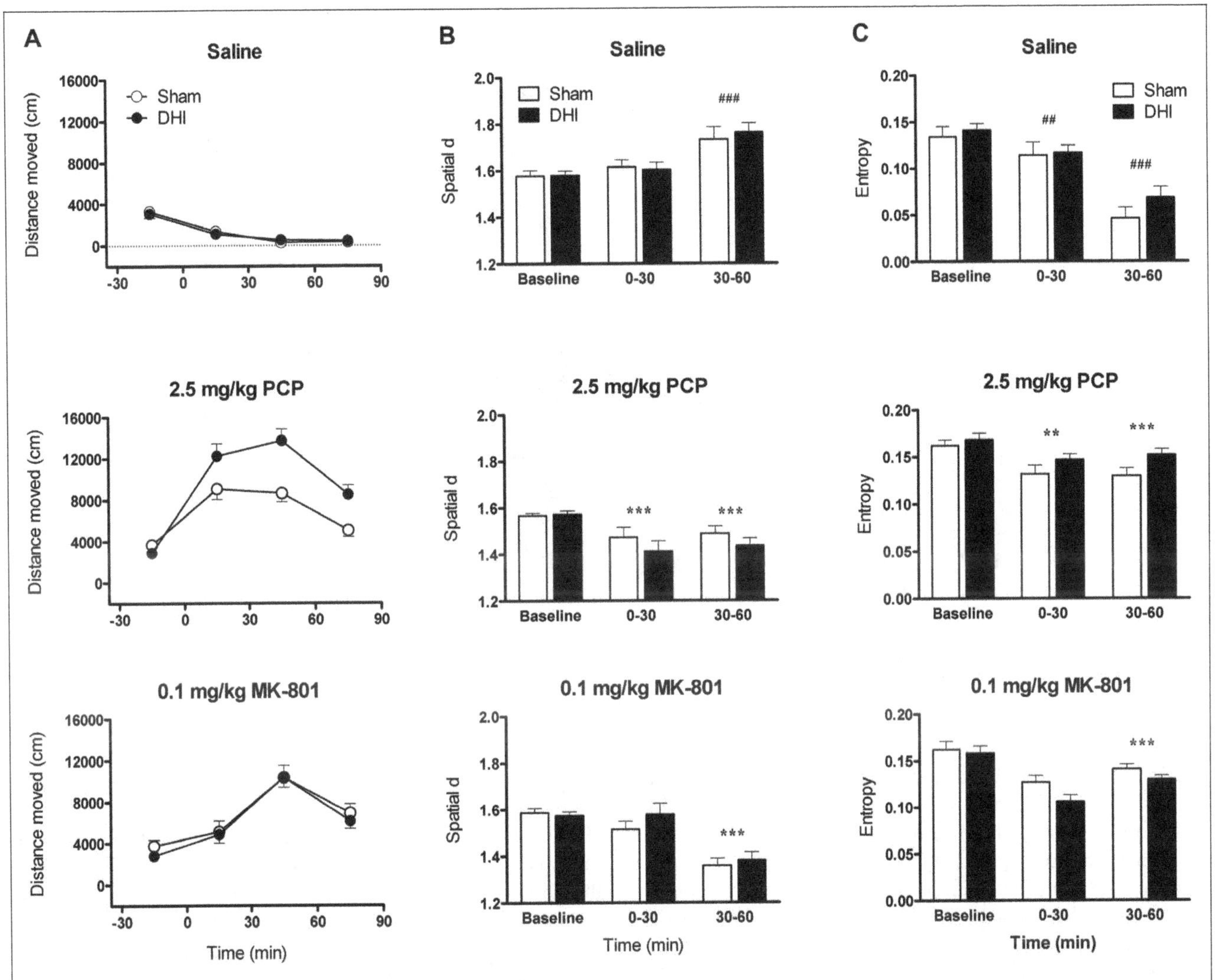

FIGURE 2 | Effect of 5,7-DHT-lesions targeting the dorsal hippocampus on qualitative aspects of locomotor hyperactivity induced by 2.5 mg/kg PCP and 0.1 mg/kg MK-801. Panels show mean **(A)** distance moved (cm), **(B)** spatial d, and **(C)** entropy in 30 min intervals ± SEM for DHI ($n = 12$) and sham-operated rats ($n = 11$) treated with saline (top), 2.5 mg/kg PCP (middle), and 0.1 mg/kg MK-801 (bottom). Total distance moved following 2.5 mg/kg PCP injection was, again, significantly higher in DHI rats compared to controls (see text for details). $^{\#\#}p < 0.01$, $^{\#\#\#}p < 0.001$ for comparison with baseline. $^{**}p < 0.01$, $^{***}p < 0.001$ for comparison with saline in respective time block.

time block (drug by time interaction: $F_{1,21} = 51.4$, $p < 0.001$; 0–30 min, $F_{1,21} = 0.024$, $p = 0.878$; 30–60 min, $F_{1,21} = 64.1$, $p < 0.001$). Interestingly, compared to sham-operated controls, overall MK-801-induced enhancement of entropy was reduced in DHI rats (drug by group interaction: $F_{1,21} = 4.6$, $p = 0.043$; **Figure 2C**, bottom panel). Serotonergic lesions targeting the dorsal hippocampus, therefore, did not alter the random nature of locomotor paths traveled following PCP treatment, yet slightly reduced the extent to which MK-801 treatment increased this factor.

DISCUSSION

There is considerable interest in the behavioral mechanism of action of PCP as it can produce a state in healthy humans analogous to symptoms in schizophrenia. Here we report that rats with 5,7-DHT-lesions targeting the dorsal hippocampus show potentiated locomotor hyperactivity following treatment with 0.5 or 2.5 mg/kg PCP, extending our earlier work by showing that the lesions are also sensitive to a five-fold lower dose (Kusljic and van den Buuse, 2004). Given the role of the hippocampus in spatial information processing, we anticipated that enhanced PCP responses in DHI rats would be associated with changes in the modulation of spatial d or entropy, yet analysis of behavioral patterns revealed no lesion effects on these variables at baseline or following PCP treatment. In contrast to PCP, DHI rats did not show a parallel enhancement of locomotor responses to MK-801, but rather a slight, but significant, reduction in MK-801-induced entropy. Thus, like lesions of serotonergic cell bodies in the MnR (Kusljic et al., 2005), 5,7-DHT-lesions targeting the dorsal hippocampus are sufficient to unmask functional differences between PCP and the more selective NMDA receptor antagonist, MK-801. Together with data from numerous locomotor activity

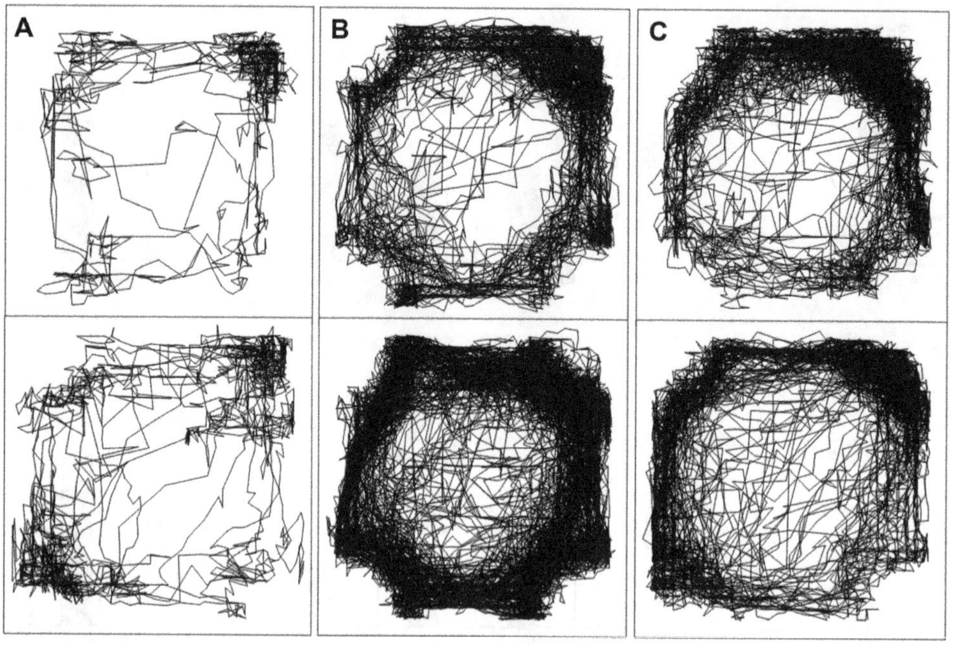

FIGURE 3 | Spatial patterns of locomotor hyperactivity shown by representative, individual sham-operated (top) and DHI (bottom) animals. Plots show activity traces in the 60–90 min time block following treatment with **(A)** saline **(B)** 2.5 mg/kg PCP and **(C)** 0.1 mg MK-801. Enhanced PCP-induced locomotor hyperactivity in DHI rats is clearly depicted by the increased density of tracings in the chamber (panel **B**, bottom).

experiments in 5,7-DHT-lesioned rats (see Adams et al., 2008 for review; Adams et al., 2009), these results indicate that serotonin projections from the MnR to the dorsal hippocampus are involved in the hyperlocomotor mechanism of action of the dissociative anesthetics, PCP and ketamine, as opposed to that of psychostimulants, like amphetamine, and in a manner seemingly independent of their ability to block NMDA receptors, or modulate spatial patterns of behavior. Like other reports (Snell et al., 1988; Hiramatsu et al., 1989; Rothman, 1994; Kapur and Seeman, 2002; Seeman et al., 2005; Seeman and Lasaga, 2005), our findings lend strength to the notion that the schizophrenomimetic effects of PCP and ketamine may not be due to NMDA receptor antagonism alone.

The differential effects of the lesions on PCP or MK-801-induced forward locomotion seem to hinge on impaired serotonergic tone in the dorsal hippocampus only, since rats with ventral hippocampus lesions in Experiment 1 showed no change in responses to either compound. In addition, dorsal hippocampus serotonin depletion appears robust in potentiating PCP responses regardless of the additional depletion observed in the ventral domain. In our early study, DHI rats showed no secondary lesion effects in the ventral hippocampus (Kusljic and van den Buuse, 2004); the asymmetric pattern of serotonin depletion observed in our DHI and VHI rats more recently has been discussed in detail elsewhere (Adams et al., 2009). However, with reduced serotonin levels in the whole hippocampus, we cannot definitively conclude that the behavioral changes are due to 5,7-DHT effects in the dorsal hippocampus only. Since entropy and spatial d was not assessed in VHI animals, it is possible that serotonin depletion in both hippocampal domains of DHI rats contributed to the reduction of MK-801-induced entropy. The ventral hippocampus also contains so-called "place cells," involved in creating an internal representation of the environment (O'Keefe and Dostrovsky, 1971; Sweatt, 2004), suggesting that it, too, participates in spatial information processing (Moser and Moser, 1998). Nevertheless, the absence of corresponding functional changes in VHI rats in Experiment 1, together with our previous work (Kusljic and van den Buuse, 2004; Adams et al., 2009), suggests that serotonin depletion in the ventral hippocampus does not largely influence drug-induced hyperlocomotion.

Neither dorsal nor ventral hippocampal lesions were found to alter baseline locomotor behavior. Given that the expression of motor deficits after 6-hydroxydopamine-lesions depends on levels of dopamine depletion being >80–90% (Koob et al., 1981; Zigmond et al., 1990), it is possible that overt effects on baseline behavior were not seen due to insufficient levels of serotonin depletion. However, some of our previous cohorts have shown >80–90% depletion of hippocampal serotonin without showing alterations in baseline activity (Kusljic and van den Buuse, 2004; Adams et al., 2009). Even so, the utility of the 30 min habituation phase to assess baseline deficits may be questioned, as activity levels soon become negligible during this period making it difficult to evaluate any change. Indeed, others report that the extent of dorsal, but not ventral, hippocampal serotonin depletion correlates with the amount of activity displayed in the dark phase (Williams and Azmitia, 1981). Observing our lesioned animals in a novel open field, potentially in the dark phase, as well as incorporating assessments of vertical activity and grooming behavior, may provide a better appraisal of baseline lesion effects on motor behavior. In the present studies, as in our previous experiments, the expression of behavioral changes due to 5,7-DHT-lesions targeting the dorsal hippocampus was found to depend on pharmacological challenge (Adams et al., 2009; Adams and van den Buuse, 2011).

Phencyclidine has previously been shown to produce biphasic effects on spatial patterns of locomotion, generating smoother paths at 2.25 mg/kg (decreasing d) and reducing the smoothness of paths (increasing d) at higher doses (6.75, 10.125 mg/kg; Krebs-Thomson et al., 1998). Using the same analytical method, we similarly found that administration of 2.5 mg/kg PCP decreased d equally in both control and DHI rats. Interestingly, pre-treatment with a 5-$HT_{2A/2C}$ agonist potentiated hyperlocomotion and further decreased spatial d in rats treated with 2.25 mg/kg PCP (Krebs-Thomson et al., 1998); together with the current data, one could speculate that 5-$HT_{2A/2C}$ receptors in the dorsal hippocampus are involved in the former, but not the latter, effect. Finding that 0.1 mg/kg MK-801 also increases locomotion while producing smoother locomotor paths (decreasing d), and that both compounds reduce the predictability of the locomotor paths traveled (increasing entropy) is novel to this study. Hippocampal NMDA receptors are vital for spatial memory and information processing, with evidence indicating that they are necessary for the acquisition, or encoding, of spatial memory but not for retrieval (Nakazawa et al., 2004; Martin and Clark, 2007). One interpretation of the increase in entropy following MK-801 or PCP treatment is that NMDA receptor blockade impairs the animals' memory of where they have previously been in the chamber, making them explore more randomly. In addition, 5,7-DHT-lesions targeting the dorsal hippocampus selectively reduced the ability of MK-801 to increase entropy, independent of its effect on locomotor activity. The mechanism underlying this more subtle effect of the lesions is unclear, but likely relates to a lesion-induced dysregulation of hippocampal NMDA receptors. Since PCP-induced entropy was not changed by the lesions, this could simply reflect the more potent and selective NMDA antagonist actions of MK-801.

Treatment with 0.1 mg/kg MK-801 and 2.5 mg/kg PCP produced equivalent levels of hyperlocomotion in control animals in both experiments. However, the maximal effect of MK-801 was seen between 30 and 60 min post-injection followed by a gradual decrease, while the peak PCP effect occurred earlier, between 15 and 30 min. The different times to onset of maximal effect of these agents corroborate previous studies (Ogren and Goldstein, 1994; Klamer et al., 2005), and may reflect differences in their temporal association to the NMDA receptor (Ogren and Goldstein, 1994). Indeed, MK-801 and PCP have similar volumes of distribution (Schwartz and Wasterlain, 1991; Shelnutt et al., 1999) and indexes of lipophilicity making them equally brain penetrant (Ault et al., 1995). In both experiments, however, the time to onset of PCP's effects in DHI rats was more rapid, and the effect more vigorous and longer lasting, which is unlikely to arise from lesion-induced changes in pharmacokinetics. Instead, altered hyperlocomotor responses to PCP, and ketamine (Adams et al., 2009), in DHI rats appear to be a quantitative enhancement of the normal motor responses to these agents. In control animals, these compounds may activate serotonergic transmission in the dorsal hippocampus in a manner such that it inhibits their own effects. Accordingly, the absence of intact serotonergic tone in the dorsal hippocampus of DHI rats unmasks this self-activated, inhibitory mechanism. This could be significant to the mechanism of action of these dissociative compounds, as the lesion-induced enhancement was observed across all tested doses of PCP (0.5, 2.5 mg/kg) and ketamine (6.25, 12.5, 25 mg/kg; Adams et al., 2009).

Mechanisms within the dorsal hippocampus through which PCP and ketamine putatively activate serotonergic transmission could be pre- or post-synaptic, or a combination of both. As hypothesized earlier (Kusljic and van den Buuse, 2004), the effect could involve reduced PCP-induced serotonin release in the dorsal hippocampus (Martin et al., 1998a). Ketamine treatment increases extracellular serotonin levels in the ventral hippocampus (Lorrain et al., 2003), yet there is a lack of data regarding its effect in the dorsal domain. Serotonin release following treatment with these agents may result directly from SERT reuptake inhibition (Hori et al., 1996; Nishimura et al., 1998; Millan et al., 1999) or indirectly via glutamatergic disinhibition (Martin et al., 1998a), whereby preferential blockade of NMDA receptors on GABAergic interneurons by NMDA receptor antagonists "disinhibits" corticolimbic circuits, causing the release of neurotransmitters (Olney et al., 1999). It follows, however, that MK-801 treatment would also disinhibit hippocampal circuits, and it was recently shown that local infusion of MK-801 increases extracellular serotonin levels in the dorsal hippocampus (Fallon et al., 2007). An alternative mechanism to explain the enhanced PCP responses may involve post-synaptic changes in serotonergic receptors. Autoradiography experiments revealed that local 5-HT_{1A} and 5-HT_{2A} receptor densities are unchanged by the lesions, yet there is a 70% increase in 5-HT_{2C} receptor densities in the dorsal hippocampus of DHI rats (Adams and van den Buuse, 2011). This finding is compelling because, unlike systemic administration, infusion of 5-HT_{2C} receptor agonists into the dorsal hippocampus stimulates locomotor activity (Takahashi et al., 2001; Stiedl et al., 2007). Thus, a simple explanation for our results would be a direct action by PCP on an upregulated 5-HT_{2C} receptor pool in the dorsal hippocampus of DHI rats. However, preliminary *in vitro* data indicate that PCP, ketamine or MK-801 do not directly bind to or activate the human 5-HT_{2C} receptor (unedited INI 5-HT_{2C} receptor isoform; Stewart and Christopoulos, Monash Institute of Pharmaceutical Sciences, Parkville, VIC, Australia, unpublished observations). While this does not exclude the possibility of a direct action on rat 5-HT_{2C} receptors, particularly in light of evidence that PCP and ketamine act directly on rat 5-HT_{2A} receptors (Nabeshima et al., 1988; Kapur and Seeman, 2002), this would have little relevance to humans. Additional locomotor behavioral experiments combining the local administration of selective ligands, such as for 5-HT_2 receptor subtypes, into the dorsal hippocampus in conjunction with systemic PCP or MK-801 treatment are required. Finally, it is also possible that downstream alterations – either intrinsic or extrinsic to the hippocampus – might be involved in altered behavioral responses in DHI rats. It is clear that there are numerous mechanisms by which 5,7-DHT-lesions targeting the dorsal hippocampus could disclose differences in the hyperlocomotor effects of PCP and MK-801; the exact reasons remain speculative without further experiments.

Building on our previous 5,7-DHT-lesion studies in rats, our data highlight an important role for serotonin projections to the dorsal hippocampus, most likely from the MnR, in the mechanism of action of the dissociative anesthetics, PCP, and ketamine, but not that of MK-801. Given the direction and sensitivity of the behavioral change in dorsal hippocampus lesioned rats, in a normal state, these compounds may activate MnR-dorsal hippocampus serotonergic transmission in manner that subsequently serves to inhibit their net hyperlocomotor effects. The importance of clarifying the pharmacology of the "NMDA receptor antagonists" in the context of understanding their schizophrenogenic properties has been emphasized before (Klamer et al., 2005; Gilmour et al., 2009; Seillier and Giuffrida, 2009), with others finding that PCP and ketamine should not be used interchangeably (Gilmour et al., 2009). Understanding of how the "NMDA receptor antagonists" exert their hyperlocomotor effects in rodents is limited and, despite the seemingly analogous outward expression of locomotor hyperactivity they elicit, it is clear that the underlying neurochemical mechanisms are different. Elucidating these differences, particularly with neurotransmitter and brain region specificity, is important in the translation of preclinical research using these compounds in the context of schizophrenia.

REFERENCES

Abi-Saab, W. M., D'Souza, D. C., Moghaddam, B., and Krystal, J. H. (1998). The NMDA antagonist model for schizophrenia: promise and pitfalls. *Pharmacopsychiatry* 31(Suppl 2), 104–109. doi: 10.1055/s-2007-979354

Adams, W., Ayton, S., and van den Buuse, M. (2009). Serotonergic lesions of the dorsal hippocampus differentially modulate locomotor hyperactivity induced by drugs of abuse in rats: implications for schizophrenia. *Psychopharmacology (Berl.)* 206, 665–676. doi: 10.1007/s00213-009-1617-1

Adams, W., Kusljic, S., and van den Buuse, M. (2008). Serotonin depletion in the dorsal and ventral hippocampus: effects on locomotor hyperactivity, prepulse inhibition and learning and memory. *Neuropharmacology* 55, 1048–1055. doi: 10.1016/j.neuropharm.2008.06.035

Adams, W., and van den Buuse, M. (2011). Hippocampal serotonin depletion facilitates the enhancement of prepulse inhibition by risperidone: possible role of 5-HT2C receptors in the dorsal hippocampus. *Neuropharmacology* 61, 458–467. doi: 10.1016/j.neuropharm.2011.03.018

Aghajanian, G. K., and Marek, G. J. (2000). Serotonin model of schizophrenia: emerging role of glutamate mechanisms. *Brain Res. Brain Res. Rev.* 31, 302–312. doi: 10.1016/S0165-0173(99)00046-6

Anis, N. A., Berry, S. C., Burton, N. R., and Lodge, D. (1983). The dissociative anaesthetics, ketamine and phencyclidine, selectively reduce excitation of central mammalian neurones by N-methyl-aspartate. *Br. J. Pharmacol.* 79, 565–575. doi: 10.1111/j.1476-5381.1983.tb11031.x

Ault, B., Miller, M. S., Kelly, M. D., Hildebrand, L. M., Earley, W. G., Luttinger, D., et al. (1995). WIN 63480, a hydrophilic TCP-site ligand, has reduced agonist-independent NMDA ion channel access compared to MK-801 and phencyclidine. *Neuropharmacology* 34, 1597–1606. doi: 10.1016/0028-3908(95)00125-5

Bast, T. (2007). Toward an integrative perspective on hippocampal function: from the rapid encoding of experience to adaptive behavior. *Rev. Neurosci.* 18, 253–281. doi: 10.1515/REVNEURO.2007.18.3-4.253

Coyle, J. T. (2006). Glutamate and schizophrenia: beyond the dopamine hypothesis. *Cell. Mol. Neurobiol.* 26, 365–384. doi: 10.1007/s10571-006-9062-8

Danysz, W., Essmann, U., Bresink, I., and Wilke, R. (1994). Glutamate antagonists have different effects on spontaneous locomotor activity in rats. *Pharmacol. Biochem. Behav.* 48, 111–118. doi: 10.1016/0091-3057(94)90506-1

Dave, K. D., Fernando, G. S., Quinn, J. L., Harvey, J. A., and Aloyo, V. J. (2004). Serotonin 5-HT2A receptors in the CA1 field of the hippocampus mediate head movements in the rabbit. *Psychopharmacology (Berl.)* 176, 287–295. doi: 10.1007/s00213-004-1887-6

Dias Soares, D., Celso Coimbra, C., and Marubayashi, U. (2007). Tryptophan-induced central fatigue in exercising rats is related to serotonin content in preoptic area. *Neurosci. Lett.* 415, 274–278. doi: 10.1016/j.neulet.2007.01.035

Fallon, S., Shearman, E., Sershen, H., and Lajtha, A. (2007). The effects of glutamate and GABA receptor antagonists on nicotine-induced neurotransmitter changes in cognitive areas. *Neurochem. Res.* 32, 535–553. doi: 10.1007/s11064-006-9113-z

Gilmour, G., Pioli, E. Y., Dix, S. L., Smith, J. W., Conway, M. W., Jones, W. T., et al. (2009). Diverse and often opposite behavioural effects of NMDA receptor antagonists in rats: implications for "NMDA antagonist modelling" of schizophrenia. *Psychopharmacology (Berl.)* 205, 203–216. doi: 10.1007/s00213-009-1530-7

Giorgetti, M., and Tecott, L. H. (2004). Contributions of 5-HT2C receptors to multiple actions of central serotonin systems. *Eur. J. Pharmacol.* 488, 1–9. doi: 10.1016/j.ejphar.2004.01.036

Halberstadt, A. L. (1995). The phencyclidine-glutamate model of schizophrenia. *Clin. Neuropharmacol.* 18, 237–249. doi: 10.1097/00002826-199506000-00004

Halberstadt, A. L., van der Heijden, I., Ruderman, M. A., Risbrough, V. B., Gingrich, J. A., Geyer, M. A., et al. (2009). 5-HT2A and 5-HT2C receptors exert opposing effects on locomotor activity in mice. *Neuropsychopharmacology* 34, 1958–1967. doi: 10.1038/npp.2009.29

Higgins, G. A., Enderlin, M., Haman, M., and Fletcher, P. J. (2003). The 5-HT2A receptor antagonist M100,907 attenuates motor and "impulsive-type" behaviours produced by NMDA receptor antagonism. *Psychopharmacology (Berl.)* 170, 309–319. doi: 10.1007/s00213-003-1549-0

Hiramatsu, M., Cho, A. K., and Nabeshima, T. (1989). Comparison of the behavioral and biochemical effects of the NMDA receptor antagonists, MK-801 and phencyclidine. *Eur. J. Pharmacol.* 166, 359–366. doi: 10.1016/0014-2999(89)90346-4

Hori, T., Suzuki, T., Baba, A., Abe, S., Yamamoto, T., Moroji, T., et al. (1996). Effects of phencyclidine metabolites on serotonin uptake in rat brain. *Neurosci. Lett.* 209, 153–156. doi: 10.1016/0304-3940(96)11617-7

Hutson, P. H., Barton, C. L., Jay, M., Blurton, P., Burkamp, F., Clarkson, R., et al. (2000). Activation of mesolimbic dopamine function by phencyclidine is enhanced by 5-HT2C/2B receptor antagonists: neurochemical and behavioural studies. *Neuropharmacology* 39, 2318–2328. doi: 10.1016/S0028-3908(00)00089-7

Javitt, D. C. (2004). Glutamate as a therapeutic target in psychiatric disorders. *Mol. Psychiatry* 9, 984–997. doi: 10.1038/sj.mp.4001551

Jentsch, J. D., and Roth, R. H. (1999). The neuropsychopharmacology of phencyclidine: from NMDA receptor hypofunction to the dopamine hypothesis of schizophrenia. *Neuropsychopharmacology* 20, 201–225. doi: 10.1016/S0893-133X(98)00060-8

Jordan, S., Chen, R., Fernalld, R., Johnson, J., Regardie, K., Kambayashi, J., et al. (2006). In vitro biochemical evidence that the psychotomimetics phencyclidine, ketamine and dizocilpine (MK-801) are inactive at cloned human and rat dopamine D2 receptors. *Eur. J. Pharmacol.* 540, 53–56. doi: 10.1016/j.ejphar.2006.04.026

Kapur, S., and Seeman, P. (2002). NMDA receptor antagonists ketamine and PCP have direct effects on the dopamine D2 and serotonin 5-HT2 receptors-implications for models of schizophrenia. *Mol. Psychiatry* 7, 837–844. doi: 10.1038/sj.mp.4001093

Klamer, D., Zhang, J., Engel, J. A., and Svensson, L. (2005). Selective interaction of nitric oxide synthase inhibition with phencyclidine: behavioural and NMDA receptor binding studies in the rat. *Behav. Brain Res.* 159, 95–103. doi: 10.1016/j.bbr.2004.10.006

Koob, G. F., Stinus, L., and Le Moal, M. (1981). Hyperactivity and hypoactivity produced by lesions to the mesolimbic dopamine system. *Behav. Brain Res.* 3, 341–359. doi: 10.1016/0166-4328(81)90004-8

Krebs-Thomson, K., Lehmann-Masten, V., Naiem, S., Paulus, M. P., and Geyer, M. A. (1998). Modulation of phencyclidine-induced changes in locomotor activity and patterns in rats by serotonin. *Eur. J. Pharmacol.* 343, 135–143. doi: 10.1016/S0014-2999(97)01557-4

Krystal, J. H., Karper, L. P., Seibyl, J. P., Freeman, G. K., Delaney, R., Bremner, J. D., et al. (1994). Subanesthetic effects of the noncompetitive NMDA antagonist, ketamine, in humans. Psychotomimetic, perceptual, cognitive, and neuroendocrine responses. *Arch. Gen. Psychiatry* 51, 199–214. doi: 10.1001/archpsyc.1994.03950030035004

Kusljic, S., Brosda, J., Norman, T. R., and van den Buuse, M. (2005). Brain serotonin depletion by lesions of the median raphe nucleus enhances the psychotomimetic action of phencyclidine, but not dizocilpine (MK-801), in rats. *Brain Res.* 1049, 217–226. doi: 10.1016/j.brainres.2005.05.017

Kusljic, S., Copolov, D. L., and van den Buuse, M. (2003). Differential role of serotonergic projections arising from the dorsal and median raphe nuclei in locomotor hyperactivity and prepulse inhibition. *Neuropsychopharmacology* 28, 2138–2147.

Kusljic, S., and van den Buuse, M. (2004). Functional dissociation between serotonergic pathways in dorsal and ventral hippocampus in psychotomimetic drug-induced locomotor hyperactivity and prepulse inhibition in rats. *Eur. J. Neurosci.* 20, 3424–3432. doi: 10.1111/j.1460-9568.2004.03804.x

Lehmann-Masten, V. D., and Geyer, M. A. (1991). Spatial and temporal patterning distinguishes the locomotor activating effects of dizocilpine and phencyclidine in rats. *Neuropharmacology* 30, 629–636. doi: 10.1016/0028-3908(91)90083-N

Lipska, B. K., and Weinberger, D. R. (2000). To model a psychiatric disorder in animals: schizophrenia as a reality test. *Neuropsychopharmacology* 23, 223–239. doi: 10.1016/S0893-133X(00)00137-8

Lodge, D., and Johnson, K. M. (1990). Noncompetitive excitatory amino acid receptor antagonists. *Trends Pharmacol. Sci.* 11, 81–86. doi: 10.1016/0165-6147(90)90323-Z

Lorrain, D. S., Schaffhauser, H., Campbell, U. C., Baccei, C. S., Correa, L. D., Rowe, B., et al. (2003). Group II mGlu receptor activation suppresses norepinephrine release in the ventral hippocampus and locomotor responses to acute ketamine challenge. *Neuropsychopharmacology* 28, 1622–1632. doi: 10.1038/sj.npp.1300238

Luby, E. D., Cohen, B. D., Rosenbaum, G., Gottlieb, J. S., and Kelley, R. (1959). Study of a new schizophrenomimetic drug – sernyl. *AMA Arch. Neurol. Psychiatry* 81, 363–369. doi: 10.1001/archneurpsyc.1959.02340150095011

Maj, J., Rogoz, Z., Skuza, G., and Wedzony, K. (1996). The synergistic effect of fluoxetine on the locomotor hyperactivity induced by MK-801, a non-competitive NMDA receptor antagonist. *J. Neural Transm.* 103, 131–146. doi: 10.1007/BF01292622

Martin, P., Carlsson, M. L., and Hjorth, S. (1998a). Systemic PCP treatment elevates brain extracellular 5-HT: a microdialysis study in awake rats. *Neuroreport* 9, 2985–2988. doi: 10.1097/00001756-199809140-00012

Martin, P., Waters, N., Schmidt, C. J., Carlsson, A., and Carlsson, M. L. (1998b). Rodent data and general hypothesis: antipsychotic action exerted through 5-HT2A receptor antagonism is dependent on increased serotonergic tone. *J. Neural Transm.* 105, 365–396. doi: 10.1007/s007020050064

Martin, S. J., and Clark, R. E. (2007). The rodent hippocampus and spatial memory: from synapses to systems. *Cell. Mol. Life Sci.* 64, 401–431. doi: 10.1007/s00018-007-6336-3

Maurel-Remy, S., Bervoets, K., and Millan, M. J. (1995). Blockade of phencyclidine-induced hyperlocomotion by clozapine and MDL 100,907 in rats reflects antagonism of 5-HT2A receptors. *Eur. J. Pharmacol.* 280, R9–R11. doi: 10.1016/0014-2999(95)00333-G

Meltzer, H. Y., Horiguchi, M., and Massey, B. W. (2011). The role of serotonin in the NMDA receptor antagonist models of psychosis and cognitive impairment. *Psychopharmacology (Berl.)* 213, 289–305. doi: 10.1007/s00213-010-2137-8

Millan, M. J., Brocco, M., Gobert, A., Joly, F., Bervoets, K., Rivet, J., et al. (1999). Contrasting mechanisms of action and sensitivity to antipsychotics of phencyclidine versus amphetamine: importance of nucleus accumbens 5-HT2A sites for PCP-induced locomotion in the rat. *Eur. J. Neurosci.* 11, 4419–4432. doi: 10.1046/j.1460-9568.1999.00858.x

Moghaddam, B., and Jackson, M. E. (2003). Glutamatergic animal models of schizophrenia. *Ann. N. Y. Acad. Sci.* 1003, 131–137. doi: 10.1196/annals.1300.065

Morris, B. J., Cochran, S. M., and Pratt, J. A. (2005). PCP: from pharmacology to modelling schizophrenia. *Curr. Opin. Pharmacol.* 5, 101–106. doi: 10.1016/j.coph.2004.08.008

Moser, M. B., and Moser, E. I. (1998). Functional differentiation in the hippocampus. *Hippocampus* 8, 608–619. doi: 10.1002/(SICI)1098-1063(1998)8:6<608::AID-HIPO3>3.0.CO;2-7

Nabeshima, T., Ishikawa, K., Yamaguchi, K., Furukawa, H., and Kameyama, T. (1988). Protection with phencyclidine against inactivation of 5-HT2 receptors by sulfhydryl-modifying reagents. *Biochem. Pharmacol.* 37, 3277–3283. doi: 10.1016/0006-2952(88)90639-9

Nakazawa, K., Mchugh, T. J., Wilson, M. A., and Tonegawa, S. (2004). NMDA receptors, place cells and hippocampal spatial memory. *Nat. Rev. Neurosci.* 5, 361–372. doi: 10.1038/nrn1385

National Health and Medical Research Council of Australia. (2004). *Australian Code of Practice for the Care and Use of Animals for Scientific Purposes.* Canberra: Australian Government Publishing Services.

Nishimura, M., Sato, K., Okada, T., Yoshiya, I., Schloss, P., Shimada, S., et al. (1998). Ketamine inhibits monoamine transporters expressed in human embryonic kidney 293 cells. *Anesthesiology* 88, 768–774. doi: 10.1097/00000542-199803000-00029

O'Keefe, J., and Dostrovsky, J. (1971). The hippocampus as a spatial map. Preliminary evidence from unit activity in the freely-moving rat. *Brain Res.* 34, 171–175. doi: 10.1016/0006-8993(71)90358-1

Ogren, S. O., and Goldstein, M. (1994). Phencyclidine- and dizocilpine-induced hyperlocomotion are differentially mediated. *Neuropsychopharmacology* 11, 167–177. doi: 10.1038/sj.npp.1380103

Olney, J. W., Newcomer, J. W., and Farber, N. B. (1999). NMDA receptor hypofunction model of schizophrenia. *J. Psychiatr. Res.* 33, 523–533. doi: 10.1016/S0022-3956(99)00029-1

Paulus, M. P., and Geyer, M. A. (1991). A temporal and spatial scaling hypothesis for the behavioral effects of psychostimulants. *Psychopharmacology (Berl.)* 104, 6–16. doi: 10.1007/BF02244547

Paulus, M. P., and Geyer, M. A. (1993). Three independent factors characterize spontaneous rat motor activity. *Behav. Brain Res.* 53, 11–20. doi: 10.1016/S0166-4328(05)80262-1

Paxinos, G., and Watson, C. (1998). *The Rat Brain in Stereotaxic Co-ordinates.* New York: Academic Press.

Rabin, R. A., Doat, M., and Winter, J. C. (2000). Role of serotonergic 5-HT2A receptors in the psychotomimetic actions of phencyclidine. *Int. J. Neuropsychopharmacol.* 3, 333–338. doi: 10.1017/S1461145700002091

Rothman, R. B. (1994). PCP site 2: a high affinity MK-801-insensitive phencyclidine binding site. *Neurotoxicol. Teratol.* 16, 343–353. doi: 10.1016/0892-0362(94)90022-1

Schwartz, P. H., and Wasterlain, C. G. (1991). Cardiac arrest and resuscitation alters the pharmacokinetics of MK-801 in the rat. *Res. Commun. Chem. Pathol. Pharmacol.* 73, 181–195.

Seeman, P., Ko, F., and Tallerico, T. (2005). Dopamine receptor contribution to the action of PCP, LSD and ketamine psychotomimetics. *Mol. Psychiatry* 10, 877–883. doi: 10.1038/sj.mp.4001682

Seeman, P., and Lasaga, M. (2005). Dopamine agonist action of phencyclidine. *Synapse* 58, 275–277. doi: 10.1002/syn.20210

Seillier, A., and Giuffrida, A. (2009). Evaluation of NMDA receptor models of schizophrenia: divergences in the behavioral effects of sub-chronic PCP and MK-801. *Behav. Brain Res.* 204, 410–415. doi: 10.1016/j.bbr.2009.02.007

Shelnutt, S. R., Gunnell, M., and Owens, S. M. (1999). Sexual dimorphism in phencyclidine in vitro metabolism and pharmacokinetics in rats. *J. Pharmacol. Exp. Ther.* 290, 1292–1298.

Small, S. A. (2002). The longitudinal axis of the hippocampal formation: its anatomy, circuitry, and role in cognitive function. *Rev. Neurosci.* 13, 183–194. doi: 10.1515/REVNEURO.2002.13.2.183

Snell, L. D., Yi, S. J., and Johnson, K. M. (1988). Comparison of the effects of MK-801 and phencyclidine on catecholamine uptake and NMDA-induced norepinephrine release. *Eur. J. Pharmacol.* 145, 223–226. doi: 10.1016/0014-2999(88)90235-X

Stiedl, O., Misane, I., Koch, M., Pattij, T., Meyer, M., and Ogren, S. O. (2007). Activation of the brain 5-HT2C receptors causes hypolocomotion without anxiogenic-like cardiovascular adjustments in mice. *Neuropharmacology* 52, 949–957. doi: 10.1016/j.neuropharm.2006.10.012

Stone, J. M., and Pilowsky, L. S. (2006). Psychopathological consequences of ketamine. *Br. J. Psychiatry* 189, 565–566. doi: 10.1192/bjp.189.6.565b

Svensson, T. H. (2000). Dysfunctional brain dopamine systems induced by psychotomimetic NMDA-receptor antagonists and the effects of antipsychotic drugs. *Brain Res. Brain Res. Rev.* 31, 320–329. doi: 10.1016/S0165-0173(99)00048-X

Sweatt, J. D. (2004). Hippocampal function in cognition. *Psychopharmacology (Berl.)* 174, 99–110. doi: 10.1007/s00213-004-1795-9

Takahashi, H., Takada, Y., Nagai, N., Urano, T., and Takada, A. (2000). Serotonergic neurons projecting to hippocampus activate locomotion. *Brain Res.* 869, 194–202. doi: 10.1016/S0006-8993(00)02385-4

Takahashi, H., Takada, Y., Urano, T., and Takada, A. (2001). Dissociation of systemic and hippocampal modulation of rat locomotor activity by 5-HT2C receptors. *Neurosci. Res.* 40, 97–103. doi: 10.1016/S0168-0102(01)00215-2

Tricklebank, M. D., Singh, L., Oles, R. J., Preston, C., and Iversen, S. D. (1989). The behavioural effects of MK-801: a comparison with antagonists acting non-competitively and competitively at the NMDA receptor. *Eur. J. Pharmacol.* 167, 127–135. doi: 10.1016/0014-2999(89)90754-1

Williams, J. H., and Azmitia, E. C. (1981). Hippocampal serotonin re-uptake and nocturnal locomotor activity after microinjections of 5,7-DHT in the fornix-fimbria. *Brain Res.* 207, 95–107. doi: 10.1016/0006-8993(81)90681-8

Zigmond, M. J., Abercrombie, E. D., Berger, T. W., Grace, A. A., and Stricker, E. M. (1990). Compensations after lesions of central dopaminergic neurons: some clinical and basic implications. *Trends Neurosci.* 13, 290–296. doi: 10.1016/0166-2236(90)90112-N

Conflict of Interest Statement: The authors declare that the research was conducted in the absence of any commercial or financial relationships that could be construed as a potential conflict of interest.

9

Antidepressant-like drug effects in juvenile and adolescent mice in the tail suspension test: relationship with hippocampal serotonin and norepinephrine transporter expression and function

Nathan C. Mitchell[1], Georgianna G. Gould[2], Corey M. Smolik[1,3], Wouter Koek[2,3†] and Lynette C. Daws[1,3 *†]

[1] Department of Physiology, University of Texas Health Science Center, San Antonio, TX, USA
[2] Department of Psychiatry, University of Texas Health Science Center, San Antonio, TX, USA
[3] Department of Pharmacology, University of Texas Health Science Center, San Antonio, TX, USA

Edited by:
Maarten Van Den Buuse, Mental Health Research Institute, Australia

Reviewed by:
Caitlin Elissa McOmish, Columbia University, USA
Terence Y. Pang, Florey Institute of Neuroscience and Mental Health, Australia
Irwin Lucki, Pennsylvania State University, USA

***Correspondence:**
Lynette C. Daws, Department of Physiology, University of Texas Health Science Center, 7703 Floyd Curl Drive, San Antonio, TX 78229-3900, USA
e-mail: daws@uthscsa.edu

† Lynette C. Daws and Wouter Koek are co-senior authors.

Depression is a major health problem for which most patients are not effectively treated. This problem is further compounded in children and adolescents where only two antidepressants [both selective serotonin reuptake inhibitors (SSRIs)] are currently approved for clinical use. Mouse models provide tools to identify mechanisms that might account for poor treatment response to antidepressants. However, there are few studies in adolescent mice and none in juvenile mice. The tail suspension test (TST) is commonly used to assay for antidepressant-like effects of drugs in adult mice. Here we show that the TST can also be used to assay antidepressant-like effects of drugs in C57Bl/6 mice aged 21 (juvenile) and 28 (adolescent) days post-partum (P). We found that the magnitude of antidepressant-like response to the SSRI escitalopram was less in P21 mice than in P28 or adult mice. The smaller antidepressant response of juveniles was not related to either maximal binding (B_{max}) or affinity (K_d) for [^{3}H]citalopram binding to the serotonin transporter (SERT) in hippocampus, which did not vary significantly among ages. Magnitude of antidepressant-like response to the tricyclic desipramine was similar among ages, as were B_{max} and K_d values for [^{3}H]nisoxetine binding to the norepinephrine transporter in hippocampus. Together, these findings suggest that juvenile mice are less responsive to the antidepressant-like effects of escitalopram than adults, but that this effect is not due to delayed maturation of SERT in hippocampus. Showing that the TST is a relevant behavioral assay of antidepressant-like activity in juvenile and adolescent mice sets the stage for future studies of the mechanisms underlying the antidepressant response in these young populations.

Keywords: antidepressant, selective serotonin reuptake inhibitor, tricyclic, serotonin transporter, norepinephrine transporter, juvenile, adolescent, depression

INTRODUCTION

Depression is a major public health problem for which most patients are not effectively treated. This problem is further compounded in children and adolescents by limited pharmacological treatment options (Bylund and Reed, 2007). The selective serotonin reuptake inhibitor (SSRI) fluoxetine is currently the only FDA approved treatment for depression in children and adolescents up to 18 years old, and escitalopram is approved for children and adolescents age 12 and older. Exacerbating the situation further, children and adolescents respond poorly to these antidepressants compared with adults (Tsapakis et al., 2008; Hetrick et al., 2009, 2010). Given the high prevalence of adolescent depression, affecting 4–8% of the population with an incidence of 25% by the end of adolescence (Kessler et al., 2001; Bujoreanu et al., 2011) and, of major concern, the high prevalence of suicide in this young population (the third leading cause of death in the 15- to 19-year age group; Reed et al., 2008), there is a clear need to understand the neural mechanisms accounting for these differences between children and adolescents on the one hand and adults on the other, with the hope to uncover targets for the development of more effective treatments. However, despite many reports showing marked differences in the antidepressant response of children and adolescents compared with adults (Bylund and Reed, 2007; Tsapakis et al., 2008; Hetrick et al., 2009, 2010; Hazell and Mirzaie, 2013) there is a paucity of studies investigating the underlying mechanisms. Thus, reasons for the age-dependency of antidepressant response remain poorly understood.

Animal models are needed to examine the mechanisms underlying age-dependent effects of antidepressants. To date, there are only a few preclinical studies of antidepressants in juvenile and early adolescent animals, and most have been conducted using rats. SSRIs were found to reduce time spent immobile in the forced swim test (FST), an index of antidepressant-like activity, in rats as young as postnatal day (P) 21 as well as in adults, whereas blockers of the norepinephrine (NE) transporter, such as the tricyclic antidepressant desipramine (DMI), were ineffective in the FST in rats younger than P28 (Pechnick et al., 2008; Reed et al., 2008). The mechanistic basis for these findings remains to be determined, but is thought to involve the delayed maturation of the NE neurotransmitter system relative to the serotonin (5-HT) system. In terms of the actual drug targets themselves, i.e., the serotonin and norepinephrine transporters (SERT and NET, respectively), information about their expression in juvenile and adolescent animals is sparse. Using quantitative autoradiography, Galineau et al. (2004) reported a triphasic profile for SERT in amygdala and hypothalamus of rats where expression peaked around P21, decreased at P28 and plateaued through P70, the oldest age tested (see also Daws and Gould, 2011). For NET, Sanders et al. (2005) also using autoradiography, reported that expression of NET in some brain regions (e.g., locus coeruleus) was much greater in rats aged P20 than in adults, while in other regions NET expression in P20 rats was either less than (e.g., CA3 region of hippocampus) or similar (e.g., cortex, CA1 and CA2 regions of hippocampus, dentate gyrus) to that of adult rats. Thus, it is not clear from studies in rats, if expression or activity of SERT and NET correlates positively with the emergence of an antidepressant-like response to SSRIs and NET blockers.

Lacking are studies in mice to probe the mechanistic basis underlying differences in antidepressant-efficacy among juveniles, adolescents, and adults. The relative ease with which mice can be genetically manipulated makes them a powerful tool for preclinical research. However, there are few studies that have used adolescent (≥P28) mice to investigate antidepressant-like response (Bourin et al., 1998; David et al., 2001a; Mason et al., 2009) and none that have used mice younger than P28. Although mice have been used to examine the consequences of antidepressant treatment during prenatal, early postnatal and adult periods, juvenile and adolescent periods remain largely unexplored. Likewise, little is known about SERT and NET expression during these juvenile and adolescent periods in mice.

The tail suspension test (TST) is a preclinical test with good predictive validity that has become one of the most widely used models for assessing antidepressant-like activity in adult mice (Cryan et al., 2005). Currently there is only one report of its use in adolescent (P35) mice. Thus, it is unknown if the TST can be used to detect antidepressant-like effects of drugs in early adolescent (P28) and juvenile (P21) mice. The goals of the present study were twofold: first, to examine if the TST can be used to measure antidepressant-like activity in P21 and P28 mice; and second, to begin to examine the relationship between antidepressant-like activity and the expression and affinity of hippocampal SERT and NET in juvenile, adolescent, and adult mice.

MATERIALS AND METHODS

ANIMALS

Juvenile (P21), early adolescent (P28), and adult (P62–90) male and female C57Bl/6 mice were obtained from an in house breeding colony (breeding pairs originally obtained from Jackson Lab). Body weights for male mice ranged from 6.6 to 9.8 g for P21, from 9.7 to 18.5 g for P28, and from 23.7 to 42.8 g for adults, and body weights for female mice ranged from 6.3 to 10.0 g for P21, from 10.8 to 15.1 g for P28, and from 19.1 to 31.3 g for adults. Animals were housed in a temperature-controlled (24°C) vivarium maintained on a 14/10-h light/dark cycle (lights on at 07:00, experiments conducted during the light period) in plastic cages (29 cm × 18 cm × 13 cm) containing rodent bedding (Sani-chips, Harlan Teklad, Madison, WI, USA) with free access to food (Rodent sterilizable diet, Harlan Teklad, Madison, WI, USA) and water. After weaning on postnatal day 21, mice were housed in groups of five with same-sex peers. All procedures were conducted in accordance with the National Institute of Health Guide for the Care and Use of Laboratory Animals (Institute of Laboratory Animal Resources, Commission on Life Sciences, National Research Council 1996), and with the Institutional Animal Care and Use Committee, The University of Texas Health Science Center at San Antonio.

TAIL SUSPENSION TEST

The TST was conducted based on the original description by Steru et al. (1985) [for a review, see (Castagne et al., 2011)]. On the day before testing, mice were moved from the colony room and housed overnight in a holding room adjoining the procedure room. On the test day, mice were placed in the procedure room and allowed 1–2 h to acclimate before receiving an injection of saline vehicle (subcutaneously [sc] or intraperitoneally [ip]), escitalopram (10 mg/kg, sc), or DMI (32 mg/kg, ip). Routes of drug administration were based on results in adult mice reported by Cryan et al. (2005) and Sanchez et al. (2003). Each mouse was tested only once (i.e., not given multiple drugs nor exposed to the TST on multiple occasions). Drugs or saline were injected 30 min before testing. Immediately before testing, the distal end of the tail was fastened to a flat aluminum (2 × 0.3 × 10 cm) bar using adhesive tape at a 90° angle to the longitudinal axis of the mouse tail and the aluminum bar, with a distance of 3–4 cm between the base of the tail and the edge of the bar. A hole opposite the taped end of the bar was used to secure the bar to a hook in the ceiling of a visually isolated white test box (40 cm × 40 cm × 40 cm). Each mouse was suspended by its tail for 6 min, allowing the ventral surface and front and hind limbs to be video-recorded using a digital camera facing the test box. Total time immobile was measured (in seconds) during the entire 6 min test period. Immobility was defined as the absence of initiated movements, and included passive swaying of the body. A mouse was excluded from the experiments if it climbed and held on to its tail or the aluminum bar for a period of 3 s or longer. In the present study no mice aged P21 or P28 were excluded. Approximately 5% of adult mice were excluded. Immobility was scored manually by observers watching the video and who were blind to the treatment. Typically two observers scored each videotape with excellent inter-observer agreement ($r^2 > 0.9$).

Initial experiments were designed to examine the utility of the TST in juvenile and adolescent mice. Male and female mice were given either a sc or ip injection of saline, corresponding to the route of administration for escitalopram and DMI, respectively. The purpose of these initial experiments was to identify possible effects of age, gender, and route of administration, as well as any interactions among these factors, on immobility in the TST. Age affected basal immobility, and did so in a similar manner in both genders after both routes of administration (see Results). Subsequent experiments investigated the two reference antidepressant drugs, escitalopram (10 mg/kg, sc) and DMI (32 mg/kg, ip), in male mice. Drug doses were selected based on preliminary data obtained in our laboratory that showed these doses to be the lowest to produce maximal effects on immobility in adult C57Bl/6J mice.

[^{3}H]CITALOPRAM AND [^{3}H]NISOXETINE SATURATION BINDING IN HIPPOCAMPAL HOMOGENATES

All binding experiments were carried out using tissue from male C57Bl/6 mice.

[^{3}H]citalopram binding to SERT

Saturation binding of [^{3}H]citalopram in membrane homogenate preparations from mouse hippocampi was carried out following the methods of D'Amato et al. (1987) with minor modifications. Briefly, male mice were decapitated, the brain removed and hippocampi collected. Hippocampi from individual mice were homogenized in 25 ml of 4°C 50 mM Tris, 120 mM NaCl, 5 mM KCl buffer (pH 7.4 at 25°C), at 2600 rpm on a Polytron tissue homogenizer (Brinkman Instruments, Westbury, NY, USA). The homogenate was centrifuged for 10 min at 30,600 × *g* at 4°C. The supernatant was discarded, and the pellet re-suspended on ice using a Potter Elvehjem glass and Teflon homogenizer in 25 ml ice-cold buffer. The homogenate was re-centrifuged for 10 min at 30,600 × *g*. The final pellet was re-suspended to yield a protein concentration of approximately 0.5–1.2 μg/μl. Protein was quantified spectrophotometrically on a plate reader (SpectraMax 190, Molecular Devices, Sunnyvale, CA, USA) using Bradford reagent (Sigma, St. Louis, MO, USA). Binding assays were run in triplicate for each hippocampal membrane homogenate preparation. Homogenates were incubated at 25°C for 1 h in buffer (50 mM Tris, 120 mM NaCl, 5 mM KCl) containing 0.1–10 nM [^{3}H]citalopram (Perkin Elmer). Non-specific binding was defined by addition of 10 μM sertraline (Pfizer). Incubation was terminated by addition of 4 ml of ice cold buffer and rapid filtration under vacuum onto Whatman GF/B filter paper strips (Brandel, Gaithersburg, MD, USA) pre-soaked in 5% polyethyleneimine (Sigma). Filters were washed twice and radioactivity trapped on the filters was measured by liquid scintillation counting using a Beckman 6500 (Beckman, Brea, CA, USA) with efficiencies of 40–65%. Binding data were analyzed by non-linear regression using GraphPad Prism 5.04.

[^{3}H]nisoxetine binding to NET

Saturation binding of [^{3}H]nisoxetine in membrane homogenate preparations from mouse hippocampi was carried out following the methods of Tejani-Butt (1992). Hippocampal homogenate preparation for [^{3}H]nisoxetine binding was as described for [^{3}H] citalopram binding, except that hippocampi were pooled from two mice to yield protein concentrations of 1.0–1.7 μg/μl, the buffer was pH 7.4 at 4°C and the final washed pellet was re-suspended in 50 mM Tris, 300 mM NaCl, 5 mM KCl (pH 7.4 at 4°C). Binding assays were carried out for 4 h at 4°C in 50 mM Tris, 300 mM NaCl, 5 mM KCl at the same volumes used for [^{3}H] citalopram binding. [^{3}H] nisoxetine concentration ranged from 0.5 to 30 nM for the saturation assays. Non-specific binding was defined with 10 μM mazindol (Sigma, St Louis, MO, USA). Data collection and analysis were the same as described for [^{3}H]citalopram binding.

STATISTICAL ANALYSIS

Statistical analyses were performed using Prism 5.04 (GraphPad, San Diego, CA, USA) and NCSS 2007 (Kaysville, UT, USA). TST data were analyzed using ANOVA, followed by Tukey's multiple comparison tests. Binding data were analyzed using Kruskal–Wallis test because of significant differences in standard deviations among age groups (Bartlett's test). All data are expressed as mean ± standard error of the mean (SEM), and $P < 0.05$ was considered statistically significant.

DRUGS

Escitalopram oxalate [Shanco International Inc. (Hazlet, NJ, USA)] and DMI hydrochloride [Sigma-Aldrich (St. Louis, MO, USA)] were dissolved in physiological saline. Escitalopram was injected sc at doses expressed as base per kilogram body weight (Sanchez et al., 2003). DMI was injected ip at doses expressed as salt per kilogram body weight. The injection volume was 10 ml/kg.

RESULTS

USE OF THE TST IN JUVENILE AND ADOLESCENT MICE

The TST is a preclinical test with good predictive validity that is widely used to detect antidepressant-like activity (Cryan and Holmes, 2005; Cryan et al., 2005), and that has been used in mice as young as P35 (Mason et al., 2009). Antidepressant-like activity in this test is defined by the ability of a drug to reduce the time a mouse spends immobile. We first examined if the TST could be used in P21 and P28 mice, given the possibility that young mice may display so little baseline immobility that the effect of a drug to reduce immobility further may not be detectible. To this end, six separate groups of mice (male and female, $n = 20$ of each gender and each age, P21, P28, or adult) received an injection of saline either sc or ip ($n = 10$ of each gender and age receiving saline sc, and $n = 10$ of each gender and age receiving saline ip) and time spent immobile in a 6 min test was quantified. There was no significant effect of gender or route of administration on immobility time, a finding that is consistent with reports for adult mice (e.g., David et al., 2001b; Jones and Lucki, 2005; Andreasen and Redrobe, 2009). There was however, a significant effect of age [$F(2, 119) = 6.63$, $P < 0.0025$]. Because there were no significant interactions among age, gender, and route of administration, data were collapsed with age as the only variable (**Figure 1**). P21 mice spent significantly less time immobile (99 ± 8 s) than P28 (123 ± 7 s) or adult mice (135 ± 6 s), and P28 mice did not differ significantly from adults. A factor that might contribute to reduced immobility time in P21 mice is their smaller size. Regression analyses of immobility time as a function of body weight for all ages and both genders, inclusive, revealed an overall positive correlation ($r = 0.24$, $P < 0.01$). However, regression analyses within each age group revealed no significant correlation between body weight and immobility time (P21, $r = -0.12$, $P = 0.46$; P28, $r = 0.23$, $P = 0.11$; adult, $r = 0.05$, $P = 0.66$, data not shown).

These data show that juvenile and adolescent mice spend sufficient time immobile in the TST that detection of a drug effect

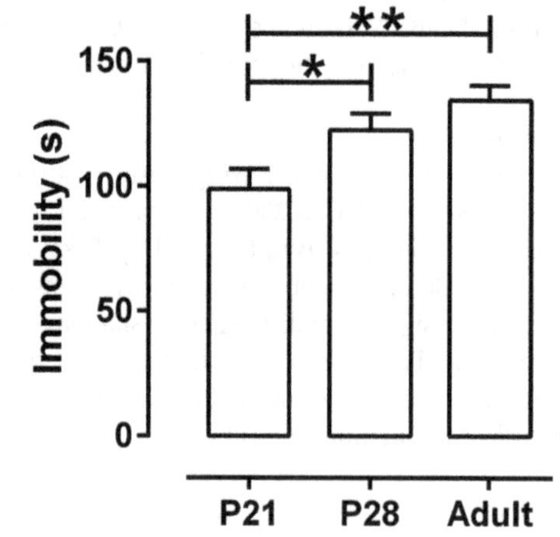

FIGURE 1 | Immobility time in the TST as a function of age. Juvenile mice (P21) spent significantly less time immobile than either adolescent (P28) or adult mice ($P > 62$). Each age group consisted of 40 animals treated with saline (20 males and 20 females, half of them treated sc and the other half ip). Because there were neither main nor interaction effects of gender and route of administration, data are shown collapsed with age as the only factor. $^*P < 0.05$, $^{**}P < 0.01$ (Tukey *post hoc* test). Data are mean and SEM.

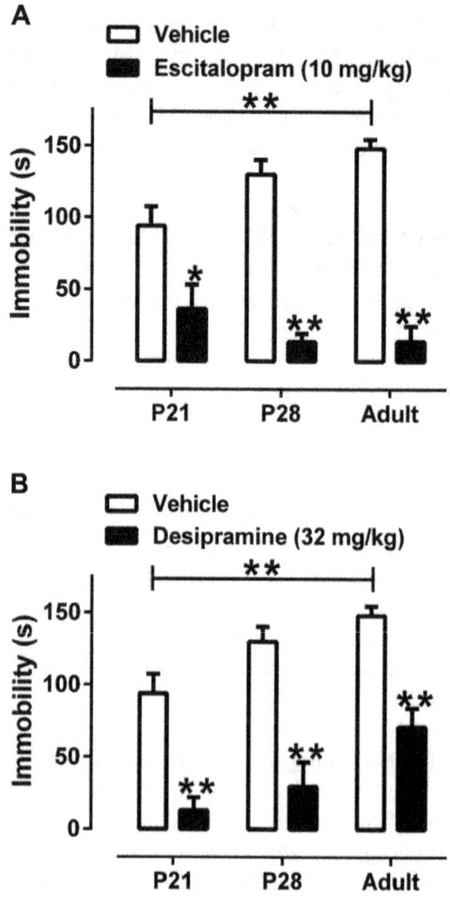

FIGURE 2 | Effect of escitalopram and DMI to reduce time spent immobile in the TST in male juvenile, adolescent, and adult mice. **(A)** Escitalopram (10 mg/kg, sc) significantly reduced immobility time in all age groups. There was a significant interaction between age and treatment revealing that escitalopram is less effective in reducing immobility time in P21 mice, compared with P28 or adult mice. **(B)** DMI (32 mg/kg, ip) significantly reduced immobility time in all age groups. Sample sizes were as follows: P21, $n = 38$ (20 saline, 8 escitalopram, 10 DMI); P28, $n = 37$ (20 saline, 8 escitalopram, 8 DMI); adult mice $n = 39$ (20 saline, 10 escitalopram, 9 DMI). There was no main effect of route of saline administration, so saline data were collapsed with age and drug as the only factors; two-way ANOVA with Tukey's *post hoc* tests, $^*P < 0.05$, $^{**}P < 0.01$. Data are mean and SEM.

to decrease immobility should be possible. To test this, juvenile and adolescent mice were treated acutely with either escitalopram (sc) or DMI (ip), two antidepressants known to produce robust effects in the TST in adult mice (Sanchez et al., 2003; O'Leary et al., 2007).

REFERENCE ANTIDEPRESSANTS REDUCE IMMOBILITY ACROSS AGES

Escitalopram (10 mg/kg, sc) and DMI (32 mg/kg, ip) reduced immobility time in the TST in all age groups [$F(1, 51) = 66.45$, $P < 0.01$] (**Figure 2**). However, the extent to which they decreased immobility differed among the age groups. For escitalopram there was a significant interaction between treatment and age [$F(2, 51) = 5.08$, $P < 0.01$] because escitalopram reduced immobility less in P21 mice than in P28 and adult mice. For DMI there was a significant effect of age [$F(2, 51) = 7.14$, $P < 0.01$] and DMI tended to reduce immobility more in P21 and P28 mice than in adults, but the interaction between treatment and age did not reach statistical significance. Sample sizes for saline-, escitalopram-, and DMI-treated mice, respectively, were 20, 8, and 10 for mice aged P21; 20, 8, and 8 for mice aged P28, and 20, 10, and 9 for adult mice. The larger sample size for saline-treated mice is due to pooling data from male mice injected with saline sc ($n = 10$) and ip ($n = 10$) for each age. These results show that the TST can be used to examine antidepressant-like drug effects in mice as young as P21. Next we investigated the relationship between the antidepressant-like effects of escitalopram and DMI and the expression of their targets, the SERT and NET, respectively, in hippocampus of P21, P28, and adult mice.

[^{3}H]CITALOPRAM AND [^{3}H]NISOXETINE SATURATION BINDING IN HIPPOCAMPUS AS A FUNCTION OF AGE

As shown in **Figures 3A,C,E** and **Table 1**, [^{3}H]citalopram saturation binding in mouse hippocampal homogenates revealed no significant difference in maximal binding (B_{max}) or affinity (K_d) values among P21 ($n = 10$), P28 ($n = 8$), and adult ($n = 9$) male mice. Likewise, [^{3}H]nisoxetine saturation binding in mouse hippocampal homogenates revealed no significant difference in B_{max} or K_d values among P21 ($n = 9$), P28 ($n = 9$), and adult ($n = 7$) male mice (**Figures 3B,D,F; Table 1**). Of note is the greater variability in K_d values for [^{3}H]citalopram binding in P21 mice, compared with their P28 and adult counterparts ($P < 0.001$, Bartlett's test). Similarly, the variance of the K_d values for [^{3}H]nisoxetine binding in young mice was greater than in adults ($P < 0.01$, Bartlett's test), suggesting that these young ages may represent a transitional period where SERT and NET are shifting toward the functional activity state of adult SERT and NET.

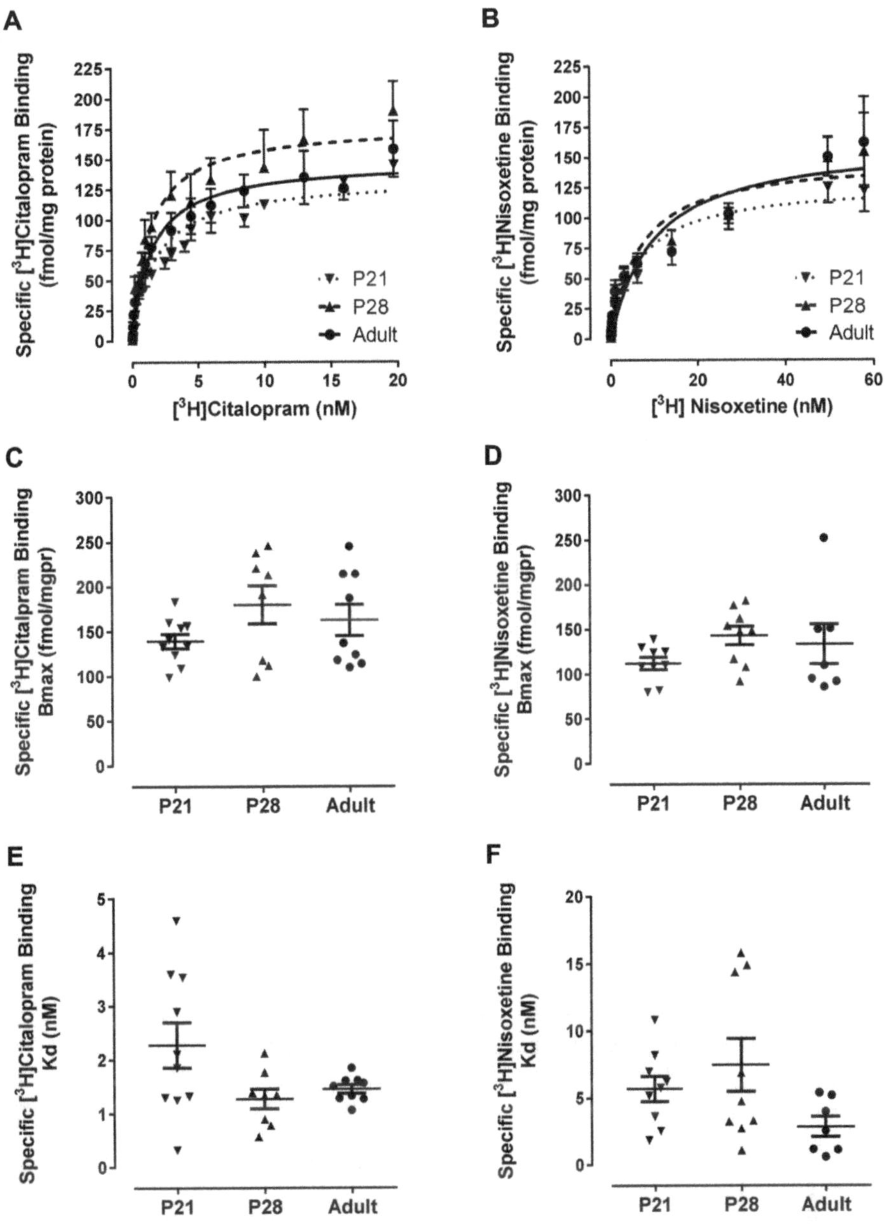

FIGURE 3 | Specific binding of [^{3}H]citalopram to SERT and [^{3}H]nisoxetine to NET in hippocampal membrane homogenates from male P21(▼) P28 (▲) and adult (•) mice. Membrane preparations were incubated with increasing concentrations of [^{3}H]citalopram or [^{3}H]nisoxetine. Non-specific binding was defined in the presence of 10 μM sertraline or 10 μM mazindol, respectively. Specific binding was obtained by subtracting non-specific binding from total binding at each ligand concentration. **(A,B)** Show saturation binding isotherms for binding of [^{3}H]citalopram or [^{3}H]nisoxetine, respectively. B_{max} and K_d values for [^{3}H]citalopram to SERT are summarized in **(C,E)**, and for [^{3}H]nisoxetine binding to NET in **(D,F)**, respectively. For [^{3}H]citalopram sample sizes were as follows: P21 $n = 10$, P28 $n = 8$, adult $n = 9$; and for [^{3}H]nisoxetine, P21 $n = 9$, P28 $n = 9$, adult $n = 7$. Data are mean and SEM.

RELATIONSHIP BETWEEN ANTIDEPRESSANT-LIKE EFFECT AND SATURATION BINDING WITH [^{3}H]CITALOPRAM AND [^{3}H]NISOXETINE IN HIPPOCAMPUS ACROSS AGE GROUPS

Data from **Figure 2** and **Table 1** are plotted in **Figure 4** and illustrate the relationship, or lack thereof, between the ability of escitalopram and DMI to produce antidepressant-like effects in the TST and the expression and affinity values for hippocampal SERT (**Figures 4A,C**) and NET (**Figures 4B,D**). TST data plotted in **Figure 4** are the immobility times for each individual escitalopram- or DMI-treated mouse, subtracted from the mean value for immobility time of the same age saline-treated mice (i.e., data from **Figure 2**). This difference provides a measure of the magnitude of antidepressant-like response that takes into account the difference in immobility times among saline-treated mice of different ages. The ability of escitalopram to produce antidepressant-like effects in the

Table 1 | Summary of B_{max} and K_d values for [^{3}H]citalopram binding to SERT and [^{3}H]nisoxetine binding to NET in male P21, P28, and adult mice.

	P21	P28	Adult
[^{3}H]Citalopram			
B_{max} (fmol/mgpr)	139 ± 8	180 ± 21	163 ± 17
K_d (nM)	2.3 ± 0.4	1.3 ± 0.2	1.5 ± 0.1
[^{3}H]Nisoxetine			
B_{max} (fmol/mgpr)	112 ± 7	143 ± 10	136 ± 23
K_d (nM)	5.7 ± 0.9	7.4 ± 2.0	2.5 ± 0.8

[^{3}H]citalopram binding n = 8–10 per group where hippocampi were from one mouse per assay. For [^{3}H]nisoxetine binding n = 7–9 per group, but where each assay was from pooled hippocampi from two mice. For each ligand, there were no significant differences in B_{max} or K_d values among ages (Kruskal–Wallis). Data are mean and SEM.

TST increased with age, but was not associated with parallel increases in either B_{max} (**Figure 4A**) or affinity of SERT for [^{3}H]citalopram (i.e., smaller K_d values; **Figure 4D**). The ability of DMI to produce antidepressant-like effects did not change significantly across age groups. Likewise, B_{max} and K_d values for [^{3}H]nisoxetine binding to NET did not vary significantly as a function of age.

DISCUSSION

The major findings of the present study are first, that the SSRI escitalopram and the NET blocker DMI produced antidepressant-like effects in mice as young as P21, the youngest age tested; second, that the magnitude of antidepressant-like response to escitalopram increased with age but was not paralleled by increasing expression or affinity of hippocampal SERT; and third that the magnitude of antidepressant-like response to the tricyclic, DMI, as well as expression and affinity of hippocampal NET, did not differ significantly among P21, P28, and adult mice. These findings support the utility of juvenile mice to study antidepressant-like activity of drugs. Moreover, our finding that juvenile mice are less sensitive to the antidepressant-like effect of escitalopram than adults, parallels clinical data reporting that, compared to adults, children have a relatively poor therapeutic response to the SSRIs, fluoxetine, and

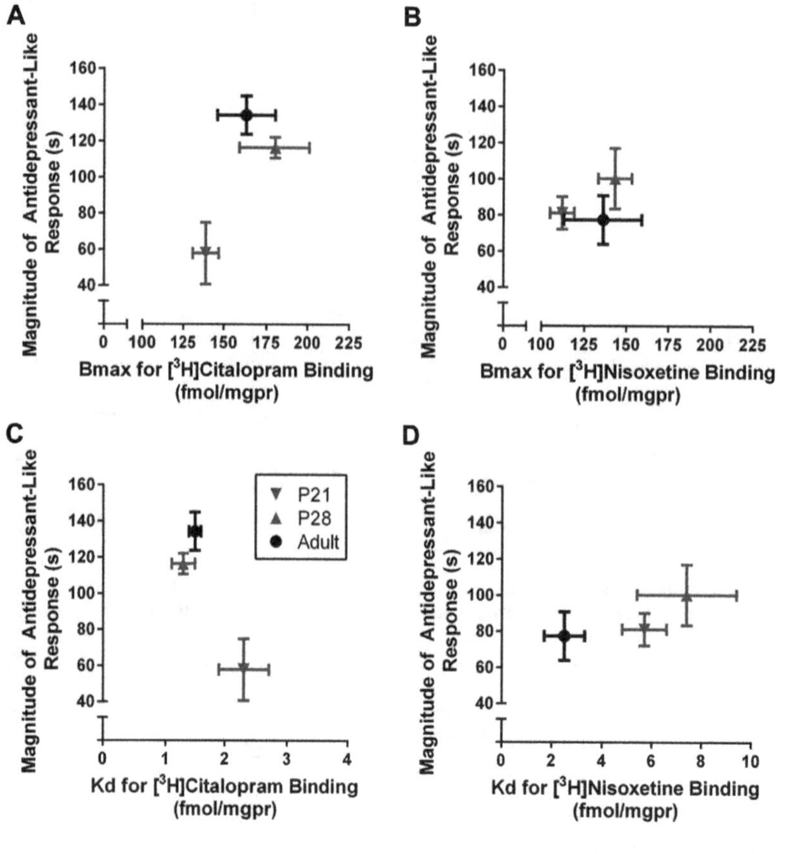

FIGURE 4 | Relationship between antidepressant-like response and hippocampal SERT and NET expression and affinity in P21, P28, and adult male mice. The magnitude of antidepressant-like response to the SERT blocker, escitalopram, increased with age but neither B_{max} **(A)** nor K_d **(C)** values for [^{3}H]citalopram binding to SERT varied significantly with age. The magnitude of antidepressant-like response to the NET blocker, DMI, as well as B_{max} **(B)** and K_d **(D)** values for [^{3}H]nisoxetine binding to NET remained relatively constant across ages. Data are re-plotted from **Figure 2** and **Table 1**. TST data from **Figure 2** are plotted on the *y*-axis as "magnitude of antidepressant-like response," defined as the immobility time for individual drug-treated mice subtracted from the mean immobility time of same aged saline-treated mice; the larger the number, the greater the antidepressant-like effect. Sample sizes are the same as reported in legends to **Figures 2,3** and **Table 1**. Data are mean and SEM.

escitalopram, the only two FDA approved antidepressants for this young population.

In rodents, postnatal days 21–27 are considered the juvenile period and postnatal days 28–42 equivalent to early adolescence (Spear, 2000; Bylund and Reed, 2007). To date only a few studies have investigated antidepressant-like activity of drugs in adolescent mice and none have studied juvenile mice. Adolescent mice (P28 or P35) were found to be sensitive to the antidepressant-like effect of both SSRIs and tricyclics in the FST (Bourin et al., 1998; David et al., 2001a,b; Mason et al., 2009). Only one study has used the TST to investigate antidepressant-like activity in adolescent mice (P35) and, as for studies using the FST, found that both SSRIs and tricyclics were effective in reducing immobility time. Consistent with these studies, we also found that both SSRI and tricyclic classes of antidepressant effectively reduced immobility time of adolescent (P28) and adult mice in the TST. Likewise, our findings in P28 and adult mice are in good agreement with reports in P28 and adult rats, where both SSRIs and tricyclic antidepressants were effective in producing antidepressant-like activity in the FST (Reed et al., 2008).

To our knowledge, this is the first report of antidepressant-like activity in P21 mice. We found that the SSRI, escitalopram, produced antidepressant-like activity in these mice; however the magnitude of this effect was less than that in adolescent (P28) or adult mice. Similarly, studies using rats aged P21 in the FST, found them to be sensitive to the antidepressant-like effects of SSRIs, including escitalopram (Reed et al., 2008). However, in this study a head-to-head comparison with P28 and adult rats was not included, making it difficult to draw conclusions as to whether the magnitude of antidepressant-like effect was less in P21 rats, compared to P28 or adult rats. Based on the present studies, where P21, P28, and adult mice were compared head-to-head, it is clear that the magnitude of escitalopram to produce antidepressant-like effects in P21 mice is less than in adult mice.

We also found that P21 mice were sensitive to the antidepressant-like effect of the tricyclic, DMI. Unlike our finding for escitalopram, the magnitude of antidepressant-like effect of DMI was similar among P21, P28, and adult mice. This finding contrasts with studies using rats, where Reed et al. (2008) found P21 rats to be insensitive to tricyclics, including DMI. Potential reasons for these differences include species (rat versus mouse), behavioral test (FST versus TST), drug dose, and route of administration. For example, the highest dose of DMI tested in studies using P21 rats was 20 mg/kg (ip; Reed et al., 2008), whereas in our studies using mice, the dose was 32 mg/kg (ip). Thus, our ability to detect antidepressant-like effects of DMI in mice as young as P21 may result in part from using a higher dose. Certainly, pharmacokinetic differences between species and across ages are also a consideration.

In the clinical setting a key difference between adult and pediatric depression is response to pharmacotherapy (Hazell et al., 1995; Kratochvil et al., 2006; Bridge et al., 2007; Bylund and Reed, 2007; Hazell and Mirzaie, 2013). The present studies using mice, as well as published reports using rats, show that like humans, juvenile mice, and rats respond differently to antidepressant drugs. While there are some apparent discrepancies in reported findings, particularly those relating to the emergence of antidepressant-like activity of DMI, there are numerous factors that may account for these; some of which have been touched on already (e.g., dose, species, test). With regard to the clinical setting, it is important to keep in mind that therapeutic benefit is also contingent upon tolerability of the drug. Thus, although tricyclics are not approved for use in children and adolescents, data from clinical trials have been mixed, with some studies reporting that tricyclics lowered depression scores in adolescents, while others found tricyclics to be therapeutically ineffective (Hazell and Mirzaie, 2013). However, consistent with the mechanism of action of tricyclic antidepressants, these drugs were more likely than placebo to produce adverse side effects, including vertigo, tremor, low blood pressure, and dry mouth. Thus, due to inconclusive demonstrations of therapeutic benefit in young humans, and the possibility of harmful side effects, or increased sensitivity to adverse side-effects in this patient population, tricyclic antidepressants are not prescribed for children and adolescents.

The key finding from the present study is that it is possible to detect antidepressant-like activity of drugs in mice as young as P21. This finding opens the door for studies geared to understanding the mechanisms underlying the relatively poor therapeutic response of young humans to SSRIs, which in turn paves the way for identifying treatments with improved therapeutic efficacy. It is worth emphasizing that essentially nothing is known about the mechanisms of antidepressant activity in juvenile and adolescent mice. Rat studies have led the way, but even then, knowledge is not extensive (for review, see Bylund and Reed, 2007) with many unknowns remaining. For example, the effect of antidepressants can be dependent on relative rates of neurotransmitter synthesis and it is not yet known if the activity of neurotransmitter synthesizing enzymes (e.g., tryptophan hydroxylase, tyrosine hydroxylase) varies during these postnatal periods in mice. Here, we began to investigate possible mechanisms underlying the divergent response of juvenile mice to SSRIs and tricyclic antidepressants by first quantifying the expression and affinity of their target proteins, SERT and NET, in hippocampus.

Hippocampus was selected for these initial studies given its importance in mood and antidepressant drug effects (Campbell and McQueen, 2004). In rats the delayed emergence of antidepressant-like activity of tricyclics is thought to be related to delayed maturation of the noradrenergic system compared with the serotonergic system (Murrin et al., 2007). As far as NET is concerned, the primary target of DMI, its expression during postnatal development in rat brain, measured using quantitative autoradiography, is age and brain region dependent. NET expression increases rapidly across brain regions between P10 and P15, and attains adult levels in some regions (e.g., cortex, CA1 and CA2 regions of hippocampus, dentate gyrus, amygdala, striatum) that are maintained into adulthood; in others regions (e.g., CA3 region of hippocampus) NET expression attains adult levels at P15, but then decreases at P20 before returning to adult levels at P25 (Sanders et al., 2005). To date there are no reports on the development of expression of NET in mouse brain over the postnatal ages studied here. Our data show that in hippocampus, NET expression was similar in P21, P28, and adult mice. Likewise, the affinity of NET for $[^3H]$nisoxetine was similar across these ages. Data from adult mouse hippocampus presented here are in general agreement with those reported by others [e.g., B_{max} 127 ± 5 fmol/mgpr and K_d 0.7 ± 0.05 nM, C57Bl/6 male mice (Csölle et al., 2013)], and in adult rat cerebral cortex [B_{max} 97 ± 12 fmol/mgpr and K_d 0.8 ± 0.11 nM (Tejani-Butt, 1992)]. Our data are also consistent with the quantitative autoradiography measures of NET in rat hippocampus reported by Sanders et al. (2005), where, with the exception of CA3 region, NET expression did not vary across juvenile, adolescent, and adult ages. Given that we carried out saturation binding assays in homogenates taken from whole hippocampus it would be unlikely we would detect any age-dependent changes in a sub-region of hippocampus (such as CA3). At the expense of anatomical resolution, our saturation binding approach afforded a measure of transporter affinity, which to our knowledge has not been previously reported for P21 or P28 mouse or rat. Our findings in mouse hippocampus show that NET expression and affinity are at adult levels by P21. Given that the antidepressant-like effects of DMI in the TST were also similar among juvenile, adolescent, and adult mice, it appears that NET expression and affinity in hippocampus parallels DMI's antidepressant efficacy in mice. It must be recognized, however, that this does not rule out the possibility that DMI's antidepressant-like activity in the TST depends on NET expression in other regions. Further studies are needed to determine the brain region(s) and mechanisms (e.g., transporters, receptors) that mediate antidepressant-like behavioral activity in the TST following administration of NET blockers, and how this may vary with age.

Even less is known about the postnatal development of expression and affinity of SERT in mice. Quantitative autoradiography studies to date indicate that in rats, SERT expression reaches adult levels between birth and P21 (Zhou et al., 2000; Galineau et al., 2004; Bylund and Reed, 2007). Consistent with these findings in rats, we found that SERT expression in hippocampus of P21 and P28 mice was similar to that in adults. We also found that the affinity of hippocampal SERT for [^{3}H]citalopram was equivalent among P21, P28, and adult mice. To our knowledge there are only two reports of [^{3}H]citalopram binding using adult C57Bl/6 mouse hippocampal homogenate preparations. Our group previously reported values in good agreement with those reported here [B_{max} 171 ± 20 fmol/mgpr; K_d 1.1 ± 0.2 nM (Gould et al., 2011)]. Another group reported a higher B_{max} (555 ± 35 fmol/mgpr) but a similar K_d (1.2 ± 0.1 nM; Csölle et al., 2013). Of note in the present study, even though statistical analyses did not reveal significant differences in affinity of hippocampal SERT for [^{3}H]citalopram among ages, the variance of the K_d values differed significantly among ages. As is clear in **Figure 3E**, K_d values varied from 0.3 to 4.6 nM in juveniles, 0.6 to 2.1 nM in adolescents and 1.0 to 1.8 nM in adults. Thus, the spread in K_d values dropped from 4.3 nM in P21 mice, to 1.5 nM in P28 mice and to 0.8 nM in adult mice. These data suggest that juvenile and adolescent periods may be critical periods in development where, although the density of SERT is at adult expression levels, the functional activity (affinity) of SERT is undergoing a transition to that of the adult. In the case of the present data, approximately half of P21 mice had K_d values in line with those of adults, and the remainder had K_d values two or more fold greater (i.e., lower affinity for [^{3}H]citalopram). Based on these initial data, it is tempting to speculate that this variability in when the "switch" from juvenile to adult SERT affinity occurs, accounts in part for the variability in individual response to SSRIs in pediatric depression.

These studies are, to our knowledge, the first to obtain B_{max} and K_d values for [^{3}H]citalopram binding to SERT and [^{3}H]nisoxetine binding to NET, two of the most prominent targets of currently available antidepressant drugs, in juvenile and adolescent mice, and the results are in agreement with the few existing reports from adult mice (Gould et al., 2011; Csölle et al., 2013). The present findings raise the possibility that, although SERT expression may be at or near adult levels in P21 mice, the large variability in affinity state of SERT for SSRIs may account, at least in part, for the lower clinical effectiveness of SSRIs in children. Showing that the TST is a relevant behavioral assay of antidepressant-like activity in juvenile (P21) and adolescent (P28) mice, sets the stage for future studies of the mechanisms underlying the antidepressant response in these young populations.

ACKNOWLEDGMENTS

The authors gratefully acknowledge the technical assistance of Mr. Steven Alvarado, Mr. Peter Campos, Ms. Sonia Cano, and Ms. Melissa Vitela. Supported by NIH grants MH064489-S1 (Lynette C. Daws), MH093320 (Lynette C. Daws and Wouter Koek), MH086708 (Georgianna G. Gould), UL1RR025767 (sub-award to Corey M. Smolik), and NARSAD (Lynette C. Daws).

REFERENCES

Andreasen, J. T., and Redrobe, J. P. (2009). Antidepressant-like effects of nicotine and mecamylamine in the mouse forced swim and tail suspension tests: role of strain, test and sex. *Behav. Pharmacol.* 20, 286–295. doi: 10.1097/FBP.0b013e32832c713e

Bourin, M., Colombel, M. C., Redrobe, J. P., Nizard, J., Hascoët, M., and Baker, G. B. (1998). Evaluation of efficacies of different classes of antidepressants in the forced swimming test in mice at different ages. *Prog. Neuropsychopharmacol. Biol. Psychiatry* 22, 343–351. doi: 10.1016/S0278-5846(98)00009-8

Bridge, J. A., Iyengar, S., Salary, C. B., Barbe, R. P., Birmaher, B., Pincus, H. A., et al. (2007). Clinical response and risk for reported suicidal ideation and suicide attempts in pediatric antidepressant treatment: a meta-analysis of randomized control trials. *JAMA* 297, 1683–1696. doi: 10.1001/jama.297.15.1683

Bujoreanu, S., Benhayon, D., and Szigethy, E. (2011). Treatment of depression in children and adolescents. *Pediatr. Ann.* 40, 548–555. doi: 10.3928/00904481-20111007-05

Bylund, D. B., and Reed, A. L. (2007). Childhood and adolescent depression: why do children and adults respond differently to antidepressant drugs? *Neurochem. Int.* 51, 246–253. doi: 10.1016/j.neuint.2007.06.025

Campbell, S., and McQueen, G. (2004). The role of the hippocampus in the pathophysiology of major depression. *J. Psychiatr. Neurosci.* 29, 417–426.

Castagne, V., Moser, P., Roux, S., and Porsolt, R. D. (2011). Rodent models of depression: forced swim and tail suspension behavioral despair tests in rats and mice. *Curr. Protoc. Neurosci.* Chapter 8, Unit 8.10A. doi: 10.1002/0471142301.ns0810as55

Csölle, C., Baranyi, M., Zsilla, G., Kittel, A., Gölöncsér, F., Illes., et al. (2013). Neurochemical changes in the mouse hippocampus underlying the antidepressant effect of genetic deletion of P2X7 receptors. *PLoS ONE* 8:e66547. doi: 10.1371/journal.pone.0066547

Cryan, J. F., and Holmes, A. (2005). The ascent of mouse: advances in modeling human depression and anxiety. *Nat. Rev. Drug Discov.* 4, 775–790. doi: 10.1038/nrd1825

Cryan, J. F., Mombereau, C., and Vassout, A. (2005). The tail suspension test a model for assessing antidepressant activity: review of pharmacological studies in mice. *Neurosci. Biobehav. Rev.* 29, 571–625. doi: 10.1016/j.neubiorev.2005.03.009

D'Amato, R. J., Largent, B. L., Snowman, A. M., and Snyder, S. H. (1987). Selective labeling of serotonin uptake sites in rat brain by [3H]citalopram contrasted to labeling of multiple sites by [3H]imipramine. *J. Pharmacol. Exp. Ther.* 242, 364–371.

David, D. J. P., Bourin, M., Hascoët, M., Colombel, M. C., Baker, G. B., and Jolliet, P. (2001a). Comparison of antidepressant activity in 4- and 40-week-old male mice in the forced swimming test: involvment of 5-HT1A and 5-HT1B receptors in old mice. *Psychopharmacology* 153, 443–449. doi: 10.1007/s00213000 0588

David, D. J. P., Dhonnchadha, B. A. N., Jolliet, P., Hascoët, M., and Bourin, M. (2001b). Are there gender differences in the temperature profile of mice after acute antidepressant administration and exposure to tow animal models of depression. *Behav. Brain Res.* 119, 203–211. doi: 10.1016/S0166-4328(00)00351-X

Daws, L. C., and Gould, G. G. (2011). Ontogeny and regulation of the serotonin transporter: providing insight into human disorders. *Pharmacol. Ther.* 131, 61–79. doi: 10.1016/j.pharmthera.2011.03.013

Galineau, L., Kodas, E., Guilloteau, D., Vilar, M. P., and Chalon, S. (2004). Ontogeny of the dopamine and serotonin transporters in the rat brain: an autoradiographic study. *Neurosci. Lett.* 363, 266–271. doi: 10.1016/j.neulet.2004.04.007

Gould, G. G., Hensler, J. G., Burke, T. F., Benno, R. H., Onaivi, E. S., and Daws, L. C. (2011). Density and function of central serotonin (5-HT) transporters, 5-HT1A and 5HT2A receptors, and effects of their targeting on BTBR T+tf/J mouse social behavior. *J. Neurochem.* 116, 291–303. doi: 10.1111/j.1471-4159.2010.07104.x

Hazell, P., and Mirzaie, M. (2013). Tricyclic drugs for depression in children and adolescents. *Cochrane Database Syst. Rev.* 6. doi: 10.1002/14651858.CD002317.pub2

Hazell, P., O'Connell, D., Heathcote, D., Robertson, J., and Henry, D. (1995). Efficacy of tricylcic drugs in treating child and adolescent depression: a meta-analysis. *BMJ* 310, 897–901. doi: 10.1136/bmj.310.6984.897

Hetrick, S. E., McKenzie, J. E., and Merry, S. N. (2010). The use of SSRIs in children and adolescents. *Curr. Opin. Psychiatr.* 23, 53–57. doi: 10.1097/YCO.0b013e328334bc92

Hetrick, S. E., Merry, S. N., McKenzie, J., Sindahl, P., and Proctor, M. (2009). Selective serotonin reuptake inhibitors (SSRIs) for depressive disorders in children and adolescents (Review). *Cochrane Database Syst. Rev.* 1–91.

Jones, M. D., and Lucki, I. (2005). Sex differences in the regulation of serotonergic transmission and behavior in 5-HT receptor knockout mice. *Neuropsychopharmacology* 30, 1039–1047. doi: 10.1038/sj.npp.1300664

Kessler, R. C., Avenevoli, S., and Reis Merikangas, K. (2001). Mood disorders in children and adolescents: an epidemiologic perspective. *Biol. Psychiatry* 49, 1002–1014. doi: 10.1016/S0006-3223(01)01129-5

Kratochvil, C., Emslie, G., Silva, S., McNulty, S., Walkup, J., Curry, J., et al. (2006). Acute time to response in the Treatment of Adolescents with Depression Study (TABS). *J. Am. Acad. Child Adolesc. Psychiatry* 45, 1412–1418. doi: 10.1097/01.chi.0000237710.73755.14

Mason, S. S., Baker, K. B., Davis, K. W., Pogorelov, V. M., Malbari, M. M., Ritter, R., et al. (2009). Differential sensitivity to SSRI and tricyclic antidepressants in juvenile and adult mice of three strains. *Eur. J. Pharmacol.* 602, 306–315. doi: 10.1016/j.ejphar.2008.11.010

Murrin, L. C., Sander, J. D., and Bylund, D. B. (2007). Comparison of the maturation of the adrenergic and serotonergic neurotransmitter systems in the brain: implications for differential drug effects on juveniles and adults. *Biochem. Pharmacol.* 73, 1225–1236. doi: 10.1016/j.bcp.2007.01.028

O'Leary, O. F., Bechtholt, A. J., Crowley, J. J., Hill, T. E., Page, M. E., and Lucki, I. (2007). Depletion of serotonin and catecholamines block the acute behavioral response to different classes of antidepressant drugs in the mouse tail suspension test. *Psychopharmacology* 192, 357–371. doi: 10.1007/s00213-007-0728-9

Pechnick, R. N., Bresee, C. J., Manalo, C. M., and Poland, R. E. (2008). Comparison of the effects of desmethylimipramine on behavior in the forced swim test in peripubertal and adult rats. *Behav. Pharmacol.* 19, 81–84. doi: 10.1097/FBP.0b013e3282f3d07f

Reed, A. L., Happe, H. K., Petty, F., and Bylund, D. B. (2008). Juvenile rats in the forced-swim test model the human response to antidepressant treatment for pediatric depression. *Psychopharmacology* 197, 433–441. doi: 10.1007/s00213-007-1052-0

Sanchez, C., Bergqvist, P. B. F., Brennum, L. T., Gupta, S., Hogg, S., Larsen, A., et al. (2003). Escitalopram, the S-(+)-enantiomer of citalopram, is a selective serotonin reuptake inhibitor with potent effects in animal models predictive of antidepressant and anxiolytic activities. *Psychopharmacology* 167, 353–362.

Sanders, J. D., Happe, H. K., Bylund, D. B., and Murrin, L. C. (2005). Development of the norepinephrine transporter in the rat CNS. *Neuroscience* 130, 107–117. doi: 10.1016/j.neuroscience.2004.09.014

Spear, L. P. (2000). The adolescent brain and age-related behavioral manifestations. *Neurosci. Behav. Rev.* 24, 417–463. doi: 10.1016/S0149-7634(00)00014-2

Steru, L., Chermat, R., Thierry, B., and Simon, P. (1985). The tail suspension test: a new method for screening antidepressants in mice. *Psychopharmacology* 85, 367–370. doi: 10.1007/BF00428203

Tejani-Butt, S. (1992). [3H]nisoxetine: a radioligand for quantitation of norepinephrine uptake sites by autoradiography or homogenate binding. *J. Pharmacol. Exp. Ther.* 260, 427–436.

Tsapakis, E. M., Soldani, F., Tondo, L., and Baldessarini, R. J. (2008). Efficacy of antidepressants in juvenile depression: meta-analysis. *Br. J. Psychiatry* 193, 10–17. doi: 10.1192/bjp.bp.106.031088

Zhou, F. C., Sari, Y., and Zhang, J. K. (2000). Expression of serotonin transporter protein in developing rat brain. *Brain Res. Dev. Brain Res.* 119, 33–45. doi: 10.1016/S0165-3806(99)00152-2

Conflict of Interest Statement: The authors declare that the research was conducted in the absence of any commercial or financial relationships that could be construed as a potential conflict of interest.

Identification of subpopulations of prairie voles differentially susceptible to peer influence to decrease high alcohol intake

Allison M. J. Anacker*† and Andrey E. Ryabinin

Department of Behavioral Neuroscience, Oregon Health & Science University, Portland, OR, USA

Edited by:
Thibault Renoir, Florey Institute of Neuroscience and Mental Health, Australia

Reviewed by:
Gregg E. Homanics, University of Pittsburgh, USA
Enrico Sanna, University of Cagliari, Italy
Terence Pang, Florey Institute of Neuroscience and Mental Health, Australia

***Correspondence:**
Allison M. J. Anacker, Department of Behavioral Neuroscience, Oregon Health & Science University, 3181 SW Sam Jackson Park Road, Mail Code L470, Portland, OR, USA
e-mail: allison.anacker@gmail.com
†

Peer influences are critical in the decrease of alcohol (ethanol) abuse and maintenance of abstinence. We previously developed an animal model of inhibitory peer influences on ethanol drinking using prairie voles and here sought to understand whether this influential behavior was due to specific changes in drinking patterns and to variation in a microsatellite sequence in the regulatory region of the vasopressin receptor 1a gene (*avpr1a*). Adult prairie voles' drinking patterns were monitored in a lickometer apparatus that recorded each lick a subject exhibited during continuous access to water and 10% ethanol during periods of isolation, pair housing of high and low drinkers, and subsequent isolation. Analysis of fluid consumption confirmed previous results that high drinkers typically decrease ethanol intake when paired with low drinkers, but that a subset of voles do not decrease. Analysis of bout structure revealed differences in the number of ethanol drinking bouts in the subpopulations of high drinkers when paired with low drinkers. Lickometer drinking patterns analyzed by visual and by cross-correlation analyses demonstrated that pair housing did not increase the rate of subjects drinking in bouts occurring at the same time. The length of the *avpr1a* microsatellite did not predict susceptibility to peer influence or any other drinking behaviors. In summary, subpopulations of high drinkers were identified, by fluid intake and number of drinking bouts, which did or did not lower their ethanol intake when paired with a low drinking peer, and these subpopulations should be explored for testing the efficacy of treatments to decrease ethanol use in groups that are likely to be responsive to different types of therapy.

Keywords: prairie vole, social behavior, alcohol, ethanol, peer pressure, vasopressin, genetics, regulatory microsatellite

INTRODUCTION

Excessive alcohol (ethanol) use in the United States contributes to over 80,000 deaths per year (apps.nccd.cdc.gov/DACH_ARDI). Therefore, it is extremely important to understand all factors contributing to excessive ethanol drinking, as well as those that contribute to decreases in drinking. Peer influences can lead to increases in ethanol drinking in some cases, and to decreases in others. Both types of influence can be crucial on the path to either alcohol abuse (Fisher et al., 2007; Park et al., 2008) or abstinence (Gordon and Zrull, 1991; Bond et al., 2003; Wu and Witkiewitz, 2008; Kelly et al., 2011). Understanding the processes by which peer influences take effect will help inform and improve prevention and treatment strategies for alcoholism.

Biological mechanisms underlying peer influence are underexplored, in large part because such influence is difficult to model in laboratory animals. Most laboratory animals do not develop selective affiliations between individual adult animals and therefore cannot model specific social interactions between peers. In contrast, individuals of socially monogamous species do form such selective affiliations. For example, socially monogamous prairie voles (*Microtus ochrogaster*) exhibit increased preference not only for their sexual partner, but also to their same-sex cage mates (Getz et al., 1981; Williams, 1992; DeVries et al., 1997a). We have previously modeled specific social influences of ethanol drinking in prairie voles. Specifically, we have shown that, depending on the experimental conditions, housing with siblings or peers can either facilitate (Anacker et al., 2011a) or inhibit ethanol drinking in these animals (Anacker et al., 2011b). Moreover, such influence on ethanol drinking is specific to same-sex peers, and not male–female pairs (Hostetler et al., 2012).

The positive (inhibitory) influence of voles drinking low doses of ethanol on voles drinking high doses of ethanol was specific to ethanol, and was not observed with other palatable fluids (Anacker et al., 2011b). The decrease in ethanol drinking did not occur when high drinking animals were housed together, indicating that the high drinkers did not decrease their intake spontaneously or due to potential anxiety associated with cohabitation, but did so because of the influence of low drinkers. Moreover, the change in intake due to this peer influence was long-lasting and maintained even after the voles were separated. However, we also observed that while some of the voles changed their drinking behaviors due to influence of their peer, others did not. It is important to understand what makes a specific individual susceptible or resistant to peer influence, in order to target prevention or treatment accordingly. Based on our previous findings showing that high and low drinkers will alter alcohol intake levels when paired together, while matched drinkers will not, here we explored the manner in which the high–low drinking pairs affect one another. We hypothesized that high drinkers' decrease in ethanol intake would be due to the development of a drinking pattern that was linked to that of a low drinking peer when they were housed together. To address this hypothesis here, we investigated features of prairie voles' drinking patterns using a lickometer system.

Reports from other laboratories have demonstrated that the establishment of social bonds in prairie voles is dependent on the neuropeptide arginine vasopressin, acting via the vasopressin 1a receptor (V1aR; Winslow et al., 1993; Carter et al., 1995; Liu et al., 2001; Nair and Young, 2006; Donaldson et al., 2010). The gene for this receptor in prairie voles (*avpr1a*) contains a microsatellite region upstream of the transcription start site, which is polymorphic (Young et al., 1997; Hammock and Young, 2002, 2004; Hammock et al., 2005; Ophir et al., 2008; Solomon et al., 2009). Studies have demonstrated that the length of the microsatellite influences gene expression and receptor levels in many brain regions, and the expression in turn affects behavior (Hammock et al., 2005; Solomon et al., 2009). Specifically, several types of social behaviors including partner preference have been correlated with microsatellite length. In addition to vasopressin's involvement in social behaviors, the neuropeptide levels are also affected by ethanol drinking and thought to play a role in the development of tolerance (Linkola et al., 1978; Hoffman et al., 1990; Inder et al., 1995; Harding et al., 1996; Rivier and Lee, 1996; Madeira and Paula-Barbosa, 1999; Silva et al., 2002). In addition, while one laboratory reported no effects of *avpr1a* deletion on ethanol intake (Caldwell et al., 2006), a more recent study found increased ethanol intake in *avpr1a* knockout mice (Sanbe et al., 2008). While studies on the role of *avpr1a* in alcohol drinking provided conflicting results, we explored whether the microsatellite length could relate to the degree of social influence on alcohol intake. Therefore, we further hypothesized that the length of the V1aR microsatellite could be correlated with ethanol drinking or the degree of social influence on ethanol drinking in prairie voles, and addressed this hypothesis in this study.

MATERIALS AND METHODS

ANIMALS

Prairie voles were bred in our colony at the Portland Veterans Affairs Medical Center Veterinary Medical Unit. All procedures were approved by the Institutional Animal Care and Use Committee and adhered to the guidelines put forth in the National Institutes of Health Guide for the Care and Use of Laboratory Animals. Voles were weaned around 21 days of age and housed in same-sex sibling pairs, with females and males housed in different rooms, until beginning the experiment. Voles were housed under 14L:10D lighting conditions and had continuous *ad libitum* access to water and food (corn, oats, and rabbit chow). Adult male and female voles ($n = 95$) were used in these studies, ranging from 58 to 95 days of age at the start of the experiment.

APPARATUS

The "lickometer" apparatus used in these experiments was a variation of that described previously (Ford et al., 2005; Anacker et al., 2011a). As before, the apparatus consisted of a metal floor (10 cm × 20 cm and 30 mm high; VWR, Tualatin, WA, USA), connected by electrical wires to metal spouts of the drinking tubes to create an open circuit through a dual lickometer device (MED Associates, Inc., St. Albans, VT, USA), which was connected to a PC. The wire bottom was positioned underneath the sipper tubes so that the animals were required to have at least one paw on the metal rack to touch the drinking spout, thereby completing the electrical circuit. Each lick exhibited by a subject was recorded by MED-PC IV software (MED Associates, Inc.) and stored for later analysis. The cage containing each apparatus was modified from the apparatus designed by Ford et al. and a schematic diagram is pictured in **Figure 1**. The plastic cage bottom that surrounded the wire rack was 16.8 cm × 27.6 cm and 5.4 cm high (Flair Plastic Products, Inc., Portland, OR, USA) and had bedding, food, and a nestlet available, so the subjects were not required to be on the wire rack when they were not drinking. The plastic cage top was 17 cm high and in addition to the holes for the drinking spouts, there were holes in the lid and openings along the bottom for air circulation (Flair Plastic Products, Inc.). The cages used for pair housing were identical except that they were twice as wide, with separate lids for each half, and a wire mesh down the center that divided the cage into two equal compartments but allowed the subjects visual, olfactory, vocal, and some tactile contact, similar to what has been described by us previously (Anacker et al., 2011a,b; Hostetler et al., 2012). Wire dividers were distant from the wire racks and drinking spouts and did not interfere with lickometer data collection.

PROCEDURE

At the beginning of the experiment, voles were placed in individual lickometer cages and given access to water in the drinking tubes for 5 days, to habituate to the apparatus. After habituation, subjects were presented with ethanol in one drinking tube (10% ethanol by volume in tap water) and water in the other, and they had continuous access to these solutions throughout the rest of the experiment. Fluid volumes were recorded every 24 h, and the position of the bottles relative to one another was counterbalanced across pairs and switched every 2 days. Fluids were replaced every 2 days. After recording fluid volumes each day, and changing fluids every second day, the lickometer recording began and continued for 22 h.

After 4 days of access to ethanol in isolation, subjects were categorized as consistent high, medium, or low drinkers, dependent on the amount of ethanol they consumed (g/kg/day) and the preference ratio for ethanol over water, using identical criteria to a previous study (Anacker et al., 2011b). Specifically, high drinking was defined as no less than 9 g/kg of ethanol per day and no less than 0.75 ethanol preference over water. Low drinking was defined as less than 5 kg/day and less than 0.5 ethanol preference. After 4 days of baseline drinking in isolation, each animal

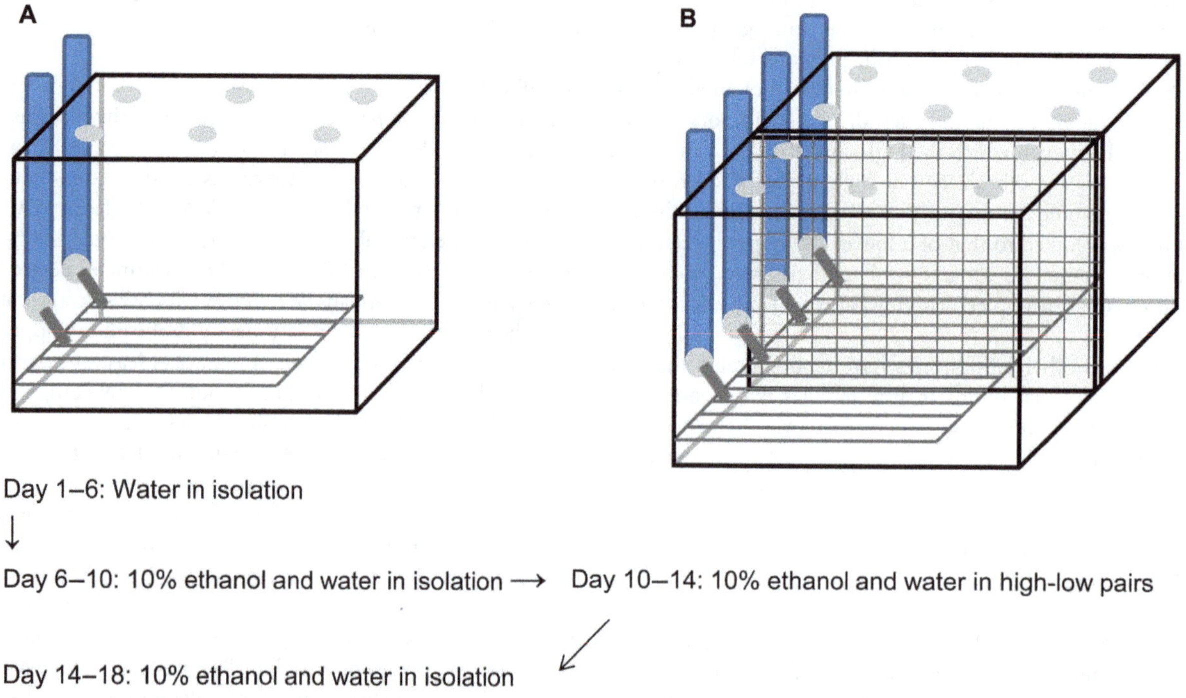

FIGURE 1 | Schematic diagram of lickometer cages and timeline. Custom-designed cages were made to house voles individually **(A)** or in pairs separated by a mesh divider **(B)**. In both cases, plastic cages with air holes in the top surrounded wire metal racks that covered most of the cage floor. Voles had to step on the wire rack to reach the metal sipper tubes to obtain fluid, completing an electrical circuit to register each lick on the drinking tube. Subjects habituated to drinking water from the tubes for 5 days prior to the start of the experiment. They then had access to 10% ethanol and water for 4 days, after which time they were categorized as high or low drinkers. High and low drinkers were paired and given access to ethanol and water for another 4 days, followed by a final 4 days of isolation with continued access to ethanol and water.

was categorized by subtracting the number of "low" scores for preference and dose from the number of "high" scores. Animals receiving a positive number were labeled "high drinkers" while those receiving negative numbers were labeled "low drinkers." Also as in other studies (Anacker et al., 2011b; Hostetler et al., 2012), high drinkers were paired with low drinkers and moved into the double cages with mesh dividers, where continuous access to ethanol and water continued for 4 days. Here, pairs were made up of same-sex, unrelated strangers. After pairing, subjects were again moved into isolation and had access to ethanol and water for a final 4 days. In this experiment, the controls similar to those used in past studies (namely high–high and low–low matched drinking pairs) were not used, since the focus of the study was on the behavioral mechanism by which the change in drinking occurs specifically in high–low pairs. Instead, subjects for comparison were generated based on individual performance in the experiment: subjects that changed their drinking level when paired were compared with those subjects that did not alter drinking.

Following the final isolation period, voles were euthanized by CO_2 inhalation, and tail tissue samples were taken for genetic analysis.

DRINKING ANALYSES

Ethanol intake and preference were calculated for each day based on fluid volumes consumed. Average measures for each housing period were compared by two-way repeated measures ANOVA with high and low drinkers as a between-subjects variable. Further analyses were done by splitting high drinkers into a group of animals that decreased their drinking level category during the 4 days of pair housing with a low drinker and a group of animals that did not, and comparing ethanol intake on each day of isolation and pair housing. Drinking data from days two and six are not presented in order to correspond with the lickometer data (see below), but data from each of these days were very consistent with the respective surrounding days. Bonferroni post-tests were used to determine specific group differences. As in a previous study (Anacker et al., 2011b), there were no sex differences in measures of alcohol consumption or the effects of pair housing on ethanol consumption and so data are presented and analyzed collapsed across sexes.

To validate the lickometer, water and ethanol volume consumed were each compared with the number of licks registered for each subject, and analyzed using a Pearson's correlation.

The lickometer data were analyzed as described previously (Ford et al., 2005) by custom software for bout frequency (number of bouts), bout size, interbout interval, bout length, lick rate, and latency to first bout. For voles with zero or one drinking bouts per day, the data could not be analyzed using this software. However, the number of bouts for these subjects was included in the group analysis. Averages were compared by repeated measures ANOVA with three groups (high drinkers that remained high, high drinkers that decreased drinking level when paired, and low drinkers) as a between-subjects variable and each day throughout isolation and pair housing as the repeated measure. Due to a power failure, lickometer data for days two and six were not collected for a subset of animals. Rather than eliminating these subjects from the entire repeated-measures analysis, those 2 days were removed. Bonferroni post-tests were used to determine specific group differences.

The lickometer data were then processed using custom-designed software (u2615, Portland, OR, USA) which first rescaled the data from 10 ms to 1 s resolution. Cumulative lick plots for each pair on the last day of isolation and pairing were examined, since the subjects would have had the most time to establish stable drinking patterns under each housing condition. The number of bouts occurring in temporal proximity ($\leq$15 min apart) was determined using a standardized visual assessment. The number of close bouts, and the number of close bouts normalized to the lowest number of bouts exhibited by one member of the pair, were compared using two-way repeated measures ANOVA with change in drinking as a between-subjects factor and housing as the repeated measure.

The data processed through u2615 were then analyzed for each pair by a cross-correlation analysis (R for Mac OS). The correlations were compared between the last day of isolation and the last day of pair housing. The presence or absence of a significant correlation for each day was noted, as well as the lag time and degree of correlation (autocorrelation function, ACF) for each significant correlation. The lag time range was limited to $\pm$10 min, in order to analyze only behaviors that occurred close together in time. This metric indicated which subject followed the other in drinking, and was examined in conjunction with individual pair data indicating which subject changed intake.

MICROSATELLITE LENGTH ANALYSIS

DNA was extracted from each subject's tail tissue sample using a DNeasy Blood and Tissue Extraction Kit (Qiagen, Valencia, CA, USA). The V1aR microsatellite sequence was amplified using a variation of a previously published PCR technique (Hammock et al., 2005). We used the same sequences of primers but the forward primer was labeled with a 5-FAM fluorophore (Eurofins MWG Operon, Huntsville, AL, USA). We also used a touchdown PCR protocol to increase the specificity of the reaction (Korbie and Mattick, 2008), with a HotStarTaq DNA polymerase (Qiagen). The reactions were heated to 94°C for 15 min to activate the polymerase, and then had 28 cycles of 30 s denaturing (94°C), 45 s annealing, and 1 min for elongation (72°C). The annealing temperature started at 71°C on the first cycle and decreased by 1°C in each of the following 12 cycles. The last 25 cycles all had an annealing temperature of 58°C. The reaction was ended by a 5 min elongation at 72°C and cooling to 4°C.

The samples were each read by a 3130xl Genetic Analyzer (Applied Biosystems, Carlsbad, CA, USA), by the Oregon Clinical and Translational Research Institute Core Laboratory at Oregon Health & Science University (OHSU). The microsatellite length was determined for each allele for each subject with approximately 3 base pair resolution.

Microsatellite allele lengths were not normally distributed due to a highly leptokurtotic sample, which could not be normalized by any transformation. Thus, correlations could not be conducted using the collected data. Instead, a median split was applied to the data and t-tests were performed to compare between animals that had short or long average microsatellite length. A number of dependent variables were tested (baseline preference and intake, change in preference and intake for high or low drinkers between isolation 1 and pairing, or pairing and isolation 2, or overall from isolation 1 to isolation 2) and a Bonferroni correction for multiple comparisons was applied to yield the corrected threshold for significance $\alpha = 0.005$.

RESULTS

High drinkers were paired with low drinkers, leading to a total of 32 pairs that completed the experiment, while medium drinkers did not continue past the initial isolation phase. Of these, 14 pairs were female and 18 pairs were male.

As expected, high drinkers had a significantly higher preference for ethanol than low drinkers (high: 0.703 $\pm$ 0.024; low: 0.372 $\pm$ 0.030; $F_{(1,62)} = 45.71$; $p < 0.0001$) and exhibited higher intakes (high: 11.7 $\pm$ 0.536 g/kg; low: 5.45 $\pm$ 0.369 g/kg; $F_{(1,62)} = 40.85$; $p < 0.0001$), in accordance with their categorization. There was a significant effect of housing conditions on preference ($F_{(1,124)} = 4.91$; $p = 0.009$) but not intake ($F_{(1,124)} = 0.82$; $p = 0.441$). As seen in our previous study (Anacker et al., 2011b), there was a significant interaction between drinking category and housing condition on preference ($F_{(1,124)} = 6.94$; $p = 0.0014$) and intake ($F_{(1,124)} = 4.48$; $p = 0.013$). Planned Bonferroni post-tests revealed that high drinkers decreased their ethanol preference from baseline (isolation 1) to paired housing and isolation 2 ($t = 3.93$ and 3.26, respectively; df = 15; $p < 0.001$), as well as the intake level ($t = 2.76$ and 2.44, respectively; df = 15; $p < 0.05$), while low drinkers did not significantly change (**Figure 2**).

Also as in the previous study (Anacker et al., 2011b), the behavior of individual animals within the high drinkers differed, and they could be subcategorized into animals that either did (15/32; ~47%; 7 female and 8 male) or did not (17/32; ~53%; 7 female and 10 male) change their drinking under social conditions. The change was defined as the subject's average drinking during pair housing meeting the criteria for a drinking level different than the baseline drinking level. While all high drinkers had greater ethanol preference and intake than low drinkers on the first and last day of the first isolation period, only those high drinkers that altered their drinking under social conditions decreased their preference and intake to the level of the low drinkers during pair housing (**Figure 3**). There was a main effect of group on ethanol preference ($F_{(2,305)} = 51.65$, $p < 0.0001$) and intake ($F_{(2,305)} = 34.47$, $p < 0.0001$), a main effect of day on preference ($F_{(5,305)} = 10.26$, $p < 0.0001$) and intake ($F_{(5,305)} = 7.66$, $p < 0.0001$), and an interaction between the group and housing on preference ($F_{(10,305)} = 6.40$, $p < 0.0001$) and intake ($F_{(10,305)} = 9.86$, $p < 0.0001$). *Post hoc* tests revealed that the low drinkers had significantly lower ethanol preference and intake than both groups of high drinkers on each day of isolation ($p < 0.001$), while during pair housing, both the low drinkers and the high group that changed had significantly lower ethanol intake than the high drinkers that did not change ($p < 0.001$). On day 4 of isolation, the high-change group had a significantly lower preference

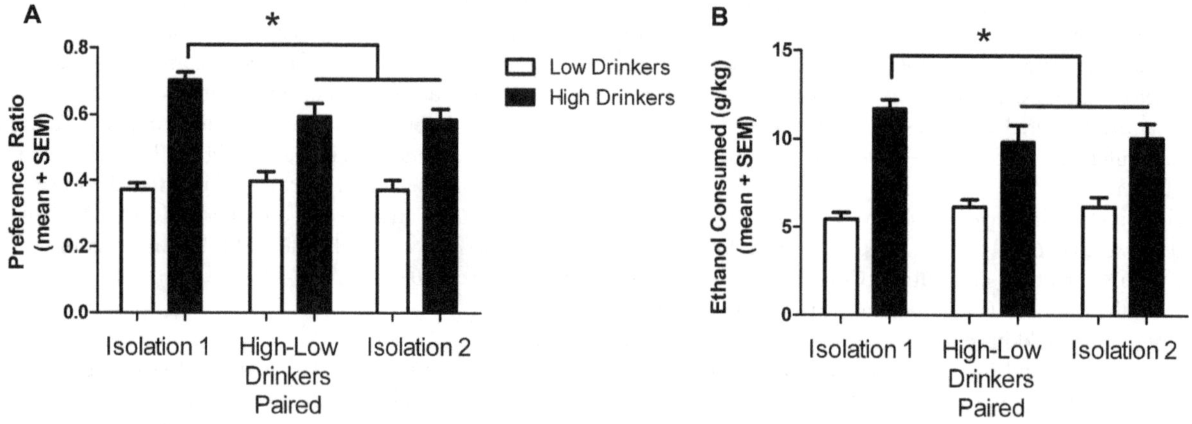

FIGURE 2 | Ethanol preference and intake in different housing conditions. Ethanol preference **(A)** and intake **(B)** by high (black) and low (white) drinkers in each housing condition. *Significant difference between isolation 1 and subsequent housing conditions for high drinkers; $p < 0.05$.

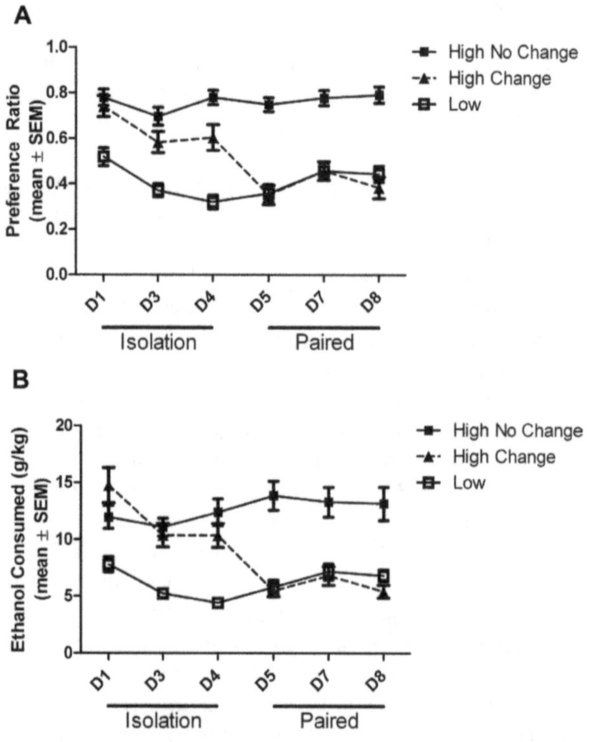

FIGURE 3 | Ethanol preference and intake across days. Ethanol preference **(A)** and intake **(B)** by high drinkers that did (black square) or did not (black triangle) change ethanol intake when paired with low drinkers (white square) is shown across days of isolation and pair housing. In isolation, both high groups are significantly higher than the low drinkers. During pair housing, the high drinkers that change intake and the low drinkers are both significantly lower than the constant high drinkers.

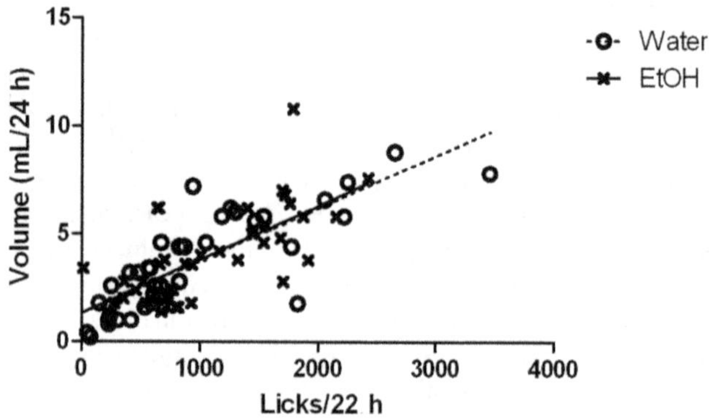

FIGURE 4 | Correlation of recorded licks with fluid volume consumed. The relationship between the number of recorded licks from each drinking tube on the *X*-axis with the volume of water (O) or ethanol (X) consumed on the *Y*-axis, for each of 4 days in isolation is graphed for one cohort of animals ($n = 10$) representative of the entire experiment. There was a strong positive correlation for both water ($r = 0.815$, $n = 40$, $p < 0.0001$) and ethanol ($r = 0.694$, $n = 40$, $p < 0.0001$).

for ethanol than the high-no change group ($p < 0.05$), while still remaining significantly higher than the low drinkers, as described above.

Volumes of ethanol and water consumed each day correlated very well with the number of licks recorded for each subject (**Figure 4**). Analysis of the bouts of ethanol consumption revealed one notable difference between high drinkers that did not change ethanol intake when paired with low drinkers, and high drinkers that did change, out of six different parameters assessed (**Figure 5**). Since the software could not analyze data from subjects with one or fewer drinking bouts, 10 low drinkers and one high drinker were not included in the analysis of other features besides the number of bouts. There was a main effect of group on the number of bouts ($F_{(2,300)} = 10.69$; $p = 0.0001$), interbout interval ($F_{(2,240)} = 5.71$; $p = 0.006$), and lick rate ($F_{(2,225)} = 5.30$; $p = 0.009$). There was also a main effect of day on the number of bouts ($F_{(5,300)} = 12.82$; $p < 0.0001$), interbout interval ($F_{(5,240)} = 5.33$; $p = 0.0001$), and lick rate ($F_{(5,225)} = 11.17$; $p < 0.0001$). Most notably, there was an interaction effect of group and day on the number of bouts ($F_{(10,300)} = 3.06$; $p = 0.001$).

Post hoc tests revealed the source of the interaction between group and day on the number of ethanol drinking bouts. The

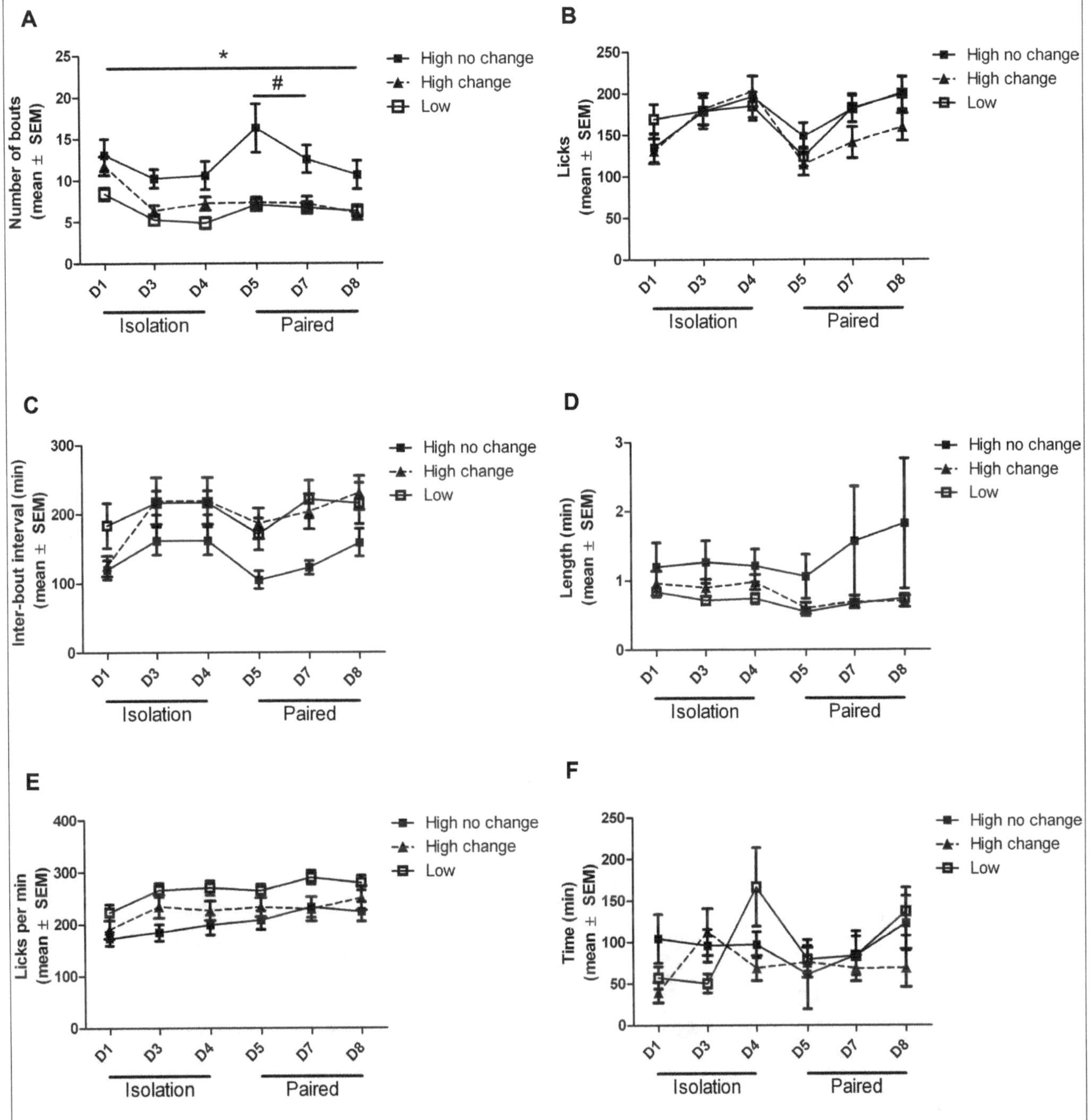

FIGURE 5 | Ethanol drinking bout features. Bout features of high drinkers that did (black triangle) or did not (black square) change ethanol intake when paired with low drinkers (white square) are shown throughout isolation and pair housing. The number of bouts of ethanol drinking **(A)**, the average length of bouts as measured by number of licks **(B)** and time **(D)**, the average time between bouts **(C)**, the rate of licks within a bout **(E)**, and the average time until the first lick was recorded **(F)** are shown for each 22 h period. **Post hoc* significant difference between high-no change group and low group; #*Post hoc* significant difference between high-no change group and high-change group.

number of bouts was significantly higher in the high-no change group than in the low group on all days ($p < 0.05$), while the high-change group was never significantly different from the low group. The high-change group did have significantly fewer drinking bouts than the high-no change group on days 5 ($p < 0.001$) and 7 ($p < 0.05$) during pair housing (**Figure 5A**).

Visual analysis of the cumulative lick graphs (**Figure 6**) revealed that while there were occurrences of ethanol drinking bouts close together in time for pairs of animals, the frequency of close bouts was not significantly different between isolation (**Figure 6A**) and pair housing (**Figure 6B**), or between pairs that did not change drinking levels compared to those who did, and there was no

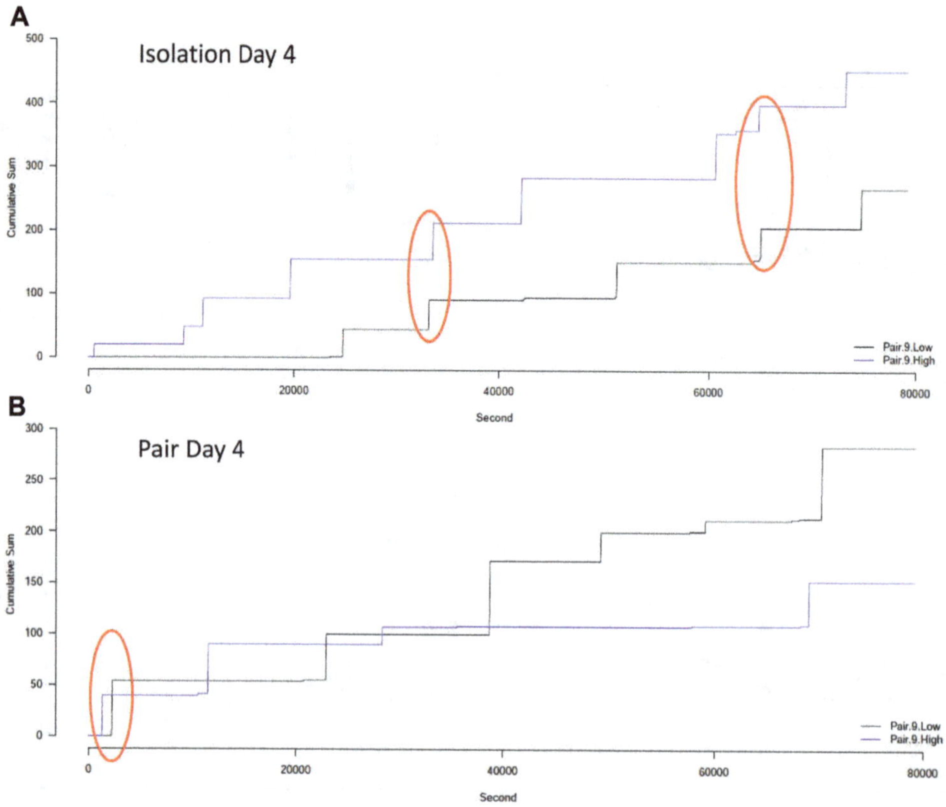

FIGURE 6 | Cumulative number of licks of ethanol over 22 h for an example pair. (A) The drinking patterns for subjects in a pair on the last day of isolation. **(B)** The drinking patterns for subjects in the same pair on the last day of pair housing. The high drinker is shown in blue and the low drinker is shown in black. Each "step up" in the graph indicates a bout of drinking while each horizontal line indicates a time when no drinking occurred. The red circle indicates bouts that occurred close together in time, within the applied threshold.

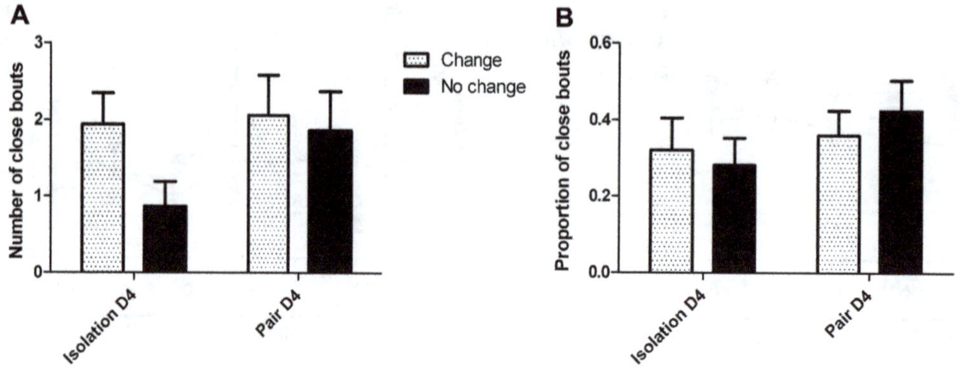

FIGURE 7 | Visual assessment of close ethanol drinking bouts between partners in isolation and pair housing. (A) The number of close bouts does not significantly differ between housing conditions or group changes, and there is no significant interaction of effects. **(B)** The proportion of close bouts relative to the lowest number of bouts one subject exhibited does not significantly differ between housing conditions or group changes, and there is no significant interaction of effects.

interaction between the two factors when either the number (**Figure 7A**) or proportion (**Figure 7B**) of close bouts was assessed.

Cross-correlation analyses revealed that over two-thirds of the pairs exhibited a significant correlation between ethanol drinking patterns regardless of whether they were physically isolated (**Figure 8A**) or housed together (**Figure 8B**). Additionally, there was no consistent difference in the presence or absence of correlations between pairs that exhibited changes in drinking behavior and those that did not (**Table 1**). Contrary to our hypothesis, there was no consistent directionality of the lag time of cross-correlations in pairs that changed their drinking level: in pairs where high drinkers changed to low drinkers, there was not a

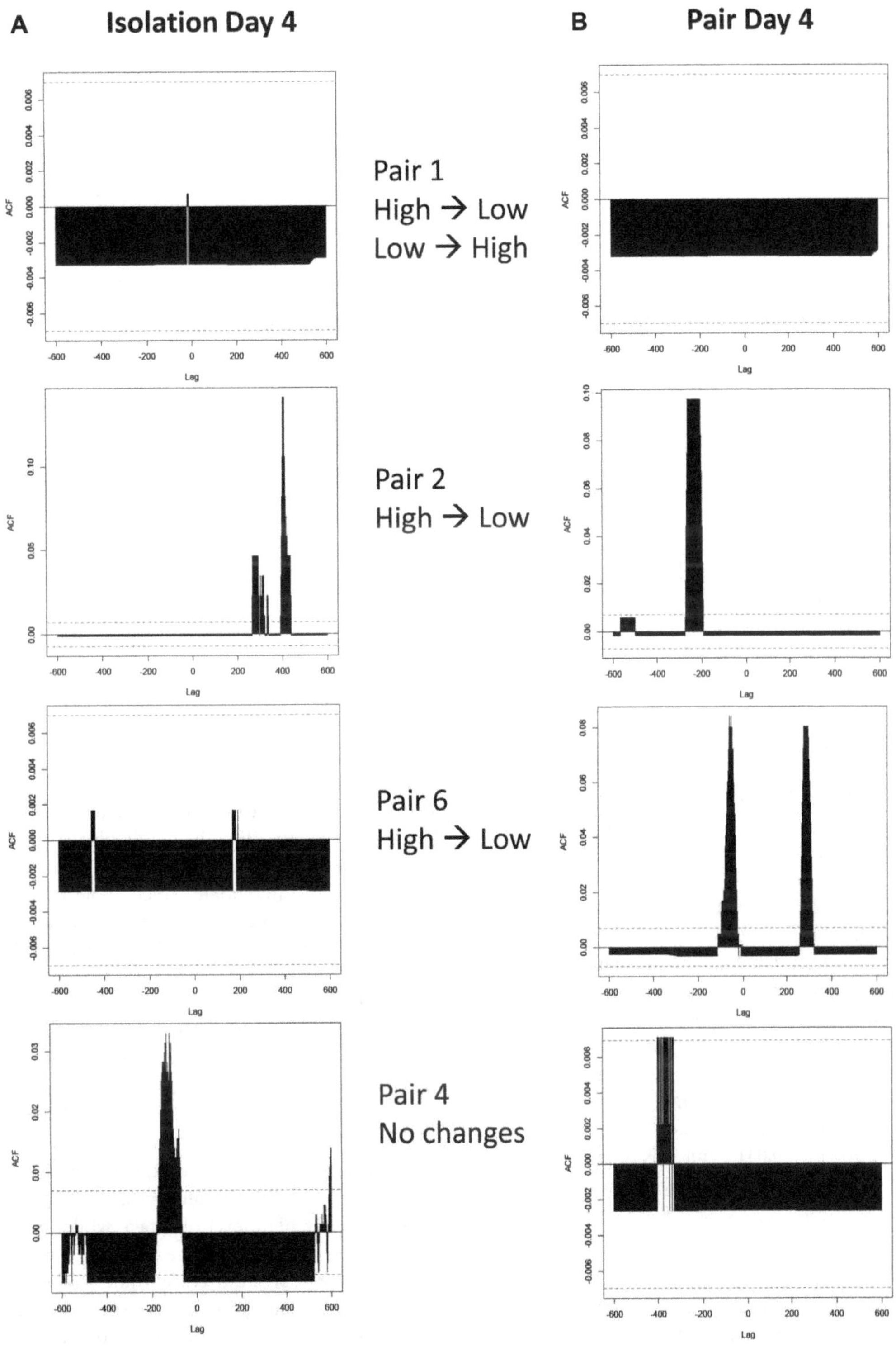

FIGURE 8 | Cross-correlations between ethanol drinking patterns of peers. (A) Correlations between high and low drinkers in isolation, before they have been housed together. **(B)** Correlations between high and low drinkers in pairs on the fourth day of pair housing. The *Y*-axis represents the strength of the correlation (autocorrelation function; ACF), while horizontal dashed lines represent the threshold for significance. The *X*-axis represents "lag" time, in seconds, between drinking events. A significant correlation at a lag time "*h*" indicates that *h* seconds after the high drinker licks, the low drinker is likely to lick; a positive *h* value indicates that the high drinker leads the low drinker, and a negative value indicates that the low drinker leads the high drinker. Pairs shown are examples of each type of pair observed: those where both subjects changed drinking levels when paired (top panels), those where the high drinker changed to match the low drinker (middle panels show two of many variations of outcomes), and those where neither subject changes (bottom panels).

Table 1 | Number of pairs exhibiting significant correlations in drinking patterns.

		Ethanol isolation 1	Ethanol pair	Water isolation 1	Water pair
Change	Correlation	11	12	14	14
	No correlation	6	5	3	3
No change	Correlation	12	12	12	15
	No correlation	3	3	3	0

The total number of pairs (32) is divided into groups where at least one subject changed the drinking pattern and those that did not (change, no change). For each group, the number of pairs exhibiting a significant correlation or not, when analyzed by the cross-correlation function within a lag time of 10 min is shown for each ethanol and water drinking patterns, in isolation and pair housing. There are clearly no significant differences between groups that did or did not change, between isolation and pairing, or between ethanol and water.

Table 2 | Effect of V1aR microsatellite length on ethanol drinking behaviors.

Behavior	*t*, df	*p* Value
Baseline preference	$t = 0.151$ df $= 57$	0.880
Baseline intake	$t = 1.37$ df $= 57$	0.176
High preference change 1	$t = 1.30$ df $= 26$	0.207
High preference change overall	$t = 2.27$ df $= 26$	**0.0314**
Low preference change 1	$t = 0.257$ df $= 29$	0.799
Low preference change overall	$t = 0.638$ df $= 29$	0.529
High intake change 1	$t = 0.166$ df $= 26$	0.870
High intake change overall	$t = 0.441$ df $= 26$	0.663
Low intake change 1	$t = 0.000571$ df $= 29$	1.00
Low intake change overall	$t = 0.0418$ df $= 29$	0.967

Subjects possessing a short or long average microsatellite length were compared for each of the behaviors listed in the column on the left. The results of the t tests are listed in the middle column, with the p value in the right. Significant ($p < 0.05$) values prior to correction are shown in bold, though no tests remained significant when the Bonferroni correction was applied ($p < 0.005$). Baseline preference and intake were based on the average ethanol (and water) intakes of the first 4 days of access, during isolation. "High" indicates a comparison between only the high drinkers, and "Low" indicates only the low drinkers. "change 1" indicates the change in drinking from the average during isolation 1 to the average during pair housing. "change overall" indicates the change in drinking from the average during isolation 1 to the average during isolation 2 following pair housing.

greater presence of a negative lag time that would indicate the low drinker "leading" the high drinker (**Figure 8B** panels 2 and 3).

There was no significant correlation between the number of close bouts by visual assessment and the strength of cross-correlations (ACF value; $r = 0.083$; $n = 19$; $p = 0.734$). However, there was a statistical trend for a positive correlation between the *proportion* of close bouts by visual assessment (number normalized to the lowest number possible for each pair) and the strength of cross-correlations ($r = 0.444$; $n = 18$; $p = 0.065$).

The region containing the V1aR microsatellite was successfully amplified and lengths were determined for 59 subjects. The rate of homozygosity was 47%. The length of the amplified region ranged from 669 to 736 base pairs. The mean, median and mode for all alleles were 703, 699, and 698 bp, respectively. The allele lengths were not normally distributed.

There was no significant difference in drinking behavior between subjects with short or long average microsatellite lengths on any measure of behavior (**Table 2**): initial ethanol preference, initial ethanol intake, change in ethanol preference or intake from isolation to pair housing, pair housing to subsequent isolation, or overall change from the beginning to the end of the experiment. There was a difference within high drinkers, where subjects with long alleles had a greater decrease in ethanol preference from the beginning to the end of the experiment than those with short alleles ($t = 2.27$; df $= 26$; $p = 0.031$), but this difference did not remain significant when adjusted for multiple comparisons.

DISCUSSION

Prairie voles drinking large amounts of ethanol paired with low drinkers in the lickometer apparatus exhibit a decrease in drinking similar to what we have previously demonstrated in home cage drinking (Anacker et al., 2011b). This previous study has already indicated that this decrease is not spontaneous but is due to social influence. The present experiments indicate that the observed changes in ethanol drinking are not dependent on peers drinking together at the same time, or following specific patterns of consumption. Accordingly, this finding is in agreement with our previous results which showed that no changes in saccharin drinking occurred when high drinkers were paired with low drinkers (Anacker et al., 2011b). Specifically, the lack of changes in saccharin drinking suggested that even if pair housing of animals could synchronize their consummatory behaviors, this synchronization is not sufficient to affect their individual drinking levels. However, there are subtle differences in the features of voles' drinking bouts that can differentiate which subjects change their intake when paired. Specifically, high drinkers that lowered their ethanol intake when paired with a low drinker exhibited a lower number of ethanol drinking bouts when paired than the high drinkers that did not change. It is interesting to note that a tendency toward a lower number of drinking bouts was present in this group even before pairing, along with gradual decreases in intake and preference across days in isolation. The high-change group showed a tendency toward a lower number of ethanol drinking bouts in isolation relative to the high drinking group, while the intake levels remained similar; this may be explained by the slight increase in the lick rate of the high-change group, which would allow them to maintain the high level of intake while decreasing the number of bouts. The high-change group also exhibited a tendency toward higher total fluid consumption relative to the high-no change group, resulting in a similar ethanol dose consumed but a lower preference in the high-change group compared to the high-no change group. This observation suggests that the pairing with a low drinker interacted with this tendency toward lower preference and lower number of bouts to produce a more robust decrease in ethanol intake. Thus, we could differentiate subpopulations of high drinkers that were and were not responsive to social influence to decrease ethanol intake, based on differences in fluid preference and on the number of drinking bouts that already existed when isolated.

These findings have potential to lead to future translational work. It is widely known that different types of therapies work for only subsets of people with alcohol use disorders (Anton et al., 2006). Some people may be responsive to social support groups, others to drug therapies, and others to cognitive or behavioral therapy, while still others benefit from a combination. It would be extremely helpful if there were tools to allow clinicians to identify these subpopulations in order to target appropriate treatment to achieve the greatest effect to decrease problem drinking. To our knowledge, there is currently no other animal model where subpopulations that are likely to be responsive to different types of treatments have been identified. If further studies identified behavioral and biological mechanisms of actions or endophenotypes that could predict the success of social influence on lowering drinking, this information could be explored to improve treatment outcomes. Future studies could also test whether the group of high drinking voles that was unresponsive to pairing with a low drinker would be more responsive to pharmacotherapy than to peer influence to decrease drinking.

Furthermore, it remains to be explored why a subset of voles was susceptible to peer influence. One possibility is that different levels of anxiety predispose particular individuals to imitate or avoid a peer. The argument could be made in either direction: higher social anxiety could lead to an increase in trying to "blend in" or to avoid contact and influence from a peer. Hostetler et al. (2012) showed that baseline anxiety-related behavior in the elevated plus maze was correlated with alcohol drinking, although the correlation was higher in isolated housing than in paired housing, and specifically in males, but it remains possible that individual differences in baseline or reactive anxiety are associated with the changes in alcohol drinking levels. While no measures of stress or anxiety levels were taken in the current study, it needs to be noted that early studies did not find effects of same-sex pairing on glucocorticoid levels (DeVries et al., 1997b). Since the initial aim of this study was to examine drinking patterns of behavior without disturbing the animals, future studies should examine different types of anxiety in relation to alcohol intake, as well as corticosterone levels. It is also possible that the voles that responded to peer influence have different social behaviors overall, which may have led them to alter their drinking behavior, for example to spend more time interacting with the partner rather than drinking. It would be interesting to explore social behaviors, e.g., in a social interaction test, to examine how they relate to propensity to alter drinking behavior in a social context.

Interestingly, specific episodes of peer influence were not detected by any comparisons of drinking patterns undertaken here. The visual assessment of the cumulative lick records and the cross-correlation analyses both indicated that subjects often have drinking bouts that are close together in time. We initially hypothesized that these coincident drinking bouts would occur more often when pairs were housed together than when they were in isolation, since they may synchronize their ultradian rhythms to be awake and feeding and drinking at the same time. However, this was not the case; nearly equal numbers of pairs had significant correlations in isolation and in paired housing.

While we found that neither cumulative lick record nor cross-correlation analyses revealed evidence of consistent patterns of linked ethanol intake in pairs, we also found that these different analyses did not exhibit strong correlations with one another. In particular, we would have expected a large number of close drinking bouts in a visual assessment of drinking patterns to be associated with a stronger ACF value in the cross-correlation, but this positive correlation did not reach statistical significance. There are many possible reasons for this. One explanation is that the lag time between bouts would have to be nearly identical within a pair in order to produce a strong ACF by cross-correlation. If the time between paired subjects' drinking bouts varied even by 30 s for each bout, it is possible that a significant ACF value would never be produced by cross-correlation: each lag time would be cataloged, but would have such a low frequency of occurrence that none would be considered significant. In this case, with animal behavior having the potential to be extremely variable even within a framework of a consistent pattern, cross-correlational analyses may not be optimal for detecting such patterns.

Given the evidence from the various types of pattern analyses performed in this study, it appears that prairie voles do not alter their ethanol drinking behavior by synchronizing their drinking patterns with those of a peer. Therefore, another mechanism must be at work to explain the peer-dependent change in drinking levels observed in the present study and previous work, where most often the high drinker decreases its intake when paired with a low drinker. Thus, it is an open question whether the low drinker is typically the dominant vole within the pair and, if so, how this may dictate ethanol intake or changes in ethanol intake. Another possible explanation is that the voles try to match one another's intoxication levels, perhaps through visual cues or vocal interactions. This explanation would address the specificity of behavioral changes observed for ethanol but not saccharin, a rewarding substance that does not lead to intoxication.

The length of the vasopressin receptor 1a (*avpr1a*) microsatellite fragment observed here was different than what has previously been reported by others. Hammock and Young (2005) and Solomon et al. (2009) reported a range of 723–760 and 703–798 base pairs, respectively, which are considerably longer and show very little overlap with our sample. Additionally, they observed between 75 and 100% heterozygosity and a normal distribution while almost half or our sample was homozygous, leading in part to a highly leptokurtic distribution. Since the subjects in our study arose from different colonies of prairie voles than the previously published findings, it is possible that they originate from a different subsample of the wild prairie vole population, and that in our colony we have a larger presence of similarly sized alleles leading to a higher frequency of particular alleles and homozygosity.

In addition to differences in allele length in the samples, the present experiment did not find effects of the microsatellite length on any measure of prairie voles' ethanol drinking behavior, or on the propensity to change ethanol intake when paired with a peer. There was an indication of an effect of the longer microsatellite length corresponding to a greater change in ethanol preference following the effect of a peer influence, but this effect did not remain significant following adjustment for multiple comparisons. Thus, this trend should only be considered suggestive of the potential for the *avpr1a* microsatellite to modulate social influence on ethanol drinking. A recent study in human adolescents demonstrated no role of a different repeat region, a variable number tandem repeat in the dopamine D4 receptor gene, in the effects of friends' drinking levels on subjects' drinking (van der Zwaluw et al., 2012).

The effects of the V1aR microsatellite length reported by others appear to be very specific to particular tests and environments. For example, microsatellite length was correlated with the receptor expression level in various brain regions, and several of these regions were then correlated with measures of partner preference in the laboratory test (Hammock et al., 2005), but not when laboratory-bred voles were tested for social monogamy in semi-natural enclosures (Ophir et al., 2008; Solomon et al., 2009), or in wild prairie voles (Mabry et al., 2011). In contrast, the length was correlated with genetic monogamy in the wild, but not in semi-natural enclosures.

One possible reason for effects that may be difficult to detect has previously been proposed by others (Ophir et al., 2008): while there are several ways in which microsatellite length may influence expression levels (Hammock and Young, 2005), it is likely that particular single nucleotide polymorphisms in *avpr1*, rather than its length, could be a better predictor gene expression and, ultimately, behavior.

CONCLUSION

The present study shows that while high drinkers decrease their ethanol intake when paired with low drinkers, it is not due to matching patterns of drinking, and the behavioral changes cannot be predicted by the length of the microsatellite polymorphism in the vasopressin receptor 1a. Other behaviors and specific genetic polymorphisms that may affect peer-influenced ethanol drinking may be studied in the future. This study demonstrates new methods for examining data from fluid consumption studies where social influences can be assessed using visual and cross-correlational analyses. Most importantly, this study shows that subpopulations of high drinkers that decrease their ethanol intake can be identified based on changes in intake levels and bout number when paired with a low drinker. This provides a model system in which the efficacy of potential therapies can be tested using groups which are likely to respond to different types of treatments. It will be important to examine whether subpopulations of human alcohol drinkers can be identified with similar means, and to explore whether they are similarly responsive to social or other types of treatments to decrease alcohol drinking; then further testing of this animal model of alcohol drinking can be used to elucidate specific mechanisms of action and responses to treatments that can inform treatment of humans with alcohol use disorders.

ACKNOWLEDGMENTS

We would like to acknowledge Dr. Jennifer Loftis and the Portland Veterans Affairs Medical Center Veterinary Medical Unit for maintenance of the prairie vole colony. Kyle Ambert designed u2615 software to process the data for these analyses and his work was sponsored in part by the Tartar Trust Fellowship Award to Allison M. J. Anacker. Dr. Matthew Ford provided assistance and advice in establishing the lickometer apparatus as well as additional software code for analyzing drinking bouts. Davelle Cocking assisted with data collection, and Ryan Bailey-Crandell and Dr. Stephen David assisted with cross-correlational analyses. We would also like to acknowledge Dr. Clive Woffendin at the OCTRI Core Laboratory. This research was funded by AA019793 to Andrey E. Ryabinin and AA020136 to Allison M. J. Anacker.

REFERENCES

Anacker, A. M., Loftis, J. M., Kaur, S., and Ryabinin, A. E. (2011a). Prairie voles as a novel model of socially facilitated excessive drinking. *Addict. Biol.* 16, 92–107. doi: 10.1111/j.1369-1600.2010.00234.x

Anacker, A. M., Loftis, J. M., and Ryabinin, A. E. (2011b). Alcohol intake in prairie voles is influenced by the drinking level of a peer. *Alcohol. Clin. Exp. Res.* 35, 1884–1890. doi: 10.1111/j.1530-0277.2011.01533.x

Anton, R. F., O'Malley, S. S., Ciraulo, D. A., Cisler, R. A., Couper, D., Donovan, D. M., et al. (2006). Combined pharmacotherapies and behavioral interventions for alcohol dependence: the COMBINE study: a randomized controlled trial. *JAMA* 295, 2003–2017. doi: 10.1001/jama.295.17.2003

Bond, J., Kaskutas, L. A., and Weisner, C. (2003). The persistent influence of social networks and alcoholics anonymous on abstinence. *J. Stud. Alcohol* 64, 579–588.

Caldwell, H. K., Stewart, J., Wiedholz, L. M., Millstein, R. A., Iacangelo, A., Holmes, A., et al. (2006). The acute intoxicating effects of ethanol are not dependent on the vasopressin 1a or 1b receptors. *Neuropeptides* 40, 325–337. doi: 10.1016/j.npep.2006.08.001

Carter, C. S., Devries, A. C., and Getz, L. L. (1995). Physiological substrates of mammalian monogamy: the prairie vole model. *Neurosci. Biobehav. Rev.* 19, 303–314. doi: 10.1016/0149-7634(94)00070-H

DeVries, A. C., Johnson, C. L., and Carter, C. S. (1997a). Familiarity and gender influence social preferences in prairie voles. *Can. J. Zool.* 75, 295–301. doi: 10.1139/z97-037

DeVries, A. C., Taymans, S. E., and Carter, C. S. (1997b). Social modulation of corticosteroid responses in male prairie voles. *Ann. N. Y. Acad. Sci.* 807, 494–497. doi: 10.1111/j.1749-6632.1997.tb51949.x

Donaldson, Z. R., Spiegel, L., and Young, L. J. (2010). Central vasopressin V1a receptor activation is independently necessary for both partner preference formation and expression in socially monogamous male prairie voles. *Behav. Neurosci.* 124, 159–163. doi: 10.1037/a0018094

Fisher, L. B., Miles, I. W., Austin, S. B., Camargo, C. A. Jr, and Colditz, G. A. (2007). Predictors of initiation of alcohol use among US adolescents: findings from a prospective cohort study. *Arch. Pediatr. Adolesc. Med.* 161, 959–966. doi: 10.1001/archpedi.161.10.959

Ford, M. M., Nickel, J. D., Phillips, T. J., and Finn, D. A. (2005). Neurosteroid modulators of GABA(A) receptors differentially modulate Ethanol intake patterns in male C57BL/6J mice. *Alcohol. Clin. Exp. Res.* 29, 1630–1640. doi: 10.1097/01.alc.0000179413.82308.6b

Getz, L. L., Carter, C. S., and Gavish, L. (1981). The mating system of the prairie vole, *Microtus ochrogaster*: field and laboratory evidence for pair-bonding. *Behav. Ecol. Sociobiol.* 8, 189–194. doi: 10.1007/BF00299829

Gordon, A. J., and Zrull, M. (1991). Social networks and recovery: one year after inpatient treatment. *J. Subst. Abuse Treat.* 8, 143–152. doi: 10.1016/0740-5472(91)90005-U

Hammock, E. A., Lim, M. M., Nair, H. P., and Young, L. J. (2005). Association of vasopressin 1a receptor levels with a regulatory microsatellite and behavior. *Genes Brain Behav.* 4, 289–301. doi: 10.1111/j.1601-183X.2005.00119.x

Hammock, E. A., and Young, L. J. (2002). Variation in the vasopressin V1a receptor promoter and expression: implications for inter- and intraspecific variation in social behaviour. *Eur. J. Neurosci.* 16, 399–402. doi: 10.1046/j.1460-9568.2002.02083.x

Hammock, E. A., and Young, L. J. (2004). Functional microsatellite polymorphism associated with divergent social structure in vole species. *Mol. Biol. Evol.* 21, 1057–1063. doi: 10.1093/molbev/msh104

Hammock, E. A., and Young, L. J. (2005). Microsatellite instability generates diversity in brain and sociobehavioral traits. *Science* 308, 1630–1634. doi: 10.1126/science.1111427

Harding, A. J., Halliday, G. M., Ng, J. L., Harper, C. G., and Kril, J. J. (1996). Loss of vasopressin-immunoreactive neurons in alcoholics is dose-related and time-dependent. *Neuroscience* 72, 699–708. doi: 10.1016/0306-4522(95)00577-3

Hoffman, P. L., Ishizawa, H., Giri, P. R., Dave, J. R., Grant, K. A.,

Liu, L. I., et al. (1990). The role of arginine vasopressin in alcohol tolerance. *Ann. Med.* 22, 269–274. doi: 10.3109/07853899009148939

Hostetler, C. M., Anacker, A. M. J., Loftis, J. M., and Ryabinin, A. E. (2012). Social housing and alcohol drinking in male–female pairs of prairie voles (*Microtus ochrogaster*). *Psychopharmacology (Berl.)* 224, 121–132. doi: 10.1007/s00213-012-2836-4

Inder, W. J., Joyce, P. R., Wells, J. E., Evans, M. J., Ellis, M. J., Mattioli, L., et al. (1995). The acute effects of oral ethanol on the hypothalamic-pituitary-adrenal axis in normal human subjects. *Clin. Endocrinol. (Oxf.)* 42, 65–71. doi: 10.1111/j.1365-2265.1995.tb02600.x

Kelly, J. F., Stout, R. L., Magill, M., and Tonigan, J. S. (2011). The role of Alcoholics Anonymous in mobilizing adaptive social network changes: a prospective lagged mediational analysis. *Drug Alcohol Depend.* 114, 119–126. doi: 10.1016/j.drugalcdep.2010.09.009

Korbie, D. J., and Mattick, J. S. (2008). Touchdown PCR for increased specificity and sensitivity in PCR amplification. *Nat. Protoc.* 3, 1452–1456. doi: 10.1038/nprot.2008.133

Linkola, J., Ylikahri, R., Fyhquist, F., and Wallenius, M. (1978). Plasma vasopressin in ethanol intoxication and hangover. *Acta Physiol. Scand.* 104, 180–187. doi: 10.1111/j.1748-1716.1978.tb06265.x

Liu, Y., Curtis, J. T., and Wang, Z. (2001). Vasopressin in the lateral septum regulates pair bond formation in male prairie voles (*Microtus ochrogaster*). *Behav. Neurosci.* 115, 910–919. doi: 10.1037/0735-7044.115.4.910

Mabry, K. E., Streatfeild, C. A., Keane, B., and Solomon, N. G. (2011). avpr1a length polymorphism is not associated with either social or genetic monogamy in free-living prairie voles. *Anim. Behav.* 81, 11–18. doi: 10.1016/j.anbehav.2010.09.021

Madeira, M. D., and Paula-Barbosa, M. M. (1999). Effects of alcohol on the synthesis and expression of hypothalamic peptides. *Brain Res. Bull.* 48, 3–22. doi: 10.1016/S0361-9230(98)00131-2

Nair, H. P., and Young, L. J. (2006). Vasopressin and pair-bond formation: genes to brain to behavior. *Physiology (Bethesda)* 21, 146–152. doi: 10.1152/physiol.00049.2005

Ophir, A. G., Campbell, P., Hanna, K., and Phelps, S. M. (2008). Field tests of cis-regulatory variation at the prairie vole avpr1a locus: association with V1aR abundance but not sexual or social fidelity. *Horm. Behav.* 54, 694–702.doi: 10.1016/j.yhbeh.2008.07.009

Park, A., Sher, K. J., and Krull, J. L. (2008). Risky drinking in college changes as fraternity/sorority affiliation changes: a person-environment perspective. *Psychol. Addict. Behav.* 22, 219–229. doi: 10.1037/0893-164X.22.2.219

Rivier, C., and Lee, S. (1996). Acute alcohol administration stimulates the activity of hypothalamic neurons that express corticotropin-releasing factor and vasopressin. *Brain Res.* 726, 1–10. doi: 10.1016/0006-8993(96)00301-0

Sanbe, A., Takagi, N., Fujiwara, Y., Yamauchi, J., Endo, T., Mizutani, R., et al. (2008). Alcohol preference in mice lacking the Avpr1a vasopressin receptor. *Am. J. Physiol. Regul. Integr. Comp. Physiol.* 294, R1482–R1490. doi: 10.1152/ajpregu.00708.2007

Silva, S. M., Madeira, M. D., Ruela, C., and Paula-Barbosa, M. M. (2002). Prolonged alcohol intake leads to irreversible loss of vasopressin and oxytocin neurons in the paraventricular nucleus of the hypothalamus. *Brain Res.* 925, 76–88. doi: 10.1016/S0006-8993(01)03261-9

Solomon, N. G., Richmond, A. R., Harding, P. A., Fries, A., Jacquemin, S., Schaefer, R. L., et al. (2009). Polymorphism at the avpr1a locus in male prairie voles correlated with genetic but not social monogamy in field populations. *Mol. Ecol.* 18, 4680–4695. doi: 10.1111/j.1365-294X.2009.04361.x

van der Zwaluw, C. S., Larsen, H., and Engels, R. C. (2012). Best friends and alcohol use in adolescence: the role of the dopamine D4 receptor gene. *Addict. Biol.* 17, 1036–1045. doi: 10.1111/j.1369-1600.2010.00305.x

Williams, J. R. (1992). Development of partner preference in female prairie voles (*Microtus ochrogaster*): the role of social and sexual experience. *Horm. Behav.* 26, 339–349. doi: 10.1016/0018-506X(92)90004-F

Winslow, J. T., Hastings, N., Carter, C. S., Harbaugh, C. R., and Insel, T. R. (1993). A role for central vasopressin in pair bonding in monogamous prairie voles. *Nature* 365, 545–548. doi: 10.1038/365545a0

Wu, J., and Witkiewitz, K. (2008). Network support for drinking: an application of multiple groups growth mixture modeling to examine client-treatment matching. *J. Stud. Alcohol Drugs* 69, 21–29.

Young, L. J., Winslow, J. T., Nilsen, R., and Insel, T. R. (1997). Species differences in V1a receptor gene expression in monogamous and nonmonogamous voles: behavioral consequences. *Behav. Neurosci.* 111, 599–605. doi: 10.1037/0735-7044.111.3.599

Conflict of Interest Statement: The authors declare that the research was conducted in the absence of any commercial or financial relationships that could be construed as a potential conflict of interest.

11

Exposure to chronic mild stress prevents kappa opioid-mediated reinstatement of cocaine and nicotine place preference

Ream Al-Hasani[1,2], Jordan G. McCall[1,3] and Michael R. Bruchas[1,2,3,4] *

[1] Basic Research Division, Department of Anesthesiology, Washington University School of Medicine, St. Louis, MO, USA
[2] Department of Anatomy and Neurobiology, Washington University School of Medicine, St. Louis, MO, USA
[3] Division of Biological and Biomedical Sciences, Washington University School of Medicine, St. Louis, MO, USA
[4] Washington University Pain Center, Washington University School of Medicine, St. Louis, MO, USA

Edited by:
Thibault Renoir, Florey Institute of Neuroscience and Mental Health, Australia

Reviewed by:
Mariela Fernanda Perez, Universidad Nacional de Cordoba, Argentina
Lynn G. Kirby, Temple University School of Medicine, USA

***Correspondence:**
Michael R. Bruchas, Basic Research Division, Department of Anesthesiology and Department of Anatomy and Neurobiology, Washington University School of Medicine, 660 South Euclid Avenue, Box 8054, St. Louis, MO 63110, USA
e-mail: bruchasm@wustl.edu

Stress increases the risk of drug abuse, causes relapse to drug seeking, and potentiates the rewarding properties of both nicotine and cocaine. Understanding the mechanisms by which stress regulates the rewarding properties of drugs of abuse provides valuable insight into potential treatments for drug abuse. Prior reports have demonstrated that stress causes dynorphin release, activating kappa opioid receptors (KOR) in monoamine circuits resulting in both potentiation and reinstatement of cocaine and nicotine conditioned place preference. Here we report that kappa opioid-dependent reinstatement of cocaine and nicotine place preference is reduced when the mice are exposed to a randomized chronic mild stress (CMS) regime prior to training in a conditioned place preference-reinstatement paradigm. The CMS schedule involves seven different stressors (removal of nesting for 24 h, 5 min forced swim stress at 15°C, 8 h food and water deprivation, damp bedding overnight, white noise, cage tilt, and disrupted home cage lighting) rotated over a 3-week period. This response is KOR-selective, as CMS does not protect against cocaine or nicotine drug-primed reinstatement. This protection from reinstatement is also observed following sub-chronic social defeat stress, where each mouse is placed in an aggressor mouse home cage for a period of 20 min over 5 days. In contrast, a single acute stressor resulted in a potentiation of KOR-induced reinstatement, as previously reported. Prior studies have shown that stress alters sensitivity to opioids and prior stress can influence the pharmacodynamics of the opioid receptor system. Together, these findings suggest that exposure to different forms of stress may cause a dysregulation of kappa opioid circuitry and that changes resulting from mild stress can have protective and adaptive effects against drug relapse.

Keywords: kappa opioid receptor, cocaine, nicotine, stress, conditioned place preference

INTRODUCTION

It is well-established that stress increases the risk of drug abuse, relapse to drug seeking, and potentiates the rewarding properties of cocaine (Covington and Miczek, 2001; McLaughlin et al., 2003; Redila and Chavkin, 2008; Bruchas et al., 2010). Previous studies have implicated a critical role for dynorphin/kappa opioid systems in the mediation of stress-induced behaviors including reinstatement of drug seeking in both place preference and self-administration animal models. Studies have shown that stress-induced reinstatement to alcohol, cocaine, and nicotine seeking is absent in kappa opioid receptor (KOR) KO and dynorphin KO mice as well as following pretreatment with KOR antagonists (Beardsley et al., 2005; Redila and Chavkin, 2008; Walker and Koob, 2008; Walker et al., 2011; Jackson et al., 2013). However, while numerous models of acute stress reinstate drug seeking through dynorphin/KOR activation, the effects of prior repeated stress exposure, and various magnitudes of stress exposure on KOR-mediated reinstatement has not been examined.

The dynorphin/KOR system is composed of prodynorphin peptides and KOR, a seven-transmembrane spanning $G_{i/o}$ protein-coupled receptor (GPCR). In addition to the classical inhibitor effects on adenylate cyclase activity, KOR also couples to mitogen-activated protein kinase pathways (Bruchas et al., 2010; Al-Hasani and Bruchas, 2011) to mediate various behavioral effects (Bruchas et al., 2011; Potter et al., 2011). It is thought that stress causes dynorphin release activating KOR within monoamine nuclei (ventral tegmental area, dorsal raphe, locus coeruleus) and their projection targets (extended amygdala, nucleus accumbens, etc.; Wise, 2004; Zhang et al., 2005; Carlezon et al., 2006; Gehrke et al., 2008; Land et al., 2008, 2009; Ebner et al., 2010; Bruchas et al., 2011; Al-Hasani et al., 2013; Graziane et al., 2013). The KOR-mediated reduction in dopamine and serotonin activity results in dysphoria-like behavior that drives reinstatement of drug seeking to relieve this negative affective state. KORs are highly regulated via G-protein-coupled receptor kinase (GRK) phosphorylation and desensitization mechanisms. In opioid receptors this cellular regulatory system acts to remove receptor-G-protein activation, and promotes tolerance, arrestin signaling and/or receptor recycling (McLaughlin et al., 2004; Al-Hasani and Bruchas, 2011; Williams et al., 2013).

Chronic mild stress (CMS) is a widely adopted animal model for inducing depression- and anxiety-like behaviors because it mimics the unpredictable intermittent stress exposure that humans experience, for complete review see Hill et al. (2012). The model utilizes repeated, randomized stress events, over the course of several weeks to mimic the unpredictable nature of mild stress experience (Elizalde et al., 2008; Peng et al., 2012; Tye et al., 2013). Numerous studies have demonstrated that various types of CMS models act to alter neurotransmitter systems including monoamine (dopamine, serotonin, and norepinephrine), gamma-aminobutyric acid (GABA), and glutamatergic transmission (Rasheed et al., 2008; Vancassel et al., 2008; Tye et al., 2013). However, the role of CMS on opioid system regulation is not as well-known, with only a few reports showing that dynorphin and enkephalin opioid neuropeptide mRNA remain relatively unchanged in CMS models in various brain regions (Bertrand et al., 1997; Bergström et al., 2008). More recent reports have shown that repeated stress can dysregulate the effects of KOR signaling within dorsal raphe serotonergic circuits (Lemos et al., 2012a) but the functional consequences of repeated stress exposure or CMS compared to acute and sub-chronic stressors on kappa opioid-dependent behaviors has not been investigated.

Here we determined how different types of exposure to stress (acute, sub-chronic, and chronic) impact subsequent kappa opioid-mediated reinstatement of cocaine and nicotine place preference. We determined how different forms of stress, including a 3-week CMS, sub-chronic social defeat stress (SDS), and acute forced swim stress (FSS), impact kappa opioid-induced reinstatement. We found that the initial cocaine and nicotine conditioned place preference were unchanged in sub-chronic stress and CMS exposure, however, KOR-induced cocaine and nicotine reinstatement was absent in mice that were pre-exposed to CMS, in contrast to acute stress, which caused potentiated KOR-reinstatement. In addition, we found that cocaine and nicotine drug-primed reinstatement is not affected by pre-exposure to stress, suggesting that this protective ablation of KOR-induced reinstatement by CMS, selectively affects KOR-mediated behavioral responses.

MATERIALS AND METHODS

ANIMAL SUBJECTS

Male C57BL/6 wild-type mice, bred locally and maintained in Washington University mouse facility (20–30 g) were used for all experiments. All mice were group-housed within the Animal Core Facility at Washington University in St. Louis, given access to food pellets and water *ad libitum,* and maintained in specific pathogen-free housing. Mice were transferred at least 1 week before testing into a colony room adjacent to the behavioral testing room to acclimatize to the study environment and prevent stress during conditioning phases. Housing rooms were illuminated on a 12-h light/dark cycle with lights on at 7 AM. All animal procedures were approved by the Animal Care and Use Committee of Washington University in St. Louis, in accordance with the National Institutes of Health *Guide for the Care and Use of Laboratory Animals.*

DRUGS

Cocaine HCl and racemic U50,488 methanesulfonate were provided by the National Institute on Drug Abuse and Drug Supply Program and in some instances Sigma Aldrich (St. Louis, MO, USA). Nicotine hydrogen tartrate salt was purchased from Sigma Aldrich (St. Louis, MO, USA), dissolved in phosphate buffered solution. The free base form of nicotine was used for calculating all injection doses. All drugs were dissolved in saline unless otherwise indicated.

CONDITIONED PLACE PREFERENCE AND REINSTATEMENT PARADIGM

Mice were trained in an unbiased, balanced three-compartment conditioning apparatus and the reinstatement of cocaine place preference (CPP) paradigm was conducted as previously described (Land et al., 2009; Bruchas et al., 2011; Al-Hasani et al., 2013). On pre-conditioning day mice were allowed free access to all three chambers for 30 min (cocaine CPP) and 20 min (nicotine CPP). Time spent in each compartment was recorded with a video camera (ZR90; Canon) and analyzed using Ethovision 8.5 (Noldus). Mice were randomly assigned to saline and drug compartments and received a saline injection in the morning (10 ml/kg, s.c.) and cocaine (15 mg/kg, s.c.) or nicotine (0.5 mg/kg, s.c.; Jackson et al., 2013) injection in the afternoon, at least 4 h after the morning training on two consecutive days for nicotine conditioning and three consecutive days for cocaine conditioning. To test for cocaine place preference the mice were allowed free access to the three compartments. Scores were calculated by subtracting the time spent in the drug-paired compartment, post-test minus the pre-test. Mice were considered to have conditioned if the conditioning score was within 15–85% of total conditioning time, approximately 50 and 80% of mice reached this criteria for nicotine and cocaine conditioning, respectively. This was followed by 2 days (nicotine) or 3 days (cocaine) of extinction training during which saline (10 ml/kg, s.c.) was injected in both the morning and afternoon prior to placement into isolated conditioning compartments. Mice were then tested for extinction of place preference with free access to all three chambers. Mice were considered to have extinguished cocaine and nicotine preference if scores fell within 15% of their initial preference scores, approximately 98% of mice met this criteria. Mice that did not meet these criteria were excluded from the study and mice that met these criteria and extinguished continued on to the reinstatement phase.

On reinstatement test day mice were injected with KOR agonist, U50,488 (5 mg/kg, i.p.), placed in their home cage for 30 min (cocaine CPP) or 20 min (nicotine CPP) as previously described (Redila and Chavkin, 2008; Land et al., 2009; Al-Hasani et al., 2013), after which they were placed in the CPP apparatus and allowed free access to all three compartments for reinstatement expression. Reinstatement was measured as time (s) in drug-paired chamber on reinstatement test day minus time spent in drug-paired chamber following extinction training. On the following day, all mice were exposed to a priming injection of cocaine (15 mg/kg, s.c.) or nicotine (0.5 mg/kg, s.c.) to test for drug-primed reinstatement and placed in the apparatus with free access to all compartments. Reinstatement scores were calculated by subtracting the time spent in the cocaine or nicotine side post-reinstatement minus the extinction test as previously described (Land et al., 2009; Bruchas et al., 2011).

ACUTE STRESS

During reinstatement (day 10) mice were subjected to FSS in which they were placed in an 18 cm deep bucket of water at 30°C and allowed to swim for upto 6 min. Mice were removed immediately if they appeared to be at risk of drowning. After a 5 min dry off and recovery period mice were injected with U50, 488 (5 mg/kg, i.p.) in the home cage for 30 min and then placed in the CPP chambers, with access to all three compartments to access reinstatement to cocaine place preference.

SUB-CHRONIC SOCIAL DEFEAT STRESS

Social defeat stress was performed as previously described (Bruchas et al., 2011). From the afternoon of the conditioning post-test (day 5) until post-extinction day (day 9) mice were placed in the home cage of an aggressor mouse for a period of 20 min in the afternoon 2 h following extinction or post-testing (typically from 4 to 6 PM). Mice were monitored carefully for severe injury during SDS and were removed if necessary. No mice met this criterion in this study. In addition, as previously described (Land et al., 2009; Bruchas et al., 2011) all mice are observed and tracked to receive similar bouts of aggression and exhibit characteristic social defeat postures (McLaughlin et al., 2006; Land et al., 2009) to ensure similar stress exposure in each treatment group. On day 10 mice were injected with U50,488 (5 mg/kg, i.p.) in the home cage and then placed in the CPP chambers 30 min later to access reinstatement to cocaine seeking. On day 11, for drug-primed reinstatement, mice were injected with cocaine (15 mg/kg, i.p.) and immediately placed in the testing chambers.

CHRONIC MILD STRESS PARADIGM

In order to model randomized mild stress exposure, we adapted a previously validated CMS paradigm. Stressors were randomly assigned during the 3-week stress period (outlined in **Table 1**) prior to conditioned place preference/reinstatement procedure. During reinstatement phase the mice were injected with U50,488 (5 mg/kg, i.p.) in the home cage (30 min) and then placed in the CPP chambers to assess reinstatement to cocaine place preference. On the following day, mice were injected with cocaine (15 mg/kg, s.c.) or nicotine (0.5 mg/kg, s.c.) priming injection and again allowed free access to all three chambers to determine drug prime-induced reinstatement of place preference.

LOCOMOTOR ACTIVITY

During the 3-day conditioning period and during reinstatement test days, locomotor activity was recorded as distance traveled (cm) throughout the 30 min period using video tracking (Canon) of animal movement and Ethovision 8.5 software analysis (Noldus). During the conditioning period the total distance (cm) on conditioning days are represented. During reinstatement post-test trials distance (cm) is represented as 5 min bins throughout the 30 min test period.

DATA ANALYSES AND STATISTICS

Data were expressed as means ± SEM. All raw data were calculated via Ethovision video tracking and then place preference or locomotor data were calculated as described. Data were normally distributed, and differences between groups were determined using Student's independent t-tests, one-way ANOVA, or two-way ANOVA as appropriate. ANOVA's were followed by *post hoc* Bonferroni comparisons if the main effect was significant at $p < 0.05$. Statistical analyses were conducted using GraphPad Prism 5.0F (GraphPad, San Diego, CA, USA).

RESULTS

ACTIVATION OF KAPPA OPIOID RECEPTORS FOLLOWING ACUTE STRESS POTENTIATES REINSTATEMENT OF COCAINE PLACE PREFERENCE

It has previously been shown that FSS is sufficient to induce reinstatement and potentiation to drug seeking in a KOR-dependent manner (McLaughlin et al., 2003; Schindler et al., 2012; Smith et al., 2012). Furthermore, stress-induced activation of KOR reinstates nicotine, alcohol, and cocaine seeking (Bruchas et al., 2010; Van Bockstaele et al., 2010; Wee and Koob, 2010; Graziane et al., 2013). In this study, we determined whether acute exposure to a single swim stress would prevent or potentiate a subsequent KOR-mediated reinstatement of CPP. Mice were subjected to cocaine conditioning, extinction, and reinstatement as described. On reinstatement day mice were exposed to swim stress for up to 6 min, were injected with KOR agonist U50,488 (5 mg/kg, i.p) 5 min following recovery, and then placed in the CPP chamber 30 min later (**Figure 1A**). Mice subjected to FSS prior to KOR activation by U50,488 showed significant and robust potentiation of reinstatement to cocaine seeking when compared to mice that were not subjected to FSS but that were injected with only U50,488 to induce reinstatement (**Figure 1B**, $n = 8$–15 (***$p < 0.001$, no stress and U50 vs. FSS and U50; one-way ANOVA, Bonferroni *post hoc* test). Locomotor activity during the reinstatement test was measured and the combination of FSS, followed by KOR-induced reinstatement to cocaine seeking showed a reduction in locomotor activity when compared to both the non-stressed group and the FSS alone group (**Figure 1C**). These data suggest that acute stress exposure induces a potentiation of KOR agonist-induced reinstatement of cocaine place preference.

SUB-CHRONIC STRESS EXPOSURE BLOCKS SUBSEQUENT KOR AGONIST-INDUCED REINSTATEMENT OF COCAINE PLACE PREFERENCE

To determine the effects of multiple rounds of stress exposure on KOR-induced reinstatement, mice were subjected to 20 min of SDS at the end of the day during extinction training and prior to the reinstatement phase. On day 10, the reinstatement test day, a single dose of U50,488 (5 mg/kg, i.p.) was administered to induce reinstatement of cocaine place preference (**Figure 2A**). Prior exposure to sub-chronic SDS resulted in a significant block of U50,488 induced reinstatement of cocaine place preference (**Figure 2B**: *$p < 0.05$, no stress and U50,488 vs. SDS and U50,488, **$p < 0.01$, SDS and U50,488 vs. SDS and cocaine; one-way ANOVA followed by Bonferroni *post hoc* test, $n = 12$–16). This inhibition of reinstatement was selective for activation of KOR because a priming injection of cocaine (15 mg/kg, s.c.) still caused significant reinstatement of cocaine CPP following exposure to

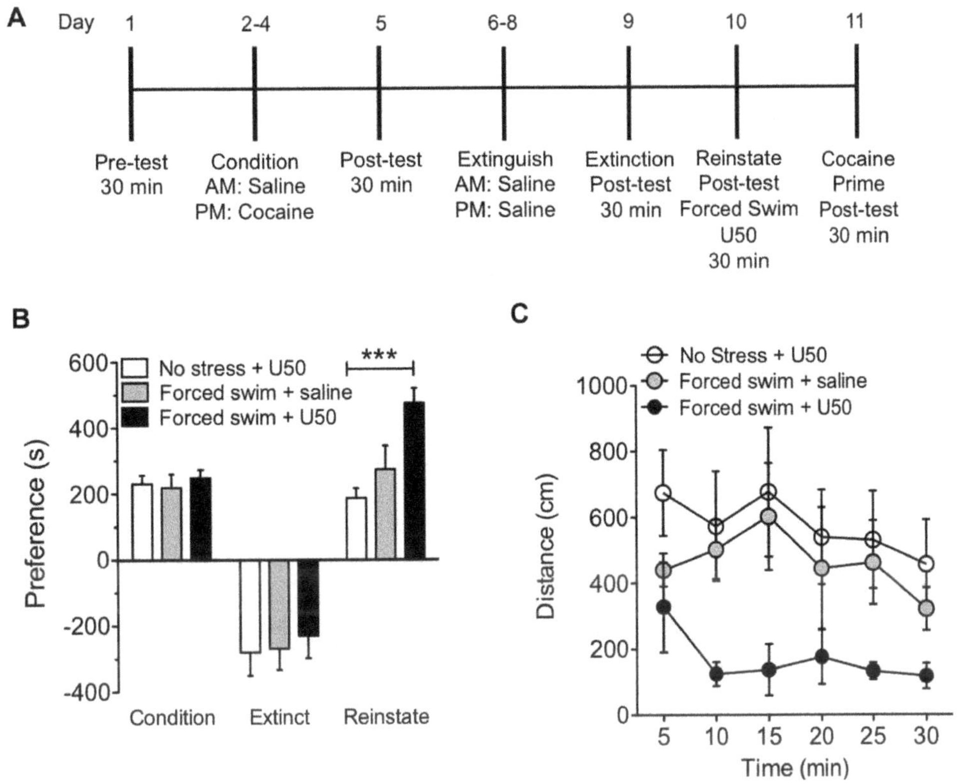

FIGURE 1 | Acute forced swim stress potentiates U50,488-induced reinstatement of cocaine place preference. (A) Timeline of cocaine place preference-reinstatement experimental paradigm. **(B)** Cocaine preference scores (day 5), calculated as post-test minus pre-test on the cocaine-paired side (condition) and U50,488-induced (5 mg/kg, i.p.) reinstatement scores (day 10) of extinguished place preference (reinstate). Data show a significant potentiation in KOR-reinstatement following forced swim stress and U50,488. Groups are defined in the figures as their final reinstatement grouping (U50 = U50,488). Data represent the mean preference (s) ± SEM, $n = 8$–15 ($^{***}p < 0.001$, no stress and U50 vs. forced swim stress and U50; one-way ANOVA followed by Bonferroni *post hoc* test). **(C)** Locomotor activity measured as distance traveled (cm) during the 30 min reinstatement trial. Data represent the mean preference (s) ± SEM, $n = 8$–15.

the sub-chronic SDS paradigm (**Figure 2B**; $^{**}p < 0.01$, SDS and U50 vs. SDS with cocaine, $n = 12$–16). We also measured locomotor activity during the 30 min reinstatement phase. Both the non-stress + U50,488 group and the SDS + U50,488 group show a similar KOR-mediated reduction in locomotor over the 30 min period, supporting the notion that prevention of reinstatement by pre-exposure to stress, is not due to additional alterations in mouse locomotor activity (**Figure 2C**). In contrast, as shown in previous studies (Reith, 1986; Tolliver et al., 1994; Giros et al., 1996; Sora et al., 1998; Zhang et al., 2002) locomotor activity was significantly elevated in mice reinstated with cocaine ($^{\#\#}p < 0.01$ and $^{\#\#\#}p < 0.005$, SDS and U50,488 vs. SDS and cocaine at 5 and 10 min time point, respectively; $^{**}p < 0.01$, no stress and U50,488 vs. SDS and U50,488 at 10 min time point; $^{***}p < 0.005$, SDS and cocaine vs. both no stress and U50 and SDS and U50,488 at 15 min; $^{****}p < 0.001$ SDS and cocaine vs. both no stress and U50 and SDS and U50,488 at 20, 25, and 30 min time points; two-way ANOVA followed by Bonferroni *post hoc* test, $n = 12$–16). Taken together, these data suggest that exposure to a sub-chronic repeated SDS causes a significant prevention of kappa agonist-induced reinstatement of cocaine place preference.

CHRONIC MILD STRESS PROTECTS AGAINST U50,488-INDUCED REINSTATEMENT TO COCAINE AND NICOTINE PLACE PREFERENCE

Kappa opioid receptor agonists and stress have been shown in numerous models to affect the magnitude of cocaine and nicotine place preference as well as cause reinstatement of cocaine and nicotine preference behavior (Redila and Chavkin, 2008; Land et al., 2009; Bruchas et al., 2010; Al-Hasani and Bruchas, 2011; Al-Hasani et al., 2013; Jackson et al., 2013). However, it is not known how repeated CMS ultimately influences cocaine and nicotine preference, or how CMS influences subsequent KOR or drug-primed reinstatement of cocaine or nicotine reinstatement. Therefore, we determined how a CMS paradigm adapted from Elizalde et al. (2008); Peng et al. (2012), and Tye et al. (2013) (**Table 1** and **Figures 3A** and **4A**) influences cocaine and nicotine conditioning, as well as KOR-induced reinstatement of cocaine and nicotine CPP. The CMS paradigm involved a random assignment of seven mild stressors during a 3-week period (see **Table 1**) prior to the cocaine or nicotine CPP/reinstatement training protocol.

There was no significant difference between the no stress and CMS-exposed groups in the magnitude of the initial cocaine (15 mg/kg, s.c.) or nicotine (0.5 mg/kg, s.c.) conditioned place preference scores. This finding suggests that exposure to CMS does

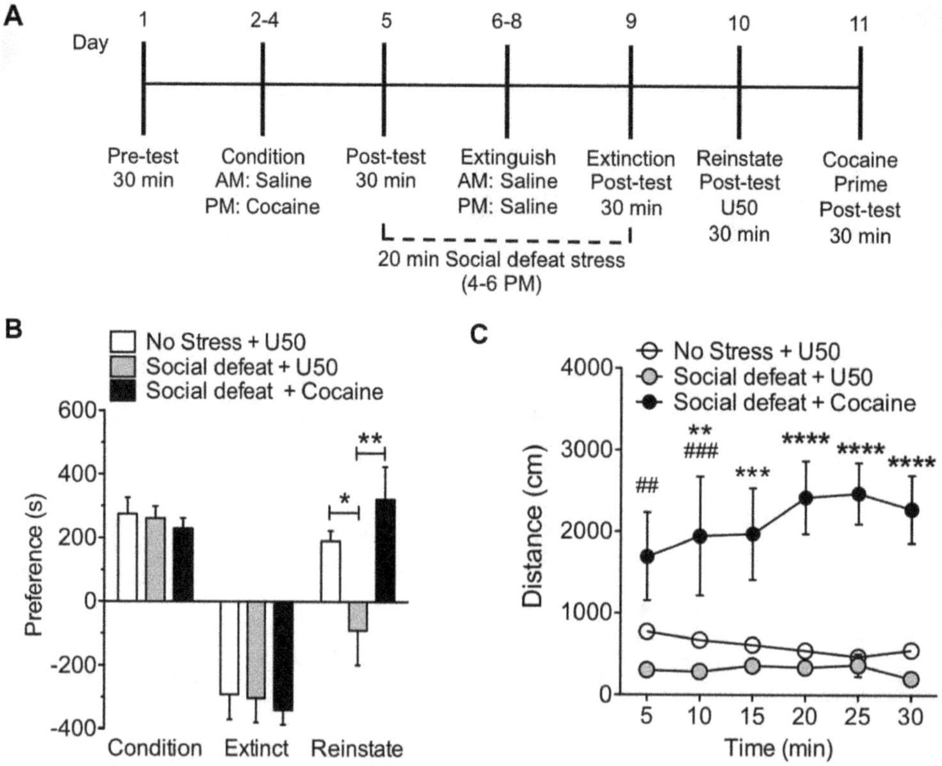

FIGURE 2 | Exposure to sub-chronic social defeat stress prevents U50,488-induced reinstatement of cocaine place preference. (A) Timeline of cocaine place preference-reinstatement experiment. **(B)** Cocaine preference scores (day 5) calculated as post-test minus pre-test on the cocaine-paired side (condition) and U50,488-induced (5 mg/kg, i.p.) reinstatement scores (day 10) of extinguished place preference (reinstate), calculated as reinstatement test day minus extinction post-test day. Groups are defined in the figures as their final reinstatement grouping (U50 = U50,488). Data show a significant attenuation in KOR-reinstatement following sub-chronic social defeat stress. Data represent the mean preference (s) ± SEM, $n = 12$–16 ($^{*}p < 0.05$, no stress and U50,488 vs. social defeat stress and U50,488, $^{**}p < 0.01$, social defeat stress and U50,488 vs. social defeat stress and cocaine; one-way ANOVA followed by Bonferroni *post hoc* test). **(C)** Locomotor activity measured as distance traveled (cm) during the 30 min reinstatement trial. Data represent the mean preference (s) ± SEM, $n = 12$–16 ($^{\#\#}p < 0.01$ and $^{\#\#\#}p < 0.005$, social defeat stress and U50,488 vs. social defeat stress and cocaine at 5 and 10 min time point, respectively; $^{**}p < 0.01$, no stress and U50,488 vs. social defeat stress and U50,488 at 10 min time point; $^{***}p < 0.005$, social defeat stress and cocaine vs. both no stress and U50 and social defeat stress and U50,488 at 15 min; $^{****}p < 0.001$ social defeat stress and cocaine vs. both no stress and U50 and social defeat stress and U50,488 at 20, 25, and 30 min time points; two-way ANOVA followed by Bonferroni *post hoc* test).

not effect the subsequent conditioned rewarding effects of cocaine or nicotine (**Figures 3B** and **4B**). Extinction rates of place preference between no stress, SDS-exposed and CMS-exposed groups were not significantly changed. In contrast, following extinction of either cocaine or nicotine place preference in CMS groups, KOR-induced reinstatement of both cocaine and nicotine place preference was significantly reduced (**Figure 3B**: $^{*}p < 0.05$, no stress and U50,488 vs. stress and U50,488; Student's t-test, $n = 7$;

Table 1 | Three-week chronic mild stress schedule.

Week	Day 1	Day 2	Day 3	Day 4	Day 5	Day 6	Day 7
1	17:00 to next day: damp bedding	4 h white noise	8 h cage tilt	Continuous light 24 h	Removal of nesting 24 h	Food and water deprivation 8 h	Swimming at 4°C for 5 min
2	Continuous light 24 h	17:00 to next day: damp bedding	Food and water deprivation 8 h	Swimming at 4°C for 5 min	8 h cage tilt	4 h white noise	Removal of nesting 24 h
3	Swimming at 4°C for 5 min	Continuous light 24 h	8 h cage tilt	Removal of nesting 24 h	4 h white noise	Food and water deprivation 8 h	17:00 to next day: damp bedding

Three weeks prior to cocaine or nicotine conditioned place preference-reinstatement paradigm the mice were randomly assigned the different stressors highlighted in the table. Paradigm is modified from Elizalde et al. (2008); Peng et al. (2012), *and* Tye et al. (2013).

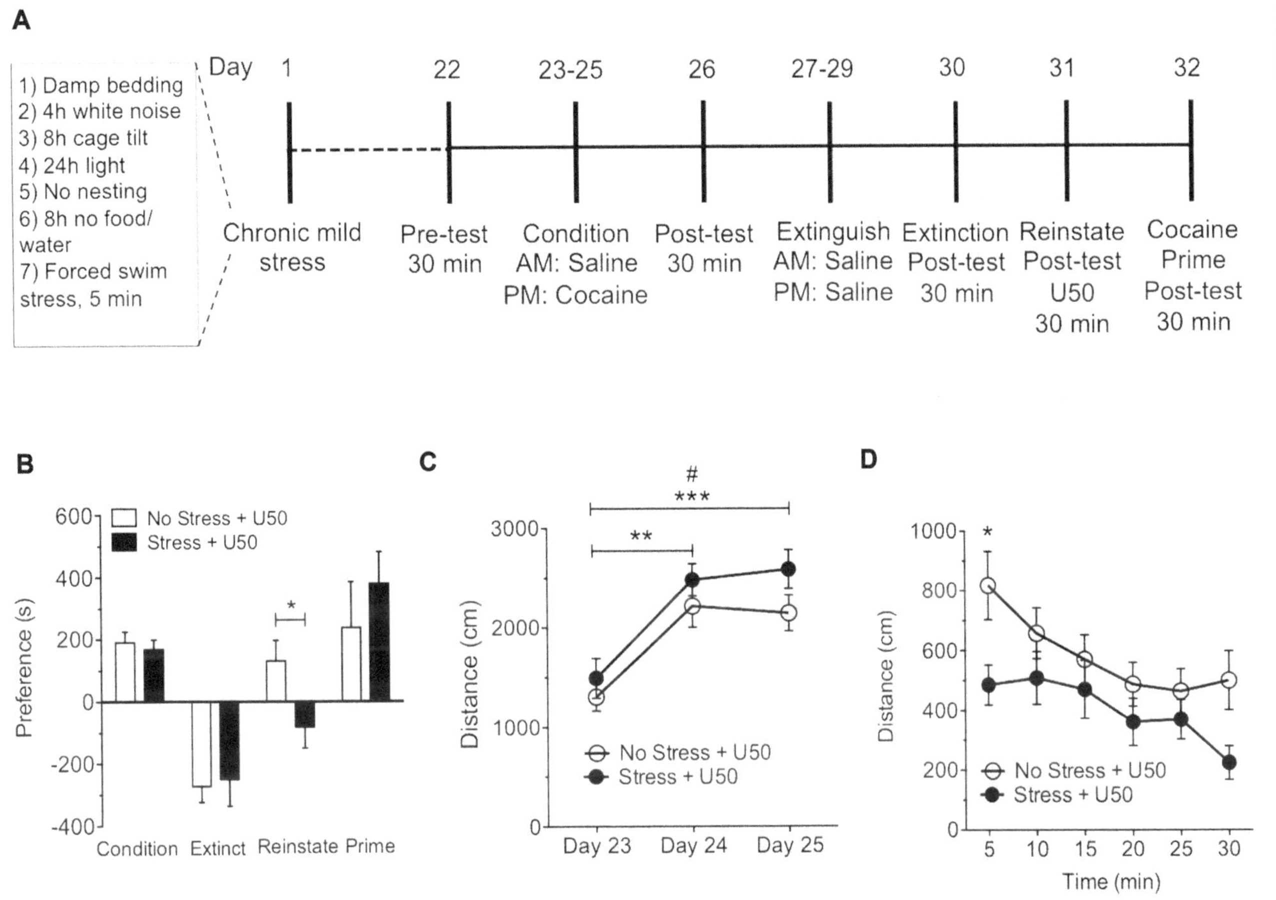

FIGURE 3 | Exposure to chronic mild stress blocks U50,488-induced but not cocaine-primed reinstatement of cocaine place preference. **(A)** Timeline of cocaine place preference-reinstatement experiment. **(B)** Cocaine preference scores (day 26), calculated as post-test minus pre-test on the cocaine-paired side (condition), U50,488-induced (5 mg/kg, i.p.) reinstatement scores (reinstate, day 31), or cocaine-induced (15 mg/kg, i.p) reinstatement (prime, day 32) of extinguished place preference. Data show a significant attenuation in U50,488-induced but not cocaine-primed reinstatement to cocaine seeking following chronic mild stress. Groups are defined in the figures as their final reinstatement grouping (U50 = U50,488).Data represent the mean preference (s) ± SEM, $n = 7$ (*$p < 0.05$, no stress and U50,488 vs. stress and U50,488; Unpaired Student's *t*-test). **(C)** Locomotor activity measured as distance traveled (cm) during three cocaine conditioning days. Data represent the mean preference (s) ± SEM, $n = 7$ ($^{\#}p < 0.05$ day 23 vs. day 25 in the no stress group; **$p < 0.01$day 23 vs. day 24 and ***$p < 0.005$ day 23 vs. day 25 between stress group; one-way ANOVA followed by Bonferroni *post hoc* test). **(D)** Locomotor activity measured as distance traveled (cm) during reinstatement. Data represent the mean preference (s) ± SEM, $n = 7$ (*$p < 0.05$ at 5 min time point in the no stress group vs. CMS group; two-way ANOVA followed by Bonferroni *post hoc* test).

Figure 4B: *$p < 0.05$, Student's t-test, $n = 5$–8. While CMS protected against U50,488-induced reinstatement it had no significant effect on cocaine or nicotine drug-primed reinstatement; indicating that this protective effect of CMS was selective for KOR agonist-induced reinstatement. Locomotor activity was measured during the 3-day conditioning period to determine if exposure to 3 weeks of CMS alters the locomotor response to nicotine (0.05 mg/kg, s.c.) and cocaine (15 mg/kg, s.c.). No significant differences in locomotor activity were found between no stress group and the CMS group following cocaine treatment (**Figure 3C**). As predicted, distance traveled significantly increased over the 3-day cocaine conditioning period, as previously shown (Zhang et al., 2002; Tzschentke, 2007; **Figure 3C:** $^{\#}p < 0.05$ day 23 vs. day 25 in the no stress group; **$p < 0.01$ day 23 vs. day 24 and ***$p < 0.005$ day 23 vs. day 25 between stress group; one-way ANOVA followed by Bonferroni *post hoc* test, $n = 7$). However, nicotine-induced elevations in locomotor activity were significantly reduced following CMS on the second and third day of nicotine conditioning (**Figure 4C:** *$p < 0.05$, no stress vs. CMS as compared to the no-CMS group; two-way ANOVA followed by Bonferroni *post hoc* test, $n = 5$–8). Locomotor activity was also measured during U50-induced reinstatement in both the nicotine and cocaine groups. In the cocaine group only at the 5 min time point was there a significant decrease in locomotor activity in the CMS group compared to the no stress group (**Figure 3D:** *$p < 0.05$; two-way ANOVA followed by Bonferroni *post hoc* test). The nicotine group showed a similar profile, locomotor activity was also significantly decreased in the CMS group compared to the no stress group at both the 5 and 10 min time point (**Figure 4D:** *$p < 0.05$; two-way ANOVA followed by Bonferroni *post hoc* test). Together, these results support the conclusion that CMS protects against subsequent KOR-mediated cocaine and nicotine reinstatement

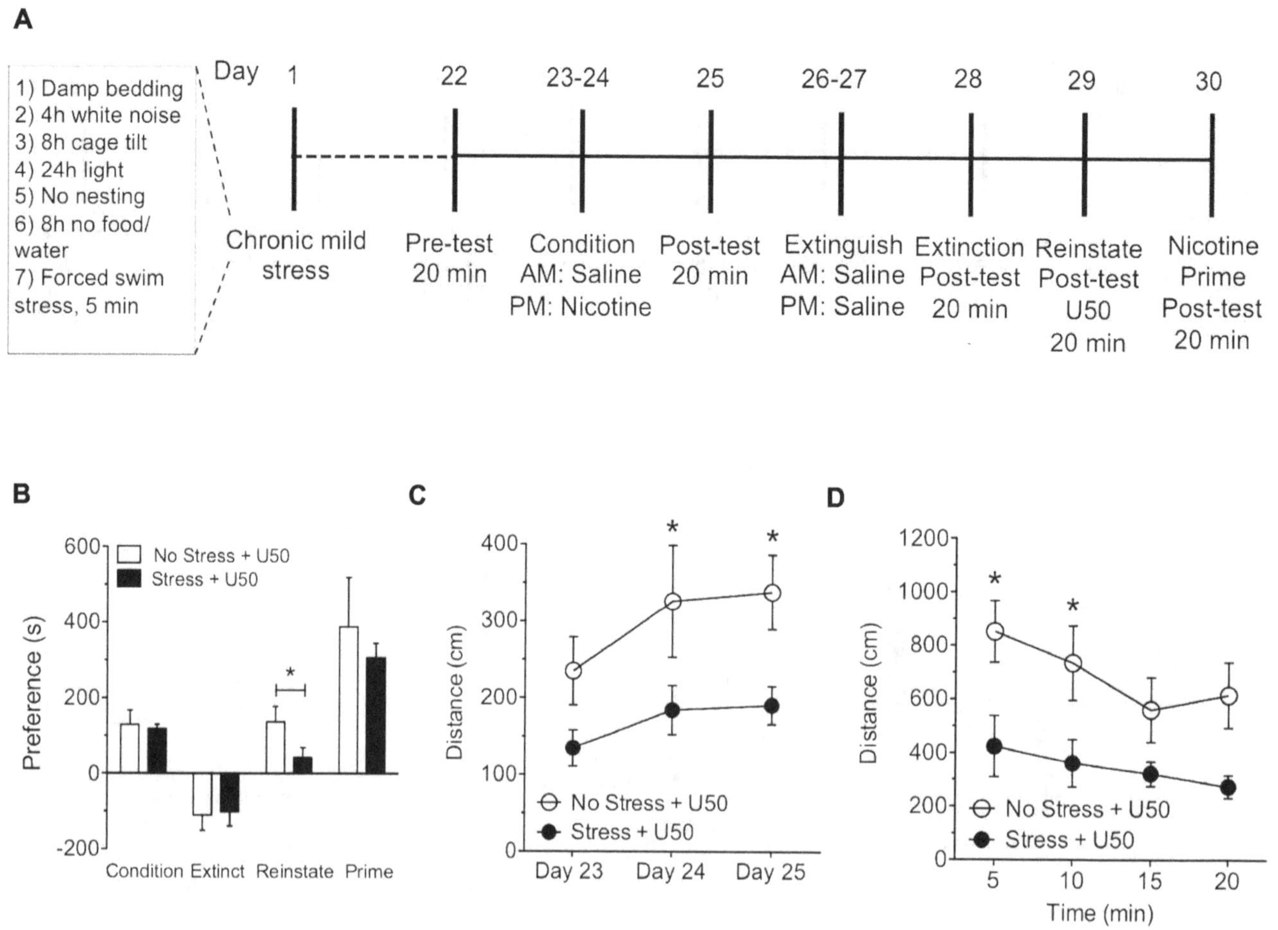

FIGURE 4 | Exposure to chronic mild stress blocks U50,488-induced but not nicotine-primed reinstatement of nicotine place preference. **(A)** Timeline of nicotine place preference-reinstatement experiment. **(B)** Nicotine preference scores (day 26), calculated as post-test minus pre-test on the nicotine-paired side(condition), U50,488-induced (5 mg/kg, i.p.; reinstate, day 31) and nicotine-induced (0.5mg/kg, i.p) reinstatement (prime, day 32) scores of extinguished place preference. Data show a significant reinstatement of nicotine place preference following U50,488 in the no stress group. Groups are defined in the figures as their final reinstatement grouping (U50 = U50,488). Data represent the mean preference (s) ± SEM, $n = 5$–8 (*$p < 0.05$, Student's *t*-test). **(C)** Locomotor activity measured as distance traveled (cm) during three cocaine conditioning days. Data represent the mean preference (s) ± SEM, $n = 5$–8 (*$p < 0.05$, no stress vs. chronic mild stress on days 24 and 25, respectively; two-way ANOVA followed by Bonferroni *post hoc* test). **(D)** Locomotor activity measured as distance traveled (cm) during reinstatement. Data represent the mean preference (s) ± SEM, $n = 5$–8 (*$p < 0.05$ at 5 min and 10 min time point in the no stress group vs. CMS group; two-way ANOVA followed by Bonferroni *post hoc* test).

and further suggests that CMS may act to regulate KOR system function.

DISCUSSION

In the present study we investigated the interactions between various types of stress paradigms and how they influence KOR-induced reinstatement of cocaine and nicotine preference. We determined the effects of a single acute stress, sub-chronic social defeat, and CMS on cocaine and nicotine conditioned place preference and KOR-induced reinstatement. Although, FSS, SDS, and CMS have all been implicated in regulating hedonic state and reward, the present report describes a previously unknown connection between prior stress exposure and KOR-mediated stress-induced behavior. Together, these findings suggest that various types of stress exposure act to influence the dynorphin/KOR-mediated reinstatement response, but they also demonstrate that prior CMS has no lasting effect on the rewarding properties of cocaine or nicotine in conditioned place preference paradigms.

Stress-induced opioid peptide release has been reported for three major opioid systems, and its release has been demonstrated to be associated with a variety of behavioral outputs including stress-induced analgesia, reinstatement, dysphoria, depression, and anxiety-like behaviors (Carlezon et al., 2006; Land et al., 2008; Bruchas et al., 2010; Chartoff et al., 2012; Al-Hasani et al., 2013). In these reports, animals are typically exposed to a single stress event (e.g., forced swim, social defeat, foot shock) and then KOR-mediated behaviors are measured following acute stress exposure (McLaughlin et al., 2003; Bruchas et al., 2011; Schindler et al., 2012). However, the stress experience over the course of an animal's lifetime is complex in nature occurring usually in multiple, randomized epochs. Therefore, the effects of CMS on KOR-mediated behavior remain an important area of investigation. Both repeated stress, and CMS models have been reported to induce dramatic changes in neural circuits and neuromodulator function (Hill et al., 2012; Lemos et al., 2012a,b; Tye et al., 2013), however, CMS effects on regulating cocaine-, nicotine-, and opioid-mediated conditioned preference behaviors is not known. Specifically, CMS-induced changes in serotonergic, noradrenergic, and dopaminergic signaling and release have all been reported (Rasheed et al., 2008; Vancassel et al., 2008; Hill et al., 2012) implicating important functions of monoamine regulation in CMS alterations of mood and reward seeking. In addition, it has been shown that repeated stress and CMS dramatically alter neuropeptidergic circuit function and impact neuropeptide modulation in subsequent stress responsivity, by either sensitizing the response or acting to facilitate desensitization. In the current report we found that following a single acute FSS, activation of KOR signaling caused potentiation of cocaine preference-reinstatement (**Figure 1**). In contrast, repeated SDS or CMS protected against subsequent KOR-mediated reinstatement (**Figures 2**, **3**, and **4**). We also found that this CMS protective effect not only influenced KOR-induced cocaine reinstatement (**Figure 3**) but it also blocked KOR-induced reinstatement of nicotine place preference (**Figure 4**), suggesting a conserved mechanism for multiple drugs of abuse. Interestingly, CMS exposure had no effect on the initial cocaine or nicotine conditioning, nor did CMS exposure impact the magnitude of drug-primed reinstatement. These findings suggest that SDS and CMS induce a type of "tolerance" to subsequent KOR activity, which has also been previously reported when administering repeated doses of KOR agonists (McLaughlin et al., 2004). Stress adaptability mechanisms are a critical consideration in our current findings because reports demonstrating that dramatic changes in neural circuit function include effects on KOR and corticotropin releasing factor (CRF) signaling following various types of repeated stress exposure (McEwen and Gianaros, 2011; Lemos et al., 2012a,b).

The precise neuronal and molecular mechanisms for SDS- and CMS-induced attenuation of KOR-induced reinstatement were not identified in this study but are important and exciting extensions of this work. There are a number of mechanisms that maybe involved in CMS-induced regulation of KOR-reinstatement. KOR regulation following repeated and high agonist-receptor occupancy has been previously reported to be mediated by GRK3 phosphorylation of serine 369 in mouse/rat KOR or serine 358 in the human KOR (Wang et al., 2003; McLaughlin et al., 2004; Bruchas et al., 2006, 2007a; Chen et al., 2007). In repeated SDS or CMS models it is possible that recurrent activation of KOR causes subsequent downregulation and desensitization of KOR signaling preventing further activation of KOR until full recovery. Furthermore, KOR regulation and deactivation (in contrast to mu-opioid receptors) take several weeks to recover as functional receptor entities (McLaughlin et al., 2004; Bruchas et al., 2007b), consistent with the CMS time course used in this study. Surprisingly the preventative effect of prior stress on KOR-mediated reinstatement did not also prevent KOR-induced decreases in locomotor activity (**Figure 2C**) suggesting that SDS acts in specific neural circuits associated with reinstatement but not locomotion. Therefore selective blockade of KORs in specific brain regions during repeated SDS, and CMS and subsequent measures of KOR-mediated behavioral responses will be required in future studies. In addition, utilizing GRK3 knockout mice, or expression of KOR-S369/358 mutants *in vivo*, and exposure to CMS are interesting extensions of this work as prior work has shown that GRK3 signaling is required for KOR-mediated behavioral effects via phosphorylation, arrestin recruitment, and p38 signaling (Bruchas et al., 2011). It has also been shown that KOR-mediated signaling to G-protein inwardly rectifying potassium channels in the serotonergic dorsal raphe nucleus (DRN) is altered following repeated stress exposure (Lemos et al., 2012a). Together, with the recent evidence that these circuits are implicated in KOR-induced reinstatement (Land et al., 2009; Bruchas et al., 2011) it is possible that CMS causes dysregulation of KOR signaling in the DRN to ultimately influence subsequent KOR-induced behavioral responses including reinstatement of drug seeking. Furthermore, CMS may cause downregulation of KOR in the locus coeruleus, a region which has recently been identified to play a key role in KOR-mediated reinstatement to cocaine place preference (Al-Hasani et al., 2013). However, these hypotheses will require further study using selective neural circuit dissection techniques.

The effects of stress on cocaine and nicotine seeking have been widely reported by numerous groups (for reviews see Koob, 2008; Aguilar et al., 2009). In the case of cocaine, it is well-established that stress and exposure to cues causes robust reinstatement of drug seeking in both animals models and human subjects (Koob and Kreek, 2007). The effects of stress on nicotine reinstatement in animal models are less well-characterized, although reports have shown that acute stress exposure potentiates nicotine-seeking behavior and reinstates drug seeking (Buczek et al., 1999; Bilkei-Gorzo et al., 2008; Plaza-Zabala et al., 2010; Yamada and Bruijnzeel, 2011; Leão et al., 2012; Smith et al., 2012). It has also been established that human subjects widely report stress as the primary reason for their continued tobacco use (Bruijnzeel, 2012). However, the effects of randomized CMS on nicotine place preference in animal models has not been previously studied, nor have mechanisms of stress on KOR-induced regulation of nicotine-induced behavior been widely explored with the exception of some recent reports implicating KOR in nicotine-induced behavior (Smith et al., 2012; Jackson et al., 2013). Our current findings build on this prior work, and for the first time show that agonist-induced KOR activation is sufficient to cause reinstatement of nicotine CPP. Additionally, our finding that KOR agonist does not promote reinstatement of nicotine CPP following CMS suggests interesting and complex interactions between CMS and dynorphin/KOR neural circuits that are conserved for both nicotine and cocaine. However, whether similar neural circuits (e.g., dopaminergic, serotonergic) are required for KOR-dependent nicotine reinstatement as compared to cocaine reinstatement will require further investigation.

In summary, we report that frequency and duration of stress differentially influences KOR-induced reinstatement of cocaine and nicotine preference. The present study shows that repeated stress or CMS prior to reinstatement prevents a KOR-induced reinstatement response, while acute exposure to stress induces potentiation of KOR-reinstatement. The wide array of recent studies investigating the interactions between stress and KOR function on reward, reinstatement, and dysphoria suggest that KOR interacts with multiple neurotransmitter systems and circuits to mediate its complex role in behavioral output. We identified previously unrecognized roles for acute, sub-chronic, and chronic stress exposure on KOR-mediated behavioral function. These findings suggest that understanding the regulation of dynorphin/KOR systems in response to various stress exposures is critical to understanding and identifying KOR as a potentially novel therapeutic target system in drug relapse, anxiety, and depression.

ACKNOWLEDGMENTS

These studies were supported by NIDA grant R01DA033396-A1, R00-DA025182 (to Michael R. Bruchas), McDonnell Center for Systems Neuroscience (MRB), NIMH F31MH101956 (Jordan G. McCall), WUSTL DBBS (Jordan G. McCall). We thank the NIDA drug program for providing U50,488 and cocaine HCl. We thank the members of the Bruchas laboratory for helpful discussion and technical assistance. We also thank Marina Picciotto (Yale) for technical advice.

REFERENCES

Aguilar, M. A., Rodríguez-Arias, M., and Miñarro, J. (2009). Neurobiological mechanisms of the reinstatement of drug-conditioned place preference. *Brain Res. Rev.* 59, 253–277. doi: 10.1016/j.brainresrev.2008.08.002

Al-Hasani, R., and Bruchas, M. R. (2011). Molecular mechanisms of opioid receptor-dependent signaling and behavior. *Anesthesiology* 115, 1363–1381. doi: 10.1097/ALN.0b013e318238bba6

Al-Hasani, R., McCall, J. G., Foshage, A. M., and Bruchas, M. R. (2013). Locus coeruleus kappa opioid receptors modulate reinstatement of cocaine place preference through a noradrenergic mechanism. *Neuropsychopharmacology* doi: 10.1038/npp.2013.151 [Epub ahead of print].

Beardsley, P. M., Howard, J. L., Shelton, K. L., and Carroll, F. I. (2005). Differential effects of the novel kappa opioid receptor antagonist, JDTic, on reinstatement of cocaine-seeking induced by footshock stressors vs cocaine primes and its antidepressant-like effects in rats. *Psychopharmacology (Berl.)* 183, 118–126. doi: 10.1007/s00213-005-0167-4

Bergström, A., Jayatissa, M. N., Mørk, A., and Wiborg, O. (2008). Stress sensitivity and resilience in the chronic mild stress rat model of depression; an in situ hybridization study. *Brain Res.* 1196, 41–52. doi: 10.1016/j.brainres.2007.12.025

Bertrand, E., Smadja, C., Mauborgne, A., Roques, B. P., and Daugé, V. (1997). Social interaction increases the extracellular levels of [Met]enkephalin in the nucleus accumbens of control but not of chronic mild stressed rats. *Neuroscience* 80, 17–20.

Bilkei-Gorzo, A., Rácz, I., Michel, K., Darvas, M., Maldonado, R., and Zimmer, A. (2008). A common genetic predisposition to stress sensitivity and stress-induced nicotine craving. *Biol. Psychiatry* 63, 164–171. doi:10.1016/j.biopsych.2007.02.010

Bruchas, M. R., Land, B. B., Aita, M., Xu, M., Barot, S. K., Li, S., et al. (2007a). Stress-induced p38 mitogen-activated protein kinase activation mediates kappa-opioid-dependent dysphoria. *J. Neurosci.* 27, 11614–11623. doi: 10.1523/JNEUROSCI.3769-07.2007

Bruchas, M. R., Yang, T., Schreiber, S., Defino, M., Kwan, S. C., Li, S., et al. (2007b). Long-acting kappa opioid antagonists disrupt receptor signaling and produce noncompetitive effects by activating c-Jun N-terminal kinase. *J. Biol. Chem.* 282, 29803–29811. doi: 10.1074/jbc.M705540200

Bruchas, M. R., Land, B. B., and Chavkin, C. (2010). The dynorphin/kappa opioid system as a modulator of stress-induced and pro-addictive behaviors. *Brain Res.* 1314, 44–55. doi: 10.1016/j.brainres.2009.08.062

Bruchas, M. R., Macey, T. A., Lowe, J. D., and Chavkin, C. (2006). Kappa Opioid Receptor Activation of p38 MAPK Is GRK3- and Arrestin-dependent in Neurons and Astrocytes. *J. Biol. Chem.* 281, 18081–18089. doi: 10.1074/jbc.M513640200

Bruchas, M. R., Schindler, A. G., Shankar, H., Messinger, D. I., Miyatake, M., Land, B. B., et al. (2011). Selective p38α MAPK deletion in serotonergic neurons produces stress resilience in models of depression and addiction. *Neuron* 71, 498–511. doi: 10.1016/j.neuron.2011.06.011

Bruijnzeel, A. W. (2012). Tobacco addiction and the dysregulation of brain stress systems. *Neurosci. Biobehav. Rev.* 36, 1418–1441. doi: 10.1016/j.neubiorev.2012.02.015

Buczek, Y., Lê, A. D., Wang, A., Stewart, J., and Shaham, Y. (1999). Stress reinstates nicotine seeking but not sucrose solution seeking in rats. *Psychopharmacology (Berl.)* 144, 183–188.

Carlezon, W. A. Jr., Béguin, C., DiNieri, J. A., Baumann, M. H., Richards, M. R., Todtenkopf, M. S., et al. (2006). Depressive-like effects of the kappa-opioid receptor agonist salvinorin A on behavior and neurochemistry in rats. *J. Pharmacol. Exp. Ther.* 316, 440–447.

Chartoff, E., Sawyer, A., Rachlin, A., Potter, D., Pliakas, A., and Carlezon, W. A. (2012). Blockade of kappa opioid receptors attenuates the development of depressive-like behaviors induced by cocaine withdrawal in rats. *Neuropharmacology* 62, 167–176. doi: 10.1016/j.neuropharm.2011.06.014

Chen, Y., Chen, C., and Liu-Chen, L.-Y. (2007). Dynorphin peptides differentially regulate the human kappa opioid receptor. *Life Sci.* 80, 1439–1448. doi: 10.1016/j.lfs.2007.01.018

Covington, H. E. III, and Miczek, K. A. (2001). Repeated social-defeat stress, cocaine or morphine. Effects on behavioral sensitization and intravenous cocaine self-administration "binges." *Psychopharmacology (Berl.)* 158, 388–398. doi: 10.1007/s002130100858

Ebner, S. R., Roitman, M. F., Potter, D. N., Rachlin, A. B., and Chartoff, E. H. (2010). Depressive-like effects of the kappa opioid receptor agonist salvinorin A are associated with decreased phasic dopamine release in the nucleus accumbens. *Psychopharmacology (Berl.)* 210, 241–252. doi: 10.1007/s00213-010-1836-5

Elizalde, N., Gil-Bea, F. J., Ramírez, M. J., Aisa, B., Lasheras, B., Del Rio, J., et al. (2008). Long-lasting behavioral effects and recognition memory deficit induced by chronic mild stress in mice: effect of antidepressant treatment. *Psychopharmacology (Berl.)* 199, 1–14. doi: 10.1007/s00213-007-1035-1

Gehrke, B. J., Chefer, V. I., and Shippenberg, T. S. (2008). Effects of acute and repeated administration of salvinorin A on dopamine function in the rat dorsal striatum. *Psychopharmacology (Berl.)* 197, 509–517. doi: 10.1007/s00213-007-1067-6

Giros, B., Jaber, M., Jones, S. R., Wightman, R. M., and Caron, M. G. (1996). Hyperlocomotion and indifference to cocaine and amphetamine in mice lacking the dopamine transporter. *Nature* 379, 606–612. doi: 10.1038/379606a0

Graziane, N. M., Polter, A. M., Briand, L. A., Pierce, R. C., and Kauer, J. A. (2013). Kappa opioid receptors regulate stress-induced cocaine seeking and synaptic plasticity. *Neuron* 77, 942–954. doi: 10.1016/j.neuron.2012.12.034

Hill, M. N., Hellemans, K. G. C., Verma, P., Gorzalka, B. B., and Weinberg, J. (2012). Neurobiology of chronic mild stress: parallels to major depression. *Neurosci. Biobehav. Rev.* 36, 2085–2117. doi: 10.1016/j.neubiorev.2012.07.001

Jackson, K. J., McLaughlin, J. P., Carroll, F. I., and Damaj, M. I. (2013). Effects of the kappa opioid receptor antagonist, norbinaltorphimine, on stress and drug-induced reinstatement of nicotine-conditioned place preference in mice. *Psychopharmacology (Berl.)* 226, 763–768. doi: 10.1007/s00213-012-2716-y

Koob, G., and Kreek, M. J. (2007). Stress, dysregulation of drug reward pathways, and the transition to drug dependence. *Am. J. Psychiatry* 164, 1149–1159. doi: 10.1176/appi.ajp.2007.05030503

Koob, G. F. (2008). A role for brain stress systems in addiction. *Neuron* 59, 11–34. doi: 10.1016/j.neuron.2008.06.012

Land, B. B., Bruchas, M. R., Lemos, J. C., Xu, M., Melief, E. J., and Chavkin, C. (2008). The dysphoric component of stress is encoded by activation of the dynorphin kappa-opioid system. *J. Neurosci.* 28, 407–414. doi: 10.1523/JNEUROSCI.4458-07.2008

Land, B. B., Bruchas, M. R., Schattauer, S., Giardino, W. J., Aita, M., Messinger, D., et al. (2009). Activation of the kappa opioid receptor in the dorsal raphe nucleus mediates the aversive effects of stress and reinstates drug seeking. *Proc. Natl. Acad. Sci. U.S.A.* 106, 19168–19173. doi: 10.1073/pnas.0910705106

Leão, R. M., Cruz, F. C., Marin, M. T., and Planeta Cda, S. (2012). Stress induces behavioral sensitization, increases nicotine-seeking behavior and leads to a decrease of CREB in the nucleus accumbens. *Pharmacol.*

Biochem. Behav. 101, 434–442. doi: 10.1016/j.pbb.2012.01.025

Lemos, J. C., Roth, C. A., Messinger, D. I., Gill, H. K., Phillips, P. E. M., and Chavkin, C. (2012a). Repeated stress dysregulates κ-opioid receptor signaling in the dorsal raphe through a p38α MAPK-dependent mechanism. *J. Neurosci.* 32, 12325–12336. doi: 10.1523/JNEUROSCI.2053-12.2012

Lemos, J. C., Wanat, M. J., Smith, J. S., Reyes, B. A. S., Hollon, N. G., Van Bockstaele, E. J., et al. (2012b). Severe stress switches CRF action in the nucleus accumbens from appetitive to aversive. *Nature* 490, 402–406. doi: 10.1038/nature11436

McEwen, B. S., and Gianaros, P. J. (2011). Stress- and allostasis-induced brain plasticity. *Annu. Rev. Med.* 62, 431–445. doi: 10.1146/annurev-med-052209-100430

McLaughlin, J. P., Land, B. B., Li, S., Pintar, J. E., and Chavkin, C. (2006). Prior activation of kappa opioid receptors by U50,488 mimics repeated forced swim stress to potentiate cocaine place preference conditioning. *Neuropsychopharmacology* 31, 787–794. doi: 10.1038/sj.npp.1300860

McLaughlin, J. P., Marton-Popovici, M., and Chavkin, C. (2003). Kappa opioid receptor antagonism and prodynorphin gene disruption block stress-induced behavioral responses. *J. Neurosci.* 23, 5674–5683.

McLaughlin, J. P., Myers, L. C., Zarek, P. E., Caron, M. G., Lefkowitz, R. J., Czyzyk, T. A., et al. (2004). Prolonged kappa opioid receptor phosphorylation mediated by G-protein receptor kinase underlies sustained analgesic tolerance. *J. Biol. Chem.* 279, 1810–1818. doi: 10.1074/jbc.M305796200

Peng, Y.-L., Liu, Y.-N., Liu, L., Wang, X., Jiang, C.-L., and Wang, Y.-X. (2012). Inducible nitric oxide synthase is involved in the modulation of depressive behaviors induced by unpredictable chronic mild stress. *J. Neuroinflammation* 9, 75. doi: 10.1186/1742-2094-9-75

Plaza-Zabala, A., Martín-García, E., de Lecea, L., Maldonado, R., and Berrendero, F. (2010). Hypocretins regulate the anxiogenic-like effects of nicotine and induce reinstatement of nicotine-seeking behavior. *J. Neurosci.* 30, 2300–2310. doi: 10.1523/JNEUROSCI.5724-09.2010

Potter, D. N., Damez-Werno, D., Carlezon, W. A. Jr., Cohen, B. M., and Chartoff, E. H. (2011). Repeted exposure to kappa-opioid receptor agonist salvinorin A modulates extracellular signal-regulated kinase and reward sensitivity. *Biol. Psychiatry* 70, 744–753. doi: 10.1016/j.biopsych.2011.05.021

Rasheed, N., Tyagi, E., Ahmad, A., Siripurapu, K. B., Lahiri, S., Shukla, R., et al. (2008). Involvement of monoamines and proinflammatory cytokines in mediating the anti-stress effects of Panax quinquefolium. *J. Ethnopharmacol.* 117, 257–262. doi: 10.1016/j.jep.2008.01.035

Redila, V. A., and Chavkin, C. (2008). Stress-induced reinstatement of cocaine seeking is mediated by the kappa opioid system. *Psychopharmacology (Berl.)* 200, 59–70. doi: 10.1007/s00213-008-1122-y

Reith, M. E. (1986). Effect of repeated administration of various doses of cocaine and WIN 35,065-2 on locomotor behavior of mice. *Eur. J. Pharmacol.* 130, 65–72. doi: 10.1016/0014-2999(86)90184-6

Schindler, A. G., Messinger, D. I., Smith, J. S., Shankar, H., Gustin, R. M., Schattauer, S. S., et al. (2012). Stress produces aversion and potentiates cocaine reward by releasing endogenous dynorphins in the ventral striatum to locally stimulate serotonin reuptake. *J. Neurosci.* 32, 17582–17596. doi: 10.1523/JNEUROSCI.3220-2.2012

Smith, J. S., Schindler, A. G., Martinelli, E., Gustin, R. M., Bruchas, M. R., and Chavkin, C. (2012). Stress-induced activation of the dynorphin/κ-opioid receptor system in the amygdala potentiates nicotine conditioned place preference. *J. Neurosci.* 32, 1488–1495. doi: 10.1523/JNEUROSCI.2980-11.2012

Sora, I., Wichems, C., Takahashi, N., Li, X. F., Zeng, Z., Revay, R., et al. (1998). Cocaine reward models: conditioned place preference can be established in dopamine- and in serotonin-transporter knockout mice. *Proc. Natl. Acad. Sci. U.S.A.* 95, 7699–7704. doi: 10.1073/pnas.95.13.7699

Tolliver, B. K., Belknap, J. K., Woods, W. E., and Carney, J. M. (1994). Genetic analysis of sensitization and tolerance to cocaine. *J. Pharmacol. Exp. Ther.* 270, 1230–1238.

Tye, K. M., Mirzabekov, J. J., Warden, M. R., Ferenczi, E. A., Tsai, H.-C., Finkelstein, J., et al. (2013). Dopamine neurons modulate neural encoding and expression of depression-related behaviour. *Nature* 493, 537–541. doi: 10.1038/nature11740

Tzschentke, T. M. (2007). Measuring reward with the conditioned place preference (CPP) paradigm: update of the last decade. *Addict. Biol.* 12, 227–462. doi: 10.1111/j.1369-1600.2007.00070.x

Van Bockstaele, E. J., Reyes, B. A. S., and Valentino, R. J. (2010). The locus coeruleus: a key nucleus where stress and opioids intersect to mediate vulnerability to opiate abuse. *Brain Res.* 1314, 162–174. doi: 10.1016/j.brainres.2009.09.036

Vancassel, S., Leman, S., Hanonick, L., Denis, S., Roger, J., Nollet, M., et al. (2008). n-3 polyunsaturated fatty acid supplementation reverses stress-induced modifications on brain monoamine levels in mice. *J. Lipid Res.* 49, 340–348. doi: 10.1194/jlr.M700328-JLR200

Walker, B. M., and Koob, G. F. (2008). Pharmacological evidence for a motivational role of kappa-opioid systems in ethanol dependence. *Neuropsychopharmacology* 33, 643–652. doi: 10.1038/sj.npp.1301438

Walker, B. M., Zorrilla, E. P., and Koob, G. F. (2011). Systemic κ-opioid receptor antagonism by nor-binaltorphimine reduces dependence-induced excessive alcohol self-administration in rats. *Addict. Biol.* 16, 116–119. doi: 10.1111/j.1369-1600.2010.00226.x

Wang, Y., Li, J.-G., Huang, P., Xu, W., and Liu-Chen, L.-Y. (2003). Differential effects of agonists on adenylyl cyclase superactivation mediated by the kappa opioid receptors: adenylyl cyclase superactivation is independent of agonist-induced phosphorylation, desensitization, internalization, and down-regulation. *J. Pharmacol. Exp. Ther.* 307, 1127–1134. doi: 10.1124/jpet.103.055814

Wee, S., and Koob, G. F. (2010). The role of the dynorphin-kappa opioid system in the reinforcing effects of drugs of abuse. *Psychopharmacology (Berl.)* 210, 121–135. doi: 10.1007/s00213-010-1825-8

Williams, J. T., Ingram, S. L., Henderson, G., Chavkin, C., von Zastrow, M., Schulz, S., et al. (2013). Regulation of μ-opioid receptors: desensitization, phosphorylation, internalization, and tolerance. *Pharmacol. Rev.* 65, 223–254. doi: 10.1124/pr.112.005942

Wise, R. A. (2004). Dopamine, learning and motivation. *Nat. Rev. Neurosci.* 5, 483–494. doi: 10.1038/nrn1406

Yamada, H., and Bruijnzeel, A. W. (2011). Stimulation of α2-adrenergic receptors in the central nucleus of the amygdala attenuates stress-induced reinstatement of nicotine seeking in rats. *Neuropharmacology* 60, 303–311. doi: 10.1016/j.neuropharm.2010.09.013

Zhang, Y., Butelman, E. R., Schlussman, S. D., Ho, A., and Kreek, M. J. (2005). Effects of the plant-derived hallucinogen salvinorin A on basal dopamine levels in the caudate putamen and in a conditioned place aversion assay in mice: agonist actions at kappa opioid receptors. *Psychopharmacology (Berl.)* 179, 551–558. doi: 10.1007/s00213-004-2087-0

Zhang, Y., Mantsch, J. R., Schlussman, S. D., Ho, A., and Kreek, M. J. (2002). Conditioned place preference after single doses or "binge" cocaine in C57BL/6J and 129/J mice. *Pharmacol. Biochem. Behav.* 73, 655–662. doi: 10.1016/S0091-3057(02)00859-6

Conflict of Interest Statement: The authors declare that the research was conducted in the absence of any commercial or financial relationships that could be construed as a potential conflict of interest.

12

Positive environmental modification of depressive phenotype and abnormal hypothalamic-pituitary-adrenal axis activity in female C57BL/6J mice during abstinence from chronic ethanol consumption

Terence Y. Pang**, Xin Du†, William A. Catchlove†, Thibault Renoir, Andrew J. Lawrence and Anthony J. Hannan

Behavioural Neurosciences Division, Florey Institute of Neuroscience and Mental Health, University of Melbourne, Melbourne, VIC, Australia

Edited by:
Laurence Lanfumey, Institut National de la Santé et de la Recherche Médicale (Inserm), France

Reviewed by:
Asha Suryanarayanan, Manchester College School of Pharmacy, USA
Etienne Sibille, University of Pittsburgh, USA

****Correspondence:***
Terence Y. Pang, Behavioural Neurosciences Division, Florey Institute of Neuroscience and Mental Health, University of Melbourne, Kennth Myer Building, Off Genetics Lane, Royal Parade, Melbourne VIC 3010, Australia
e-mail: terence.pang@florey.edu.au

† These authors have contributed equally to this work.

Depression is a commonly reported co-morbidity during rehabilitation from alcohol use disorders and its presence is associated with an increased likelihood of relapse. Interventions which impede the development of depression could be of potential benefit if incorporated into treatment programs. We previously demonstrated an ameliorative effect of physical exercise on depressive behaviors in a mouse model of alcohol abstinence. Here, we show that environmental enrichment (cognitive and social stimulation) has a similar beneficial effect. The hypothalamic-pituitary-adrenal (HPA) axis is a key physiological system regulating stress responses and its dysregulation has been separably implicated in the pathophysiology of depression and addiction disorders. We performed a series of dexamethasone challenges and found that mice undergoing 2 weeks of alcohol abstinence had significantly greater corticosterone and ACTH levels following a DEX-CRH challenge compared to water controls. Environmental enrichment during alcohol abstinence corrected the abnormal DEX-CRH corticosterone response despite a further elevation of ACTH levels. Examination of gene expression revealed abstinence-associated alterations in glucocorticoid receptor (*Gr*), corticotrophin releasing hormone (*Crh*) and pro-opiomelanocortin (*Pomc1*) mRNA levels which were differentially modulated by environmental enrichment. Overall, our study demonstrates a benefit of environmental enrichment on alcohol abstinence-associated depressive behaviors and HPA axis dysregulation.

Keywords: alcohol, abstinence, depression, environmental enrichment, HPA axis, dexamethasone, GR, pomc1

INTRODUCTION

One of the biggest impediments to recovery programs for alcohol use disorders is the development of psychological disturbances by patients, such as post-dependent dysphoric syndromes. This is a significant issue to be addressed because the presence of co-morbid psychiatric conditions such as depression and anxiety during abstinence is linked to a greater probability of relapse (Pelc et al., 2002). However, attempts to improve rehabilitation rates are hindered by the uncertainty over the precise causes of abstinence-associated psychopathology. Numerous studies of rodent models have provided evidence that withdrawal from exposure to addictive compounds elicit depression-related behavioral phenotypes (reviewed by Renoir et al., 2012). Not dissimilar, depression-related behavioral changes also feature in rodents withdrawn from alcohol and include anhedonia and helplessness, similar to the major aspects of clinical depression (Rasmussen et al., 2001; Stevenson et al., 2009; Fukushiro et al., 2012; Pang et al., 2013). Several studies have established that the withdrawal phase itself is marked by specific cellular and molecular changes in the brain (Crews et al., 2004; Nixon and Crews, 2004; Aberg et al., 2005; He et al., 2009; Stevenson et al., 2009). Recently, Vendruscolo and colleagues proposed that the phases of acute withdrawal and protracted abstinence are distinct within themselves, marked by differences in hypothalamic-pituitary-adrenal (HPA) axis activity and expression levels of the glucocorticoid receptor (Vendruscolo et al., 2012).

The HPA axis is the key physiological system that regulates circulating levels of adrenal stress hormones (cortisol, corticosterone). Dysregulation of HPA axis activity is separably implicated in the pathology of addiction disorders (see reviews by Sinha, 2008; Picciotto et al., 2010; Picetti et al., 2013) and depression (see reviews by Braquehais et al., 2012; Laryea et al., 2012; Lopresti et al., 2013). Modification of HPA axis signaling can alter drug seeking behavior (Deroche-Gamonet et al., 2003; Pastor et al., 2008; Wang et al., 2008). There have been few examinations of HPA axis regulation in a clinical population of alcoholics or those undergoing rehabilitation. However, the early evidence is that HPA axis activity is dysregulated during alcohol withdrawal. The biphasic nature of withdrawal proposed by Vendruscolo is consistent with the finding that recovering alcoholics have increased levels of cortisol and ACTH levels initially, which typically normalize upon completion of a rehabilitation program (Hundt et al., 2001). While an increase in ACTH levels is indicative of anterior pituitary dysfunction, a recent report indicated increased methylation of the *pomc1* gene promoter region in alcohol dependent patients (Muschler et al., 2010) which translates to suppression of gene expression and a predicted reduction in ACTH levels. The conflicting implications of these studies demonstrate that further work is required to better understand the nature of HPA axis pathology during abstinence from alcohol.

The development of non-pharmacological interventions for the treatment of addiction and depression are highly attractive as simple and low-cost approaches. We previously demonstrated that mice abstinent from alcohol display depression-related behaviors which are ameliorated by engaging in physical exercise (wheel-running) provided during the period of abstinence (Pang et al., 2013). Other groups have reported that environmental enrichment, a paradigm of social and cognitive stimulation, has the capacity for non-drug modification of addiction-related behaviors (Solinas et al., 2008; Chauvet et al., 2009; Nader et al., 2012). Furthermore, environmental enrichment can exert antidepressive effects on behavior in several models of depression (Pang et al., 2009; Hendriksen et al., 2012; Lehmann et al., 2013; Stuart et al., 2013), possibly through HPA axis modulation (Du et al., 2012). Therefore, we sought to investigate whether environmental enrichment could exert a corrective effect on the depressive phenotype of a mouse model of alcohol abstinence.

MATERIALS AND METHODS

MICE

Six-week old female C57BL/6J mice were purchased from Animal Resources Centre (Murdoch, WA, Australia) and housed at the Florey Neuroscience Laboratories (University of Melbourne, VIC, Australia) in a temperature-controlled environment on a 12:12 h light-dark cycle with food and water provided *ad libitum*. All the behavioral studies were conducted at the Integrative Neuroscience Facility (INF). All experiments were approved by the Howard Florey Institute animal ethics committee in accordance with the recommended guidelines set by the National Health and Medical Research Council (NHMRC) of Australia.

ETHANOL SELF-ADMINISTRATION

From 8 weeks of age, mice were allowed to self-administer 10% (v/v) ethanol solution (two bottle free-choice) for a period of six weeks as previously published (Pang et al., 2013). An alternative source of untreated water was freely available at all times (see **Figure 1A** for study schematic). The placements of the ethanol- and water-containing bottles were randomly alternated throughout the experiment to avoid location preference bias. The control group only had access to normal tap water provided in two drink bottles. All mice were single-housed during the first 6 weeks of this study and daily fluid intake was recorded. Consistent with our previous publication (Pang et al., 2013), mice did not differ in total daily fluid intake (data not shown). Ethanol consuming mice showed high preference >85%, averaging 15–18 g/kg alcohol per day. There was no difference in weight gain across the six weeks. After six weeks of free-choice ethanol drinking, the ethanol solution-containing drink bottle was removed for two weeks prior to commencement of behavioral testing. Water-drinking mice were provided a single bottle of water during this period. Mice were randomly allocated to continue being maintained in standard-housing (Alc Abstn SH) or undergo environmental enrichment (Alc Abstn EE). Mice undergoing enrichment were re-grouped 4–6 mice per cage since social stimulation was part of the enrichment paradigm. Enriched mice were housed in larger cages supplemented with shredded paper, tunnels and objects of varying textures and shapes. The configuration of the cage was changed every 3 days. Behavioral testing commenced after 14 days of abstinence; separate cohorts of mice were used for the DEX combinatorial challenges which were conducted on the 15th day of abstinence.

SACCHARIN PREFERENCE TEST (SPT)

Mice (10 per group) were single-housed over a 12 h overnight period and provided the opportunity to consume 0.1% (w/v) saccharin solution or tap water (Short et al., 2006). The total volume of fluid intake was recorded, and preference ratio was determined by calculating the volume of saccharin solution consumed as a proportion of total fluid intake. Enriched mice were re-grouped in their enrichment cages after the test.

FORCED-SWIM TEST (FST)

Mice (10 per group) were individually placed into beakers (17 cm diameter) of water (23–25°C) filled to a depth such that tails would not be in contact with the bottom of the beaker. Each test lasted for a total of 5 mins and was video recorded for subsequent scoring by an experimenter who was blind to treatment and housing conditions of the mice. The total immobility time adopted by each mouse over the final 4 mins of the test was recorded.

DEXAMETHASONE CHALLENGES

The dexamethasone suppression test (DST) involved a single i.p. injection of dexamethasone (DEX) (0.1 mg/kg body weight; Sigma-Aldrich, St. Louis, MO, USA) between 0800–1000H. Six hours later, mice were killed and trunk blood collected for corticosterone analysis. For the DEX-CRH and DEX-ACTH challenges, mice were treated according as per the DST. Six hours after DEX administration, mice received CRH (i.p., 20 mg/kg body weight; Sigma-Aldrich) or ACTH (i.p., 50 μg/100 g body weight; Prospec, Rehovot, Israel). Thirty mins post-CRH/ACTH injections, mice (4–6 per group) were killed and trunk blood collected for corticosterone analysis.

QUANTIFICATION OF SERUM CORTICOSTERONE AND ACTH LEVELS

For basal levels of corticosterone, non-stress mice were killed between 0900–1100H for blood collection. Post-stress levels were determined with blood samples collected from mice exposed to 10 mins of forced-swim stress performed between 0900–1100H then killed immediately after. Briefly, mice were killed by cervical dislocation and trunk blood was collected, allowed to coagulate at room temperature for 30 mins before being centrifuged at 1070 rcf for 15 mins. Serum was collected and stored at −20°C until quantification of corticosterone was performed. Corticosterone was quantified using EIA (Cayman Chemical, Ann Arbor, MI, USA) according to the manufacturer's instructions. Serum ACTH levels were determined using a Milliplex Mouse Bone Panel 2A kit (Millipore, St. Charles, MO, USA) as per the manufacturer's recommendations. Samples were read on a Luminex 100 instrument. These analyses were performed by Cardinal Bioresearch (New Farm, QLD, Australia).

TISSUE COLLECTION, SAMPLE PREPARATION AND SEMI-QUANTITATIVE REAL-TIME PCR

Mice (5–6 per group) were killed via cervical dislocation and brains were removed for microdissection of the relevant regions. Adrenal glands were harvested. All tissue was snap frozen in liquid nitrogen and stored at –80°C. Tissue was disrupted using a bioruptor and RNA was isolated using RNeasy RNA Mini kits (Qiagen, Melbourne, VIC, Australia) according to the manufacturer's instructions. Extracted RNA was stored at –80°C. Sample was reverse transcribed into cDNA using SuperScript®VILO™ cDNA synthesis kit (Invitrogen, Mulgrave, VIC, Australia) according to the manufacturer's instructions. cDNA products were stored at –20°C until further use. cDNA was amplified using the SYBR Green JumpStart Taq Ready Mix (Sigma, Castle Hill, NSW, Australia) based on the manufacturer's instructions [primer sequences are provided in Du et al. (2012)]. Efficiency curves and optimal reaction volumes for all primer pairs were determined. Glucocorticoid receptor (GR, nr3c1) and mineralocorticoid receptor (MR, nr3c2) expression was measured in the hypothalamus and pituitary. CRH expression was measured in the hypothalamus and proopiomelanocotin (POMC1) and dopamine receptor D2 (Drd2) expression was measured in the pituitary gland. Real-time quantitative PCR was carried out using the Applied Biosystems 7500 Fast Real-time PCR system sequence detection software version 1.4 (Applied Biosystems, Foster City, CA, USA). Cyclophilin was used as an endogenous control for the hypothalamus and pituitary analyses. Each sample and housekeeping control was run in duplicate.

STATISTICAL ANALYSIS

Statistical analyses were performed using SPSS statistics 17.0 and graphical data was generated with GraphPad Prism 5.0. Data was analysed with one or two-way analysis of variance (ANOVA) and where a significant difference was detected, followed up with *post-hoc* Bonferroni *t*-tests to determine specific between-group differences. In all cases, the significance level was set at $p < 0.05$.

RESULTS

ETHANOL ABSTINENCE-ASSOCIATED DEPRESSIVE PHENOTYPE IS CORRECTED BY ENVIRONMENTAL ENRICHMENT

Saccharin preference test

One-way ANOVA revealed a significant difference in saccharin preference between the groups [$F_{(2, 29)} = 44.6$, $p < 0.001$] (**Figure 1B**). Standard-housed alcohol abstinent (Alc Abstn) mice had decreased saccharin preference compared to water controls ($p < 0.001$). Environmentally enriched Alc Abstn mice had significantly greater saccharin preference compared to the

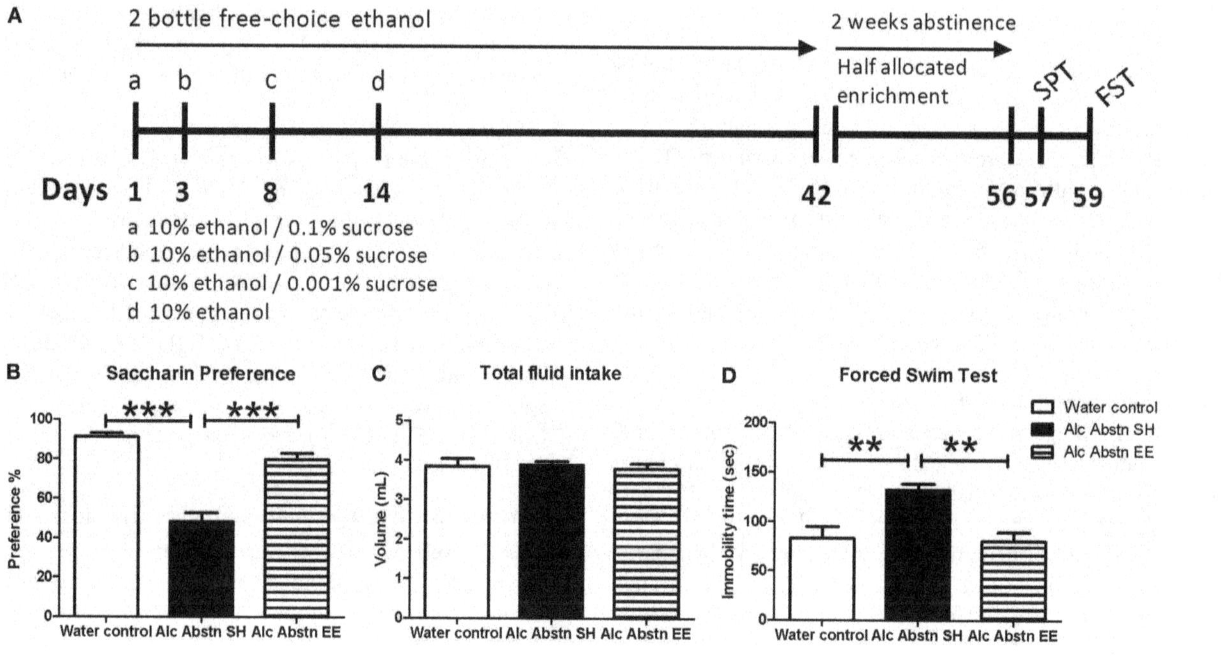

FIGURE 1 | Environmentally enriched alcohol abstinent mice do not display pro-depressive behaviors. (A) Schematic representation of experimental design leading up to behavioral testing. An identical design was used in the lead up to the DEX combinatorial challenges. **(B)** Reduced saccharin preference associated with alcohol abstinence was not observed in the enriched group. **(C)** Differences in saccharin preference test were not due to change in total fluid consumption. **(D)** Alcohol abstinent mice recorded significantly greater immobility times in the forced-swim test compared to water controls and enriched abstinent mice. Alc Abstn SH: 2 week alcohol abstinence in standard housing conditions; Alc Abstn EE: 2 week alcohol abstinence in environmentally enriched housing conditions. 10 mice per group. 1-way ANOVA followed by *post-hoc* Bonferroni's *t*-test: $^{**}p < 0.01$; $^{***}p < 0.001$.

standard-housed Alc Abstn group ($p < 0.001$), but not different to controls. There was no significant difference in total fluid consumption during the test [$F_{(2, 29)} = 0.131$, $p = 0.818$] (**Figure 1C**).

Forced swim test

One-way ANOVA revealed a significant difference between the groups for total immobility time in the FST [$F_{(2, 29)} = 10.29$, $p < 0.001$] (**Figure 1D**). *Post-hoc* testing showed that the standard-housed Alc Abstn mice averaged greater immobility times than water controls ($p < 0.01$). Environmentally enriched Alc Abstn mice had significantly reduced FST immobility times compared to the standard-housed group ($p < 0.01$), but not different to controls.

ETHANOL ABSTINENCE IS ASSOCIATED WITH ABNORMAL DEX-CRH RESPONSE

Quantification of serum corticosterone levels after forced-swim stress revealed an overall effect of stress ($F_{(1, 14)} = 45.6$, $p < 0.001$) with no difference between the treatment groups [$F_{(1, 14)} = 0.0652$, $p = 0.80$] (**Figure 2A**). There were no apparent differences in baseline and post-stress corticosterone levels. We examined HPA axis activity in further detail by conducting the dexamethasone suppression challenge in combination with CRH and ACTH. There were no significant differences in serum corticosterone levels between water controls and alcohol abstinent mice following DEX and DEX-ACTH treatments (**Figure 2B**). However, alcohol abstinent mice had significantly higher serum corticosterone levels compared to water controls following the DEX-CRH challenge ($p < 0.01$). Serum ACTH levels did not differ between the groups after DEX challenge, but was significantly higher in alcohol abstinent mice compared to water controls after DEX-CRH challenge ($p < 0.05$) (**Figure 2C**).

ENVIRONMENTAL ENRICHMENT MODIFIES DEX-CRH RESPONSE OF ALCOHOL ABSTINENT MICE

Having found a specific difference in corticosterone response in the DEX-CRH challenge, we repeated the DEX-CRH challenge, and included a group of Alc Abstn mice that had undergone environmental enrichment during the abstinence period. There was no significant difference between the three groups in the DEX challenge [$F_{(2, 17)} = 2.82$, $p = 0.09$] (**Figure 3A**). However, one-way ANOVA detected a significant difference between the groups in the DEX-CRH challenge [$F_{(2, 17)} = 26.12$, $p < 0.001$].

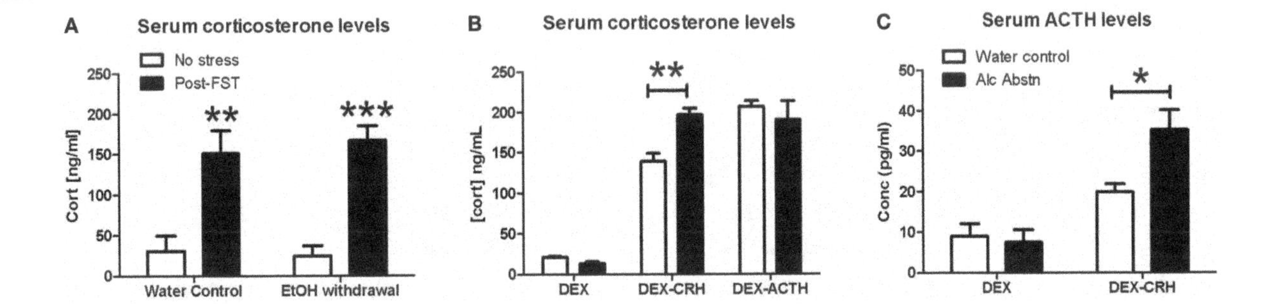

FIGURE 2 | Alcohol abstinence associated with abnormal DEX-CRH response. (A) No significant difference in serum corticosterone levels at baseline and immediately following forced-swim stress. **(B)** Similar levels of serum corticosterone after DEX and DEX-ACTH challenges. Alcohol abstinent mice had significantly higher corticosterone levels compared to water controls in the DEX-CRH challenge. **(C)** Serum ACTH levels were similar after DEX challenge but alcohol abstinent mice have significantly higher levels of ACTH after the DEX-CRH challenge. 4–6 mice per group. Two or one-way ANOVA followed by *post-hoc* Bonferroni's *t*-test: *$p < 0.05$, **$p < 0.01$, ***$p < 0.001$.

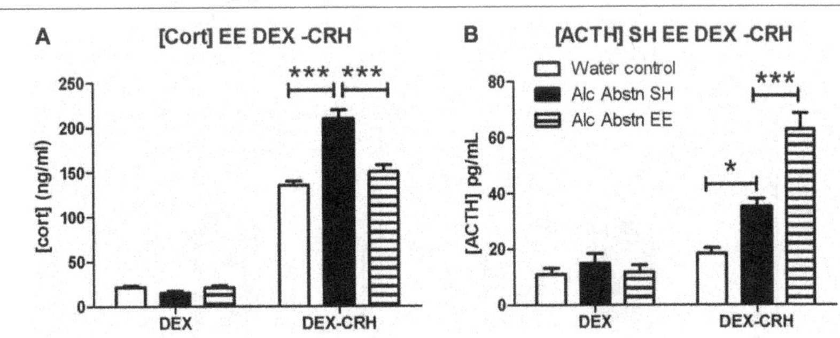

FIGURE 3 | Environmental enrichment modifies DEX-CRH response of alcohol abstinent mice. (A) Serum corticosterone levels did not differ between the groups in the DEX challenge. In the DEX-CRH challenge, Alc Abstn mice had significantly higher levels of corticosterone compared to water controls and the environmentally enriched abstinent mice. **(B)** The three groups had similar ACTH levels following the DEX challenge. However, following DEX-CRH, enriched Alc Abstn mice responded with even greater levels of ACTH compared to the standard-housed Alc Abstn group. Alc Abstn SH: 2 week alcohol abstinence in standard housing conditions; Alc Abstn EE: 2 week alcohol abstinence in environmentally enriched housing conditions. 6 mice per group. One-way ANOVA followed by *post-hoc* Bonferroni's *t*-test: *$p < 0.05$; ***$p < 0.001$.

Post-hoc Bonferroni's *t*-test showed that serum corticosterone levels of standard-housed Alc Abstn mice were significantly greater than water controls ($p < 0.001$) and environmentally enriched Alc Abstn mice ($p < 0.001$).

Serum ACTH levels did not differ between the groups in the DEX challenge [$F_{(2, 17)} = 0.51, p = 0.61$] (**Figure 3B**). ACTH levels differed significantly between the groups in the DEX-CRH challenge [$F_{(2, 17)} = 32.64$, $p < 0.001$]. Similar to the data in **Figure 2C**, standard-housed Alc Abstn mice had higher ACTH levels than water controls ($p < 0.05$). Surprisingly, environmentally enriched Alc Abstn mice had significantly higher levels of ACTH compared to standard-housed Alc Abstn mice ($p < 0.001$).

MODIFIED GENE EXPRESSION DURING ETHANOL ABSTINENCE: EFFECTS OF ENVIRONMENTAL ENRICHMENT

Withdrawal from an acute binge-like ethanol intake is associated with stress hyper-reactivity manifesting as enhanced CORT and ACTH responses to stress (Buck et al., 2011). The findings that Alc Abstn mice respond with significantly higher levels of corticosterone and ACTH in the DEX-CRH challenge is further evidence of HPA axis hyperactivity. To gain a better appreciation of this pathophysiology, we examined the mRNA levels of key regulatory genes involved in HPA axis function, namely the glucocorticoid receptor (GR), mineralocorticoid receptor (MR), crh, pomc1 (the precursor of ACTH) and dopamine 2 receptor (drd2). A previous study had demonstrated the dynamic nature of GR mRNA expression which differs between a state of acute withdrawal (down-regulation) and protracted abstinence (up-regulation) (Vendruscolo et al., 2012). We examined pituitary drd2 gene expression due to evidence of dopamine D2 receptor-mediated regulation of pomc1 mRNA levels (Cote et al., 1986; Pardy et al., 1990).

In the hypothalamus, GR mRNA levels were significantly different between the groups [$F_{(2, 14)} = 9.288$, $p = 0.003$] (**Figure 4A**). *Post-hoc* Bonferroni showed that GR gene expression was significantly greater in the standard-housed Alc Abstn group compared to both the water controls ($p < 0.01$) and the environmentally enriched Alc Abstn group ($p < 0.05$). In contrast, there was no significant difference in MR gene expression between the groups [$F_{(2, 14)} = 0.429, p = 0.661$] (**Figure 4B**).

GR mRNA levels were also significantly different between the groups in the pituitary [$F_{(2, 14)} = 6.389, p = 0.013$] (**Figure 4C**). *Post-hoc* testing showed greater MR gene expression in the standard-housed Alc Abstn group ($p < 0.05$) and environmentally enriched Alc Abstn group ($p < 0.05$) compared to water controls. Similarly, but in contrast to the findings in the hypothalamus, pituitary MR mRNA levels significantly differed between the groups [$F_{(2, 14)} = 6.973, p = 0.01$] (**Figure 4D**) with both standard-housed ($p < 0.05$) and environmentally enriched Alc Abstn ($p < 0.05$) groups having higher expression levels compared to the water control group.

Crh gene expression was also significantly different between the groups [$F_{(2, 14)} = 17.72$, $p < 0.001$] (**Figure 5A**). *Post-hoc* testing showed significantly reduced *Crh* mRNA levels in the standard-housed Alc Abstn group ($p < 0.001$) and

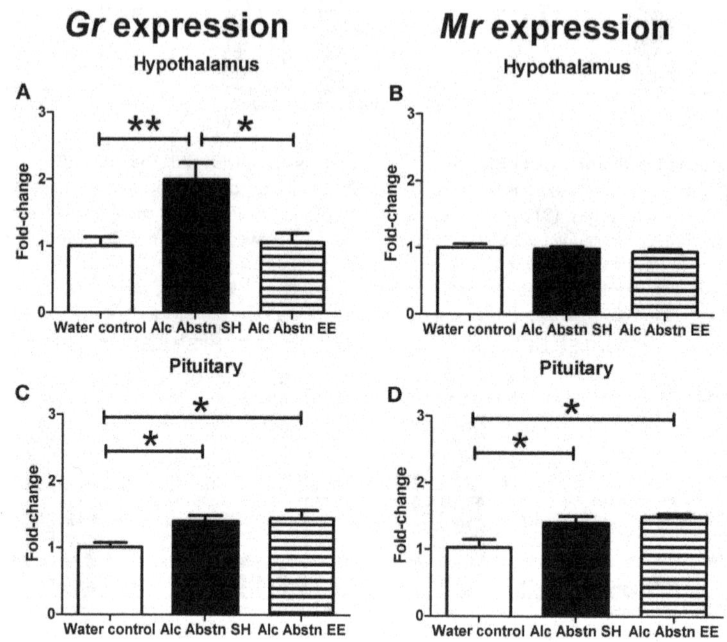

FIGURE 4 | Differential effects of environmental enrichment on steroid hormone receptors. (A) An up-regulation of GR expression in the hypothalamus of Alc Abstn mice is not observed in the group exposed to enrichment. **(B)** No observable change to hypothalamic MR expression. **(C)** Up-regulation of pituitary GR expression in Alc Abstn mice is maintained in the enriched group. **(D)** In contrast to the hypothalamus, pituitary MR expression was increased with alcohol abstinence, and this persisted in the enriched group. Alc Abstn SH: 2 week alcohol abstinence in standard housing conditions; Alc Abstn EE: 2 week alcohol abstinence in environmentally enriched housing conditions. Five mice per group. One-way ANOVA followed by *post-hoc* Bonferroni's *t*-test: $^{*}p < 0.05$, $^{**}p < 0.01$.

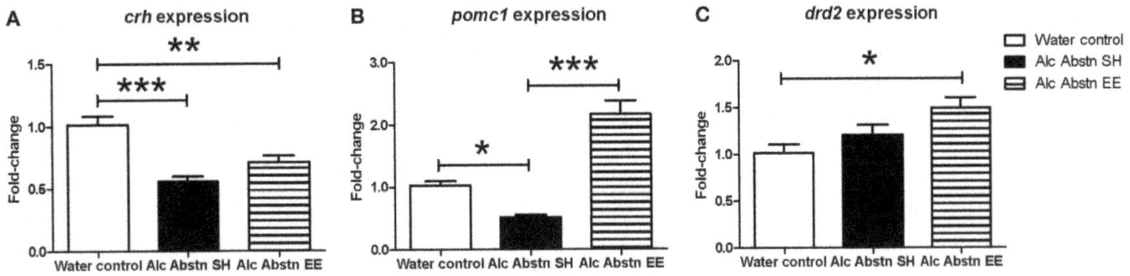

FIGURE 5 | Differential effects of enrichment on hypothalamic and pituitary gene expression. (A) Hypothalamic *Crh* expression was significantly reduced in the standard-housed Alc abstn group, and unaltered by enrichment. **(B)** Pituitary *pomc1* expression was significantly reduced in the standard-housed Alc Abstn group but was significantly elevated in the enriched group. **(C)** Pituitary *Drd2* expression was not significantly altered by alcohol abstinence. Alc Abstn SH: 2 week alcohol abstinence in standard housing conditions; Alc Abstn EE: 2 week alcohol abstinence in environmentally enriched housing conditions. 5–6 mice per group. 1-way ANOVA followed by *post-hoc* Bonferroni's *t*-test: $^*p < 0.05$, $^{**}p < 0.01$, $^{***}p < 0.001$.

environmentally enriched Alc Abstn group ($p < 0.01$) compared to water controls.

In the pituitary, *pomc1* gene expression was significantly different between the groups [$F_{(2, 14)} = 45.78, p < 0.001$] (**Figure 5B**). The expression level in standard-housed Alc Abstn mice was 0.51 fold compared to the water control group ($p < 0.05$). *pomc1* gene expression was significantly increased in environmentally enriched Alc Abstn mice when compared to water control ($p < 0.001$) and standard-housed Alc abstn ($p < 0.001$) groups. There was a significant difference in *drd2* gene expression between the groups [$F_{(2, 14)} = 5.05, p = 0.0238$] (**Figure 5C**) with *post-hoc* analysis revealing no significant difference between controls and standard-housed Alc Abstn mice, but a significant elevation in environmentally enriched Alc Abstn mice compared to controls ($p < 0.05$).

DISCUSSION

Our study has provided further evidence that the expression levels of key centrally-expressed regulators of HPA activity are altered during abstinence from self-administration of alcohol. More specifically, we noted an up-regulation of the two major adrenal steroid receptors in the brain, with the observed effect on GR consistent with previous reports (Vendruscolo et al., 2012). We also observed a region-specific effect of abstinence since MR was up-regulated in the pituitary but remained unaffected in the hypothalamus. Additionally, hypothalamic expression of crh and pituitary expression of pomc1 were down-regulated. The collective data suggest suppression of HPA axis activity during abstinence following chronic alcohol consumption. Given the current evidence implicating HPA axis pathophysiology as a feature of clinical depression, our findings support the hypothesis that dysregulation of the HPA axis is a key event for the development of abstinence-related depression which we have replicated in a mouse model.

FUNCTIONAL CHARACTERIZATION OF HPA AXIS PATHOLOGY DURING ALCOHOL ABSTINENCE

This is the first study attempting to functionally characterize pathophysiology of the HPA axis during abstinence from alcohol in mice. By performing the DEX challenge in combination with CRH and ACTH administration, we interrogated steroid receptor-mediated suppression of corticosterone levels as well as pituitary and adrenal function. It was important to determine the response to DEX because DEX non-suppression is a reported feature of clinical depression associated with high levels of stress (Fountoulakis et al., 2004) and a smaller suppressive response to DEX has been linked to GR polymorphisms which increase risk for depression (see review by Manenschijn et al., 2009). However no significant difference in basal and post-DEX corticosterone levels between the abstinent and control groups were observed suggesting that suppression of HPA axis activity via down-stream signaling from GR is likely to be normative in abstinent animals. In contrast, we found a significantly greater corticosterone response of abstinent animals compared to controls in the DEX-CRH challenge, matched by an exaggerated elevation of ACTH. These suggest a pathological pituitary response initiated by CRH signaling in abstinent animals. The pathology is likely to be limited to the pituitary since direct stimulation of the adrenals to elicit corticosterone secretion in the DEX-ACTH challenge yielded comparable results.

As far as we are aware, this is the first time an abnormal DEX-CRH response has been reported in a mouse model of alcohol abstinence. However, our findings are consistent with the limited available clinical data. Hundt et al. also performed the DEX-CRH challenge on 19 alcoholic inpatients and reported significantly elevated cortisol and ACTH responses (Hundt et al., 2001). Interestingly, upon completion of the withdrawal program, the DEX-CRH responses of patients were largely normalized. It is important to note that another clinical study has reported that during the acute phase of withdrawal, a pathological DEX-CRH response is limited to increased cortisol levels but not ACTH (Zimmermann et al., 2003). Thus, given that we observed an increased ACTH response in the DEX-CRH test, our study design of 2 weeks abstinence accurately models protracted, not acute, abstinence. The molecular mechanisms involved in the normalization of a pathological DEX-CRH response following protracted alcohol abstinence are presently unknown and will require further investigation. Elucidating the precise signaling pathways involved could contribute to pharmacotherapies which facilitate rehabilitative efforts.

ENVIRONMENTAL ENRICHMENT CORRECTS ABSTINENCE-RELATED DEPRESSIVE BEHAVIORS

The corrective effect of environmental enrichment on saccharin preference and FST immobility suggests that cognitive and social stimulation imparts benefits in ameliorating withdrawal-associated depressive behaviors. Independent groups have demonstrated that environmental enrichment is a modifier of addiction-related neurobiology by preventing the incubation of cocaine craving (Chauvet et al., 2012) and attenuating cocaine seeking behavior (Thiel et al., 2009). Enrichment has also been reported to elicit a blunted ACTH response to stress associated with nicotine withdrawal (Skwara et al., 2012). Our study is the first to demonstrate a benefit of environmental enrichment on the depression-related behavioral phenotype associated with alcohol abstinence and extends our previous work on physical exercise as a potential anti-depressive intervention (Pang et al., 2013).

GLUCOCORTICOID RECEPTOR GENE EXPRESSION IS UP-REGULATED DURING PROTECTED ALCOHOL ABSTINENCE

Our data also indicated that a variety of molecular regulators of the HPA axis are differentially susceptible to modulation by environmental enrichment. Prior to this study, the regulation of GR gene expression by enrichment in the context of alcohol abstinence had not been investigated. Indeed, despite the positive effects of enrichment in the context of addiction, little is known about the potential molecular mechanisms underlying those effects. Our findings of increased GR gene expression are in agreement with elevated corticosterone concentrations in the brain after a period of ethanol withdrawal (Little et al., 2008). A GR-selective effect of environmental enrichment (sparing MR) in normative mice has previously been reported (Olsson et al., 1994) and this gene-specific effect of enrichment was observed in our examination of the hypothalamus. However, a previous study had found that GR protein levels are decreased after acute (24 h) withdrawal of ethanol (Roy et al., 2002) which is in contrast to the increased GR expression we observed in the hypothalamus and pituitary. This conflicting finding could reflect the differential regulation of the glucocorticoid receptor (both gene and protein levels) during acute withdrawal and after a prolonged period of withdrawal. A more definitive understanding of GR regulation under these different conditions would require future studies that directly compare GR mRNA and protein levels. Roy and colleagues had proposed that diminished GR function in hypothalamus was likely to be the underlying pathology responsible for HPA axis dysfunction during ethanol exposure and withdrawal. While that might be true during the acute phase of withdrawal, our findings together with Vendruscolo et al. (2012) indicate that it is in fact an up-regulation of GR expression during protracted alcohol abstinence that underlies HPA axis pathology. This was further supported by our observation that environmentally enriched abstinent mice had normative levels of GR in the hypothalamus.

ENVIRONMENTAL ENRICHMENT CORRECTS ABSTINENCE-RELATED ABNORMAL DEX-CRH RESPONSE AND GENE EXPRESSION

It is known that chronic alcohol consumption leads to prolonged activation of the HPA axis, persistent increases in circulating cortisol/corticosterone levels and culminating in dysregulation of *crh* gene expression which itself is a crucial factor in mediating chronic alcohol-related neuroadaptations (see review by Heilig and Koob, 2007). Our finding of decreased hypothalamic *crh* gene expression after protracted abstinence following chronic ethanol consumption is consistent with previous reports (Falco et al., 2009; Silva and Madeira, 2012). However, it is likely that the down-regulation of *crh* is a key pathological change during the process of chronic alcohol consumption which persists once alcohol is withdrawn (Richardson et al., 2008). To date, there has only been one study examining the modulation of *crh* expression by environmental enrichment which reported a non-significant increase in the hypothalamus (Francis et al., 2002). Consistent with that, we did not observe any significant effect of environmental enrichment on *crh* expression in the alcohol abstinent group. One implication of this result is that the beneficial effect of environmental enrichment in correcting the abnormal DEX-CRH response of abstinent mice is downstream of the hypothalamus, and that possibility is supported by our work which described peripheral effects of enrichment on adrenal secretion of corticosterone (Du et al., 2012).

The non-effect of enrichment on hypothalamic *crh* expression is in marked contrast to the surprising up-regulation of pituitary *pomc1* expression, further highlighting the specific nature of enrichment effects on gene expression. A previous study of rats maintained on a 7-week dark-phase ethanol consumption paired with daytime withdrawal reported a suppression of pomc1 mRNA levels by the end of a 3-week gradual ethanol withdrawal procedure (Rasmussen et al., 2000). That finding is consistent with our data on the alcohol abstinent mice which is not surprising given the somewhat similar design of the studies. This is the first report of an enrichment-associated up-regulation of *pomc1* which is consistent with the further elevation of ACTH levels in this group for the DEX-CRH challenge. However, the increased gene expression and greater functional output do not corroborate with the normalization of corticosterone levels following DEX-CRH. At the present time, we are only able to speculate on the mechanisms which could account for this apparent inconsistency. It is possible that the corrective effect of enrichment lies downstream of ACTH, i.e., exposure to environmental enrichment modifies the expression pattern of ACTH receptors located peripherally in the adrenal cortex. This possibility is supported by a study that described enrichment-mediated alterations of the temporal profile of HPA axis activity (Moncek et al., 2004).

ARGININE VASOPRESSION AS A POTENTIAL MODIFIER OF HPA AXIS IN ALCOHOL ABSTINENCE

Another potential modifier of ACTH is the stress-responsive arginine vasopressin (AVP) which is implicated in high-alcohol drinking behavior (Zhou et al., 2011a). AVP is reportedly increased after protracted abstinence from cocaine (Zhou et al., 2011b) but has yet to be investigated thoroughly in the context of alcohol abstinence. Interestingly, naloxone administration (an opioid receptor antagonist commonly used to diminish alcohol craving) has been reported to result in an up-regulation of AVP expression. However, the mechanism of AVP-dependent ACTH release is likely to involve multiple signaling pathways

(Perdona et al., 2012). Regulation by AVP could account for our observation of an apparent dissociation between ACTH and corticosterone levels since control-like corticosterone levels were elicited from enriched abstinent mice in the DEX-CRH challenge despite the presence of more exaggerated ACTH levels. Further work will be required to determine if AVP-mediated signaling is involved in imparting the corrective effects of environmental enrichment in the DEX-CRH challenge.

In summary, our study has provided molecular and functional evidence of pituitary pathology in protracted abstinence from alcohol. Environmental enrichment was able to prevent the development of abstinence-associated depression-related behaviors and corrected the pathological DEX-CRH corticosterone response. Further studies investigating the precise molecular mechanisms underlying the benefits of enrichment could uncover novel therapeutic targets to facilitate rehabilitation from alcoholism.

ACKNOWLEDGMENTS

Xin Du was supported by a Melbourne Research Scholarship (University of Melbourne). Andrew J. Lawrence is a Principal Research Fellow of the NHMRC. This work was supported by Project Grant funding (Anthony J. Hannan) from the NHMRC and an ARC Future Fellowship (Anthony J. Hannan). This work was supported by the Victorian Government through the Operational Infrastructure Scheme.

REFERENCES

Aberg, E., Hofstetter, C. P., Olson, L., and Brene, S. (2005). Moderate ethanol consumption increases hippocampal cell proliferation and neurogenesis in the adult mouse. *Int. J. Neuropsychopharmacol.* 8, 557–567. doi: 10.1017/S1461145705005286

Braquehais, M. D., Picouto, M. D., Casas, M., and Sher, L. (2012). Hypothalamic-pituitary-adrenal axis dysfunction as a neurobiological correlate of emotion dysregulation in adolescent suicide. *World J. Pediatr.* 8, 197–206. doi: 10.1007/s12519-012-0358-0

Buck, H. M., Hueston, C. M., Bishop, C., and Deak, T. (2011). Enhancement of the hypothalamic-pituitary-adrenal axis but not cytokine responses to stress challenges imposed during withdrawal from acute alcohol exposure in Sprague-Dawley rats. *Psychopharmacology (Berl).* 218, 203–215. doi: 10.1007/s00213-011-2388-z

Chauvet, C., Goldberg, S. R., Jaber, M., and Solinas, M. (2012). Effects of environmental enrichment on the incubation of cocaine craving. *Neuropharmacology* 63, 635–641. doi: 10.1016/j.neuropharm.2012.05.014

Chauvet, C., Lardeux, V., Goldberg, S. R., Jaber, M., and Solinas, M. (2009). Environmental enrichment reduces cocaine seeking and reinstatement induced by cues and stress but not by cocaine. *Neuropsychopharmacology* 34, 2767–2778. doi: 10.1038/npp.2009.127

Cote, T. E., Felder, R., Kebabian, J. W., Sekura, R. D., Reisine, T., and Affolter, H. U. (1986). D-2 dopamine receptor-mediated inhibition of pro-opiomelanocortin synthesis in rat intermediate lobe. Abolition by pertussis toxin or activators of adenylate cyclase. *J. Biol. Chem.* 261, 4555–4561.

Crews, F. T., Nixon, K., and Wilkie, M. E. (2004). Exercise reverses ethanol inhibition of neural stem cell proliferation. *Alcohol* 33, 63–71.

Deroche-Gamonet, V., Sillaber, I., Aouizerate, B., Izawa, R., Jaber, M., Ghozland, S., et al. (2003). The glucocorticoid receptor as a potential target to reduce cocaine abuse. *J. Neurosci.* 23, 4785–4790.

Du, X., Leang, L., Mustafa, T., Renoir, T., Pang, T. Y., and Hannan, A. J. (2012). Environmental enrichment rescues female-specific hyperactivity of the hypothalamic-pituitary-adrenal axis in a model of Huntington's disease. *Transl. Psychiatry* 2:e133. doi: 10.1038/tp.2012.58

Falco, A. M., Bergstrom, H. C., Bachus, S. E., and Smith, R. F. (2009). Persisting changes in basolateral amygdala mRNAs after chronic ethanol consumption. *Physiol. Behav.* 96, 169–173. doi: 10.1016/j.physbeh.2008.09.019

Fountoulakis, K., Iacovides, A., Fotiou, F., Karamouzis, M., Demetriadou, A., and Kaprinis, G. (2004). Relationship among Dexamethasone Suppression Test, personality disorders and stressful life events in clinical subtypes of major depression: an exploratory study. *Ann. Gen. Hosp. Psychiatry* 3:15. doi: 10.1186/1475-2832-3-15

Francis, D. D., Diorio, J., Plotsky, P. M., and Meaney, M. J. (2002). Environmental enrichment reverses the effects of maternal separation on stress reactivity. *J. Neurosci.* 22, 7840–7843.

Fukushiro, D. F., Saito, L. P., Mari-Kawamoto, E., Aramini, T. C., Costa, J. M., Josino, F. S., et al. (2012). Withdrawal from repeated treatment with ethanol induces a protracted decrease in novelty-seeking behavior and enhancement of environmental habituation in mice. *Pharmacol. Biochem. Behav.* 101, 132–137. doi: 10.1016/j.pbb.2011.12.013

He, J., Overstreet, D. H., and Crews, F. T. (2009). Abstinence from moderate alcohol self-administration alters progenitor cell proliferation and differentiation in multiple brain regions of male and female P rats. *Alcohol. Clin. Exp. Res.* 33, 129–138. doi: 10.1111/j.1530-0277.2008.00823.x

Heilig, M., and Koob, G. F. (2007). A key role for corticotropin-releasing factor in alcohol dependence. *Trends Neurosci.* 30, 399–406. doi: 10.1016/j.tins.2007.06.006

Hendriksen, H., Meulendijks, D., Douma, T. N., Bink, D. I., Breuer, M. E., Westphal, K. G., et al. (2012). Environmental enrichment has antidepressant-like action without improving learning and memory deficits in olfactory bulbectomized rats. *Neuropharmacology* 62, 270–277. doi: 10.1016/j.neuropharm.2011.07.018

Hundt, W., Zimmermann, U., Pottig, M., Spring, K., and Holsboer, F. (2001). The combined dexamethasone-suppression/CRH-stimulation test in alcoholics during and after acute withdrawal. *Alcohol. Clin. Exp. Res.* 25, 687–691. doi: 10.1111/j.1530-0277.2001.tb02268.x

Laryea, G., Arnett, M. G., and Muglia, L. J. (2012). Behavioral studies and genetic alterations in corticotropin-releasing hormone (crh) neurocircuitry: insights into human psychiatric disorders. *Behav. Sci. (Basel)* 2, 135–171. doi: 10.3390/bs2020135

Lehmann, M. L., Brachman, R. A., Martinowich, K., Schloesser, R. J., and Herkenham, M. (2013). Glucocorticoids orchestrate divergent effects on mood through adult neurogenesis. *J. Neurosci.* 33, 2961–2972. doi: 10.1523/JNEUROSCI.3878-12.2013

Little, H. J., Croft, A. P., O'callaghan, M. J., Brooks, S. P., Wang, G., and Shaw, S. G. (2008). Selective increases in regional brain glucocorticoid: a novel effect of chronic alcohol. *Neuroscience* 156, 1017–1027. doi: 10.1016/j.neuroscience.2008.08.029

Lopresti, A. L., Hood, S. D., and Drummond, P. D. (2013). A review of lifestyle factors that contribute to important pathways associated with major depression: diet, sleep and exercise. *J. Affect Disord.* 148, 12–27. doi: 10.1016/j.jad.2013.01.014

Manenschijn, L., Van Den Akker, E. L., Lamberts, S. W., and Van Rossum, E. F. (2009). Clinical features associated with glucocorticoid receptor polymorphisms. An overview. *Ann. N.Y. Acad. Sci.* 1179, 179–198. doi: 10.1111/j.1749-6632.2009.05013.x

Moncek, F., Duncko, R., Johansson, B. B., and Jezova, D. (2004). Effect of environmental enrichment on stress related systems in rats. *J. Neuroendocrinol.* 16, 423–431. doi: 10.1111/j.1365-2826.2004.01173.x

Muschler, M. A., Hillemacher, T., Kraus, C., Kornhuber, J., Bleich, S., and Frieling, H. (2010). DNA methylation of the POMC gene promoter is associated with craving in alcohol dependence. *J. Neural Transm.* 117, 513–519. doi: 10.1007/s00702-010-0378-7

Nader, J., Claudia, C., Rawas, R. E., Favot, L., Jaber, M., Thiriet, N., et al. (2012). Loss of environmental enrichment increases vulnerability to cocaine addiction. *Neuropsychopharmacology* 37, 1579–1587. doi: 10.1038/npp.2012.2

Nixon, K., and Crews, F. T. (2004). Temporally specific burst in cell proliferation increases hippocampal neurogenesis in protracted abstinence from alcohol. *J. Neurosci.* 24, 9714–9722. doi: 10.1523/JNEUROSCI.3063-04.2004

Olsson, T., Mohammed, A. H., Donaldson, L. F., Henriksson, B. G., and Seckl, J. R. (1994). Glucocorticoid receptor and NGFI-A gene expression are induced in the hippocampus after environmental enrichment in adult rats. *Brain Res. Mol. Brain Res.* 23, 349–353. doi: 10.1016/0169-328X(94)90246-1

Pang, T. Y., Du, X., Zajac, M. S., Howard, M. L., and Hannan, A. J. (2009). Altered serotonin receptor expression is associated with depression-related behavior in the R6/1 transgenic mouse model of Huntington's disease. *Hum. Mol. Genet.* 18, 753–766. doi: 10.1093/hmg/ddn385

Pang, T. Y., Renoir, T., Du, X., Lawrence, A. J., and Hannan, A. J. (2013). Depression-related behaviours displayed by female C57BL/6J mice during abstinence from chronic ethanol consumption are rescued by wheel-running. *Eur. J. Neurosci.* 37, 1803–1810. doi: 10.1111/ejn.12195

Pardy, K., Carter, D., and Murphy, D. (1990). Dopaminergic mediation of physiological changes in proopiomelanocortin messenger ribonucleic acid expression in the neurointermediate lobe of the rat pituitary. *Endocrinology* 126, 2960–2964. doi: 10.1210/endo-126-6-2960

Pastor, R., McKinnon, C. S., Scibelli, A. C., Burkhart-Kasch, S., Reed, C., Ryabinin, A. E., et al. (2008). Corticotropin-releasing factor-1 receptor involvement in behavioral neuroadaptation to ethanol: a urocortin1-independent mechanism. *Proc. Natl. Acad. Sci. U.S.A.* 105, 9070–9075. doi: 10.1073/pnas.0710181105

Pelc, I., Ansoms, C., Lehert, P., Fischer, F., Fuchs, W. J., Landron, F., et al. (2002). The European NEAT program: an integrated approach using acamprosate and psychosocial support for the prevention of relapse in alcohol-dependent patients with a statistical modeling of therapy success prediction. *Alcohol. Clin. Exp. Res.* 26, 1529–1538. doi: 10.1111/j.1530-0277.2002.tb02452.x

Perdona, E., Arban, R., and Griffante, C. (2012). Distinct receptor subtypes mediate arginine vasopressin-dependent ACTH release and intracellular calcium mobilization in rat pituitary cells. *Eur. J. Pharmacol.* 679, 16–23. doi: 10.1016/j.ejphar.2012.01.003

Picciotto, M. R., Brabant, C., Einstein, E. B., Kamens, H. M., and Neugebauer, N. M. (2010). Effects of galanin on monoaminergic systems and HPA axis: potential mechanisms underlying the effects of galanin on addiction- and stress-related behaviors. *Brain Res.* 1314, 206–218. doi: 10.1016/j.brainres.2009.08.033

Picetti, R., Schlussman, S. D., Zhou, Y., Ray, B., Ducat, E., Yuferov, V., et al. (2013). Addictions and stress: clues for cocaine pharmacotherapies. *Curr. Pharm. Des.* [Epub ahead of print].

Rasmussen, D. D., Boldt, B. M., Bryant, C. A., Mitton, D. R., Larsen, S. A., and Wilkinson, C. W. (2000). Chronic daily ethanol and withdrawal: 1. Long-term changes in the hypothalamo-pituitary-adrenal axis. *Alcohol. Clin. Exp. Res.* 24, 1836–1849. doi: 10.1111/j.1530-0277.2000.tb01988.x

Rasmussen, D. D., Mitton, D. R., Green, J., and Puchalski, S. (2001). Chronic daily ethanol and withdrawal: 2. Behavioral changes during prolonged abstinence. *Alcohol. Clin. Exp. Res.* 25, 999–1005. doi: 10.1111/j.1530-0277.2001.tb02308.x

Renoir, T., Pang, T. Y., and Lanfumey, L. (2012). Drug withdrawal-induced depression: serotonergic and plasticity changes in animal models. *Neurosci. Biobehav. Rev.* 36, 696–726. doi: 10.1016/j.neubiorev.2011.10.003

Richardson, H. N., Lee, S. Y., O'dell, L. E., Koob, G. F., and Rivier, C. L. (2008). Alcohol self-administration acutely stimulates the hypothalamic-pituitary-adrenal axis, but alcohol dependence leads to a dampened neuroendocrine state. *Eur. J. Neurosci.* 28, 1641–1653. doi: 10.1111/j.1460-9568.2008.06455.x

Roy, A., Mittal, N., Zhang, H., and Pandey, S. C. (2002). Modulation of cellular expression of glucocorticoid receptor and glucocorticoid response element-DNA binding in rat brain during alcohol drinking and withdrawal. *J. Pharmacol. Exp. Ther.* 301, 774–784. doi: 10.1124/jpet.301.2.774

Short, J. L., Ledent, C., Drago, J., and Lawrence, A. J. (2006). Receptor crosstalk: characterization of mice deficient in dopamine D1 and adenosine A2A receptors. *Neuropsychopharmacology* 31, 525–534. doi: 10.1038/sj.npp.1300852

Silva, S. M., and Madeira, M. D. (2012). Effects of chronic alcohol consumption and withdrawal on the response of the male and female hypothalamic-pituitary-adrenal axis to acute immune stress. *Brain Res.* 1444, 27–37. doi: 10.1016/j.brainres.2012.01.013

Sinha, R. (2008). Chronic stress, drug use, and vulnerability to addiction. *Ann. N.Y. Acad. Sci.* 1141, 105–130. doi: 10.1196/annals.1441.030

Skwara, A. J., Karwoski, T. E., Czambel, R. K., Rubin, R. T., and Rhodes, M. E. (2012). Influence of environmental enrichment on hypothalamic-pituitary-adrenal (HPA) responses to single-dose nicotine, continuous nicotine by osmotic mini-pumps, and nicotine withdrawal by mecamylamine in male and female rats. *Behav. Brain Res.* 234, 1–10. doi: 10.1016/j.bbr.2012.06.003

Solinas, M., Chauvet, C., Thiriet, N., El Rawas, R., and Jaber, M. (2008). Reversal of cocaine addiction by environmental enrichment. *Proc. Natl. Acad. Sci. U.S.A.* 105, 17145–17150. doi: 10.1073/pnas.0806889105

Stevenson, J. R., Schroeder, J. P., Nixon, K., Besheer, J., Crews, F. T., and Hodge, C. W. (2009). Abstinence following alcohol drinking produces depression-like behavior and reduced hippocampal neurogenesis in mice. *Neuropsychopharmacology* 34, 1209–1222. doi: 10.1038/npp.2008.90

Stuart, S. A., Butler, P., Munafo, M. R., Nutt, D. J., and Robinson, E. S. (2013). A translational rodent assay of affective biases in depression and antidepressant therapy. *Neuropsychopharmacology.* doi: 10.1038/npp.2013.69. [Epub ahead of print].

Thiel, K. J., Sanabria, F., and Neisewander, J. L. (2009). Synergistic interaction between nicotine and social rewards in adolescent male rats. *Psychopharmacology (Berl).* 204, 391–402. doi: 10.1007/s00213-009-1470-2

Vendruscolo, L. F., Barbier, E., Schlosburg, J. E., Misra, K. K., Whitfield, T. W. Jr., Logrip, M. L., et al. (2012). Corticosteroid-dependent plasticity mediates compulsive alcohol drinking in rats. *J. Neurosci.* 32, 7563–7571. doi: 10.1523/JNEUROSCI.0069-12.2012

Wang, X. Y., Zhao, M., Ghitza, U. E., Li, Y. Q., and Lu, L. (2008). Stress impairs reconsolidation of drug memory via glucocorticoid receptors in the basolateral amygdala. *J. Neurosci.* 28, 5602–5610. doi: 10.1523/JNEUROSCI.0750-08.2008

Zhou, Y., Colombo, G., Carai, M. A., Ho, A., Gessa, G. L., and Kreek, M. J. (2011a). Involvement of arginine vasopressin and V1b receptor in alcohol drinking in Sardinian alcohol-preferring rats. *Alcohol. Clin. Exp. Res.* 35, 1876–1883. doi: 10.1111/j.1530-0277.2011.01532.x

Zhou, Y., Litvin, Y., Piras, A. P., Pfaff, D. W., and Kreek, M. J. (2011b). Persistent increase in hypothalamic arginine vasopressin gene expression during protracted withdrawal from chronic escalating-dose cocaine in rodents. *Neuropsychopharmacology* 36, 2062–2075. doi: 10.1038/npp.2011.97

Zimmermann, U., Hundt, W., Spring, K., Grabner, A., and Holsboer, F. (2003). Hypothalamic-pituitary-adrenal system adaptation to detoxification in alcohol-dependent patients is affected by family history of alcoholism. *Biol. Psychiatry* 53, 75–84. doi: 10.1016/S0006-3223(02)01444-0

Conflict of Interest Statement: The authors declare that the research was conducted in the absence of any commercial or financial relationships that could be construed as a potential conflict of interest.

13

Controversies about the enhanced vulnerability of the adolescent brain to develop addiction

Aurélien Bernheim*[1]*, Olivier Halfon*[2]*, Benjamin Boutrel*[1,2]**

[1] *Center for Psychiatric Neuroscience, Division of Child and Adolescent Psychiatry, Lausanne University Hospital, Lausanne, Switzerland*
[2] *Division of Child and Adolescent Psychiatry, Lausanne University Hospital, Lausanne, Switzerland*

Edited by:
Laurence Lanfumey, Institut National de la Santé et de la Recherche Médicale, France

Reviewed by:
Sara Morley-Fletcher, Centre National de la Recherche Scientifique, University Lille, France
Jorge Mario Rodríguez-Fernandez, Yale University, USA

****Correspondence:***
Benjamin Boutrel, Center for Psychiatric Neuroscience, Division of Child and Adolescent Psychiatry, Lausanne University Hospital, CH-1008 Lausanne, Switzerland
e-mail: benjamin.boutrel@chuv.ch

Adolescence, defined as a transition phase toward autonomy and independence, is a natural time of learning and adjustment, particularly in the setting of long-term goals and personal aspirations. It also is a period of heightened sensation seeking, including risk taking and reckless behaviors, which is a major cause of morbidity and mortality among teenagers. Recent observations suggest that a relative immaturity in frontal cortical neural systems may underlie the adolescent propensity for uninhibited risk taking and hazardous behaviors. However, converging preclinical and clinical studies do not support a simple model of frontal cortical immaturity, and there is substantial evidence that adolescents engage in dangerous activities, including drug abuse, despite knowing and understanding the risks involved. Therefore, a current consensus considers that much brain development during adolescence occurs in brain regions and systems that are critically involved in the perception and evaluation of risk and reward, leading to important changes in social and affective processing. Hence, rather than naive, immature and vulnerable, the adolescent brain, particularly the prefrontal cortex, should be considered as prewired for expecting novel experiences. In this perspective, thrill seeking may not represent a danger but rather a window of opportunities permitting the development of cognitive control through multiple experiences. However, if the maturation of brain systems implicated in self-regulation is contextually dependent, it is important to understand which experiences matter most. In particular, it is essential to unveil the underpinning mechanisms by which recurrent adverse episodes of stress or unrestricted access to drugs can shape the adolescent brain and potentially trigger life-long maladaptive responses.

Keywords: drug addiction, adolescence, impulsivity, brain imaging, animal models

INTRODUCTION

A common consideration on addiction disorders acknowledges that individual characteristics may predispose to drug addiction; meanwhile excessive drug intake still is considered to influence personal traits and promote compulsive drug consumption (Swendsen and Le Moal, 2011). The vast majority of drug users are teenagers and young adults or began consuming during adolescence (O'Loughlin et al., 2009). In particular, a recent report of the National Survey on Drug Use and Health indicated that 31.2% of people below the age of 25 had consumed illicit drugs during the past month, while only 6.3% of older people acknowledged to do so (Substance Abuse and Mental Health Services Administration, 2010). The younger teenagers start using drugs, the more severe signs of drug addiction are. Among people in the USA that tried marijuana before the age of 14, 12.6% developed signs of drug abuse or dependence, while only 2.1% of those experiencing marijuana after the age of 18 suffered from severe signs of dependence (Substance Abuse and Mental Health Services Administration, 2010).

Adolescent risk-taking and reckless behavior is a major public health concern that increases the odds of poor lifetime outcomes, including loss of control over drug use. Compelling evidence based on imaging technologies have shown that brain circuitries involved in affective and cognitive processes interact dynamically across development. At the cellular level, these changes correspond with the marked overproduction of axons and synapses in early puberty, and rapid pruning in later adolescence and young adulthood. The current consensus considers that patterns of neural connection among systems of emotion, motivation and cognitive processes related to the pursuit of long-term goals undergo a natural reorganization and a set of maturational refinements during adolescence (Gogtay et al., 2004; Giedd, 2008). In contrast to the relatively early and rapid changes in affective systems that appear to be linked to pubertal maturation, another set of cognitive skills and competence in self-control seem to develop gradually across adolescence and continue to mature long after puberty is over (Dahl, 2008). This key observation may explain why adolescence is characterized by an imbalance between the relative influences of motivational and control systems on behavior (Somerville et al., 2011). As a consequence, the adolescent brain is a tempted brain as long as the development of executive functions including relevant decision making and planning, abstract reasoning and response inhibition remains unfinished (Dahl, 2008).

In this perspective, taking drugs during adolescence may interfere with the normal brain development, and may increase the vulnerability to abuse drugs later during adulthood (Andersen, 2003; Crews et al., 2007). Despite the growing number of prevention campaigns, drug consumption in adolescents remains quite stable over the past years. Strikingly, a relevant communication released in 1952 already acknowledged that "*drug addiction in adolescence is not a new phenomenon*" (Zimmering et al., 1952), and the ultimate question was already clearly identified "*However, there is still the question of why, under apparently similar external conditions, some boys will try the drugs and others won't, why some go down the road of addiction while others give up the drug* (. . .)." Sixty years later, this question remains partially unanswered. Animal models, especially rodents, have contributed to a better comprehension of the juvenile state. In particular, converging evidence has pointed out to an enhanced vulnerability to drug abuse in adolescents, but questions and controversies remain regarding the relevance of the different animal models and the interpretation of the data (Schramm-Sapyta et al., 2009). Interestingly, these authors conclude that even if an increased recreational drug use is usually observed during adolescence, evidence relating to pathological drug seeking and taking still is lacking. In this review, we try to summarize the biological factors relevant to adolescent driving risks and we discuss the clinical observations in the light of preclinical findings linking impulsivity and emotional reactivity to initiation of drug use and risks of abuse.

PUBERTY AND ADOLESCENCE

Risk taking during adolescence is the product of an interaction between heightened stimulation seeking and an immature self-regulatory system that is not yet able to modulate reward-seeking impulses (Steinberg and Morris, 2001; Steinberg, 2004, 2005). A consensus could put adolescents at risk for emotional and behavioral disorders. Nevertheless, increased risk and novelty seeking can be beneficial for learning novel strategies for survival (Kelley et al., 2004). Indeed, from an anthropologic perspective, some types of risk taking can be viewed as an adaptive willingness to demonstrate bravery in order to acquire a better social status. In many situations, it seems that adolescent do not become more fearless after puberty but rather they may become more highly motivated to act boldly despite their fears, particularly when they perceive that acting in a brave or reckless way might bring them increased recognition by peers (Dahl, 2008).

The period of adolescence is a time of considerable change, as sex-specific pubertal hormones bring about changes in physical stature, reproductive organs and other secondary sexual characteristics. Neuroendocrine changes during puberty influence behavioral and emotional development (Waylen and Wolke, 2004). Since testosterone cross the blood brain barrier (Pardridge and Mietus, 1979), it contributes to the cortical pruning during adolescence, especially in frontal and temporal lobes (Witte et al., 2010; Nguyen et al., 2013). This observation is of interest and may explain sexual dimorphism in gray matter and its behavioral consequences (Neufang et al., 2009; Paus et al., 2010; Bramen et al., 2012).

A classical strategy to assess this influence is to select adolescents of similar age, but experiencing different stage of puberty. Mid-late puberty adolescents differ from adolescents in early puberty in their emotional regulation of startle response and postauricular reflex, two physiological measure of defensive and appetitive motivation (Quevedo et al., 2009). Similar results have been reported with mid/late puberty adolescents displaying an enhanced pupil dilatation in response to emotional words (Silk et al., 2009).

GRADUAL EMERGENCE OF COGNITIVE SELF-CONTROL DURING ADOLESCENCE: INSIGHT FROM NEUROIMAGING

The adolescent behavior, marked by intense affective expression and impulsive responses, has long been studied, but the most recent imaging technologies have contributed to a better knowledge of the developing brain during adolescence. In particular, it has been shown that proportion of gray matter decreases whereas white matter increases during transition from childhood to young adulthood (Paus et al., 1999; Lenroot and Giedd, 2006). Whereas the enhanced myelination follows a quite linear pattern all over the brain, with only slight local variations, the diminution of gray matter, also called synaptic pruning, is more selective. Hence, myelination is not only considered as an electrical insulator that increases the speed of neuronal signal transmission, but also as a key process that modulates the timing and synchrony of neuronal firing patterns that convey meaning in the brain (Giedd, 2008). The main neurobiological changes that account for risky behaviors in adolescence occur in the mesocorticolimbic system, particularly in the prefrontal structures (Chambers et al., 2003; Crews et al., 2007; Crews and Boettiger, 2009). Studies comparing adult and adolescent cortical function indicate that adolescent process information differently, often enlisting different brain regions than adults. Difficulty with executive cognitive functioning and behavioral self-control, including difficulties with planning, attention, foresight, abstract reasoning, judgment, and self-monitoring have been reported in adolescents, and several functional magnetic resonance imaging (fMRI) studies have examined the functional neuroanatomy underlying executive processing in children, adolescent and adults (Luna et al., 2010). This growing body of evidence supports the idea that frontostriatal systems undergo significant remodeling in the period from adolescence to young adulthood. Specifically, protracted development of prefrontal cortex (PFC), in concert with an amplified motivational drive mediated by the striatum, is thought to be critical to increased novelty seeking and suboptimal decision making that leads to risky behavior and experimental drug use. Assuming that orbitofrontal cortex (OFC) is critical to making value decisions, individual differences in the development of this region might increase or decrease sensitivity to reward through suboptimal computation of incentive value based on reward magnitude coded by the striatum. Conversely, reduced orbitofrontal modulation of striatal-mediated motivational drive could lead to increased novelty seeking and impulsive choice. In either case, significant imbalance in the neurodevelopmental trajectory of this circuit could lead to loss of self-control during a vulnerable period (Yurgelun-Todd, 2007).

The immature connections between the PFC, the nucleus accumbens (Nacc) and the amygdala have been proposed to largely influence goal-directed behaviors in adolescents (Galvan et al., 2006; Ernst et al., 2009). In particular, it has been shown that teenagers engage the orbitofrontal cortex to a much lesser extent compared to adults when facing risky choices. Similarly, adolescents have been also shown to display a decreased and uncoordinated neuronal processing in the OFC during simple reward-related behavior (Sturman and Moghaddam, 2011). These types of observation may partially explain the increased propensity for reckless behaviors during adolescence (Eshel et al., 2007). Finally, in order to emphasize the adolescent brain immaturity upon reward expectations, compelling evidence recently demonstrated a linear reduction of insular activation along with age, with early adolescents displaying the higher activation and late adolescents exhibiting the most reduced signal while gambling in a slot machine task (Van Leijenhorst et al., 2010).

Several epidemiological researches support the idea that adolescence is the life period with the highest rate of impulsive behavior (Steinberg et al., 2008; Romer et al., 2009). Steinberg and colleagues described a linear decrease of impulsivity from the age of 10–30: using different age cohorts, steeper delay discounting and weaker performances on the IOWA gambling task (IGT) have been reported in adolescents, compared to adults (Steinberg et al., 2009; Cauffman et al., 2010). A longitudinal study using the IGT in adolescents aged from 11 to 18 confirmed this result by showing that performance improved continuously with age (Overman et al., 2004). These observations are thought to mirror the maturation of the PFC, which allows the transition from impulsive to more controlled choices. Conversely, an inverted-U shape curve for sensation seeking has been reported as well, with a peak around age 14 (Steinberg et al., 2008). Again, the dissociation between the progressive development of impulse control and the non-linear development of the reward system may result in a misbalance that enhances impulsive choices for reward (Ernst et al., 2009).

Converging fMRI studies exploring decision-making tasks have shown that adolescents and adults share many similarities in neurocircuitry activation, but they also display intriguing differences. A greater response in the left Nacc was reported in teenagers while adults displayed an increased activation in the left amygdala (Ernst et al., 2005). Galvan et al. (2006) also reported enhanced Nacc response to reward in adolescent compared to adults, as well as reduced activation in areas of the frontal cortex. Most recently, in a study examining risk taking in monetary decision-making, it has been shown that adolescents displayed a reduced activation in regions of the OFC compared with adults, and reduced activity in these frontal brain regions was correlated with greater risk-taking tendencies in teens (Eshel et al., 2007). These findings suggest that adolescents engage relatively fewer prefrontal regulatory processes than adults when making decisions. Consequently teenagers may be more prone to risk taking in certain situations. In other words, reduced prefrontal cognitive control may authorize a greater influence of affective systems that dictate decision making and behavior which, in turn, increases adolescent vulnerability to social and peer contexts that activate strong feelings (Dahl, 2008).

In a recent study aiming at assessing adolescent and adult behaviors in a video driving game, it has been shown that adolescent participants took more risks, focused more on the benefits than the costs of risky behavior, and made riskier decisions when surrounded by peers compared to adults (Gardner and Steinberg, 2005). These findings confirm that adolescents may be more prone to peer influences on risky decision-making, and that peer influence (and other social-context variables) may play an important role in explaining reckless behaviors during adolescence. Interestingly, it has been established that young adolescents, categorized as highly resistant to peer influence, displayed enhanced brain connectivity, especially in the frontal cortex, compared to adolescents categorized as highly influenced by peers (Grosbras et al., 2007). Resistance to peer influence has also been positively correlated with ventral striatum activation, but negatively correlated with activation in the amygdala (Pfeifer et al., 2011). Specific pattern of cortical activation in adolescents has been reported by using mentalizing, face recognition and theory of mind tasks. For example, early adolescents aged from 10 to 14 engaged more their medial PFC than adults to analyze the intent of a drawing (sincere or ironic), despite similar performance on the task (Wang et al., 2006). This might reflect a greater effort for the youngsters to perceive social emotional situations they are not yet used to, while adults analyze these situations more effectively, based upon previous experiences.

Noteworthy, adolescence also represents a particular period of emotional perception and regulation. Cognition and decision-making processes in adolescents are highly influenced by their emotional state, a phenomenon called hot cognition (in opposition to cool cognition, in which decision-making occurs under low emotional level). Adolescents also seem to be more sensitive to stressful stimuli. The rate of cortisol release after a stressful task displayed a linear increase with age, in young adolescents aged from 9 to 15 years (Gunnar et al., 2009; Stroud et al., 2009). Presenting fearful faces, induced a higher reactivity of the amygdala in adolescents compared with children and adults (Hare et al., 2008). Interestingly, the habituation of amygdala activity to these fearful faces was lower in subjects screened for high trait anxiety. This enhanced sensitivity to stressful stimuli, together with a higher proportion of hot cognition, constitutes another support for adolescents' reckless behaviors when coping with anxiogenic situations.

ARE TEENS MORE VULNERABLE TO DRUG ABUSE THAN ADULTS?

Higher impulsivity is considered to promote drug first use, and eventually may lead to an increased vulnerability to develop drug addiction, defined as a loss of control over drug consumption and a compulsive pattern of drug use (Belin et al., 2008). Impulsivity is not easily defined (Evenden, 1999; Chamberlain and Sahakian, 2007), but a broad definition would include lack of attention, difficulty to suppress or control a behavioral response, pronounced novelty-seeking behavior, inability to anticipate consequences, difficulty to plan actions or reduced problem-solving strategies as key features. Because adolescents display more impulsive behaviors, the link between impulsivity and drug consumption has been extensively studied.

Converging studies using self-report questionnaire in teens demonstrated that impulsivity during adolescence was predictive of drug use and gambling (Romer et al., 2009), smoking initiation (O'Loughlin et al., 2009) and later alcohol abuse (Ernst et al., 2006; von Diemen et al., 2008). Reciprocally, impulsivity appeared to be exaggerated in adolescents with alcohol use disorders compared to healthy control (Soloff et al., 2000). Further, a study assessing genetic polymorphism has also demonstrated that a particular allele (A1) from the Taq1a polymorphism of the dopamine D2 receptor gene was positively correlated with alcohol and drug use (Esposito-Smythers et al., 2009). Concomitantly, impulsive carriers of the allele reported significantly more alcohol and drug-related problems than impulsive non-carriers. These findings highlight the interaction between vulnerability factors in the propensity to develop psychiatric troubles.

Cognitive impulsivity, defined as an inability to consider future outcomes, is a subdivision of impulsivity that takes into account emotional subjective representation of a delayed outcome. This concept is known as the discounting value of a reward (Rachlin, 1992). The use of the delay discounting, which offers to choose between immediate low rewards and future higher rewards, has contributed to better understand the neurobiological underpinnings of economic choice and decision-making. Adolescent tobacco smokers were found to be more impulsive than their non-smoker couterparts in a delay discounting task, and more prone to novelty seeking (Peters et al., 2011). Interestingly, the same group of adolescent smokers showed a marked decrease of striatal activation during a reward anticipation paradigm, which was positively correlated with smoking frequency. It is important to note that the increased impulsiveness reported in adolescent smokers might be a consequence, and not a predictor, of the addicted behavior. Studies comparing current and ex-smokers suggested that enhanced delay discounting curve concerns only current smoker (Bickel et al., 1999, 2008). However, other studies revealed that cognitive impulsivity could constitute a possible predictor of later substance use. Naïve adolescents, having a first cigarette smoking experience, were more impulsive in a delay discounting task (Reynolds and Fields, 2012). Nicotine intoxication is most likely not responsible for such results; it may rather reflect a personality trait shared by most of the adolescent smokers. Higher propensity to impulsive choices was also found to be predictive of the first ecstasy use in females (Schilt et al., 2009), and was also associated with binge drinking (Xiao et al., 2009).

It has been suggested that impulsivity represents a good index to predict the outcome of a smoking-cessation program: adolescents screened for higher impulsive trait significantly failed to maintain abstinence compared their non-impulsive counterparts (Krishnan-Sarin et al., 2007). Cognitive therapies targeting impulsivity, as reviewed elsewhere (Moeller et al., 2001), may constitute untapped opportunities for developing new approach to develop effective self-control in adolescents. This may contribute to prevent reckless behaviors occurring during this period of important morbidity.

MODELING THE ADOLESCENT VULNERABILITY TO DRUG ABUSE

Brain development in juvenile rodents has been reported to display similar patterns resembling those of human beings, suggesting that the rodent model might be relevant to study the neurobiological underpinnings of teenage brain maturation (Spear, 2000). The juvenile period in rodents lasts from day 28 to day 42 after birth, but these limits, a bit restrictive, are usually extended to include a larger period from day 25 to day 55 (Tirelli et al., 2003). Neuroanatomical studies have described a massive synaptic pruning of dopamine receptors during adolescence in rodents (Andersen et al., 2000): D1 and D2 receptors density increased in the Nacc, the striatum and the PFC until the age of 40 days, and then progressively declined during early adulthood. Conversely, D3 receptors increased until 60 days (Stanwood et al., 1997). Another study revealed an increase of dopamine fibers in the medial PFC soon after weaning (Benes et al., 2000), that was in part controlled by the serotoninergic system: neonatal lesion of the raphe nucleus led to an increase of dopamine (DA) fibers sprouting from the ventral tegmental area (VTA) and the substantia nigra. Additionally, glutamatergic innervations from the PFC to the Nacc (Brenhouse et al., 2008) and to the amygdala (Cunningham et al., 2002) has been shown to follow a linear sprouting from weaning age to early adulthood. Dopaminergic modulation during adolescence appeared to be not entirely functional: the effects of D1 and D2 agonist on GABAergic interneurons in the PFC were weaker in adolescent, suggesting an uncompleted maturation of this modulatory system (Tseng and O'Donnell, 2007).

Behavioral studies comparing juvenile and adult rodents revealed that mice displayed a greater preference for a novel environment (Adriani et al., 1998), and enhanced impulsive responses compared to adults in a delay discounting task (Adriani and Laviola, 2003). Juvenile rodents also expressed a higher level of social interaction since social interactions were found to be more rewarding in juvenile than in adults rodents in a conditioned place preference (CPP) paradigm (Douglas et al., 2004). In line with this observation, a study reported that juvenile rats had lesser activation of dopamine signaling in the Nacc when facing non-social stimuli, but a more persistent response to social stimuli compared with adults (Robinson et al., 2011). This might reflect the importance of social interaction in juvenile animals.

In the elevated plus maze, adolescent rats spent a reduced period of time in the open arms, indicating a higher anxiety (Doremus et al., 2003; Estanislau and Morato, 2006; Lynn and Brown, 2010) although mice displayed a reversed profile (Macrì et al., 2002). Similar observations were reported using a contextual fear conditioning: adolescent rats froze significantly more than adults (Anagnostaras et al., 1999; Brasser and Spear, 2004; Esmoris-Arranz et al., 2008), but again adolescent mice froze less than adults (Pattwell et al., 2011).

With regards to the aversive effects of drugs, it has been shown that nicotine, ethanol, THC, amphetamine and cocaine induced less aversive effects in adolescent than in adult animals. In addition, conditioned taste aversion performed with a non-addictive substance (lithium chloride that induces abdominal pain after i.p. injections) is reduced in adolescent rats suggesting that insensitivity to aversive effects may be a generalized feature of adolescence (Philpot et al., 2003; Wilmouth and Spear, 2004; Schramm-Sapyta et al., 2006, 2007; Quinn et al., 2008; Drescher et al., 2011).

Meanwhile, several studies have reported increased reward sensitivity in juvenile animals. Nicotine and alcohol were found to be more rewarding in young rodents compared with adults (Philpot et al., 2003; Brielmaier et al., 2007; Kota et al., 2007; Torres et al.,

2008; Spear and Varlinskaya, 2010). Similarly, increased sweetened condensed milk consumption (relative to body weight) was observed in adolescent rats compared with older ones. This behavioral observation was correlated with an increased c-fos expression in the Nacc core and the dorsal striatum (Friemel et al., 2010). Investigations assessing the effect of psychostimulants in adolescent rats using a CPP task remain a bit controversial, but a greater reward sensitivity in adolescents rats, particularly at lower doses, has been claimed in specific conditions (Badanich et al., 2006; Brenhouse et al., 2008; Zakharova et al., 2009).

FACTORS INFLUENCING DRUG ABUSE IN ADOLESCENT RODENTS

Motor impulsivity refers to behavioral disinhibition and loss of impulse control, without necessary integration of emotional processing (Brunner and Hen, 1997). In animals, many behavioral tests have been shaped to assess this form of impulsivity, such as the five-choice serial reaction time task (5-CSRTT) and the differential reinforcement of low-rate (DRL). To our knowledge, the only study comparing impulsivity in non-treated normal adult and adolescent rats revealed that the latter were more impulsive in a DRL schedule (Andrzejewski et al., 2011). Prenatal exposure to nicotine has been shown to increase impulsivity in a 5-CSRTT during adolescence (Schneider et al., 2012), and chronic exposure to nicotine in adolescent rats produced long-lasting increase of motor impulsivity during adulthood (Counotte et al., 2009, 2011). In this study, nicotine chronic treatment was able to induce more impulsive behaviors on the 5-CSRTT when occurred during adolescence than during adulthood. This specific alteration, which did not affect cognitive impulsivity in a delay discounting task, has been correlated with a stronger nicotine-induced dopamine release in the PFC in adolescent rats. Similarly, impulsive adolescents, screened with the latency to approach a novel object, displayed an enhanced DA response to a cocaine challenge compared to non-impulsive adolescents or impulsive young adults (Stansfield and Kirstein, 2005).

However, prenatal treatment with nicotine, shown to alter motor impulsivity, failed to alter behavioral responses in a delay-discounting task (Schneider et al., 2012). While the influence between cognitive impulsivity and drug-seeking behaviors has been well established in humans, supplementary observations will be necessary to understand how it works in rodents. Diergaarde et al. (2008) have proposed that, at least in adult rats, motor impulsivity may be related to the initiation of drug seeking, while cognitive impulsivity may be associated with a decreased ability to suppress an acquired nicotine-seeking behavior and increased vulnerability to relapse. Ultimately, motor impulsivity, but not cognitive impulsivity might be more appropriate to assess drug-seeking vulnerability in juvenile rats.

Some basal differences of Hypothalamo-Pituitary-Adrenal (HPA) axis regulation may underlie an increased sensitivity to stressful stimuli in adolescent rodents. After an acute stress, adolescent rats displayed a higher adrenocorticotropic hormone (ACTH) and corticosterone release compared to adults (Romeo et al., 2006a,b). After a 30-min chronic restraint stress every day during 7 days, juvenile rats exhibited higher corticosterone levels immediately after the stressor, but corticosterone levels return to baseline values faster in adolescent than in adult rats (Romeo et al., 2006a). Male rats have been found to be more sensitive than females to the deleterious effects of maternal separation on PFC thickness (Spivey et al., 2009). Given the relations between stress and drug-seeking behaviors (Shaham et al., 2000; Koob and Le Moal, 2001), this increased sensitivity of the stress system may explain why some adolescents persist in drug abuse. A chronic cocaine treatment during adolescence increased several measures of anxiety when animals had become adults (Stansfield and Kirstein, 2005), which may further explain this persistence.

Compared to controls, rats stressed for 7 consecutive days during adolescence showed higher nicotine-induced enhancement of locomotor activity; this effect was not reported when stress occurred during adulthood (Cruz et al., 2008). Adolescent rats exposed to either a chronic restraint stress or a multiple-stress protocol showed higher locomotor response to cocaine challenge, and higher basal corticosterone level as well (Lepsch et al., 2005). Social stresses during adolescence increased behavioral sensitization to amphetamine (Mathews et al., 2008), but opposite effects were also reported (Kabbaj et al., 2002). Maternal separation was shown to increase impulsivity and reward-seeking behaviors (Colorado et al., 2006). Three hours of maternal separation between PND 0 and PND 14 increased the locomotor sensitization to cocaine, which was associated with an increase in D3R mRNA in the Nacc shell (Brake et al., 2004). Nevertheless, another study found no effect using a chronic social isolation on the locomotor response to psychostimulants either in adolescent or adult male rats (McCormick et al., 2005).

THE JUVENILE RODENT MODEL: PROMISES AND PITFALLS

Most studies point out to an increased drug-seeking behavior in juvenile rodents, suggesting work hypotheses to explain why teens are at risk to lose control over drug intake. First, enhanced sensitivity to drug reward and two, lowered drug-induced aversive side effects provide a good rationale for studying juvenile rats vulnerability to drug abuse. However, no animal study has so far directly demonstrated an increased susceptibility to compulsive drug intake when first drug intoxication occurs during adolescence. Some methodological issues may also promote some misinterpretations, such as the lack of appropriate adult controls. As mentioned above, rats and mice appear to exhibit opposite anxiety profiles, with juvenile rats more anxious and juvenile mice less anxious than adults (Macrì et al., 2002; Lynn and Brown, 2010). Importantly, a few studies illustrated behavioral differences between early, mid and late adolescence (Tirelli et al., 2003; Wilkin et al., 2012), but most studies actually used juvenile rats of different ages that differed from one lab to the other. Further, the lack of consideration of social influence on drug consumption and related behavior may constitute another important confounding factor. Indeed, social interactions have been shown to highly influence risky behaviors and drug abuse. In particular, it has been reported that social interaction linked to a suboptimal cocaine dose could produce a CPP (Thiel et al., 2008). Meanwhile, the presence of counterparts decreased the aversive effect of ethanol in a conditioned taste aversion paradigm in male adolescent rats, but not in adults (Vetter-O'Hagen et al., 2009).

Ventral tegmental area dopaminergic neurons have been claimed to fire at a higher rate in adolescent rats, which is consistent with the hypothesis of adolescent vulnerability to drug abuse (McCutcheon et al., 2012). In line with this observation, a higher drug-induced dopamine release has been reported in adolescent rodents (Laviola et al., 2001; Walker and Kuhn, 2008). However, behavioral response to drugs does not fit with this conclusion. In particular, subchronic treatment with psychostimulants failed to induce an increased locomotor sensitization in adolescent rats (Frantz et al., 2007). Of particular importance, Frantz et al. (2007) reported similar dopamine release in the Nacc between adolescents and adults rats treated with psychostimulants. Conversely, one study reported a locomotor sensitization to cocaine in juvenile mice and not in adults (Camarini et al., 2008); however, a cocaine challenge performed 10 days after this experiment showed a lower dopamine release in the Nacc of juvenile mice, despite a faster onset peak. Further studies will be necessary to determine the relation between DA release and locomotor sensitization to psychostimulants in adolescent rats.

Although stress and impulsivity have been shown separately to promote drug use, a few studies established cross-regulations between both. Intracerebroventricular injections of corticotropin-releasing factor (CRF) did not increase impulsivity in the 5-CSRTT, but increased accuracy responding (Ohmura et al., 2009). A chronic treatment with corticosterone during adolescence failed to affect premature responses in this task, and even decreased the number of impulsive behaviors in a Stop signal task (Torregrossa et al., 2012). More studies are needed to fully understand this interaction, which is considered as a key element exaggerating the emergence of psychiatric disorders in human (Fox et al., 2010; Somer et al., 2012; Hamilton et al., 2013).

Another source of controversy is the conjecture according to which the juvenile rodents would exhibit reduced self-control and increased attraction to cues predicting reward (Ernst et al., 2009; Burton et al., 2011). In opposition with this statement, juvenile rats were shown to display a lower cue-induced reinstatement of cocaine intake (Anker and Carroll, 2010). Further contrasting with the above mentioned conjecture, juvenile mice (26–27 days) were shown to exhibit enhanced flexibility compared to adults in an odor-cue based procedure (Johnson and Wilbrecht, 2011). Given the immaturity of the PFC in juvenile rats, as well as the key role of this structure in cognitive flexibility (Baxter et al., 2000; Schoenbaum et al., 2006; Gruber et al., 2010), this result might appear counterintuitive. Nonetheless, an enhanced flexibility of adolescents might help to promote a switch between a large number of options, such as quitting drug intake in favor of a less detrimental behavior. It therefore tends to alleviate the omnipresence of vulnerability elements in juvenile rodents, since cognitive flexibility is mandatory to acquire a behavioral repertoire necessary for survival and autonomy.

It is important to acknowledge that only a minority of youngsters experiencing recreational drugs will later develop clinical symptoms of drug addiction and dependence, although the contribution of fundamental research using animal models remains quite limited to support this assertion. A current consensus suggests that interindividual variations in brain maturation might explain excessive behavioral outputs. Of particular interest, recent evidence demonstrated that first, individuals with pronounced impulsive traits displayed a thinner cortex (Shaw et al., 2011) and second, the activation of the mesolimbic neurocircuitry of adolescents trained to gamble in a monetary incentive task correlated positively with their psychosocial and behavioral difficulties (Bjork et al., 2011). The authors of this study elegantly acknowledge that correlation most likely does not imply causality but, nonetheless, these observations suggest that increased engagement in problematic behaviors may partly result from mesolimbic sensitivity to reward-predictive cues. And they conclude that increased mesolimbic sensitivity may represent a trait that, in line with the general immaturity of the adolescent brain, could partly explain behavior-related injury or death in "at-risk" adolescents (Bjork et al., 2011).

Some external factors, like sociodemographic status or familial environment, have also been considered to play a role in this variability. Adverse events in childhood were shown to be predictive of later alcohol dependence (Pilowsky et al., 2009). Converging evidence has established the negative influence of parental misconducts (including substance use disorders) on children propensity to develop similar disorders (Verdejo-Garcia et al., 2008). Gene polymorphisms among adolescents with alcohol-related disorders have been proposed to explain interindividual differences in attentional bias toward alcohol (Pieters et al., 2011), or in stress responsivity to drugs (Kreek et al., 2005). Although genetic factors have been thought to explain between 30 and 60% of addictive disorders (Kreek et al., 2005), gene influence mainly depends on interaction with environmental factors. In particular, a gene polymorphism was shown to be closely related to alcoholism in adults, and also in a subpopulation of adolescents that were exposed to high psychosocial stress during childhood (Clarke et al., 2011). A similar correlation has been found with a specific genotype of the serotonin transporter (Kaufman et al., 2007). In adolescents diagnosed for anxiety disorders, depression, or in healthy controls, amygdala pattern of activation in response to emotional faces was dependent of the pathology diagnosed (Beesdo et al., 2009).

CONCLUSION

Risk taking and sensation seeking have long been considered hallmarks of typical adolescent behavior and, meanwhile, have been thought to represent vulnerability factors for developing substance abuse disorders. Strikingly, despite a large number of preclinical investigations delineating the brain circuitries underpinning enhanced impulsiveness and increased emotional reactivity constitutive of an extended behavioral repertoire, very few studies support a specific vulnerability of juvenile rodents to lose control over drugs of abuse. A provocative statement would argue that science should better see the adult world with adolescent eyes, rather than seeing the adolescent world using an adult watch. Indeed, juvenile behaviors present adaptive benefits to acquire appropriate skills for survival in absence of parental protection. Meanwhile, it is true that these externalizing behaviors make adolescents, or at least a subset of teens, more vulnerable to reckless conducts and potential injuries. Objectively, the adolescent brain is prewired for sensation seeking and risk taking which, in line with the heightened motivation for reward, often leads to careless behaviors.

The development of self-regulatory competence is a normative process (that depends on both brain maturation and social experiences) at the end of which young adults have acquired the aptitude to better regulate their emotions and impulsiveness.

A major aim for future researches consists in finding endophenotypes and vulnerability markers of substance use disorders and drug abuse. It has been recently demonstrated that people suffering from substance abuse disorders shared with their non-addict siblings similar behavioral traits, including high impulsivity and sensation-seeking (Ersche et al., 2010). This study also revealed that abnormal prefrontal and striatal connectivity might underpin risks of drug addiction (Ersche et al., 2012). In complement, converging evidence have revealed that interindividual differences arise from heterogeneity in the PFC function (George and Koob, 2010). Therefore, deeper investigations assessing PFC interindividual adaptations during adolescence are required to understand how only specific developmental trajectories can lead to drug addiction. In particular, understanding whether (and if true, how) deficient brain maturation processes might be responsible for sustained reward seeking and poor decision-making (meaning persistence in risk taking despite adverse consequences) is of the highest importance to better protect "at-risk" young adults. A current consensus already acknowledges that the developing adolescent brain is fragile and vulnerable to neurobiological insults concomitant to drug abuse, in particular those related to alcohol intoxication (Crews et al., 2004). But, further preclinical and clinical studies focusing on the adolescent PFC are required to better understand how genes, environment, stress and individual temperament interact together to shape the neurobiological mechanisms underpinning the vulnerability to lose control over reward seeking, and potentially excessive drug taking, during the transition from the adolescent world to the adult universe.

REFERENCES

Adriani, W., Chiarotti, F., and Laviola, G. (1998). Elevated novelty seeking and peculiar d-amphetamine sensitization in periadolescent mice compared with adult mice. *Behav. Neurosci.* 112, 1152–1166. doi: 10.1037/0735-7044.112.5.1152

Adriani, W., and Laviola, G. (2003). Elevated levels of impulsivity and reduced place conditioning with d-amphetamine: two behavioral features of adolescence in mice. *Behav. Neurosci.* 117, 695–703. doi: 10.1037/0735-7044.117.4.695

Anagnostaras, S. G., Maren, S., Sage, J. R., Goodrich, S., and Fanselow, M. S. (1999). Scopolamine and Pavlovian fear conditioning in rats: dose-effect analysis. *Neuropsychopharmacology* 21, 731–744. doi: 10.1016/S0893-133X(99)00083-4

Andersen, S. L. (2003). Trajectories of brain development: point of vulnerability or window of opportunity? *Neurosci. Biobehav. Rev.* 27, 3–18. doi: 10.1016/S0149-7634(03)00005-8

Andersen, S. L., Thompson, A. T., Rutstein, M., Hostetter, J. C., and Teicher, M. H. (2000). Dopamine receptor pruning in prefrontal cortex during the periadolescent period in rats. *Synapse* 37, 167–169. doi: 10.1002/1098-2396(200008)37:2<167::AID-SYN11>3.0.CO;2-B

Andrzejewski, M. E., Schochet, T. L., Feit, E. C., Harris, R., Mckee, B. L., and Kelley, A. E. (2011). A comparison of adult and adolescent rat behavior in operant learning, extinction, and behavioral inhibition paradigms. *Behav. Neurosci.* 125, 93–105. doi: 10.1037/a0022038

Anker, J. J., and Carroll, M. E. (2010). Reinstatement of cocaine seeking induced by drugs, cues, and stress in adolescent and adult rats. *Psychopharmacology (Berl.)* 208, 211–222. doi: 10.1007/s00213-009-1721-2

Badanich, K. A., Adler, K. J., and Kirstein, C. L. (2006). Adolescents differ from adults in cocaine conditioned place preference and cocaine-induced dopamine in the nucleus accumbens septi. *Eur. J. Pharmacol.* 550, 95–106. doi: 10.1016/j.ejphar.2006.08.034

Baxter, M. G., Parker, A., Lindner, C. C., Izquierdo, A. D., and Murray, E. A. (2000). Control of response selection by reinforcer value requires interaction of amygdala and orbital prefrontal cortex. *J. Neurosci.* 20, 4311–4319.

Beesdo, K., Lau, J. Y., Guyer, A. E., Mcclure-Tone, E. B., Monk, C. S., Nelson, E. E., et al. (2009). Common and distinct amygdala-function perturbations in depressed vs anxious adolescents. *Arch. Gen. Psychiatry* 66, 275–285. doi: 10.1001/archgenpsychiatry.2008.545

Belin, D., Mar, A. C., Dalley, J. W., Robbins, T. W., and Everitt, B. J. (2008). High impulsivity predicts the switch to compulsive cocaine-taking. *Science* 320, 1352–1355. doi: 10.1126/science.1158136

Benes, F. M., Taylor, J. B., and Cunningham, M. C. (2000). Convergence and plasticity of monoaminergic systems in the medial prefrontal cortex during the postnatal period: implications for the development of psychopathology. *Cereb. Cortex* 10, 1014–1027. doi: 10.1093/cercor/10.10.1014

Bickel, W. K., Odum, A. L., and Madden, G. J. (1999). Impulsivity and cigarette smoking: delay discounting in current, never, and ex-smokers. *Psychopharmacology (Berl.)* 146, 447–454. doi: 10.1007/PL00005490

Bickel, W. K., Yi, R., Kowal, B. P., and Gatchalian, K. M. (2008). Cigarette smokers discount past and future rewards symmetrically and more than controls: is discounting a measure of impulsivity? *Drug Alcohol Depend.* 96, 256–262. doi: 10.1016/j.drugalcdep.2008.03.009

Bjork, J. M., Smith, A. R., Chen, G., and Hommer, D. W. (2011). Psychosocial problems and recruitment of incentive neurocircuitry: exploring individual differences in healthy adolescents. *Dev. Cogn. Neurosci.* 1, 570–577. doi: 10.1016/j.dcn.011.07.005

Brake, W. G., Zhang, T. Y., Diorio, J., Meaney, M. J., and Gratton, A. (2004). Influence of early postnatal rearing conditions on mesocorticolimbic dopamine and behavioural responses to psychostimulants and stressors in adult rats. *Eur. J. Neurosci.* 19, 1863–1874. doi: 10.1111/j.1460-9568.2004.03286.x

Bramen, J. E., Hranilovich, J. A., Dahl, R. E., Chen, J., Rosso, C., Forbes, E. E., et al. (2012). Sex matters during adolescence: testosterone-related cortical thickness maturation differs between boys and girls. *PLoS ONE* 7:e33850. doi: 10.1371/journal.pone.0033850

Brasser, S. M., and Spear, N. E. (2004). Contextual conditioning in infants, but not older animals, is facilitated by CS conditioning. *Neurobiol. Learn. Mem.* 81, 46–59. doi: 10.1016/S1074-7427(03)00068-6

Brenhouse, H. C., Sonntag, K. C., and Andersen, S. L. (2008). Transient D1 dopamine receptor expression on prefrontal cortex projection neurons: relationship to enhanced motivational salience of drug cues in adolescence. *J. Neurosci.* 28, 2375–2382. doi: 10.1523/JNEUROSCI.5064-07.2008

Brielmaier, J. M., Mcdonald, C. G., and Smith, R. F. (2007). Immediate and long-term behavioral effects of a single nicotine injection in adolescent and adult rats. *Neurotoxicol. Teratol.* 29, 74–80. doi: 10.1016/j.ntt.2006.09.023

Brunner, D., and Hen, R. (1997). Insights into the neurobiology of impulsive behavior from serotonin receptor knockout mice. *Ann. N. Y. Acad. Sci.* 836, 81–105. doi: 10.1111/j.1749-6632.1997.tb52356.x

Burton, C. L., Noble, K., and Fletcher, P. J. (2011). Enhanced incentive motivation for sucrose-paired cues in adolescent rats: possible roles for dopamine and opioid systems. *Neuropsychopharmacology* 36, 1631–1643. doi: 10.1038/npp.2011.44

Camarini, R., Griffin, W. C. III, Yanke, A. B., Rosalina Dos Santos, B., and Olive, M. F. (2008). Effects of adolescent exposure to cocaine on locomotor activity and extracellular dopamine and glutamate levels in nucleus accumbens of DBA/2J mice. *Brain Res.* 1193, 34–42. doi: 10.1016/j.brainres.2007.11.045

Cauffman, E., Shulman, E. P., Steinberg, L., Claus, E., Banich, M. T., Graham, S., et al. (2010). Age differences in affective decision making as indexed by performance on the Iowa Gambling Task. *Dev. Psychol.* 46, 193–207. doi: 10.1037/a0016128

Chamberlain, S. R., and Sahakian, B. J. (2007). The neuropsychiatry of impulsivity. *Curr. Opin. Psychiatry* 20, 255–261. doi: 10.1097/YCO.0b013e3280ba4989

Chambers, R. A., Taylor, J. R., and Potenza, M. N. (2003). Developmental neurocircuitry of motivation in adolescence: a critical period of addiction vulnerability. *Am. J. Psychiatry* 160, 1041–1052. doi: 10.1176/appi.ajp.160.6.1041

Clarke, T. K., Laucht, M., Ridinger, M., Wodarz, N., Rietschel, M.,

Maier, W., et al. (2011). KCNJ6 is associated with adult alcohol dependence and involved in gene × early life stress interactions in adolescent alcohol drinking. *Neuropsychopharmacology* 36, 1142–1148. doi: 10.1038/npp.2010.247

Colorado, R. A., Shumake, J., Conejo, N. M., Gonzalez-Pardo, H., and Gonzalez-Lima, F. (2006). Effects of maternal separation, early handling, and standard facility rearing on orienting and impulsive behavior of adolescent rats. *Behav. Processes* 71, 51–58. doi: 10.1016/j.beproc.2005.09.007

Counotte, D. S., Smit, A. B., Pattij, T., and Spijker, S. (2011). Development of the motivational system during adolescence, and its sensitivity to disruption by nicotine. *Dev. Cogn. Neurosci.* 1, 430–443. doi: 10.1016/j.dcn.2011.05.010

Counotte, D. S., Spijker, S., Van De Burgwal, L. H., Hogenboom, F., Schoffelmeer, A. N., De Vries, T. J., et al. (2009). Long-lasting cognitive deficits resulting from adolescent nicotine exposure in rats. *Neuropsychopharmacology* 34, 299–306. doi: 10.1038/npp.2008.96

Crews, F., He, J., and Hodge, C. (2007). Adolescent cortical development: a critical period of vulnerability for addiction. *Pharmacol. Biochem. Behav.* 86, 189–199. doi: 10.1016/j.pbb.2006.12.001

Crews, F. T., and Boettiger, C. A. (2009). Impulsivity, frontal lobes and risk for addiction. *Pharmacol. Biochem. Behav.* 93, 237–247. doi: 10.1016/j.pbb.2009.04.018

Crews, F. T., Collins, M. A., Dlugos, C., Littleton, J., Wilkins, L., Neafsey, E. J., et al. (2004). Alcohol-induced neurodegeneration: when, where and why? *Alcohol Clin. Exp. Res.* 28, 350–364. doi: 10.1097/01.ALC.0000113416.65546.01

Cruz, F. C., Delucia, R., and Planeta, C. S. (2008). Effects of chronic stress on nicotine-induced locomotor activity and corticosterone release in adult and adolescent rats. *Addict. Biol.* 13, 63–69. doi: 10.1111/j.1369-1600.2007.00080.x

Cunningham, M. G., Bhattacharyya, S., and Benes, F. M. (2002). Amygdalo-cortical sprouting continues into early adulthood: implications for the development of normal and abnormal function during adolescence. *J. Comp. Neurol.* 453, 116–130. doi: 10.1002/cne.10376

Dahl, R. E. (2008). Biological, developmental, and neurobehavioral factors relevant to adolescent driving risks. *Am. J. Prev. Med.* 35, S278-284. doi: 10.1016/j.amepre.2008.06.013

Diergaarde, L., Pattij, T., Poortvliet, I., Hogenboom, F., De Vries, W., Schoffelmeer, A. N., et al. (2008). Impulsive choice and impulsive action predict vulnerability to distinct stages of nicotine seeking in rats. *Biol. Psychiatry* 63, 301–308. doi: 10.1016/j.biopsych.2007.07.011

Doremus, T. L., Brunell, S. C., Varlinskaya, E. I., and Spear, L. P. (2003). Anxiogenic effects during withdrawal from acute ethanol in adolescent and adult rats. *Pharmacol. Biochem. Behav.* 75, 411–418. doi: 10.1016/S0091-3057(03)00134-5

Douglas, L. A., Varlinskaya, E. I., and Spear, L. P. (2004). Rewarding properties of social interactions in adolescent and adult male and female rats: impact of social versus isolate housing of subjects and partners. *Dev. Psychobiol.* 45, 153–162. doi: 10.1002/dev.20025

Drescher, C., Foscue, E. P., Kuhn, C. M., and Schramm-Sapyta, N. L. (2011). Individual differences in cocaine conditioned taste aversion are developmentally stable and independent of locomotor effects of cocaine. *Dev. Cogn. Neurosci.* 1, 600–605. doi: 10.1016/j.dcn.2011.05.004

Ernst, M., Luckenbaugh, D. A., Moolchan, E. T., Leff, M. K., Allen, R., Eshel, N., et al. (2006). Behavioral predictors of substance-use initiation in adolescents with and without attention-deficit/hyperactivity disorder. *Pediatrics* 117, 2030–2039. doi: 10.1542/peds.2005-0704

Ernst, M., Nelson, E. E., Jazbec, S., Mcclure, E. B., Monk, C. S., Leibenluft, E., et al. (2005). Amygdala and nucleus accumbens in responses to receipt and omission of gains in adults and adolescents. *Neuroimage* 25, 1279–1291. doi: 10.1016/j.neuroimage.2004.12.038

Ernst, M., Romeo, R. D., and Andersen, S. L. (2009). Neurobiology of the development of motivated behaviors in adolescence: a window into a neural systems model. *Pharmacol. Biochem. Behav.* 93, 199–211. doi: 10.1016/j.pbb.2008.12.013

Ersche, K. D., Jones, P. S., Williams, G. B., Turton, A. J., Robbins, T. W., and Bullmore, E. T. (2012). Abnormal brain structure implicated in stimulant drug addiction. *Science* 335, 601–604. doi: 10.1126/science.1214463

Ersche, K. D., Turton, A. J., Pradhan, S., Bullmore, E. T., and Robbins, T. W. (2010). Drug addiction endophenotypes: impulsive versus sensation-seeking personality traits. *Biol. Psychiatry* 68, 770–773. doi: 10.1016/j.biopsych.2010.06.015

Eshel, N., Nelson, E. E., Blair, R. J., Pine, D. S., and Ernst, M. (2007). Neural substrates of choice selection in adults and adolescents: development of the ventrolateral prefrontal and anterior cingulate cortices. *Neuropsychologia* 45, 1270–1279. doi: 10.1016/j.neuropsychologia.2006.10.004

Esmoris-Arranz, F. J., Mendez, C., and Spear, N. E. (2008). Contextual fear conditioning differs for infant, adolescent, and adult rats. *Behav. Processes* 78, 340–350. doi: 10.1016/j.beproc.2008.01.010

Esposito-Smythers, C., Spirito, A., Rizzo, C., Mcgeary, J. E., and Knopik, V. S. (2009). Associations of the DRD2 TaqIA polymorphism with impulsivity and substance use: preliminary results from a clinical sample of adolescents. *Pharmacol. Biochem. Behav.* 93, 306–312. doi: 10.1016/j.pbb.2009.03.012

Estanislau, C., and Morato, S. (2006). Behavior ontogeny in the elevated plus-maze: prenatal stress effects. *Int. J. Dev. Neurosci.* 24, 255–262. doi: 10.1016/j.ijdevneu.2006.03.001

Evenden, J. L. (1999). Varieties of impulsivity. *Psychopharmacology (Berl.)* 146, 348–361. doi: 10.1007/PL00005481

Fox, H. C., Bergquist, K. L., Peihua, G., and Rajita, S. (2010). Interactive effects of cumulative stress and impulsivity on alcohol consumption. *Alcohol. Clin. Exp. Res.* 34, 1376–1385. doi: 10.1111/j.1530-0277.2010.01221.x

Frantz, K. J., O'Dell, L. E., and Parsons, L. H. (2007). Behavioral and neurochemical responses to cocaine in periadolescent and adult rats. *Neuropsychopharmacology* 32, 625–637. doi: 10.1038/sj.npp.1301130

Friemel, C. M., Spanagel, R., and Schneider, M. (2010). Reward sensitivity for a palatable food reward peaks during pubertal developmental in rats. *Front. Behav. Neurosci.* 4:39. doi: 10.3389/fnbeh.2010.00039

Galvan, A., Hare, T. A., Parra, C. E., Penn, J., Voss, H., Glover, G., et al. (2006). Earlier development of the accumbens relative to orbitofrontal cortex might underlie risk-taking behavior in adolescents. *J. Neurosci.* 26, 6885–6892. doi: 10.1523/JNEUROSCI.1062-06.2006

Gardner, M., and Steinberg, L. (2005). Peer influence on risk taking, risk preference, and risky decision making in adolescence and adulthood: an experimental study. *Dev. Psychol.* 41, 625–635. doi: 10.1037/0012-1649.41.4.625

George, O., and Koob, G. F. (2010). Individual differences in prefrontal cortex function and the transition from drug use to drug dependence. *Neurosci. Biobehav. Rev.* 35, 232–247. doi: 10.1016/j.neubiorev.2010.05.002

Giedd, J. N. (2008). The teen brain: insights from neuroimaging. *J. Adolesc. Health* 42, 335–343. doi: 10.1016/j.jadohealth.2008.01.007

Gogtay, N., Giedd, J. N., Lusk, L., Hayashi, K. M., Greenstein, D., Vaituzis, A. C., et al. (2004). Dynamic mapping of human cortical development during childhood through early adulthood. *Proc. Natl. Acad. Sci. U.S.A.* 101, 8174–8179. doi: 10.1073/pnas.0402680101

Grosbras, M. H., Jansen, M., Leonard, G., Mcintosh, A., Osswald, K., Poulsen, C., et al. (2007). Neural mechanisms of resistance to peer influence in early adolescence. *J. Neurosci.* 27, 8040–8045. doi: 10.1523/JNEUROSCI.1360-07.2007

Gruber, A. J., Calhoon, G. G., Shusterman, I., Schoenbaum, G., Roesch, M. R., and O'Donnell, P. (2010). More is less: a disinhibited prefrontal cortex impairs cognitive flexibility. *J. Neurosci.* 30, 17102–17110. doi: 10.1523/JNEUROSCI.4623-10.2010

Gunnar, M. R., Wewerka, S., Frenn, K., Long, J. D., and Griggs, C. (2009). Developmental changes in hypothalamus-pituitary-adrenal activity over the transition to adolescence: normative changes and associations with puberty. *Dev. Psychopathol.* 21, 69–85. doi: 10.1017/S0954579409000054

Hamilton, K. R., Ansell, E. B., Reynolds, B., Potenza, M. N., and Sinha, R. (2013). Self-reported impulsivity, but not behavioral choice or response impulsivity, partially mediates the effect of stress on drinking behavior. *Stress* 16, 3–15. doi: 10.3109/10253890.2012.671397

Hare, T. A., Tottenham, N., Galvan, A., Voss, H. U., Glover, G. H., and Casey, B. J. (2008). Biological substrates of emotional reactivity and regulation in adolescence during an emotional go-nogo task. *Biol. Psychiatry* 63, 927–934. doi: 10.1016/j.biopsych.2008.03.015

Johnson, C., and Wilbrecht, L. (2011). Juvenile mice show greater flexibility in multiple choice reversal learning than adults. *Dev. Cogn. Neurosci.* 1, 540–551. doi: 10.1016/j.dcn.2011.05.008

Kabbaj, M., Isgor, C., Watson, S. J., and Akil, H. (2002). Stress during adolescence alters behavioral sensitization to amphetamine. *Neuroscience* 113, 395–400. doi: 10.1016/S0306-4522(02)00188-4

Kaufman, J., Yang, B. Z., Douglas-Palumberi, H., Crouse-Artus, M., Lipschitz, D., Krystal, J. H., et al. (2007). Genetic and environmental predictors of early alcohol use. *Biol. Psychiatry* 61, 1228–1234. doi: 10.1016/j.biopsych.2006.06.039

Kelley, A. E., Schochet, T., and Landry, C. F. (2004). Risk taking and novelty seeking in adolescence: introduction to part I. *Ann. N. Y. Acad. Sci.* 1021, 27–32. doi: 10.1196/annals.1308.003

Koob, G. F., and Le Moal, M. (2001). Drug addiction, dysregulation of reward, and allostasis. *Neuropsychopharmacology* 24, 97–129. doi: 10.1016/S0893-133X(00)00195-0

Kota, D., Martin, B. R., Robinson, S. E., and Damaj, M. I. (2007). Nicotine dependence and reward differ between adolescent and adult male mice. *J. Pharmacol. Exp. Ther.* 322, 399–407. doi: 10.1124/jpet.107.121616

Kreek, M. J., Nielsen, D. A., Butelman, E. R., and Laforge, K. S. (2005). Genetic influences on impulsivity, risk taking, stress responsivity and vulnerability to drug abuse and addiction. *Nat. Neurosci.* 8, 1450–1457. doi: 10.1038/nn1583

Krishnan-Sarin, S., Reynolds, B., Duhig, A. M., Smith, A., Liss, T., Mcfetridge, A., et al. (2007). Behavioral impulsivity predicts treatment outcome in a smoking cessation program for adolescent smokers. *Drug Alcohol Depend.* 88, 79–82. doi: 10.1016/j.drugalcdep.2006.09.006

Laviola, G., Pascucci, T., and Pieretti, S. (2001). Striatal dopamine sensitization to D-amphetamine in periadolescent but not in adult rats. *Pharmacol. Biochem. Behav.* 68, 115–124. doi: 10.1016/S0091-3057(00)00430-5

Lenroot, R. K., and Giedd, J. N. (2006). Brain development in children and adolescents: insights from anatomical magnetic resonance imaging. *Neurosci. Biobehav. Rev.* 30, 718–729. doi: 10.1016/j.neubiorev.2006.06.001

Lepsch, L. B., Gonzalo, L. A., Magro, F. J., Delucia, R., Scavone, C., and Planeta, C. S. (2005). Exposure to chronic stress increases the locomotor response to cocaine and the basal levels of corticosterone in adolescent rats. *Addict. Biol.* 10, 251–256. doi: 10.1080/13556210500269366

Luna, B., Padmanabhan, A., and O'Hearn, K. (2010). What has fMRI told us about the development of cognitive control through adolescence? *Brain Cogn.* 72, 101–113. doi: 10.1016/j.bandc.2009.08.005

Lynn, D. A., and Brown, G. R. (2010). The ontogeny of anxiety-like behavior in rats from adolescence to adulthood. *Dev. Psychobiol.* 52, 731–739. doi: 10.1002/dev.20468

Macrì, S., Adriani, W., Chiarotti, F., and Laviola, G. (2002). Risk taking during exploration of a plus-maze is greater in adolescent than in juvenile or adult mice. *Anim. Behav.* 64, 541–546. doi: 10.1006/anbe.2002.4004

Mathews, I. Z., Mills, R. G., and McCormick, C. M. (2008). Chronic social stress in adolescence influenced both amphetamine conditioned place preference and locomotor sensitization. *Dev. Psychobiol.* 50, 451–459. doi: 10.1002/dev.20299

McCormick, C. M., Robarts, D., Kopeikina, K., and Kelsey, J. E. (2005). Long-lasting, sex- and age-specific effects of social stressors on corticosterone responses to restraint and on locomotor responses to psychostimulants in rats. *Horm. Behav.* 48, 64–74. doi: 10.1016/j.yhbeh.2005.01.008

McCutcheon, J. E., Conrad, K. L., Carr, S. B., Ford, K. A., Mcgehee, D. S., and Marinelli, M. (2012). Dopamine neurons in the ventral tegmental area fire faster in adolescent rats than in adults. *J. Neurophysiol.* 108, 1620–1630. doi: 10.1152/jn.00077.2012

Moeller, F. G., Barratt, E. S., Dougherty, D. M., Schmitz, J. M., and Swann, A. C. (2001). Psychiatric aspects of impulsivity. *Am. J. Psychiatry* 158, 1783–1793. doi: 10.1176/appi.ajp.158.11.1783

Neufang, S., Specht, K., Hausmann, M., Gunturkun, O., Herpertz-Dahlmann, B., Fink, G. R., et al. (2009). Sex differences and the impact of steroid hormones on the developing human brain. *Cereb. Cortex* 19, 464–473. doi: 10.1093/cercor/bhn100

Nguyen, T. V., Mccracken, J., Ducharme, S., Botteron, K. N., Mahabir, M., Johnson, W., et al. (2013). Testosterone-related cortical maturation across childhood and adolescence. *Cereb. Cortex* 23, 1424–1432. doi: 10.1093/cercor/bhs125

O'Loughlin, J., Karp, I., Koulis, T., Paradis, G., and Difranza, J. (2009). Determinants of first puff and daily cigarette smoking in adolescents. *Am. J. Epidemiol.* 170, 585–597. doi: 10.1093/aje/kwp179

Ohmura, Y., Yamaguchi, T., Futami, Y., Togashi, H., Izumi, T., Matsumoto, M., et al. (2009). Corticotropin releasing factor enhances attentional function as assessed by the five-choice serial reaction time task in rats. *Behav. Brain Res.* 198, 429–433. doi: 10.1016/j.bbr.2008.11.025

Overman, W. H., Frassrand, K., Ansel, S., Trawalter, S., Bies, B., and Redmond, A. (2004). Performance on the IOWA card task by adolescents and adults. *Neuropsychologia* 42, 1838–1851. doi: 10.1016/j.neuropsychologia.2004.03.014

Pardridge, W. M., and Mietus, L. J. (1979). Transport of steroid hormones through the rat blood-brain barrier. Primary role of albumin-bound hormone. *J. Clin. Invest.* 64, 145–154. doi: 10.1172/JCI109433

Pattwell, S. S., Bath, K. G., Casey, B. J., Ninan, I., and Lee, F. S. (2011). Selective early-acquired fear memories undergo temporary suppression during adolescence. *Proc. Natl. Acad. Sci. U.S.A.* 108, 1182–1187. doi: 10.1073/pnas.1012975108

Paus, T., Nawaz-Khan, I., Leonard, G., Perron, M., Pike, G. B., Pitiot, A., et al. (2010). Sexual dimorphism in the adolescent brain: role of testosterone and androgen receptor in global and local volumes of grey and white matter. *Horm. Behav.* 57, 63–75. doi: 10.1016/j.yhbeh.2009.08.004

Paus, T., Zijdenbos, A., Worsley, K., Collins, D. L., Blumenthal, J., Giedd, J. N., et al. (1999). Structural maturation of neural pathways in children and adolescents: in vivo study. *Science* 283, 1908–1911. doi: 10.1126/science.283.5409.1908

Peters, J., Bromberg, U., Schneider, S., Brassen, S., Menz, M., Banaschewski, T., et al. (2011). Lower ventral striatal activation during reward anticipation in adolescent smokers. *Am. J. Psychiatry* 168, 540–549. doi: 10.1176/appi.ajp.2010.10071024

Pfeifer, J. H., Masten, C. L., Moore, W. E. III, Oswald, T. M., Mazziotta, J. C., Iacoboni, M., et al. (2011). Entering adolescence: resistance to peer influence, risky behavior, and neural changes in emotion reactivity. *Neuron* 69, 1029–1036. doi: 10.1016/j.neuron.2011.02.019

Philpot, R. M., Badanich, K. A., and Kirstein, C. L. (2003). Place conditioning: age-related changes in the rewarding and aversive effects of alcohol. *Alcohol. Clin. Exp. Res.* 27, 593–599. doi: 10.1111/j.1530-0277.2003.tb04395.x

Pieters, S., Van Der Vorst, H., Burk, W. J., Schoenmakers, T. M., Van Den Wildenberg, E., Smeets, H. J., et al. (2011). The effect of the OPRM1 and DRD4 polymorphisms on the relation between attentional bias and alcohol use in adolescence and young adulthood. *Dev. Cogn. Neurosci.* 1, 591–599. doi: 10.1016/j.dcn.2011.07.008

Pilowsky, D. J., Keyes, K. M., and Hasin, D. S. (2009). Adverse childhood events and lifetime alcohol dependence. *Am. J. Public Health* 99, 258–263. doi: 10.2105/AJPH.2008.139006

Quevedo, K. M., Benning, S. D., Gunnar, M. R., and Dahl, R. E. (2009). The onset of puberty: effects on the psychophysiology of defensive and appetitive motivation. *Dev. Psychopathol.* 21, 27–45. doi: 10.1017/S0954579409000030

Quinn, H. R., Matsumoto, I., Callaghan, P. D., Long, L. E., Arnold, J. C., Gunasekaran, N., et al. (2008). Adolescent rats find repeated Delta(9)-THC less aversive than adult rats but display greater residual cognitive deficits and changes in hippocampal protein expression following exposure. *Neuropsychopharmacology* 33, 1113–1126. doi: 10.1038/sj.npp.1301475

Rachlin, H. (1992). Diminishing marginal value as delay discounting. *J. Exp. Anal. Behav.* 57, 407–415. doi: 10.1901/jeab.1992.57-407

Reynolds, B., and Fields, S. (2012). Delay discounting by adolescents experimenting with cigarette smoking. *Addiction* 107, 417–424. doi: 10.1111/j.1360-0443.2011.03644.x

Robinson, D. L., Zitzman, D. L., Smith, K. J., and Spear, L. P. (2011). Fast dopamine release events in the nucleus accumbens of early adolescent rats. *Neuroscience* 176, 296–307. doi: 10.1016/j.neuroscience.2010.12.016

Romeo, R. D., Bellani, R., Karatsoreos, I. N., Chhua, N., Vernov, M., Conrad, C. D., et al. (2006a). Stress history and pubertal development interact to shape hypothalamic-pituitary-adrenal axis plasticity. *Endocrinology* 147, 1664–1674. doi: 10.1210/en.2005-1432

Romeo, R. D., Karatsoreos, I. N., and Mcewen, B. S. (2006b). Pubertal maturation and time of day differentially affect behavioral and neuroendocrine responses following an acute stressor. *Horm. Behav.* 50, 463–468. doi: 10.1016/j.yhbeh.2006.06.002

Romer, D., Betancourt, L., Giannetta, J. M., Brodsky, N. L., Farah, M., and Hurt, H. (2009). Executive cognitive functions and impulsivity as correlates of risk taking and problem behavior in preadolescents. *Neuropsychologia* 47, 2916–2926. doi: 10.1016/j.neuropsychologia.2009.06.019

Schilt, T., Goudriaan, A. E., Koeter, M. W., Van Den Brink, W., and Schmand, B. (2009). Decision making as a predictor of first ecstasy use: a prospective study. *Psychopharmacology (Berl.)* 203, 519–527. doi: 10.1007/s00213-008-1398-y

Schneider, T., Bizarro, L., Asherson, P. J., and Stolerman, I. P. (2012). Hyperactivity, increased nicotine consumption and impaired performance in the five-choice serial reaction time task in adolescent rats prenatally exposed to nicotine. *Psychopharmacology (Berl.)* 223, 401–415. doi: 10.1007/s00213-012-2728-7

Schoenbaum, G., Setlow, B., Saddoris, M. P., and Gallagher, M. (2006). Encoding changes in orbitofrontal cortex in reversal-impaired aged rats. *J. Neurophysiol.* 95, 1509–1517. doi: 10.1152/jn.01052.2005

Schramm-Sapyta, N. L., Cha, Y. M., Chaudhry, S., Wilson, W. A., Swartzwelder, H. S., and Kuhn, C. M. (2007). Differential anxiogenic, aversive, and locomotor effects of THC in adolescent and adult rats. *Psychopharmacology (Berl.)* 191, 867–877. doi: 10.1007/s00213-006-0676-9

Schramm-Sapyta, N. L., Morris, R. W., and Kuhn, C. M. (2006). Adolescent rats are protected from the conditioned aversive properties of cocaine and lithium chloride. *Pharmacol. Biochem. Behav.* 84, 344–352. doi: 10.1016/j.pbb.2006.05.026

Schramm-Sapyta, N. L., Walker, Q. D., Caster, J. M., Levin, E. D., and Kuhn, C. M. (2009). Are adolescents more vulnerable to drug addiction than adults? Evidence from animal models. *Psychopharmacology (Berl.)* 206, 1–21. doi: 10.1007/s00213-009-1585-5

Shaham, Y., Erb, S., and Stewart, J. (2000). Stress-induced relapse to heroin and cocaine seeking in rats: a review. *Brain Res. Brain Res. Rev.* 33, 13–33. doi: 10.1016/S0165-0173(00)00024-2

Shaw, P., Gilliam, M., Liverpool, M., Weddle, C., Malek, M., Sharp, W., et al. (2011). Cortical development in typically developing children with symptoms of hyperactivity and impulsivity: support for a dimensional view of attention deficit hyperactivity disorder. *Am. J. Psychiatry* 168, 143–151. doi: 10.1176/appi.ajp.2010.10030385

Silk, J. S., Siegle, G. J., Whalen, D. J., Ostapenko, L. J., Ladouceur, C. D., and Dahl, R. E. (2009). Pubertal changes in emotional information processing: pupillary, behavioral, and subjective evidence during emotional word identification. *Dev. Psychopathol.* 21, 7–26. doi: 10.1017/S0954579409000029

Soloff, P. H., Lynch, K. G., and Moss, H. B. (2000). Serotonin, impulsivity, and alcohol use disorders in the older adolescent: a psychobiological study. *Alcohol. Clin. Exp. Res.* 24, 1609–1619. doi: 10.1111/j.1530-0277.2000.tb01961.x

Somer, E., Ginzburg, K., and Kramer, L. (2012). The role of impulsivity in the association between childhood trauma and dissociative psychopathology: mediation versus moderation. *Psychiatry Res.* 196, 133–137. doi: 10.1016/j.psychres.2011.08.010

Somerville, L. H., Hare, T., and Casey, B. J. (2011). Frontostriatal maturation predicts cognitive control failure to appetitive cues in adolescents. *J. Cogn. Neurosci.* 23, 2123–2134. doi: 10.1162/jocn.2010.21572

Spear, L. P. (2000). The adolescent brain and age-related behavioral manifestations. *Neurosci. Biobehav. Rev.* 24, 417–463. doi: 10.1016/S0149-7634(00)00014-2

Spear, L. P., and Varlinskaya, E. I. (2010). Sensitivity to ethanol and other hedonic stimuli in an animal model of adolescence: implications for prevention science? *Dev. Psychobiol.* 52, 236–243. doi: 10.1002/dev.20457

Spivey, J. M., Shumake, J., Colorado, R. A., Conejo-Jimenez, N., Gonzalez-Pardo, H., and Gonzalez-Lima, F. (2009). Adolescent female rats are more resistant than males to the effects of early stress on prefrontal cortex and impulsive behavior. *Dev. Psychobiol.* 51, 277–288. doi: 10.1002/dev.20362

Stansfield, K. H., and Kirstein, C. L. (2005). Neurochemical effects of cocaine in adolescence compared to adulthood. *Brain Res. Dev. Brain Res.* 159, 119–125. doi: 10.1016/j.devbrainres.2005.07.005

Stanwood, G. D., Mcelligot, S., Lu, L., and Mcgonigle, P. (1997). Ontogeny of dopamine D3 receptors in the nucleus accumbens of the rat. *Neurosci. Lett.* 223, 13–16. doi: 10.1016/S0304-3940(97)13396-1

Steinberg, L. (2004). Risk taking in adolescence: what changes, and why? *Ann. N. Y. Acad. Sci.* 1021, 51–58. doi: 10.1196/annals.1308.005

Steinberg, L. (2005). Cognitive and affective development in adolescence. *Trends Cogn. Sci.* 9, 69–74. doi: 10.1016/j.tics.2004.12.005

Steinberg, L., Albert, D., Cauffman, E., Banich, M., Graham, S., and Woolard, J. (2008). Age differences in sensation seeking and impulsivity as indexed by behavior and self-report: evidence for a dual systems model. *Dev. Psychol.* 44, 1764–1778. doi: 10.1037/a0012955

Steinberg, L., Graham, S., O'Brien, L., Woolard, J., Cauffman, E., and Banich, M. (2009). Age differences in future orientation and delay discounting. *Child Dev.* 80, 28–44. doi: 10.1111/j.1467-8624.2008.01244.x

Steinberg, L., and Morris, A. S. (2001). Adolescent development. *Annu. Rev. Psychol.* 52, 83–110. doi: 10.1146/annurev.psych.52.1.83

Stroud, L. R., Foster, E., Papandonatos, G. D., Handwerger, K., Granger, D. A., Kivlighan, K. T., et al. (2009). Stress response and the adolescent transition: performance versus peer rejection stressors. *Dev. Psychopathol.* 21, 47–68. doi: 10.1017/S0954579409000042

Sturman, D. A., and Moghaddam, B. (2011). Reduced neuronal inhibition and coordination of adolescent prefrontal cortex during motivated behavior. *J. Neurosci.* 31, 1471–1478. doi: 10.1523/JNEUROSCI.4210-10.2011

Substance Abuse and Mental Health Services Administration. (2010). *Results from the 2009 National Survey on Drug Use and Health*, Vol. I, *Summary of National Findings* (Office of Applied Studies, NSDUH Series H-38A, HHS Publication No. SMA 10-4586 Findings). Rockville, MD: Substance Abuse and Mental Health Services Administration.

Swendsen, J., and Le Moal, M. (2011). Individual vulnerability to addiction. *Ann. N. Y. Acad. Sci.* 1216, 73–85. doi: 10.1111/j.1749-6632.2010.05894.x

Thiel, K. J., Okun, A. C., and Neisewander, J. L. (2008). Social reward-conditioned place preference: a model revealing an interaction between cocaine and social context rewards in rats. *Drug Alcohol Depend.* 96, 202–212. doi: 10.1016/j.drugalcdep.2008.02.013

Tirelli, E., Laviola, G., and Adriani, W. (2003). Ontogenesis of behavioral sensitization and conditioned place preference induced by psychostimulants in laboratory rodents. *Neurosci. Biobehav. Rev.* 27, 163–178. doi: 10.1016/S0149-7634(03)00018-6

Torregrossa, M. M., Xie, M., and Taylor, J. R. (2012). Chronic corticosterone exposure during adolescence reduces impulsive action but increases impulsive choice and sensitivity to yohimbine in male Sprague-Dawley rats. *Neuropsychopharmacology* 37, 1656–1670. doi: 10.1038/npp.2012.11

Torres, O. V., Tejeda, H. A., Natividad, L. A., and O'Dell, L. E. (2008). Enhanced vulnerability to the rewarding effects of nicotine during the adolescent period of development. *Pharmacol. Biochem. Behav.* 90, 658–663. doi: 10.1016/j.pbb.2008.05.009

Tseng, K. Y., and O'Donnell, P. (2007). Dopamine modulation of prefrontal cortical interneurons changes during adolescence. *Cereb. Cortex* 17, 1235–1240. doi: 10.1093/cercor/bhl034

Van Leijenhorst, L., Zanolie, K., Van Meel, C. S., Westenberg, P. M., Rombouts, S. A., and Crone, E. A. (2010). What motivates the adolescent? Brain regions mediating reward sensitivity across adolescence. *Cereb. Cortex* 20, 61–69. doi: 10.1093/cercor/bhp078

Verdejo-Garcia, A., Lawrence, A. J., and Clark, L. (2008). Impulsivity as a vulnerability marker for substance-use disorders: review of findings from high-risk research, problem gamblers and genetic association studies. *Neurosci. Biobehav. Rev.* 32, 777–810. doi: 10.1016/j.neubiorev.2007.11.003

Vetter-O'Hagen, C., Varlinskaya, E., and Spear, L. (2009). Sex differences in ethanol intake and sensitivity to aversive effects during adolescence and adulthood. *Alcohol Alcohol.* 44, 547–554. doi: 10.1093/alcalc/agp048

von Diemen, L., Bassani, D. G., Fuchs, S. C., Szobot, C. M., and Pechansky, F. (2008). Impulsivity, age of first alcohol use and substance use disorders among male adolescents: a population based case-control study. *Addiction* 103, 1198–1205. doi: 10.1111/j.1360-0443.2008.02223.x

Walker, Q. D., and Kuhn, C. M. (2008). Cocaine increases stimulated dopamine release more in periadolescent than adult rats. *Neurotoxicol. Teratol.* 30, 412–418. doi: 10.1016/j.ntt.2008.04.002

Wang, A. T., Lee, S. S., Sigman, M., and Dapretto, M. (2006). Developmental changes in the neural basis of interpreting communicative intent. *Soc. Cogn. Affect. Neurosci.* 1, 107–121. doi: 10.1093/scan/nsl018

Waylen, A., and Wolke, D. (2004). Sex 'n' drugs 'n' rock 'n' roll: the meaning and social consequences of pubertal timing. *Eur. J. Endocrinol.* 151(Suppl. 3), U151–U159. doi: 10.1530/eje.0.151U151

Wilkin, M. M., Waters, P., McCormick, C. M., and Menard, J. L. (2012). Intermittent physical stress during early- and mid-adolescence differentially alters rats' anxiety- and depression-like behaviors in adulthood. *Behav. Neurosci.* 126, 344–360. doi: 10.1037/a0027258

Wilmouth, C. E., and Spear, L. P. (2004). Adolescent and adult rats' aversion to flavors previously paired with nicotine. *Ann. N. Y. Acad. Sci.* 1021, 462–464. doi: 10.1196/annals.1308.065

Witte, A. V., Savli, M., Holik, A., Kasper, S., and Lanzenberger, R. (2010). Regional sex differences in grey matter volume are associated with sex hormones in the young adult human brain. *Neuroimage* 49, 1205–1212. doi: 10.1016/j.neuroimage.2009.09.046

Xiao, L., Bechara, A., Grenard, L. J., Stacy, W. A., Palmer, P., Wei, Y., et al. (2009). Affective decision-making predictive of Chinese adolescent drinking behaviors. *J. Int. Neuropsychol. Soc.* 15, 547–557. doi: 10.1017/S1355617709090808

Yurgelun-Todd, D. (2007). Emotional and cognitive changes during adolescence. *Curr. Opin. Neurobiol.* 17, 251–257. doi: 10.1016/j.conb.2007.03.009

Zakharova, E., Leoni, G., Kichko, I., and Izenwasser, S. (2009). Differential effects of methamphetamine and cocaine on conditioned place preference and locomotor activity in adult and adolescent male rats. *Behav. Brain Res.* 198, 45–50. doi: 10.1016/j.bbr.2008.10.019

Zimmering, P., Toolan, J., Safrin, R., and Wortis, S. B. (1952). Drug addiction in relation to problems of adolescence. *Am. J. Psychiatry* 109, 272–278.

Conflict of Interest Statement: The authors declare that the research was conducted in the absence of any commercial or financial relationships that could be construed as a potential conflict of interest.

14

Mind and body: how the health of the body impacts on neuropsychiatry

Thibault Renoir[1]*, Kyoko Hasebe[2] and Laura Gray[2]*

[1] *Melbourne Brain Centre, Florey Institute of Neuroscience and Mental Health, University of Melbourne, Melbourne, VIC, Australia*
[2] *School of Medicine, Deakin University, Geelong, VIC, Australia*

Edited by:
Maarten Van Den Buuse, Mental Health Research Institute, Australia

Reviewed by:
Sulev Kõks, University of Tartu, Estonia
Jean-Philippe Guilloux, Université Paris Sud, France

****Correspondence:***
Thibault Renoir, Melbourne Brain Centre, Florey Institute of Neuroscience and Mental Health, University of Melbourne, Melbourne, VIC, Australia
e-mail: tibo.renoir@gmail.com;
Laura Gray, School of Medicine, Deakin University, Locked Bag 20000, Geelong, VIC 3220, Australia
e-mail: l.gray@deakin.edu.au

It has long been established in traditional forms of medicine and in anecdotal knowledge that the health of the body and the mind are inextricably linked. Strong and continually developing evidence now suggests a link between disorders which involve Hypothalamic-Pituitary-Adrenal axis (HPA) dysregulation and the risk of developing psychiatric disease. For instance, adverse or excessive responses to stressful experiences are built into the diagnostic criteria for several psychiatric disorders, including depression and anxiety disorders. Interestingly, peripheral disorders such as metabolic disorders and cardiovascular diseases are also associated with HPA changes. Furthermore, many other systemic disorders associated with a higher incidence of psychiatric disease involve a significant inflammatory component. In fact, inflammatory and endocrine pathways seem to interact in both the periphery and the central nervous system (CNS) to potentiate states of psychiatric dysfunction. This review synthesizes clinical and animal data looking at interactions between peripheral and central factors, developing an understanding at the molecular and cellular level of how processes in the entire body can impact on mental state and psychiatric health.

Keywords: mind-body interactions, psychiatric diseases, stress response, HPA axis, mood disorders, peripheral disorders, inflammatory processes

INTRODUCTION

The concept that our mind and our mental processes are influenced by the health of our bodies is intuitively appealing and central to many approaches to health and wellbeing. However, there has been a recent explosion of clinical and physiological evidence to support this theory, shifting a "commonsense" approach to health toward a clinically useful and pharmacologically targetable model. We are now moving toward mechanistic models for the interactions between peripheral and central factors, gaining an understanding at the molecular and cellular level of how processes in the entire body can impact on mental state and psychiatric health. Although good evidence exists for these associations in many psychiatric disorders, in this review we will focus on depression, for which the evidence is perhaps most compelling.

Some epidemiological associations between corporeal disorders and psychological ill-health are well established. The link between coronary artery disease and depression, for example, has been extensively investigated (Nemeroff and Musselman, 2000; Rugulies, 2002; Barth et al., 2004), and it appears that not only are the two disorders strongly associated but that depression is a predictor of poor cardiovascular outcome. Such epidemiological evidence reinforces the widely held notion that the sadness of depression both co-occurs with and potentiates cardiac disease. However, we are now moving toward an understanding of the shared molecular processes which may underpin the link between these disorders.

Although evidence of psychiatric and peripheral comorbidities abounds in the literature, there is also growing interest in the more subtle variations in physiological function which may be antecedents of overt illness but which may be sufficient to modulate CNS processes and mental state. In this review we will focus on several of the major pathways implicated in the aetiology of depression which may mediate the links between the mind and body.

SYSTEMIC DISORDERS ASSOCIATED WITH DEPRESSION

Strikingly, a recent study conducted in the United States indicated that of middle aged or older adults meeting diagnostic criteria for a major depressive disorder, two thirds reported comorbid cardiovascular disease (González and Tarraf, 2013). Up to 20% of patients with coronary heart disease meet diagnostic criteria for major depression, and up to 47% report significant and long-lasting depressive symptoms (Bush et al., 2005; Carney and Freedland, 2008). Recent reports have indicated that this effect is not restricted to individuals with cardiovascular disease, as patients undergoing rehabilitation for pulmonary disease were even more likely than cardiac patients to exhibit clinically significant depression and psychological distress (Serber et al., 2012). Cardiovascular risk factors are pathologically relevant even prior to diagnosis. Studies of patients with long-term depressive or anxiety disorders revealed elevated incidence of sub-clinical cardiovascular disease, as measured by a variety of parameters including plaque deposition and arterial stiffness

(Seldenrijk et al., 2013), and blood pressure, glucose, body mass index (BMI), diet, and physical activity (Kronish et al., 2012). Interestingly, and relevant to sex differences often observed in the context of anxiety and depressive disorders [for which prevalence can be as twice higher in women compared to men, see Bekker and van Mens-Verhulst (2007); Kimbro et al. (2012)], significant depressive symptoms are more common in younger women with peripheral arterial disease than in other gender-age groups (Smolderen et al., 2010). Also, recent meta-analysis of cardiovascular risk factors and depression in later life demonstrated relatively strong associations between depression and diabetes, cardiovascular disease and stroke (Valkanova and Ebmeier, 2013).

These findings also highlight the relationship between diabetes and psychiatric health. Meta-analytic evidence suggests that patients with depression have an elevated risk of developing type two diabetes (Knol et al., 2006; Mommersteeg et al., 2013), and conversely that patients with diabetes have significantly increased risk of developing depression (Anderson et al., 2001; Rotella and Mannucci, 2013). A longitudinal study revealed that the incidence of diabetes was highest in individuals with the greatest number of depressive symptoms (Carnethon et al., 2003), and a large community-based study demonstrated that diabetes was associated with an increased risk of depression (de Jonge et al., 2006). This bi-directional relationship is suggestive of convergent pathological processes rather than a simplistic cause and effect relationship. Interestingly, some clinical studies have hypothesized that the doubled rates of depression in female diabetic patients could help explain the high prevalence of coronary heart disease in women with diabetes (Clouse et al., 2003).

Autoimmune disease, for example rheumatoid arthritis, is also associated with markedly elevated risk of depression (Margaretten et al., 2011a; Covic et al., 2012). Notably, there appears to be a strong correlation between the severity of rheumatoid arthritis and the incidence of depression, with a recent meta-analysis demonstrating that those with the most severe form of arthritic disease have a six-fold higher incidence of depression relative to those with the mildest form Godha et al. (2010).

Clearly the impact of declining quality of life associated with severe systemic disease cannot be overlooked. However, these findings and the many others describing strong associations with psychiatric disease and peripheral illness do provoke the question of whether there are fundamental mechanisms in common. How does the health of the body affect the health of the mind, and what are the underlying pathological processes which underpin this relationship? Although we do not yet have a full understanding of the complexities of the bidirectional relationship between body and brain, convergent evidence suggests that the endocrine response to stress (via the HPA axis), and immune dysregulation (via inflammatory pathways), may be playing a central role.

STRESS RESPONSIVITY AND THE HYPOTHALAMIC-PITUITARY-ADRENAL AXIS

The most well established example of mind-body interaction is the link between psychological stress and psychological ill-health. In fact, adverse or excessive responses to stressful experiences are built into the diagnostic criteria for several psychiatric disorders, including depression and anxiety disorders. The body's response to stress is mediated by the hypothalamic-pituitary-adrenal (HPA) axis, by which stressful stimuli modulate the activity of a tightly regulated cycle of circulating hormones. Stress *per se* is not necessarily problematic; the body is well equipped to respond to stressful stimuli and to some extent stress is necessary for normal function. However, excessive or prolonged stress, or perturbations in the function or regulation of the HPA axis may result in abnormal changes in hormones circulating through both the periphery and the CNS. As previously mentioned, women are twice as likely as men to suffer from stress-related psychiatric disorders and there is evidence that sex differences in stress responses could account for this sex bias (Bangasser and Valentino, 2012).

The HPA axis is the primary circuit that mediates the physiological response to stress and regulates the level of circulating glucocorticoid hormones (e.g., CORT: cortisol in humans, corticosterone in rodents). Arginine vasopressin (AVP) and corticotrophin-releasing hormone (CRH, also originally referred to as CRF for corticotrophin-releasing factor) are synthesised and released from the paraventricular nucleus (PVN) of the hypothalamus, and are arguably the highest order regulators of the HPA axis activity within the central nervous system (CNS). These neuro-hormones act synergistically to stimulate adrenocorticotrophin (ACTH) secretion from the anterior pituitary, culminating in increased levels of circulating CORT. The HPA axis is modulated by a negative feedback loop encompassing the hippocampus, hypothalamus and anterior pituitary. Following CORT secretion into the peripheral blood circulation, CORT passes through the plasma membrane of cells, particularly in the pituitary, hypothalamus, and hippocampus where it binds to the glucocorticoid receptor (GR). Finally, glucocorticoid catabolism involves 5α-reductase type 1 (predominantly a liver enzyme) and 11β-hydroxysteroid dehydrogenase type 2 (in kidney).

The psychological determinants of an individual's response to stress are important predictors of outcome, although this area is beyond the scope of this review [reviewed comprehensively by Liu and Alloy (2010)]. However, physiological variations in HPA axis function and related pathways may also modulate the response to stress and alter the threshold for psychiatric disorders. Despite substantial limitations in the objective assessment of stress, multiple studies have documented an association between stressful life experiences and depression (Kendler and Gardner, 2010). Interesting examples of HPA axis dysfunction modulating psychiatric health come from Cushing's syndrome and Addison's disease, states of hyper- and hypo-cortisolemia, respectively. Cushing's syndrome is associated with a high prevalence of psychopathology, primarily depressive symptoms but also mania and anxiety (Pereira et al., 2010). Addison's disease has been less extensively investigated but appears to be associated with an increased risk of a variety of psychiatric symptoms, including depression, delusions, hallucinations, and anxiety (Anglin et al., 2006). In both disorders it should be borne in mind that adrenal dysfunction can also lead to electrolyte and metabolic abnormalities which can also contribute to CNS disturbances. Nonetheless, the fact that treatment of the hyper- or hypo-cortisolaemia resolves the psychiatric symptoms in most cases strongly suggests that changes in adrenal corticosteroids are a primary driving force for the psychiatric symptoms (even though this is not the sole determining factor, as half of subjects with Cushing's do not develop depressive symptoms). Therapeutic administration of high doses of corticosteroids has been associated with the development of a manic behavioral state (Warrington and Bostwick, 2006; Kenna et al., 2011; Fardet et al., 2012). These observations also highlight a critical pathway by which HPA axis function may alter mental state. Corticosteroids are generally prescribed in cases of uncontrolled inflammatory disease, and act as powerful anti-inflammatory factors. As we will discuss below, inflammatory states are strongly linked to perturbations in psychiatric health. More subtle variations in HPA axis function have been directly associated with psychiatric disorders, in particular depression. A recent meta-analysis described the magnitude of the difference between depressed and non-depressed group in cortisol, ACTH and CRH levels. Looking at 361 studies, the results show that overall depression is associated with small-to-moderate elevations in ACTH and cortisol and a reduction in CRH levels (Stetler and Miller, 2011). However, in older people, the association between cortisol and major depression was U-shaped (Bremmer et al., 2007). Another large cohort study revealed significant associations between major depressive disorders and specific HPA axis indicators, such as a higher cortisol awakening response in MDD patients compared to controls (Vreeburg et al., 2009). Those modest but significant differences were also observed in patients with anxiety disorders (Vreeburg et al., 2010).

In line with clinical findings, the circadian pattern of corticosterone has been reported to be disrupted in rodent models of depression (Touma et al., 2009; Bonilla-Jaime et al., 2010). In rats, chronic stress induces a depressive-like phenotype, associated with dysregulation of the HPA axis and reductions in dopaminergic and serotonergic transmissions in the PFC (Mizoguchi et al., 2008). Affective-like behavioral deficits have been reported in mouse mutants with altered HPA axis function [see Renoir et al. (2013) for review]. Chronic treatment with corticosterone as well as isolation rearing increase the depressive-like behavior in GR-dependent and independent manners (Ago et al., 2008). Chronic elevation of corticosterone creates a vulnerability to a depression-like syndrome that is associated with increased expression of the serotonin synthetic enzyme tryptophan hydroxylase 2 (tph2), similar to that observed in depressed patients (Donner et al., 2012). Interestingly, the effects of chronic corticosterone administration in animal models have also been studied in the context of affective and systemic disorders. In that regard, chronic corticosterone in mice was found to induce anxiety/depression-like behaviors (David et al., 2009) as well as decrease sucrose consumption in a model of anhedonia (Gourley et al., 2008). Chronic antidepressant treatment reversed those behavioral impairments. Furthermore, relevant to the relationship between stress and metabolic syndrome, 4-wk exposure to high doses of corticosterone in mice, has been found to increase weight gain and plasma insulin levels as well as reduce home-cage locomotion (Karatsoreos et al., 2010).

Using a chronic mild stress (CMS) paradigm, in which mice were housed individually and alternatively submitted to unpredictable "mild" stressors (such as periods of continuous overnight illumination, short periods of food/water deprivation etc.), Palumbo et al. (2010) found that mice subjected to the CMS procedure exhibited an increase in serum corticosterone levels during the first few weeks of exposure. However, these elevated corticosterone levels returned to baseline levels after 6 weeks of CMS. Similarly, Adzic et al. (2009) reported reduced CORT levels in chronically isolated rats (for 21 days), whereas CORT was increased after an acute 30-min immobilization stress. Altered circadian activity of the HPA axis has also been reported in a CMS rat model of depression (Christiansen et al., 2012). Interestingly, this study suggests a recovery of diurnal corticosterone rhythm after 8 weeks of CMS. Taken together, these observations suggest an adaptive capacity for the HPA axis to cope with prolonged stress.

The effects of chronic stress on HPA axis function have been widely studied in both animal models and clinical populations. Many of those investigations have focused on the negative feedback part of the HPA axis (mainly mediated by the GR). Such feedback is efficiently probed by the established combined dexamethasone-suppression/corticotrophin-releasing hormone stimulation (dex/CRH) test (Ising et al., 2007). Altered dex/CRH test are seen in major depression (Mokhtari et al., 2013) as well as in chronic stress conditions. For example, over-commitment in chronically work-stressed teachers was significantly associated with blunted response to the dex/CRH challenge (Wolfram et al., 2013). Further regression analyses showed that low social support at work and high job strain were associated with more cortisol suppression after the dexamethasone suppression test (Holleman et al., 2012). In rodents, social isolation decreased the feedback sensitivity of the HPA axis to dexamethasone (Evans et al., 2012). Another animal study reported that socially deprived mice had increased adrenal weights as well as a greater increase in corticosterone levels in response to acute stress (Berry et al., 2012). Interestingly, those chronic stress-induced HPA axis dysfunctions were associated with depressive/anxiety-like behavior as well as impaired hippocampal plasticity (i.e., altered hippocampal neurogenesis and reduction in BDNF levels) (Berry et al., 2012; Evans et al., 2012).

Polymorphisms in genes controlling the activity of the HPA axis are also associated with differential risk of psychiatric disease. Polymorphisms in the GR gene have been associated with major depression in multiple cohorts (van West et al., 2005; van Rossum et al., 2006) [but also see Zou et al. (2010); Zimmermann et al. (2011)]. Interestingly, some GR polymorphisms are also a predictor of the HPA axis response to psychosocial tests (Kumsta et al., 2007) and have been found to be associated with the extent of stress hormone dysregulation in major depression (Menke et al., 2013). Genotype-phenotype associations have also been identified in terms of response to antidepressant response (Ellsworth et al., 2013). Evidence of gene-environment interactions in the stress response and psychiatric susceptibility comes from a study of the corticotrophin-releasing factor receptor (CRF-R) (Bradley et al., 2008). Individuals with a particular CRF-R genotype who had experienced child abuse had enhanced risk of depression as adults, an observation repeated in two ethnically different populations. Overall, studies suggest that the degree of HPA axis hyperactivity can vary considerably across psychiatric patient groups, likely due to genetic and environmental factors during early development or adult life. In that regard, two separate studies reported that polymorphisms of the FKBP5 gene that potentially modify the sensitivity of the GR are associated with an increased likelihood of adult depression for individuals exposed to adverse life events (Zimmermann et al., 2011) and childhood physical abuse (Appel et al., 2011). Genes involved in other pathways may also potentiate an aversive response to stress. A landmark early study described an association between a variant in the serotonin transporter gene and the response to stressful life experiences (Caspi et al., 2003). This functional variant in a major target of antidepressant therapies is associated with an elevated response to fearful stimuli, elevated hormonal responses to stress, and increased risk of depression in response to stress exposure (Lesch et al., 1996; Hariri et al., 2002; Jabbi et al., 2007). Variants in multiple genes in the serotonergic pathway have also been associated with altered behavioral phenotypes in animal models [reviewed in Holmes (2008)]. Critically, changes in circulating corticosteroids can regulate the activity of the rate-limiting serotonin synthetic enzyme tryptophan hydroxylase 2 in the brain (Clark et al., 2005, 2007). In rodent models, acute restraint stress up-regulates serotonin production in the amygdala (Mo et al., 2008), whilst chronic administration of ACTH to disrupt HPA axis function results in an increased level of serotonin in the prefrontal cortex in response to acute stress (Walker et al., 2013). Taken together these findings demonstrate that alterations in HPA axis function can directly impact on CNS systems known to be associated with psychiatric disease.

PERIPHERAL DISORDERS ASSOCIATED WITH HPA CHANGES AND PSYCHIATRIC DISEASE

A wealth of evidence is now emerging to illustrate the link between stress and risk factors for physiological disorders, in particular metabolic disorders. Hyperactivity of the HPA axis and hypercortisolaemia is associated with the metabolic syndrome (Anagnostis et al., 2009). Similarly, both chronic stress and chronic treatment with glucocorticoids are associated with central adiposity, dyslipidaemia, atrophy of skeletal muscles, insulin resistance, and glucose intolerance: a suite of symptoms remarkably resemblant of the metabolic syndrome itself (Kyrou and Tsigos, 2009; van Raalte et al., 2009).

Elevations of circulating glucocorticoids have also been linked with an increased risk of depression in those with metabolic disorder (Vogelzangs et al., 2009), and relative insensitivity to the dexamethasone suppression test has been documented in patients with this disorder (Kazakou et al., 2012). On the other hand, disturbances in fatty acid metabolism have been observed in cohort studies of depression (Assies et al., 2010). Fatty acid levels appear to have a bidirectional relationship with HPA axis activity, with glucocorticoids modulating fatty acid metabolism (Brenner et al., 2001; Macfarlane et al., 2008), and supplementation of polyunsaturated fatty acids reducing cortisol levels in both healthy subjects (Delarue et al., 2003) and in those with depression (Jazayeri et al., 2010; Mocking et al., 2012). A study examining this relationship in more detail has shown that the circadian changes in cortisol have a different association with the major fatty acid forms in major depression patients compared to controls (Mocking et al., 2013). Other studies have demonstrated both changes in visceral fat levels and adrenal gland volume in women with major depressive disorders (Ludescher et al., 2008). Some of these associations appear to have developmental antecedents, with exposure to dietary high fat in the perinatal period being linked with both altered HPA axis function and mood changes (Sasaki et al., 2013).

If metabolic disorders are considered as a spectrum, then diabetes is arguably positioned as the end point of this decline in function. Chronic stress and sustained dysregulation of corticosteroid production are strongly associated with the development of type 2 diabetes mellitus in both human cohorts and in animal models (Chan et al., 2003; Rosmond, 2005; Reagan et al., 2008; Anagnostis et al., 2009; Matthews and Hanley, 2011). As an example in mice, streptozotocin (STZ)-induced diabetes resulted in increased depressive-like behavior as well as increased corticosterone levels (Ho et al., 2012). The convergence of the associations between HPA axis dysfunction and both diabetes and depression is striking, with compelling evidence for links between the two disorders and this central underlying risk factor [reviewed in Champaneri et al. (2010)].

Dysfunction of HPA signaling also appears to interact with the autonomic nervous system to influence cardiovascular function. Components of the HPA axis act outside the hypothalamus to regulate sympathetic outflow, and thus heart rate. Elevated heart rate has been associated with depression in multiple studies (Forbes and Chaney, 1980; Carney et al., 1993, 2000; Lechin et al., 1995), and is a strong predictor of multiple parameters of cardiovascular disease, including myocardial ischaemia, arrhythmias, hypertension, and cardiac failure (Dyer et al., 1980; Kannel et al., 1987; Palatini and Julius, 1997). Depression is associated with an increased risk of mortality in patients with cardiovascular disease (Mann and Thakore, 1999), and this increased risk is strongly linked with hypercortisolaemia (Jokinen and Nordstrom, 2009). In healthy subjects, cortisol and ACTH response to the Dex/CRH test were negatively associated with central adiposity and blood pressure and positively associated with HDL cholesterol, strong risk factors for cardiovascular disease (Tyrka et al., 2012).

Taken together, these studies speak to the accumulating evidence suggesting a link between disorders which involve HPA dysregulation and the risk of developing psychiatric disease. This is illustrative of the bidirectional relationship between peripheral illness and mental health: HPA axis changes may be either contributors to or consequences of peripheral disorders but also have the capacity to modulate brain function and predispose to psychiatric disease.

PHARMACOLOGICAL TARGETING OF THE HPA AXIS

The GR antagonist mifepristone has been tested as an adjunctive treatment for psychiatric disorders (Schatzberg and Lindley, 2008). Most recently, a randomized controlled trial of adjunctive mifepristone in patients with bipolar disorder demonstrated alterations in cortisol levels which were correlated with improvements on neuropsychological tests of working memory (Watson et al., 2012). An earlier, smaller scale trial by the same group showed improvements in both neurocognitive function and depression rating scores (Young et al., 2004). However, a similar study in schizophrenia showed alterations in plasma cortisol but no significant change in symptoms (Gallagher et al., 2005). These mixed findings do highlight the potential utility of therapeutics targeting HPA axis function, but also are suggestive of the heterogeneity in the role of the HPA axis across, and potentially also within, psychiatric disorder diagnoses. The main challenge in pharmacological targeting of the HPA axis is that blockage of all GR-dependent processes could ultimately lead to counteractive effects such as elevated endogenous corticosterone levels. In that context, a newly developed high-affinity GR ligand (C108297) shows promising characteristics in rats (Zalachoras et al., 2013). Indeed, C108297 displays partial agonistic activity for suppression of CRH gene expression and potently enhances GR-dependent memory consolidation. This compound, which does not lead to disinhibition of the HPA axis, could help in dissecting the molecular signaling pathways underlying stress-related disorders. In recent years, other therapeutic strategies interacting at different levels of the HPA axis have been developed. Those include agents acting on CRH-R1 receptor and adrenal steroidogenesis as well as modulators of the 11β-hydroxysteroid dehydrogenase type (11β-HSD1), the enzyme regulating cortisol metabolism (Thomson and Craighead, 2008; Martocchia et al., 2011).

In patients who were successfully treated with fluoxetine, the secretion of cortisol decreased (Piwowarska et al., 2012). Furthermore, recent data suggest that GR levels in lymphocytes could be used to predict response to antidepressant treatment in major depressive patients (Rojas et al., 2011). However, it should be noted that GR levels seemed inconsistent over time in this study. Also, measuring cortisol levels in depressed patients before and following treatment with SSRI, Keating et al. (2013) concluded that that stress physiology was unlikely to be a key factor in the response to antidepressant treatment. The variation in findings from these studies may reflect differing modes of activity of the different antidepressant drug classes, superimposed on a heterogeneous patient population. This was illustrated in a study examining changes in daily cortisol patterns in patients using SSRIs, tricyclic antidepressants, other therapeutics or no medications (Manthey et al., 2011). A complex pattern emerged, with some antidepressants suppressing the morning peak in cortisol, and others altering the response to the dexamethasone suppression test. However, the challenges inherent to measuring a circulating factor which is both diurnally regulated and acutely sensitive to environmental cues should not be underestimated.

IMMUNE DYSREGULATION, INFLAMMATION AND PSYCHIATRIC HEALTH

There is strong evidence that peripheral growth factors, pro-inflammatory cytokines, endocrine factors, and metabolic markers contribute to the pathophysiology of major depressive disorders and antidepressant response (Schmidt et al., 2011). Similarly, many of the systemic disorders associated with a higher incidence of psychiatric disease involve a significant inflammatory component. In fact, as our understanding of the aetiology of these disorders deepens, it has become apparent that there is significant overlap between the factors driving peripheral inflammatory disease and psychiatric disorders. Elevations of pro-inflammatory cytokines have been observed in both clinical populations and animal models of heart failure (Levine et al., 1990; Francis et al., 2003), after coronary surgery (Hennein et al., 1994), and following heart transplants (Azzawi and Hasleton, 1999). Importantly, the pathogenesis of atherosclerosis is intrinsically inflammatory (Koenig, 2001), with elevated local and circulating pro-inflammatory cytokines. In addition, the acute-phase marker C-reactive protein (CRP) is strongly associated with cardiovascular disease (van Holten et al., 2013), and can be used as a diagnostic or prognostic factor. As discussed above, cardiovascular disease is strongly associated with changes in psychiatric health, in particular depression.

Cardiovascular disease is in turn closely linked with obesity, dyslipidemia, diabetes and metabolic disease. The elevated frequency of anxiety and depression in these disorders may in part underlie the association between cardiovascular and psychiatric risk factors. In studies of diabetic patient cohorts, the inflammatory marker CRP was consistently predictive of direct associations between depression severity, lipid profiles and obesity levels (van Reedt Dortland et al., 2013). Similarly, increased risk of depression in a cohort of patients with diabetes was associated with a higher BMI, illustrating the link between depression and poor control of cardiovascular risk factors (Kimbro et al., 2012). Obesity itself is considered to be a state of low-grade inflammation, and is linked with elevated depressive symptoms. In addition, in a longitudinal study CRP levels at baseline were statistically associated with depression scores (Daly, 2013).

Other disease states involving inflammatory processes are associated with elevated risk of depression. Major depression is the most common psychiatric manifestation of multiple sclerosis, with an incidence approaching 50% (Lo Fermo et al., 2010). Likewise, although the incidence rate varies significantly between studies, an elevated incidence of depression has been documented in systemic lupus erythematosus (Palagini et al., 2013) and rheumatoid arthritis (Dickens et al., 2002). Common to all of these disorders is an autoimmune-mediated elevation of inflammatory signaling, with increased circulating pro-inflammatory cytokines observed in the periphery and in the CNS. Large case-control studies have described increased rates of anxiety and depression in patients with inflammatory bowel disease (Kurina et al., 2001; Ananthakrishnan et al., 2013a,b). Altered gut permeability to enteric bacteria has also been associated with depression. Translocation of bacterial allergens [in particular lipopolysaccharide (LPS)], stimulates a systemic immune response characterized by elevated IgM and IgA antibodies reactive to the bacteria. Individuals with chronic depression are more likely to display increased LPS-reactive IgM and IgA than control subjects, indicating that elevated gut permeability may be potentiating a systemic inflammatory state (Maes et al., 2008, 2012a).

The case for altered peripheral inflammation in psychiatric disease is strong, perhaps most so for major depression. Individuals with clinically classifiable major depression exhibit a wide range of changes in inflammatory markers, including elevated cytokines, chemokines, and acute phase proteins, findings which have been replicated in several meta-analyses and which in some studies appear to be correlated with specific depressive symptoms (Miller et al., 2009). There appears to be a shift in the function of the immune system in depression, with an increase in pro-inflammatory cytokines accompanied by a decrease in cellular immunity (Zorrilla et al., 2001; Dowlati et al., 2010). The strength of these findings is heightened by a positive correlation between the elevations in pro-inflammatory cytokines and the severity of depression rating scores (Howren et al., 2009). A recent longitudinal population-based study demonstrated strong associations between depressive symptoms and elevated levels of the pro-inflammatory cytokine IL-6 and CRP (Lu et al., 2013). Notably, heightened IL-6, CRP and depressive symptoms were all predictive of reduced pulmonary function, in a cohort with no known history of obstructive pulmonary disease. This large study highlights the substantial cross-over between inflammatory disease and depressive symptomatology. However, there may be differences between sub-populations in depression, with some individuals more likely to display an inflammatory pathophysiology. Although the number of patients classified as suffering atypical depression is relatively low, these patients may be more likely to show high levels of inflammatory markers such as CRP (Hickman et al., 2013). Part of the population variance may result from polymorphisms in the CRP gene. The association between CRP levels and depressive symptoms may be moderated by CRP gene haplotype, in a complex manner which may underpin some of the variations in other association studies (Halder et al., 2010). Patients receiving therapeutic administration of cytokines for cancer or chronic viral infections, [in particular interferon (IFN)-alpha and interleukin-2] frequently experience psychiatric symptoms, including the development of frank major depression in a significant proportion of patients (Capuron et al., 2004; Raison et al., 2005). IFN-alpha stimulates both peripheral and central release of pro-inflammatory cytokines, a fact which underpins the behavioral effects of this cytokine and highlights the capacity for systemic immune signals to regulate CNS processes (Capuron et al., 2000, 2001, 2002, 2003, 2004; Raison et al., 2005; Eller et al., 2009; Alavi et al., 2012; Birerdinc et al., 2012; Udina et al., 2012).

Of particular relevance to the treatment of depressive disorders is the emerging evidence that at least part of the therapeutic efficacy of currently available antidepressants may result from their concomitant anti-inflammatory effects. Although the response rate and efficacy of current antidepressants is far from universal, at least some patient populations derive significant benefit from these medications. However, the previously accepted notion that modulation of synaptic monoamines represents the sum total of the therapeutic effects of these drugs has now come into question. Recent studies have shown that selective-serotonin-reuptake inhibitor medications can suppress immune cell activation and release of inflammatory cytokines in the periphery and *ex-vivo* (Diamond et al., 2006; Taler et al., 2007; Branco-de-Almeida et al., 2011). Notably, this immune-regulatory effect is not restricted only to the periphery, but can also affect microglia, the immune cells of the CNS (Hashioka et al., 2007; Horikawa et al., 2010). A recent meta-analysis of human depression studies showed that antidepressant treatment at least partially ameliorates the elevations of pro-inflammatory cytokines associated with the disorder (Hannestad et al., 2011). Although it is clear that drug discovery in psychiatric disease needs to look beyond established drug classes, these findings emphasize the potential clinical utility of targeting inflammatory function in depression. Finally, potential sex-differences have been suggested when assessing the effects of LPS on cytokine gene expression. Indeed, females had increased hippocampal levels of IL-6 of TNF-α with respect to males after repeated administration of LPS (Tonelli et al., 2008).

MECHANISMS OF IMMUNE MODULATION OF PSYCHIATRIC FUNCTION

Historically the CNS was regarded as a "privileged" site with regards to the immune system, with little immune communication across the blood-brain barrier except in cases of frank CNS infection. However, it is now clear that the brain is sensitive to peripheral immune stimuli and can respond with activation of central immune cells and local production of inflammatory cytokines. Microglia are the CNS equivalent of macrophages, releasing cytokines upon activation and facilitating a central immune response, even in the absence of peripheral immune cell migration into the CNS. The brain's response to peripheral inflammatory stimuli can be seen most clearly in the pattern of behavioral changes which reliably results from systemic infection, administration of synthetic bacterial wall components or administration of cytokines (Dantzer, 2004; Pucak and Kaplin, 2005). Termed "sickness behavior," this encompasses changes in motor activity, consummatory behavior, social interaction, circadian rhythms, and responsivity to hedonic and aversive stimuli. The parallels between these behavioral changes and aspects of depression have been well noted and have been a prompt for extensive research.

Systemic administration of synthetic bacterial endotoxin, or LPS, induces a well-established pattern of peripheral inflammation. However, multiple studies have now also demonstrated that systemic inflammation activates CNS microglia, including in non-human primates (Henry et al., 2008; Hannestad et al., 2012). In mice, systemic LPS causes microglial activation and synthesis of cytokines (Puntener et al., 2012). Microglia form close contacts with synaptic structures and appear to regulate synaptic strength (Wake et al., 2009). These cells also express multiple neurotransmitter receptors and are therefore acutely responsive to neuronal signaling (Kettenmann et al., 2011). Activated microglia are also a key source of reactive oxygen species, contributing to a status of inflammation-induced oxidative stress in the CNS (Dringen, 2005). Oxidative stress, driven both peripherally and centrally, is strongly associated with psychiatric aetiology.

Reduced plasma L-tryptophan, the precursor for serotonin, is a potential biomarker of "vulnerability to depression" (Maes et al., 1993). Indeed, tryptophan depletion is widely used to study the contribution of reduced serotonin transmission to the pathogenesis of major depressive disorder (Van der Does, 2001) and also relevant in the context of immune activation (Kurz et al., 2011). The depressive symptomatology associated with immunomodulatory therapy may be mediated in part by changes in tryptophan metabolism. Pro-inflammatory cytokines such as IFN-γ, IFN-α, and TNF-α, and reactive oxygen species, induce activation of the enzyme, indolamine 2, 3 dioxygenase (IDO) in microglia, which metabolizes tryptophan via the kyneurenine pathway (Maes, 1999; Wichers et al., 2005; Dantzer et al., 2008; Maes et al.,

2012b). This shifts the balance of tryptophan toward kynurenine and away from serotonin, reducing serotonin bioavailability (Capuron et al., 2002, 2003; Vignau et al., 2009). Notably, in the CNS only microglia further metabolize kynurenine to quinolinic acid, which exerts neurotoxic effects (Guillemin et al., 2005; Soczynska et al., 2012). Patients treated with IFN-α for hepatitis C infection developed depressive symptoms including negative moods that were correlated with increased levels of kynurenine (Wichers et al., 2005). In addition, analysis of plasma tryptophan and kynurenine pathway metabolites in patients with major depression showed increased rates of tryptophan degradation compared to normal control subjects (Myint et al., 2007). Taken together, these findings indicate that cytokine-induced microglial activation can mediate changes in neurotransmitters and other bioactive metabolites which may underpin mood disorders. Also, recent data indicate that cognitive impairments (as well as the decline in neurogenesis observed during ageing) can be in part attributed to dysregulation in blood-borne factors such as changes in peripheral CCL11 chemokine levels (Villeda et al., 2011). These findings support the crosstalk between peripheral molecular processes to central effects related to cognitive and emotional function.

PHARMACOLOGICAL TARGETING OF INFLAMMATORY PATHWAYS

Several of the therapies for the inflammatory disorder rheumatoid arthritis potentiate the effects of antidepressant therapies (Margaretten et al., 2011b). Such drugs target pro-inflammatory cytokine pathways, for example TNF-α antagonists such as etanercept. This particular drug is also commonly used in the treatment of the inflammatory skin condition psoriasis, and large-scale studies of this drug have indicated that patients with psoriasis receiving this drug show reduced depression scores relative to placebo (although the level of depressive symptoms in these patients was relatively low overall, and would not constitute a diagnosis of major depression) (Tyring et al., 2006). Interestingly, follow-up studies indicated that the change in depression score was independent of disease state (Krishnan et al., 2007). Drugs with a similar TNF-α antagonist activity have also shown antidepressant activity in trials in patients with other inflammatory conditions, including Crohn's disease and ankylosing spondylitis (Persoons et al., 2005; Ertenli et al., 2012).

Critically, a recent study of the TNF-α antagonist infliximab in otherwise healthy patients with major depression demonstrated that the antidepressant activity of this drug was dependent on the level of inflammatory markers at baseline (Raison et al., 2013). This study demonstrated that depressed patients with higher levels of the inflammatory markers TNF-α and CRP showed a decrease in depression rating scores over the course of the study. It is also worth noting that the patients in this study were poorly responsive to classical antidepressant therapy, which may indicate that a sub-population exists in whom inflammation is correlated with both poor antidepressant response and efficacy of anti-inflammatory medication. A second recent study also demonstrated that patients with depression who experienced a decline in symptoms with infliximab treatment also showed elevated inflammatory gene expression in peripheral immune cells (Mehta et al., 2013). Response to infliximab was also associated with reductions in the expression of other genes involved with innate immune activation. Agents such as infliximab are too large to cross the blood-brain barrier, and therefore the amelioration of depressive symptoms is more likely associated with resolution of peripheral inflammation than direct effects of the drug in the brain. However, as we have discussed above, CNS microglia are acutely sensitive to circulating cytokine levels and so their level of activity may well be modulated by anti-inflammatory treatment.

The developing focus on inflammatory function in depression has spurred trials of other anti-inflammatory drugs as adjuncts to antidepressant treatment. A large-scale longitudinal population study revealed that statin users were less likely than non-users to have depression at baseline (Otte et al., 2012). Statin users who did not have depressive symptoms at baseline were also less likely to develop depression during the follow-up period. Statins are commonly prescribed to individuals who have had a cardiac event or intervention. A prospective study in this population showed that prescription of statins reduced the likelihood of developing depression by up to 79% (Stafford and Berk, 2011). A large community study also documented reduced exposure to statins and aspirin (another non-steroidal anti-inflammatory agent) in women with major depressive disorder (Pasco et al., 2010). Likewise, women who were exposed to these agents were also less likely to develop depression over the course of the study. Similar results were also observed in a large population-based cohort of elderly patients, with statins exerting a protective effect against the development of depressive symptoms (Feng et al., 2008). Notably, this study also documented a positive correlation between the use of systemic corticosteroids and depression.

The cyclooxygenase-2 (COX-2) inhibitor celecoxib is a non-steroidal anti-inflammatory drug used widely in the treatment of pain, particularly related to arthritic conditions. This drug has been found to improve depressive symptoms when administered in conjunction with the antidepressants sertraline (Abbasi et al., 2012), reboxetine (Muller et al., 2006), and fluoxetine (Akhondzadeh et al., 2009). However, it should be noted that other trials have resulted in conflicting findings, with several showing no beneficial effect of celecoxib in depression (Musil et al., 2011; Fields et al., 2012). The discrepancies in these study results are potentially reflective of the complexity of the inflammatory pathways, in which COX-2 and many other key molecules may play multiple roles. In the brain, COX-2 has anti-inflammatory and neuroprotective effects (Minghetti, 2004), and COX-2 deficient mice show increased neuronal damage, microglial reactivity and oxidative stress markers (Aid et al., 2008). Hence targeting of inflammatory pathways in depression requires careful investigation of both peripheral and central responsivity. COX-2, in particular, may not be the most appropriate target for adjunct therapies in depression [reviewed in Maes (2012)]. In addition, modulation of immune and inflammatory signaling necessitates caution with regard to the potential of lowering defenses to opportunistic infection and malignancy. Long term use of immune-modifying drugs has been associated with increased incidence of serious infections and cancer (Bongartz et al., 2006; Atzeni et al., 2012; van Dartel et al., 2013). This raises the possibility that agents which directly regulate the CNS rather than peripheral inflammatory response, or have more mild anti-inflammatory effects, may be more appropriate targets for the pharmacotherapy of depression.

Still peripherally-active, but arguably milder in effect, are the non-steroidal anti inflammatory medications, including aspirin. Animal studies using aspirin have shown moderate but discernible effects on depressive behavior (Brunello et al., 2006; Wang et al., 2011). Preliminary clinical trials have correlated this, showing a synergistic effect of co-therapy with antidepressants and aspirin (Mendlewicz et al., 2006). However, perhaps more compelling is the result from a large-scale longitudinal cohort study, which documented an association between aspirin use and lowered risk of depression (Pasco et al., 2010). Echoing this is a cross-sectional study which demonstrated that men with elevated plasma homocysteine, a marker of cardiovascular risk, had a reduced risk of depression if they had been taking aspirin (Almeida et al., 2012).

Minocycline, a second-generation tetracycline derivative, has recently attracted significant attention for its potential efficacy as an antidepressant. This well characterized drug has potent anti-inflammatory and neuroprotective effects which are independent of its antibiotic efficacy (Pae et al., 2008; Dean et al., 2012). Most importantly, minocycline readily crosses the blood brain barrier and is known to inhibit microglial activation (Pae et al., 2008; Dean et al., 2012). Studies in mice have demonstrated that minocycline attenuated the elevations in CNS IL-1β, IL-6, and IDO induced by bacterial endotoxins (Henry et al., 2008). This study also showed that pre-treatment with minocycline prevented the development of depressive-like behavioral endophenotypes, and normalized the kynurenine/tryptophan ratio in the plasma and brain (Henry et al., 2008). These findings clearly indicate that minocycline has effects on microglia through inhibition of the synthesis of pro-inflammatory cytokines and IDO up-regulation, and that these may flow through to ameliorate mood states. Echoing this, a small open-label study reported minocycline (150 mg/kg/day) in combination with serotonin reuptake inhibitor contributed to ameliorate depressive mood and psychotic symptoms in patients with psychotic unipolar depression (Miyaoka et al., 2012).

The developing appreciation of the role of inflammatory function in depression has highlighted the potential role of dietary sources of anti-inflammatory species. Deficiencies of the anti-oxidant and anti-inflammatory Coenzyme Q10 (CoQ10) have been associated with depressed mood (Maes et al., 2009), and a preliminary study of supplementation with CoQ10 showed an amelioration of depression scores in a cohort with bipolar disorder (Forester et al., 2012). Several studies in pre-clinical models have shown potential antidepressant effects of omega 3 fatty acids (Watanabe et al., 2004), and conversely, deficient diets during prenatal development have been associated with persistent changes in mood state (Chen and Su, 2013). Compounding this, altered lipid profiles have been described in the cortex of patients with mood disorders (Tatebayashi et al., 2012). Large-scale population assays have shown associations between dietary lipid profiles and the risk of depression (Hoffmire et al., 2012). Although the outcomes of clinical trials using omega 3 supplementation are still under some debate, recent meta-analyses have pointed to some degree of improved outcome in depressed patients (Lin and Su, 2007; Bloch and Hannestad, 2012; Martins et al., 2012). Intriguingly, omega 3 fatty acids have received particular attention for the treatment of depressive symptoms post-myocardial infarction (Gilbert et al., 2013; Siddiqui and Harvey, 2013). In such cases, the anti-inflammatory effects of this lipid may be ameliorating both the peripheral inflammatory state and the secondary central inflammation.

INTERFACES BETWEEN HPA AXIS AND IMMUNE DYSFUNCTION

Whilst it is clear that both inflammation and HPA dysfunction are associated with psychiatric pathology, these two systems interact at multiple levels and may together constitute a synergistic effect on neuronal function. Across the spectrum of systemic disorders associated with peripheral inflammation and an increased risk of depression, many are also associated with elevated susceptibility to, or worsening symptoms in response to stress. A large scale longitudinal study showed an association between inflammatory bowel disease (Crohn's disease and ulcerative colitis) and depressive symptoms (Ananthakrishnan et al., 2013b). These disorders are strongly associated with perceived life stress, with time to relapse predicted by stress levels (Triantafillidis et al., 2013). Studies of metabolic syndrome, diabetes and associated cardiovascular diseases have shown that not only is this suite of disorders associated with increased risk of depression and a low-grade inflammatory state, but that chronic stress is a strong promoting factor [reviewed in Kyrou and Tsigos (2009)]. These interactions may have developmental antecedents, with exposure to a high fat diet in early life being associated with both altered HPA axis function, inflammatory regulation and disordered behavioral profiles in later life (Sasaki et al., 2013). Nonetheless, the question remains as to how these complex systems interact in both the periphery and CNS, and by what mechanisms these systems modulate neuronal function and mood.

Synthetic glucocorticoids are used therapeutically at supra-physiological levels for their anti-inflammatory effects. However, when examining the relationship between the HPA axis and the immune system in physiological or pathophysiological states, the situation appears more complex. Glucocorticoids modulate the immune system through binding to receptors expressed by immune cells, which down-regulates transcription of pro-inflammatory genes and up-regulates production of anti-inflammatory cytokines (Barnes, 2006; Leonard, 2006). Glucocorticoids also regulate the circulating numbers, tissue distribution and activity profile of lymphocytes in a time-dependent manner [comprehensively reviewed in Dhabhar (2009)]. Compared to acute stress, chronic stress appears to suppress some of the protective aspects of immune regulation, whilst enhancing the drive to a pro-inflammatory state. The complexity of these interactions is reflective of the fact that chronic stimulation of the HPA axis may not in fact result in a hypercortisolaemic state; given the capacity of the HPA axis for negative feedback regulation, the baseline cortisol levels in chronic stress may actually be lower than normal. Glucocorticoids can be used therapeutically as immuno-suppressants but in some experimental models appear to have pro-inflammatory effects. Part of this discrepancy may come from differences between *in vivo* and *in vitro* models, however in addition the complexities of chronic stress in an animal model should not be overlooked. Chronic stress may appear to increase or decrease circulating glucocorticoids depending on the method of stress and the method of glucocorticoid measurement employed. An animal with chronic down-regulation of HPA axis responsivity, for example, may respond to the acute stress of blood collection or some forms of euthanasia with an overshoot of normal glucocorticoid response, giving the impression of elevated circulating hormone levels in response to the chronic stress.

Immune activation may also feed back to modulate glucocorticoid sensitivity. Production of cytokines also up-regulates expression of the GR and modulates the sensitivity of the HPA axis to negative feedback (Arzt et al., 2000). Elevation of pro-inflammatory cytokines, including IL-2, appears to inhibit nuclear translocation of the GR and suppress glucocorticoid signaling (Goleva et al., 2009; Schewitz et al., 2009). Likewise, administration of IL-1 up-regulates HPA axis activity (Dunn, 2000). Systemic exposure to pro-inflammatory stimuli such as bacterial LPS induces secretion of CRH, therefore activating the HPA axis (Sternberg, 2006). These studies illustrate the complex bidirectional interactions between HPA axis function and regulation of inflammation. Potential sex-differences have been suggested when assessing the effects of LPS on stress response. Indeed, female rats showed a higher LPS-induced corticosterone release compared to male animals (Tonelli et al., 2008). The relationship between HPA axis activity and inflammation may also be regionally specific. The peripheral response to stress and HPA activation is likely to be qualitatively, quantitatively and temporally distinct from that observed in the CNS. In a mouse model of chronic stress, increases in basal inflammatory markers were observed in multiple brain regions (Barnum et al., 2012). Chronic unpredictable stress can also up-regulate the response to peripheral inflammatory stimuli, mediated by glucocorticoid signaling (Munhoz et al., 2006). This differs somewhat to the concept of glucocorticoid signaling as immunosuppressive, and highlights the need for further investigation of the nexus between HPA and immune function in the brain. Microglia represents the critical interface point between the activity of the HPA axis, circulating inflammatory signals and the brain's inflammatory response. Microglial number and morphological changes associated with activation can be increased by chronic stress in animal models (Nair and Bonneau, 2006; Tynan et al., 2010). Blockade of glucocorticoid signaling can block stress-induced sensitization of microglial inflammatory responses (Frank et al., 2011), and microglial activation can be primed by *in vivo* exposure to glucocorticoids (Nair and Bonneau, 2006) or chronic stress (Farooq et al., 2012). Within the CNS, the balance between pro- and anti-inflammatory responses to peripheral immune stimuli is modulated by the density of microglial cells (Pintado et al., 2011).

The relationship between microglial activation and the stress response has been most comprehensively investigated in animal models. Repeated exposure to restraint stress induced microglial activation in male C57BL/6 mice, as measured by the degree of proliferation of microglia (Nair and Bonneau, 2006). The increase in microglial number was positively correlated with elevation of serum corticosterone levels induced by stress exposure. Similarly, chronic restraint stress caused a significant increase in activated microglia and number of microglia in multiple brain regions (Tynan et al., 2010; Hinwood et al., 2012), and inescapable stress potentiates the microglial response to immune stimuli (Frank et al., 2012). However, high doses of glucocorticoid agonists suppress the microglial production of inflammatory cytokines (Chantong et al., 2012). These differential responses may be reflective of central vs. peripheral differences, in addition to switching from a pro- to anti-inflammatory response to physiological vs. pharmacological levels of glucocorticoids. Nonetheless, the consensus from these studies is that microglia are acutely sensitive to both HPA axis function and inflammatory signals, and act as an inflection point between peripheral and central responses to these stimuli. As discussed above, the activation state of the microglial population has direct effects on neuronal function, via secondary cytokine production, reactive oxygen species production, neurotoxic effects and modulation of neurotransmitter production.

CONCLUSIONS

It has long been established in traditional forms of medicine and in anecdotal knowledge that the health of the body and the mind are inextricably linked. Although strong associations between somatic illnesses and psychiatric disturbances have routinely been described in the literature, it is only recently that western medicine has sought to, or indeed had the means to, investigate the mechanisms underlying these associations. Strong and continually developing evidence now suggests that converging disruptions to inflammatory and endocrine pathways may interact in both the periphery and the CNS to potentiate states of psychiatric dysfunction, in particular depressed mood. Further evidence highlights the potential role of the CNS inflammatory

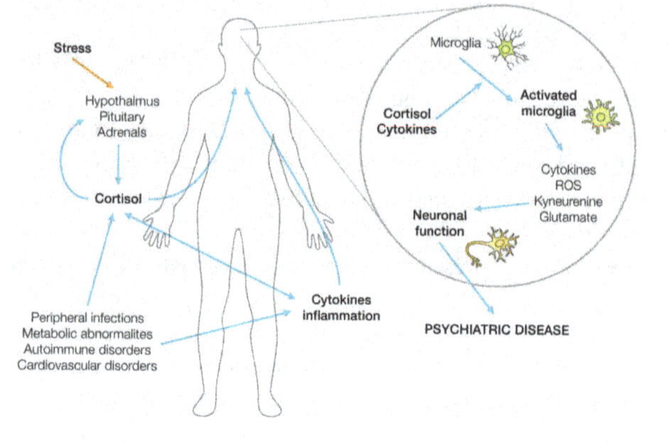

FIGURE 1 | Biological mechanisms by which peripheral dysfunction may impact on neuronal function and therefore psychiatric state. Schematic illustration of the potential role of the CNS inflammatory cells, microglia, as a critical nexus between HPA axis activity, inflammation, and neuronal dysfunction.

cells, microglia, as a critical nexus between HPA axis activity, inflammation and neuronal dysfunction (**Figure 1**). Aspects of these pathways may therefore present as possible targets for therapeutic interventions for psychiatric disease or psychiatric complications of somatic disease. Even more efficacious may be targeting multiple aspects of these pathways or convergence points such as central microglial cells.

In this review we have focused on the biological mechanisms by which peripheral dysfunction may impact on neuronal function and therefore psychiatric state. However, we do not wish to discount the psychological influence of ill health on mental function. Clearly the psychological stresses associated with chronic illness or suboptimal health may themselves potentiate, perpetuate and exacerbate psychiatric disease. An effective clinical approach to integrated patient management therefore may need to target the HPA axis dysfunction, inflammatory changes or other pathological processes associated with peripheral disorders, but also approach the psychological health of the patient.

REFERENCES

Abbasi, S. H., Hosseini, F., Modabbernia, A., Ashrafi, M., and Akhondzadeh, S. (2012). Effect of celecoxib add-on treatment on symptoms and serum IL-6 concentrations in patients with major depressive disorder: randomized double-blind placebo-controlled study. J. Affect. Disord. 141, 308–314. doi: 10.1016/j.jad.2012.03.033

Adzic, M., Djordjevic, J., Djordjevic, A., Niciforovic, A., Demonacos, C., Radojcic, M., et al. (2009). Acute or chronic stress induce cell compartment-specific phosphorylation of glucocorticoid receptor and alter its transcriptional activity in Wistar rat brain. J. Endocrinol. 202, 87–97. doi: 10.1677/joe-08-0509

Ago, Y., Arikawa, S., Yata, M., Yano, K., Abe, M., Takuma, K., et al. (2008). Antidepressant-like effects of the glucocorticoid receptor antagonist RU-43044 are associated with changes in prefrontal dopamine in mouse models of depression. Neuropharmacology 55, 1355–1363. doi: 10.1016/j.neuropharm.2008.08.026

Aid, S., Langenbach, R., and Bosetti, F. (2008). Neuroinflammatory response to lipopolysaccharide is exacerbated in mice genetically deficient in cyclooxygenase-2. J. Neuroinflammation 5, 17. doi: 10.1186/1742-2094-5-17

Akhondzadeh, S., Jafari, S., Raisi, F., Nasehi, A. A., Ghoreishi, A., Salehi, B., et al. (2009). Clinical trial of adjunctive celecoxib treatment in patients with major depression: a double blind and placebo controlled trial. Depress. Anxiety 26, 607–611. doi: 10.1002/da.20589

Alavi, M., Grebely, J., Matthews, G. V., Petoumenos, K., Yeung, B., Day, C., et al. (2012). Effect of pegylated interferon-alpha-2a treatment on mental health during recent hepatitis C virus infection. J. Gastroenterol. Hepatol. 27, 957–965. doi: 10.1111/j.1440-1746.2011.07035.x

Almeida, O. P., Flicker, L., Yeap, B. B., Alfonso, H., McCaul, K., and Hankey, G. J. (2012). Aspirin decreases the risk of depression in older men with high plasma homocysteine. Transl. Psychiatry 2:e151. doi: 10.1038/tp.2012.79

Anagnostis, P., Athyros, V. G., Tziomalos, K., Karagiannis, A., and Mikhailidis, D. P. (2009). The pathogenetic role of cortisol in the metabolic syndrome: a hypothesis. J. Clin. Endocrinol. Metab. 94, 2692–2701. doi: 10.1210/jc.2009-0370

Ananthakrishnan, A. N., Gainer, V. S., Cai, T., Perez, R. G., Cheng, S. C., Savova, G., et al. (2013a). Similar risk of depression and anxiety following surgery or hospitalization for Crohn's disease and ulcerative colitis. Am. J. Gastroenterol. 108, 594–601. doi: 10.1038/ajg.2012.471

Ananthakrishnan, A. N., Khalili, H., Pan, A., Higuchi, L. M., de Silva, P., Richter, J. M., et al. (2013b). Association between depressive symptoms and incidence of Crohn's disease and ulcerative colitis: results from the Nurses' Health Study. Clin. Gastroenterol. Hepatol. 11, 57–62. doi: 10.1016/j.cgh.2012.08.032

Anderson, R. J., Freedland, K. E., Clouse, R. E., and Lustman, P. J. (2001). The prevalence of comorbid depression in adults with diabetes: a meta-analysis. Diabetes Care 24, 1069–1078. doi: 10.2337/diacare.24.6.1069

Anglin, R. E., Rosebush, P. I., and Mazurek, M. F. (2006). The neuropsychiatric pro- file of Addison's disease: revisiting a forgotten phenomenon. J. Neuropsychiatry Clin. Neurosci. 18, 450–459. doi: 10.1176/appi.neuropsych.18.4.450

Appel, K., Schwahn, C., Mahler, J., Schulz, A., Spitzer, C., Fenske, K., et al. (2011). Moderation of adult depression by a polymorphism in the FKBP5 gene and childhood physical abuse in the general population. Neuropsychopharmacology 36, 1982–1991. doi: 10.1038/npp.2011.81

Arzt, E., Kovalovsky, D., Igaz, L. M., Costas, M., Plazas, P., Refojo, D., et al. (2000). Functional cross-talk among cytokines, T-cell receptor, and glucocorticoid receptor transcriptional activity and action. Ann. N.Y. Acad. Sci. 917, 672–677. doi: 10.1111/j.1749-6632.2000.tb05433.x

Assies, J., Pouwer, F., Lok, A., Mocking, R. J., Bockting, C. L., Visser, I., et al. (2010). Plasma and erythrocyte fatty acid patterns in patients with recur- rent depression: a matched case-control study. PLoS ONE 5:e10635. doi: 10.1371/journal.pone.0010635

Atzeni, F., Sarzi-Puttini, P., Botsios, C., Carletto, A., Cipriani, P., Favalli, E. G., et al. (2012). Long-term anti-TNF therapy and the risk of serious infections in a cohort of patients with rheumatoid arthritis: comparison of adalimumab, etanercept and infliximab in the GISEA registry. Autoimmun. Rev. 12, 225–229. doi: 10.1016/j.autrev.2012.06.008

Azzawi, M., and Hasleton, P. (1999). Tumour necrosis factor alpha and the cardiovascular system: its role in cardiac allograft rejection and heart disease. Cardiovasc. Res. 43, 850–859. doi: 10.1016/S0008-6363(99) 00138-8

Bangasser, D. A., and Valentino, R. J. (2012). Sex differences in molecular and cel- lular substrates of stress. Cell. Mol. Neurobiol. 32, 709–723. doi: 10.1007/s10571-012-9824-4

Barnes, P. J. (2006). How corticosteroids control inflammation: Quintiles Prize Lecture 2005. Br. J. Pharmacol. 148, 245–254. doi: 10.1038/sj.bjp.0706736

Barnum, C. J., Pace, T. W., Hu, F., Neigh, G. N., and Tansey, M. G. (2012). Psychological stress in adolescent and adult mice increases neuroinflammation and attenuates the response to LPS challenge. J. Neuroinflammation 9, 9. doi: 10.1186/1742-2094-9-9

Barth, J., Schumacher, M., and Herrmann-Lingen, C. (2004). Depression as a risk factor for mortality in patients with coronary heart disease: a meta-analysis. Psychosom. Med. 66, 802–813. doi: 10.1097/01.psy.0000146332.53619.b2

Bekker, M. H., and van Mens-Verhulst, J. (2007). Anxiety disorders: sex differences in prevalence, degree, and background, but gender-neutral treatment. Gend. Med. 4(Suppl. B), S178–S193. doi: 10.1016/S1550-8579(07)80057-X

Berry, A., Bellisario, V., Capoccia, S., Tirassa, P., Calza, A., Alleva, E., et al. (2012). Social deprivation stress is a triggering factor for the emergence of anxiety- and depression-like behaviours and leads to reduced brain BDNF levels in C57BL/6J mice. Psychoneuroendocrinology 37, 762–772. doi: 10.1016/j.psyneuen.2011.09.007

Birerdinc, A., Afendy, A., Stepanova, M., Younossi, I., Baranova, A., and Younossi, Z. M. (2012). Gene expression profiles associated with depression in patients with chronic hepatitis C (CH-C). Brain Behav. 2, 525–531. doi: 10.1002/brb3.72

Bloch, M. H., and Hannestad, J. (2012). Omega-3 fatty acids for the treatment of depression: systematic review and meta-analysis. Mol. Psychiatry 17, 1272–1282. doi: 10.1038/mp.2011.100

Bongartz, T., Sutton, A. J., Sweeting, M. J., Buchan, I., Matteson, E. L., and Montori, V. (2006). Anti-TNF antibody therapy in rheumatoid arthritis and the risk of serious infections and malignancies: systematic review and meta-analysis of rare harmful effects in randomized controlled trials. JAMA 295, 2275–2285. doi: 10.1001/jama.295.19.2275

Bonilla-Jaime, H., Retana-Marquez, S., Arteaga-Silva, M., Hernandez-Gonzalez, M., and Vazquez-Palacios, G. (2010). Circadian activity of corticosterone in an animal model of depression: response to muscarinic cholinergic stimulation. Physiol. Behav. 100, 311–315. doi: 10.1016/j.physbeh.2010.03.002

Bradley, R. G., Binder, E. B., Epstein, M. P., Tang, Y., Nair, H. P., Liu, W., et al. (2008). Influence of child abuse on adult depression: moderation by the corticotropin-releasing hormone receptor gene. Arch. Gen. Psychiatry 65, 190–200. doi: 10.1001/archgenpsychiatry.2007.26

Branco-de-Almeida, L. S., Kajiya, M., Cardoso, C. R., Silva, M. J., Ohta, K., Rosalen, P. L., et al. (2011). Selective serotonin reuptake inhibitors attenuate the antigen presentation from dendritic cells to effector T lymphocytes. FEMS Immunol. Med. Microbiol. 62, 283–294. doi: 10.1111/j.1574-695X.2011. 00816.x

Bremmer, M. A., Deeg, D. J., Beekman, A. T., Penninx, B. W., Lips, P., and Hoogendijk, W. J. (2007). Major depression in late life is associated with both hypo- and hypercortisolemia. Biol. Psychiatry 62, 479–486. doi: 10.1016/j.biopsych.2006.11.033

Brenner, R. R., Ayala, S., and Garda, H. A. (2001). Effect of dexamethasone on the fatty acid composition of total liver microsomal lipids and phosphatidylcholine molecular species. Lipids 36, 1337–1345. doi: 10.1007/s11745-001-0850-1

Brunello, N., Alboni, S., Capone, G., Benatti, C., Blom, J. M., Tascedda, F., et al. (2006). Acetylsalicylic acid accelerates the antidepressant effect of fluoxetine in the chronic escape deficit model of depression. Int. Clin. Psychopharmacol. 21, 219–225. doi: 10.1097/00004850-200607000-00004

Bush, D. E., Ziegelstein, R. C., Patel, U. V., Thombs, B. D., Ford, D. E., Fauerbach, J. A., et al. (2005). Post-myocardial infarction depression. Evidence Report/Technology Assessment 123, 1–8.

Capuron, L., Neurauter, G., Musselman, D. L., Lawson, D. H., Nemeroff, C. B., Fuchs, D., et al. (2003). Interferon-alpha–induced changes in trypto- phan metabolism: relationship to depression and paroxetine treatment. Biol. Psychiatry 54, 906–914. doi: 10.1016/S0006-322300173-2

Capuron, L., Ravaud, A., and Dantzer, R. (2000). Early depressive symptoms in cancer patients receiving interleukin 2 and/or interferon alfa-2b therapy. J. Clin. Oncol. 18, 2143–2151.

Capuron, L., Ravaud, A., Gualde, N., Bosmans, E., Dantzer, R., Maes, M., et al. (2001). Association between immune activation and early depres- sive symptoms in cancer patients treated with interleukin-2-based therapy. Psychoneuroendocrinology 26, 797–808. doi: 10.1016/S0306-4530(01)00030-0

Capuron, L., Ravaud, A., Miller, A. H., and Dantzer, R. (2004). Baseline mood and psychosocial characteristics of patients developing depressive symptoms during interleukin-2 and/or interferon-alpha cancer therapy. Brain Behav. Immun. 18, 205–213. doi: 10.1016/j.bbi.2003.11.004

Capuron, L., Ravaud, A., Neveu, P. J., Miller, A. H., Maes, M., and Dantzer, R. (2002). Association between decreased serum tryptophan concentrations and depressive symptoms in cancer patients undergoing cytokine therapy. Mol. Psychiatry 7, 468–473. doi: 10.1038/sj.mp.4000995

Carnethon, M. R., Kinder, L. S., Fair, J. M., Stafford, R. S., and Fortmann, S. P. (2003). Symptoms of depression as a risk factor for incident diabetes: findings from the national health and nutrition examination epidemiologic follow-up study, 1971-1992. Am. J. Epidemiol. 158, 416–423. doi: 10.1093/aje/kwg172

Carney, R. M., and Freedland, K. E. (2008). Depression in patients with coronary heart disease. Am. J. Med.121, S20–S27. doi: 10.1016/j.amjmed.2008.09.010

Carney, R. M., Freedland, K. E., Rich, M. W., Smith, L. J., and Jaffe, A. S. (1993). Ventricular tachycardia and psychiatric depression in patients with coronary artery disease. Am. J. Med. 95, 23–28. doi: 10.1016/0002-9343(93)90228-H

Carney, R. M., Freedland, K. E., Stein, P. K., Skala, J. A., Hoffman, P., and Jaffe, A. S. (2000). Change in heart rate and heart rate variability during treatment for depression in patients with coronary heart disease. Psychosom. Med. 62, 639–647.

Caspi, A., Sugden, K., Moffitt, T. E., Taylor, A., Craig, I. W., Harrington, H., et al. (2003). Influence of life stress on depression: moderation by a polymorphism in the 5-HTT Gene. Science 301, 386–389. doi: 10.1126/science.1083968

Champaneri, S., Wand, G. S., Malhotra, S. S., Casagrande, S. S., and Golden, S. H. (2010). Biological basis of depression in adults with diabetes. Curr. Diab. Rep. 10, 396–405. doi: 10.1007/s11892-010-0148-9

Chan, O., Inouye, K., Riddell, M. C., Vranic, M., and Matthews, S. G. (2003). Diabetes and the hypothalamo-pituitary-adrenal (HPA) axis. Minerva Endocrinol. 28, 87–102.

Chantong, B., Kratschmar, D. V., Nashev, L. G., Balazs, Z., and Odermatt, A. (2012). Mineralocorticoid and glucocorticoid receptors differentially regulate NF-kappaB activity and pro-inflammatory cytokine production in murine BV-2 microglial cells. J. Neuroinflammation 9, 260. doi: 10.1186/1742-2094-9-260

Chen, H. F., and Su, H. M. (2013). Exposure to a maternal n-3 fatty acid-deficient diet during brain development provokes excessive hypothalamic-pituitary-adrenal axis responses to stress and behavioral indices of depression and anxiety in male rat offspring later in life. J. Nutr. Biochem. 24, 70–80. doi: 10.1016/j.jnutbio.2012.02.006

Christiansen, S., Bouzinova, E. V., Palme, R., and Wiborg, O. (2012). Circadian activity of the hypothalamic-pituitary-adrenal axis is differentially affected in the rat chronic mild stress model of depression. Stress (Amsterdam, Netherlands) 15, 647–657. doi: 10.3109/10253890.2011.654370

Clark, J. A., Flick, R. B., Pai, L. Y., Szalayova, I., Key, S., Conley, R. K., et al. (2007). Glucocorticoid modulation of tryptophan hydroxylase-2 protein in raphe nuclei and 5-hydroxytryptophan concentrations in frontal cortex of C57/Bl6 mice. Mol. Psychiatry 13, 498–506. doi: 10.1038/sj.mp.4002041

Clark, J. A., Pai, L.-Y., Flick, R. B., and Rohrer, S. P. (2005). Differential hormonal regulation of tryptophan hydroxylase-2 mRNA in the murine dorsal raphe nucleus. Biol. Psychiatry 57, 943–946. doi: 10.1016/j.biopsych.2005.01.013

Clouse, R. E., Lustman, P. J., Freedland, K. E., Griffith, L. S., McGill, J. B., and Carney, R. M. (2003). Depression and coronary heart dis- ease in women with diabetes. Psychosom. Med. 65, 376–383. doi: 10.1097/01.PSY.0000041624.96580.1F

Covic, T., Cumming, S. R., Pallant, J. F., Manolios, N., Emery, P., Conaghan, P. G., et al. (2012). Depression and anxiety in patients with rheumatoid arthritis: prevalence rates based on a comparison of the Depression, Anxiety and Stress Scale (DASS) and the hospital, Anxiety and Depression Scale (HADS). BMC Psychiatry 12:6. doi: 10.1186/1471-244x-12-16

Daly, M. (2013). The relationship of C-reactive protein to obesity-related depressive symptoms: a longitudinal study. Obesity (Silver Spring, Md) 21, 248–250. Epub 2013/02/14. doi: 10.1002/oby.20051

Dantzer, R. (2004). Cytokine-induced sickness behaviour: a neuroimmune response to activation of innate immunity. Eur. J. Pharmacol. 500, 399–411. doi: 10.1016/j.ejphar.2004.07.040

Dantzer, R., O'Connor, J. C., Freund, G. G., Johnson, R. W., and Kelley, K. W. (2008). From inflammation to sickness and depression: when the immune system subjugates the brain. Nat. Rev. Neurosci. 9, 46–56. doi: 10.1038/nrn2297

David, D. J., Samuels, B. A., Rainer, Q., Wang, J. W., Marsteller, D., Mendez, I., et al. (2009). Neurogenesis-dependent and-independent effects of fluoxetine in an animal model of anxiety/depression. Neuron 62, 479–493. doi: 10.1016/j.neuron.2009.04.017

Dean, O. M., Data-Franco, J., Giorlando, F., and Berk, M. (2012). Minocycline: therapeutic potential in psychiatry. CNS drugs 26, 391–401. doi: 10.2165/11632000-000000000-00000

de Jonge, P., Roy, J. F., Saz, P., Marcos, G., and Lobo, A. (2006). Prevalent and incident depression in community-dwelling elderly persons with diabetes mel- litus: results from the ZARADEMP project. Diabetologia 49, 2627–2633. doi: 10.1007/s00125-006-0442-x

Delarue, J., Matzinger, O., Binnert, C., Schneiter, P., Chioléro, R., and Tappy, L. (2003). Fish oil prevents the adrenal activation elicited by mental stress in healthy men. Diabetes Metab. 29, 289–295. doi: 10.1016/S1262-36367 0039-3

Dhabhar, F. S. (2009). Enhancing versus suppressive effects of stress on immune function: implications for immunoprotection and immunopathology. Neuroimmunomodulation 16, 300–317. doi: 10.1159/000216188

Diamond, M., Kelly, J. P., and Connor, T. J. (2006). Antidepressants sup- press production of the Th1 cytokine interferon-gamma, independent of monoamine transporter blockade. Eur. Neuropsychopharmacol. 16, 481–490. doi: 10.1016/j.euroneuro.2005.11.011

Dickens, C., McGowan, L., Clark-Carter, D., and Creed, F. (2002). Depression in rheumatoid arthritis: a systematic review of the literature with meta-analysis. Psychosom. Med. 64, 52–60.

Donner, N. C., Montoya, C. D., Lukkes, J. L., and Lowry, C. A. (2012). Chronic non-invasive corticosterone administration abolishes the diurnal pattern of tph2 expression. Psychoneuroendocrinology 37, 645–661. doi: 10.1016/j.psyneuen.2011.08.008

Dowlati, Y., Herrmann, N., Swardfager, W., Liu, H., Sham, L., Reim, E. K., et al. (2010). A meta-analysis of cytokines in major depression. Biol. Psychiatry 67, 446–457. doi: 10.1016/j.biopsych.2009.09.033

Dringen, R. (2005). Oxidative and antioxidative potential of brain microglial cells. Antioxid. Redox Signal. 7, 1223–1233. doi: 10.1089/ars.2005.7.1223

Dunn, A. J. (2000). Cytokine activation of the HPA axis. Ann. N.Y. Acad. Sci. 917, 608–617. doi: 10.1111/j.1749-6632.2000.tb05426.x

Dyer, A. R., Persky, V., Stamler, J., Paul, O., Shekelle, R. B., Berkson,

D. M., et al. (1980). Heart rate as a prognostic factor for coronary heart disease and mortality: findings in three Chicago epidemiologic studies. Am. J. Epidemiol. 112, 736–749.

Eller, T., Vasar, V., Shlik, J., and Maron, E. (2009). The role of IL-2 and soluble IL-2R in depression and antidepressant response. Curr. Opin. Invest. Drugs (London, England: 2000) 10, 638–643.

Ellsworth, K. A., Moon, I., Eckloff, B. W., Fridley, B. L., Jenkins, G. D., Batzler, A., et al. (2013). FKBP5 genetic variation: association with selective serotonin reup- take inhibitor treatment outcomes in major depressive disorder. Pharmacogenet. Genomics 23, 156–166. doi: 10.1097/FPC.0b013e32835dc133

Ertenli, I., Ozer, S., Kiraz, S., Apras, S. B., Akdogan, A., Karadag, O., et al. (2012). Infliximab, a TNF-alpha antagonist treatment in patients with anky-losing spondylitis: the impact on depression, anxiety and quality of life level. Rheumatol. Int. 32, 323–330. doi: 10.1007/s00296-010-1616-x

Evans, J., Sun, Y., McGregor, A., and Connor, B. (2012). Allopregnanolone regulates neurogenesis and depressive/anxiety-like behaviour in a social isolation rodent model of chronic stress. Neuropharmacology 63, 1315–1326. doi: 10.1016/j.neuropharm.2012.08.012

Fardet, L., Petersen, I., and Nazareth, I. (2012). Suicidal behavior and severe neuropsychiatric disorders following glucocorticoid therapy in primary care. Am. J. Psychiatry 169, 491–497. doi: 10.1176/appi.ajp.2011.11071009

Farooq, R. K., Isingrini, E., Tanti, A., Le Guisquet, A.-M., Arlicot, N., Minier, F., et al. (2012). Is unpredictable chronic mild stress (UCMS) a reliable model to study depression-induced neuroinflammation. Behav. Brain Res. 231, 130–137. doi: 10.1016/j.bbr.2012.03.020

Feng, L., Tan, C. H., Merchant, R. A., and Ng, T. P. (2008). Association between depressive symptoms and use of HMG-CoA reductase inhibitors (statins), cor- ticosteroids and histamine H(2) receptor antagonists in community-dwelling older persons: cross-sectional analysis of a population-based cohort. Drugs Aging 25, 795–805. doi: 10.2165/00002512-200825090-00005

Fields, C., Drye, L., Vaidya, V., and Lyketsos, C. (2012). Celecoxib or naproxen treatment does not benefit depressive symptoms in persons age 70 and older: findings from a randomized controlled trial. Am. J. Geriatric Psychiatry 20, 505–513. doi: 10.1097/JGP.0b013e318227f4da

Forbes, L. M., and Chaney, R. H. (1980). Cardiovascular changes during acute depression. Psychosomatics 21, 472–477. doi: 10.1016/S0033-318273657-5

Forester, B. P., Zuo, C. S., Ravichandran, C., Harper, D. G., Du, F., Kim, S., et al. (2012). Coenzyme Q10 effects on creatine kinase activity and mood in geriatric bipolar depression. J. Geriatric Psychiatry Neurology 25, 43–50. doi: 10.1177/0891988712436688

Francis, J., Weiss, R. M., Johnson, A. K., and Felder, R. B. (2003). Central mineralo-corticoid receptor blockade decreases plasma TNF-alpha after coronary artery ligation in rats. Am. J. Physiol. Regul. Integr. Comp. Physiol. 284, R328–R335. doi: 10.1152/ajpregu.00376.2002

Frank, M. G., Thompson, B. M., Watkins, L. R., and Maier, S. F. (2012). Glucocorticoids mediate stress-induced priming of microglial pro-inflammatory responses. Brain Behav. Immun. 26, 337–345. doi: 10.1016/j.bbi.2011.10.005

Frank, M. G., Watkins, L. R., and Maier, S. F. (2011). Stress- and glucocorticoid-induced priming of neuroinflammatory responses: potential mechanisms of stress-induced vulnerability to drugs of abuse. Brain Behav. Immun. 25(Suppl. 1), S21–S28. doi: 10.1016/j.bbi.2011.01.005

Gallagher, P., Watson, S., Smith, M. S., Ferrier, I. N., and Young, A. H. (2005). Effects of adjunctive mifepristone (RU-486) administration on neurocognitive function and symptoms in schizophrenia. Biol. Psychiatry 57, 155–161. doi: 10.1016/j.biopsych.2004.10.017

Gilbert, K., Arseneault-Breard, J., Flores Monaco, F., Beaudoin, A., Bah, T. M.,

Tompkins, T. A., et al. (2013). Attenuation of post-myocardial infarction depression in rats by n-3 fatty acids or probiotics starting after the onset of reperfusion. Br. J. Nutr. 109, 50–56. doi: 10.1017/S0007114512003807

Godha, D., Shi, L., and Mavronicolas, H. (2010). Association between tendency towards depression and severity of rheumatoid arthritis from a national representative sample: the Medical Expenditure Panel Survey. Curr. Med. Res. Opin. 26, 1685–1690. doi: 10.1185/03007991003795808

Goleva, E., Li, L. B., and Leung, D. Y. (2009). IFN-gamma reverses IL-2- and IL-4-mediated T-cell steroid resistance. Am. J. Resp. Cell Mol. Biol. 40, 223–230. doi: 10.1165/rcmb.2007-0327OC

González, H. M., and Tarraf, W. (2013). Comorbid cardiovascular disease and major depression among ethnic and racial groups in the United States. Int. Psychogeriatrics 25, 833–841. doi: 10.1017/S1041610212002062

Gourley, S. L., Wu, F. J., and Taylor, J. R. (2008). Corticosterone regulates pERK1/2 map kinase in a chronic depression model. Ann. N.Y. Acad. Sci. 1148, 509–514. doi: 10.1196/annals.1410.076

Guillemin, G. J., Smythe, G., Takikawa, O., and Brew, B. J. (2005). Expression of indoleamine 2, 3-dioxygenase and production of quinolinic acid by human microglia, astrocytes, and neurons. Glia 49, 15–23. doi: 10.1002/glia.20090

Halder, I., Marsland, A. L., Cheong, J., Muldoon, M. F., Ferrell, R. E., and Manuck, S. B. (2010). Polymorphisms in the CRP gene moderate an association between depressive symptoms and circulating levels of C-reactive protein. Brain Behav. Immun. 24, 160–167. doi: 10.1016/j.bbi.2009.09.014

Hannestad, J., DellaGioia, N., and Bloch, M. (2011). The effect of antide-pressant medication treatment on serum levels of inflammatory cytokines: a meta-analysis. Neuropsychopharmacology 36, 2452–2459. doi: 10.1038/npp.2011.132

Hannestad, J., Gallezot, J.-D., Schafbauer, T., Lim, K., Kloczynski, T., Morris, E. D., et al. (2012). Endotoxin-induced systemic inflammation activates microglia: [11C]PBR28 positron emission tomography in nonhuman primates. Neuroimage 63, 232–239. doi: 10.1016/j.neuroimage.2012.06.055

Hariri, A. R., Mattay, V. S., Tessitore, A., Kolachana, B., Fera, F., Goldman, D., et al. (2002). Serotonin transporter genetic variation and the response of the human amygdala. Science 297, 400–403 doi: 10.1126/science.1071829

Hashioka, S., Klegeris, A., Monji, A., Kato, T., Sawada, M., McGeer, P. L., et al. (2007). Antidepressants inhibit interferon-gamma-induced microglial production of IL-6 and nitric oxide. Exp. Neurol. 206, 33–42. doi: 10.1016/j.expneurol.2007.03.022

Hennein, H. A., Ebba, H., Rodriguez, J. L., Merrick, S. H., Keith, F. M., Bronstein, M. H., et al. (1994). Relationship of the proinflammatory cytokines to myocardial ischemia and dysfunction after uncomplicated coronary revascularization. J. Thorac. Cardiovasc. Surg. 108, 626–635.

Henry, C. J., Huang, Y., Wynne, A., Hanke, M., Himler, J., Bailey, M. T., et al. (2008). Minocycline attenuates lipopolysaccharide (LPS)-induced neuroinflammation, sickness behavior, and anhedonia. J. Neuroinflammation 5, 15. doi: 10.1186/1742-2094-5-15

Hickman, R. J., Khambaty, T., and Stewart, J. C. (2013). C-reactive protein is elevated in atypical but not nonatypical depression: data from the National Health and Nutrition Examination Survey (NHANES) 1999-2004. J. Behav. Med. doi: 10.1007/s10865-013-9510-0

Hinwood, M., Tynan, R. J., Charnley, J. L., Beynon, S. B., Day, T. A., and Walker, F. R. (2012). Chronic stress induced remodeling of the prefrontal cortex: structural re-organization of microglia and the inhibitory effect of minocycline. Cereb. Cortex 24, 1058–1068. doi: 10.1093/cercor/bhs151

Ho, N., Balu, D. T., Hilario, M. R., Blendy, J. A., and Lucki, I. (2012). Depressive phenotypes evoked by experimental diabetes are reversed by insulin. Physiol. Behav. 105, 702–708. doi: 10.1016/j.physbeh.2011.09.003

Hoffmire, C. A., Block, R. C., Thevenet-Morrison, K., and van Wijngaarden, E. (2012). Associations between omega-3 poly-unsaturated fatty acids from fish consumption and severity of depressive symptoms: an analysis of the 2005-2008 National Health and Nutrition Examination Survey. Prostaglandins Leukotrienes Essential Fatty Acids 86, 155–160. doi: 10.1016/j.plefa.2012.03.003

Holleman, M., Vreeburg, S. A., Dekker, J. J., and Penninx, B. W. (2012). The relationships of working conditions, recent stressors and childhood trauma with salivary cortisol levels. Psychoneuroendocrinology 37, 801–809. doi: 10.1016/j.psyneuen.2011.09.012

Holmes, A. (2008). Genetic variation in cortico-amygdala serotonin function and risk for stress-related disease. Neurosci. Biobehav. Rev. 32, 1293–1314. doi: 10.1016/j.neubiorev.2008.03.006

Horikawa, H., Kato, T. A., Mizoguchi, Y., Monji, A., Seki, Y., Ohkuri, T., et al. (2010). Inhibitory effects of SSRIs on IFN-gamma induced microglial activation through the regulation of intracellular calcium. Prog. Neuropsychopharmacol. Biol. Psychiatry 34, 1306–1316. doi: 10.1016/j.pnpbp.2010.07.015

Howren, M. B., Lamkin, D. M., and Suls, J. (2009). Associations of depression with C-reactive protein, IL-1, and IL-6: a meta-analysis. Psychosom. Med. 71, 171–186. doi: 10.1097/PSY.0b013e3181907c1b

Ising, M., Horstmann, S., Kloiber, S., Lucae, S., Binder, E. B., Kern, N., et al. (2007). Combined dexamethasone/corticotropin releasing hormone test predicts treat- ment response in major depression- a potential biomarker. Biol. Psychiatry 62, 47–54. doi: 10.1016/j.biopsych.2006.07.039

Jabbi, M., Korf, J., Kema, I. P., Hartman, C., van der Pompe, G., Minderaa, R. B., et al. (2007). Convergent genetic modulation of the endocrine stress response involves polymorphic variations of 5-HTT, COMT and, MAOA. Mol. Psychiatry 12, 483–490. doi: 10.1038/sj.mp.4001975

Jazayeri, S., Keshavarz, S. A., Tehrani-Doost, M., Djalali, M., Hosseini, M., Amini, H., et al. (2010). Effects of eicosapentaenoic acid and fluoxetine on plasma cortisol, serum interleukin-1beta and interleukin-6 concentrations in patients with major depressive disorder. Psychiatry Res. 178, 112–115. doi: 10.1016/j.psychres.2009.04.013

Jokinen, J., and Nordstrom, P. (2009). HPA axis hyperactivity and cardiovascular mortality in mood disorder inpatients. J. Affect. Disord. 116, 88–92. doi: 10.1016/j.jad.2008.10.025

Kannel, W. B., Kannel, C., Paffenbarger, Jr. R. S., and Cupples, L. A. (1987). Heart rate and cardiovascular mortality: the Framingham Study. Am. Heart J. 113, 1489–1494. doi: 10.1016/0002-8703(87)90666-1

Karatsoreos, I. N., Bhagat, S. M., Bowles, N. P., Weil, Z. M., Pfaff, D. W., and McEwen, B. S. (2010). Endocrine and physiological changes in response to chronic corticosterone: a potential model of the metabolic syndrome in mouse. Endocrinology 151, 2117–2127. doi: 10.1210/en.2009-1436

Kazakou, P., Kyriazopoulou, V., Michalaki, M., Ierodiakonou, V., Psyrogiannis, A., and Habeos, I. (2012). Activated hypothalamic pituitary adrenal axis in patients with metabolic syndrome. Horm. Metab. Res. 44, 839–844. doi: 10.1055/s-0032- 1311632

Keating, C., Dawood, T., Barton, D. A., Lambert, G. W., and Tilbrook, A. J. (2013). Effects of selective serotonin reuptake inhibitor treatment on plasma oxytocin and cortisol in major depressive disorder. BMC Psychiatry 13:124. doi: 10.1186/1471-244x-13-124

Kendler, K. S., and Gardner, C. O. (2010). Dependent stressful life events and prior depressive episodes in the prediction of major depression: the problem of causal inference in psychiatric epidemiology. Arch. Gen. Psychiatry 67, 1120–1127. doi: 10.1001/archgenpsychiatry.2010.136

Kenna, H. A., Poon, A. W., de los Angeles, C. P., and Koran, L. M. (2011). Psychiatric complications of treatment with corticosteroids: review with case report. Psychiatry Clin. Neurosci. 65, 549–560. doi: 10.1111/j.1440-1819.2011.02260.x

Kessler, R. C., Berglund, P., Demler, O., Jin, R., Merikangas, K. R., and Walters, E. E. (2005). Lifetime prevalence and age-of-onset distributions of DSM-IV disorders in the National Comorbidity Survey Replication. Arch. Gen. Psychiatry 62, 593–602. doi: 10.1001/archpsyc.62.6.593

Kettenmann, H., Hanisch, U.-K., Noda, M., and Verkhratsky, A. (2011). Physiology of Microglia. Physiol. Rev. 91, 461–553. doi: 10.1152/physrev.00011.2010

Kimbro, L. B., Steers, W. N., Mangione, C. M., Duru, O. K., and Ettner, S. L. (2012). The association of depression and the cardiovascular risk factors of blood pressure, HbA1c, and body mass index among patients with diabetes: results from the translating research into action for diabetes study. Int. J. Endocrinol. 2012, 747460. doi: 10.1155/2012/747460

Knol, M. J., Twisk, J. W., Beekman, A. T., Heine, R. J., Snoek, F. J., and Pouwer, F. (2006). Depression as a risk factor for the onset of type 2 diabetes mellitus. A meta-analysis. Diabetologia 49, 837–845. doi: 10.1007/s00125-006-0159-x

Koenig, W. (2001). Inflammation and coronary heart disease: an overview. Cardiol. Rev. 9, 31–35. doi: 10.1097/00045415-200101000-00007

Krishnan, R., Cella, D., Leonardi, C., Papp, K., Gottlieb, A. B., Dunn, M., et al. (2007). Effects of etanercept therapy on fatigue and symptoms of depression in subjects treated for moderate to severe plaque psoriasis for up to 96 weeks. Br. J. Dermatol. 157, 1275–1277. doi: 10.1111/j.1365-2133.2007.08205.x

Kronish, I. M., Carson, A. P., Davidson, K. W., Muntner, P., and Safford, M. M. (2012). Depressive symptoms and cardiovascular health by the ameri- can heart association's definition in the reasons for geographic and racial differences in stroke (REGARDS) study. PLoS ONE 7:e52771. doi: 10.1371/jour- nal.pone.0052771

Kumsta, R., Entringer, S., Koper, J. W., van Rossum, E. F. C., Hellhammer, D. H., and Wüst, S. (2007). Sex specific associations between common glucocorticoid receptor gene variants and hypothalamus-pituitary-adrenal axis responses to psychosocial stress. Biol. Psychiatry 62, 863–869. doi: 10.1016/j.biopsych.2007.04.013

Kurina, L. M., Goldacre, M. J., Yeates, D., and Gill, L. E. (2001). Depression and anxiety in people with inflammatory bowel disease. J. Epidemiol. Commun. Health 55, 716–720. doi: 10.1136/jech.55.10.716

Kurz, K., Schroecksnadel, S., Weiss, G., and Fuchs, D. (2011). Association between increased tryptophan degradation and depression in cancer patients. Curr. Opin. Clin. Nutr. Metab. Care 14, 49–56. doi: 10.1097/MCO.0b013e328340d849

Kyrou, I., and Tsigos, C. (2009). Stress hormones: physiological stress and regulation of metabolism. Curr. Opin. Pharmacol. 9, 787–793. doi: 10.1016/j.coph.2009.08.007

Lechin, F., van der Dijs, B., Orozco, B., Lechin, M. E., Baez, S., Lechin, A. E., et al. (1995). Plasma neurotransmitters, blood pressure, and heart rate during supine-resting, orthostasis, and moderate exercise conditions in major depressed patients. Biol. Psychiatry 38, 166–173. doi: 10.1016/0006-3223(94)00258-5

Leonard, B. E. (2006). HPA and immune axes in stress: involvement of the serotonergic system. Neuroimmunomodulation 13, 268–276. doi: 10.1159/000104854

Lesch, K.-P., Bengel, D., Heils, A., Sabol, S. Z., Greenberg, B. D., Petri, S., et al. (1996). Association of anxiety-related traits with a polymorphism in the serotonin transporter gene regulatory region. Science 274, 1527–1531. doi: 10.1126/science.274.5292.1527

Levine, B., Kalman, J., Mayer, L., Fillit, H. M., and Packer, M. (1990). Elevated circulating levels of tumor necrosis factor in severe chronic heart failure. N. Eng. J. Med. 323, 236–241. doi: 10.1056/NEJM199007263230405

Lin, P. Y., and Su, K. P. (2007). A meta-analytic review of double-blind, placebo-controlled trials of antidepressant efficacy of omega-3 fatty acids. J. Clin. Psychiatry 68, 1056–1061. doi: 10.4088/JCP.v68n0712

Liu, R. T., and Alloy, L. B. (2010). Stress generation in depression: a systematic review of the empirical literature and recommendations for future study. Clin. Psychol. Rev. 30, 582–593. doi: 10.1016/j.cpr.2010.04.010

Lo Fermo, S., Barone, R., Patti, F., Laisa, P., Cavallaro, T. L., Nicoletti, A., et al. (2010). Outcome of psychiatric symptoms presenting at onset of multiple scle- rosis: a retrospective study. Multiple Sclerosis (Houndmills, Basingstoke, England) 16, 742–748. doi: 10.1177/1352458510365157

Lu, Y., Feng, L., Feng, L., Nyunt, M. S., Yap, K. B., and Ng, T. P. (2013). Systemic inflammation, depression and obstructive pulmonary function: a population- based study. Respir. Res. 14, 53. doi: 10.1186/1465-9921-14-53

Ludescher, B., Najib, A., Baar, S., Machann, J., Schick, F., Buchkremer, G., et al. (2008). Increase of visceral fat and adrenal gland volume in women with depression: preliminary results of a morphometric MRI study. Int. J. Psychiatry Med. 38, 229–240. doi: 10.2190/PM.38.3.a

Macfarlane, D. P., Forbes, S., and Walker, B. R. (2008). Glucocorticoids and fatty acid metabolism in humans: fuelling fat redistribution in the metabolic syndrome. J. Endocrinol. 197, 189–204. doi: 10.1677/JOE-08-0054

Maes, M. (1999). Major depression and activation of the inflammatory response system. Adv. Exp. Med. Biol. 461, 25–46. doi: 10.1007/978-0-585-37970-8_2

Maes, M. (2012). Targeting cyclooxygenase-2 in depression is not a viable therapeutic approach and may even aggravate the pathophysiology underpinning depression. Metab. Brain Dis. 27, 405–413. doi: 10.1007/s11011-012-9326-6

Maes, M., Kubera, M., Leunis, J. C., and Berk, M. (2012a). Increased IgA and IgM responses against gut commensals in chronic depression: further evidence for increased bacterial translocation or leaky gut. J. Affect. Disord. 141, 55–62. Epub 2012/03/14. doi: 10.1016/j.jad.2012.02.023

Maes, M., Berk, M., Goehler, L., Song, C., Anderson, G., Galecki, P., et al. (2012b). Depression and sickness behavior are Janus-faced responses to shared inflammatory pathways. BMC Med. 10:66. doi: 10.1186/1741-701 5-10-66

Maes, M., Kubera, M., and Leunis, J. C. (2008). The gut-brain barrier in major depression: intestinal mucosal dysfunction with an increased translocation of LPS from gram negative enterobacteria (leaky gut) plays a role in the inflamma- tory pathophysiology of depression. Neuro Endocrinol. Lett. 29, 117–124.

Maes, M., Meltzer, H. Y., Scharpe, S.,

Bosmans, E., Suy, E., De Meester, I., t al. (1993). Relationships between lower plasma L-tryptophan levels and immune-inflammatory variables in depression. Psychiatry Res. 49, 151–165. doi: 10.1016/0165-1781(93)90102-M

Maes, M., Mihaylova, I., Kubera, M., Uytterhoeven, M., Vrydags, N., and Bosmans, E. (2009). Lower plasma Coenzyme Q10 in depression: a marker for treatment resistance and chronic fatigue in depression and a risk factor to cardiovascular disorder in that illness. Neuro Endocrinol. Lett. 30, 462–469.

Mann, J. N., and Thakore, J. H. (1999). Melancholic depression and abdominal fat distribution: a mini-review. Stress 3, 1–15. doi: 10.3109/10253899909001108

Manthey, L., Leeds, C., Giltay, E. J., van Veen, T., Vreeburg, S. A., Penninx, B. W., et al. (2011). Antidepressant use and salivary cortisol in depressive and anxiety disorders. Eur. Neuropsychopharmacol. 21, 691–699. doi: 10.1016/j.euroneuro.2011.03.002

Margaretten, M., Barton, J., Julian, L., Katz, P., Trupin, L., Tonner, C., et al. (2011a). Socioeconomic determinants of disability and depression in patients with rheumatoid arthritis. Arthritis Care Res. 63, 240–246. doi: 10.1002/acr.20345

Margaretten, M., Julian, L., Katz, P., and Yelin, E. (2011b). Depression in patients with rheumatoid arthritis: description, causes and mechanisms. Int. J. Clin. Rheumatol. 6, 617–623. doi: 10.2217/ijr.11.6

Martins, J. G., Bentsen, H., and Puri, B. K. (2012). Eicosapentaenoic acid appears to be the key omega-3 fatty acid component associated with efficacy in major depressive disorder: a critique of Bloch and Hannestad and updated meta-analysis. Mol. Psychiatry 17, 1144–1149. discussion 63–67. doi: 10.1038/mp.2012.25

Martocchia, A., Curto, M., Toussan, L., Stefanelli, M., and Falaschi, P. (2011). Pharmacological strategies against glucocorticoid-mediated brain damage during chronic disorders. Recent Pat. CNS Drug Discov. 6, 196–204. doi: 10.2174/157488911796958020

Matthews, L. C., and Hanley, N. A. (2011). The stress of starvation: gluco-corticoid restraint of beta cell development. Diabetologia 54, 223–226. doi: 10.1007/s00125-010-1963-x

Mehta, D., Raison, C. L., Woolwine, B. J., Haroon, E., Binder, E. B., Miller, A. H., et al. (2013). Transcriptional signatures related to glucose and lipid metabolism predict treatment response to the tumor necrosis factor antagonist infliximab in patients with treatment-resistant depression. Brain Behav. Immun. 31, 205–215. doi: 10.1016/j.bbi.2013.04.004

Mendlewicz, J., Kriwin, P., Oswald, P., Souery, D., Alboni, S., and Brunello, N. (2006). Shortened onset of action of antidepressants in major depression using acetylsalicylic acid augmentation: a pilot open-label study. Int. Clin. Psychopharmacol. 21, 227–231. doi: 10.1097/00004850-200607000-00005

Menke, A., Klengel, T., Rubel, J., Bruckl, T., Pfister, H., Lucae, S., et al. (2013). Genetic variation in FKBP5 associated with the extent of stress hormone dysregulation in major depression. Genes Brain Behav. 12, 289–296. doi: 10.1111/gbb.12026

Miller, A. H., Maletic, V., and Raison, C. L. (2009). Inflammation and its discon- tents: the role of cytokines in the pathophysiology of major depression. Biol. Psychiatry 65, 732–741. doi: 10.1016/j.biopsych.2008.11.029

Minghetti, L. (2004). Cyclooxygenase-2 (COX-2) in inflammatory and degenerative brain diseases. J. Neuropathol. Exp. Neurol. 63, 901–910.

Miyaoka, T., Wake, R., Furuya, M., Liaury, K., Ieda, M., Kawakami, K., et al. (2012). Minocycline as adjunctive therapy for patients with unipolar psychotic depression: an open-label study. Prog. Neuropsychopharmacol. Biol. Psychiatry 37, 222–226. doi: 10.1016/j.pnpbp.2012.02.002

Mizoguchi, K., Shoji, H., Ikeda, R., Tanaka, Y., and Tabira, T. (2008). Persistent depressive state after chronic stress in rats is accompanied by HPA axis dysreg- ulation and reduced prefrontal dopaminergic neurotransmission. Pharmacol. Biochem. Behav. 91, 170–175. doi: 10.1016/j.pbb.2008.07.002

Mo, B., Feng, N., Renner, K., and Forster, G. (2008). Restraint stress increases serotonin release in the central nucleus of the amygdala via activation of corticotropin-releasing factor receptors. Brain Res. Bull. 76, 493–498. doi: 10.1016/j.brainresbull.2008.02.011

Mocking, R. J., Assies, J., Bot, M., Jansen, E. H., Schene, A. H., and Pouwer, F. (2012). Biological effects of add-on eicosapentaenoic acid supplementation in diabetes mellitus and co-morbid depression: a randomized controlled trial. PLoS ONE 7:e49431. doi: 10.1371/journal.pone.0049431

Mocking, R. J., Ruhe, H. G., Assies, J., Lok, A., Koeter, M. W., Visser, I., et al. (2013). Relationship between the hypothalamic-pituitary-adrenal-axis and fatty acid metabolism in recurrent depression. Psychoneuroendocrinology. doi: 10.1016/j.psyneuen.2013.01.013

Mokhtari, M., Arfken, C., and Boutros, N. (2013). The DEX/CRH test for major depression: a potentially useful diagnostic test. Psychiatry Res. 208, 131–139. doi: 10.1016/j.psychres.2012.09.032

Mommersteeg, P. M., Herr, R., Pouwer, F., Holt, R. I., and Loerbroks, A. (2013). The association between diabetes and an episode of depressive symptoms in the 2002 World Health Survey: an analysis of 231, 797 individuals from 47 countries. Diabetic Med. 30:e208–214. doi: 10.1111/dme.12193

Muller, N., Schwarz, M. J., Dehning, S., Douhe, A., Cerovecki, A., Goldstein-Muller, B., et al. (2006). The cyclooxygenase-2 inhibitor celecoxib has therapeutic effects in major depression: results of a double-blind, randomized, placebo controlled, add-on pilot study to reboxetine. Mol. Psychiatry 11, 680–684. doi: 10.1038/sj.mp.4001805

Munhoz, C. D., Lepsch, L. B., Kawamoto, E. M., Malta, M. B., Lima Lde, S., Avellar, M. C., et al. (2006). Chronic unpredictable stress exacer- bates lipopolysaccharide-induced activation of nuclear factor-kappaB in the frontal cortex and hippocampus via glucocorticoid secretion. J. Neurosci. 26, 3813–3820. doi: 10.1523/JNEUROSCI.4398-05.2006

Musil, R., Schwarz, M. J., Riedel, M., Dehning, S., Cerovecki, A., Spellmann, I., et al. (2011). Elevated macrophage migration inhibitory factor and decreased transforming growth factor-beta levels in major depression—No influence of celecoxib treatment. J. Affect. Disord. 134, 217–225. doi: 10.1016/j.jad.2011. 05.047

Myint, A-M., Kim, Y. K., Verkerk, R., Scharpé, S., Steinbusch, H., and Leonard, B. (2007). Kynurenine pathway in major depression: evidence of impaired neuroprotection. J. Affect. Disord. 98, 143–151. doi: 10.1016/j.jad.2006.07.013

Nair, A., and Bonneau, R. H. (2006). Stress-induced elevation of glucocorti- coids increases microglia proliferation through NMDA receptor activation. J. Neuroimmunol. 171, 72–85. doi: 10.1016/j.jneuroim.2005.09.012

Nemeroff, C. B., and Musselman, D. L. (2000). Are platelets the link between depression and ischemic heart disease. Am. Heart J. 140(4, Supplement), S57– S62. doi: 10.1067/mhj.2000.109978

Otte, C., Zhao, S., and Whooley, M. A. (2012). Statin use and risk of depression in patients with coronary heart disease: longitudinal data from the heart and soul study. J. Clin. Psychiatry 73, 610–615. doi: 10.4088/JCP.11m07038

Pae, C. U., Marks, D. M., Han, C., and Patkar, A. A. (2008). Does minocy- cline have antidepressant effect. Biomed. Pharmacother. 62, 308–311. doi: 10.1016/j.biopha.2007.12.005

Palagini, L., Mosca, M., Tani, C., Gemignani, A., Mauri, M., and Bombardieri, S. (2013). Depression and systemic lupus erythematosus: a systematic review. Lupus 22, 409–416. doi: 10.1177/0961203313477227

Palatini, P., and Julius, S. (1997). Association of tachycardia with morbidity and mortality: pathophysiological considerations. J. Hum. Hypertens. 11(Suppl. 1), S19–S27.

Palumbo, M. L., Canzobre, M. C., Pascuan, C. G., Rios, H., Wald, M., and Genaro, A. M. (2010). Stress induced cognitive deficit is differentially modu- lated in BAL-B/c and C57Bl/6 mice: correlation with Th1/Th2 balance after stress exposure. J. Neuroimmunol. 218, 12–20. doi: 10.1016/j.jneuroim.2009.11.005

Pasco, J. A., Jacka, F. N., Williams, L. J., Henry, M. J., Nicholson, G. C., Kotowicz, M. A., et al. (2010). Clinical implications of the cytokine hypothesis of depres- sion: the association between use of statins and aspirin and the risk of major depression. Psychother. Psychosom. 79, 323–325. doi: 10.1159/000319530

Pereira, A. M., Tiemensma, J., and Romijn, J. A. (2010). Neuropsychiatric disorders in Cushing's syndrome. Neuroendocrinology 92(Suppl. 1), 65–70. doi: 10.1159/000314317

Persoons, P., Vermeire, S., Demyttenaere, K., Fischler, B., Vandenberghe, J., Van Oudenhove, L., et al. (2005). The impact of major depressive disorder on the short- and long-term outcome of Crohn's disease treatment with infliximab. Aliment. Pharmacol. Ther. 22, 101–110. doi: 10.1111/j.1365-2036.2005.02535.x

Pintado, C., Revilla, E., Vizuete, M. L., Jimenez, S., Garcia-Cuervo, L., Vitorica, J., et al. (2011). Regional difference in inflammatory response to LPS-injection in the brain: role of microglia cell density. J. Neuroimmunol. 238, 44–51. doi: 10.1016/j.jneuroim.2011.06.017

Piwowarska, J., Chimiak, A., Matsumoto, H., Dziklinska, A., Radziwon-Zaleska, M., Szelenberger, W., et al. (2012). Serum cortisol concentration in patients with major depression after treatment with fluoxetine. Psychiatry Res. 198, 407–411. doi: 10.1016/j.psychres.2012.01.029

Pucak, M. L., and Kaplin, A. I. (2005). Unkind cytokines: current evidence for the potential role of cytokines in immune-mediated depression. Int. Rev. Psychiatry 17, 477–483. doi: 10.1080/02646830500381757

Puntener, U., Booth, S., Perry, V., and Teeling, J. (2012). Long-term impact of systemic bacterial infection on the cerebral vasculature and microglia. J. Neuroinflammation 9, 146. doi: 10.1186/1742-2094-9-146

Raison, C. L., Broadwell, S. D., Borisov, A. S., Manatunga, A. K., Capuron, L., Woolwine, B. J., et al. (2005). Depressive symptoms and viral clearance in patients receiving interferon-alpha and ribavirin for hepatitis, C. Brain Behav. Immun. 19, 23–27. doi: 10.1016/j.bbi.2004.05.001

Raison, C. L., Rutherford, R. E., Woolwine, B. J., Shuo, C., Schettler, P., Drake, D. F., et al. (2013). A randomized controlled trial of the tumor necrosis factor antagonist infliximab for treatment-resistant depression: the role of baseline inflammatory biomarkers. JAMA Psychiatry 70, 31–41. doi: 10.1001/2013.jamapsychi- atry.4

Reagan, L. P., Grillo, C. A., and Piroli, G. G. (2008). The As and Ds of stress: metabolic, morphological and behavioral consequences. Eur. J. Pharmacol. 585, 64–75. doi: 10.1016/j.ejphar.2008.02.050

Renoir, T., Pang, T. Y., and Hannan, A. J. (2013). Effects of environmental manipulations in genetically targeted animal models of affective disorders. Neurobiol. Dis. 57, 12–27. doi: 10.1016/j.nbd.2012.04.003

Rojas, P. S., Fritsch, R., Rojas, R. A., Jara, P., and Fiedler, J. L. (2011). Serum brain- derived neurotrophic factor and glucocorticoid receptor levels in lymphocytes as markers of antidepressant response in major depressive patients: a pilot study. Psychiatry Res. 189, 239–245. doi: 10.1016/j.psychres.2011.04.032

Rosmond, R. (2005). Role of stress in the pathogenesis of the metabolic syndrome. Psychoneuroendocrinology 30, 1–10. doi: 10.1016/j.psyneuen.2004.05.007

Rotella, F., and Mannucci, E. (2013). Diabetes mellitus as a risk factor for depression. A meta-analysis of longitudinal studies. Diabetes Res. Clin. Pract. 99, 98–104. doi: 10.1016/j.diabres.2012.11.022

Rugulies, R. (2002). Depression as a predictor for coronary heart disease: a review and meta-analysis. Am. J. Prev. Med. 23, 51–61. doi: 10.1016/S0749-379700439- 7

Sasaki, A., de Vega, W. C., St-Cyr, S., Pan, P., and McGowan, P. O. (2013). Perinatal high fat diet alters glucocorticoid signaling and anxiety behavior in adulthood. Neuroscience 240, 1–12. doi: 10.1016/j.neuroscience.2013.02.044

Schatzberg, A. F., and Lindley, S. (2008). Glucocorticoid antagonists in neuropsychiatric [corrected] disorders. Eur. J. Pharmacol. 583, 358–364. doi: 10.1016/j.ejphar.2008.01.001

Schewitz, L. P., Lee, R. W., Dayan, C. M., and Dick, A. D. (2009). Glucocorticoids and the emerging importance of T cell subsets in steroid refractory diseases. Immunopharmacol. Immunotoxicol. 31, 1–22. doi: 10.1080/08923970802334848

Schmidt, H. D., Shelton, R. C., and Duman, R. S. (2011). Functional biomarkers of depression: diagnosis, treatment, and pathophysiology. Neuropsychopharmacology 36, 2375–2394. doi: 10.1038/npp.2011.151

Seldenrijk, A., van Hout, H. P. J., van Marwijk, H. W. J., de Groot, E., Gort, J., Rustemeijer, C., et al. (2013). Sensitivity to depression or anxiety and subclinical cardiovascular disease. J. Affect. Disord. 146, 126–131. doi: 10.1016/j.jad.2012.06.026

Serber, E. R., Edwards-Hampton, S. A., Yeager, B., Clair, M., Taylor, M., Galloway, S. K., et al. (2012). Prevalence of chest pain, depression, somatization, anxiety, global distress, and substance use among cardiac and pulmonary rehabilitation patients. Pain Res. Treat. 2012, 4. doi: 10.1155/2012/138680

Siddiqui, R. A., and Harvey, K. A. (2013). Dietary interventions with n-3 fatty acids or probiotics targeting post-myocardial infarction depression. Br. J. Nutr. 109, 1–3. doi: 10.1017/S0007114512004254

Smolderen, K. G., Spertus, J. A., Vriens, P. W., Kranendonk, S., Nooren, M., and Denollet, J. (2010). Younger women with symptomatic peripheral arterial dis- ease are at increased risk of depressive symptoms. J. Vasc. Surg. 52, 637–644. doi: 10.1016/j.jvs.2010.04.025

Soczynska, J. K., Mansur, R. B., Brietzke, E., Swardfager, W., Kennedy, S. H., Woldeyohannes, H. O., et al. (2012). Novel therapeutic targets in depression: minocycline as a candidate treatment. Behav. Brain Res. 235, 302–317. doi: 10.1016/j.bbr.2012.07.026

Stafford, L., and Berk, M. (2011). The use of statins after a cardiac intervention is associated with reduced risk of subsequent depression: proof of concept for the inflammatory and oxidative hypotheses of depression. J. Clin. Psychiatry 72, 1229–1235. doi: 10.4088/JCP.09m05825blu

Sternberg, E. M. (2006). Neural regulation of innate immunity: a coordinated nonspecific host response to pathogens. Nat. Rev. Immunol. 6, 318–328. doi: 10.1038/nri1810

Stetler, C., and Miller, G. E. (2011). Depression and hypothalamic-pituitary-adrenal activation: a quantitative summary of four decades of research. Psychosom. Med. 73, 114–126. doi: 10.1097/PSY.0b013e31820ad12b

Taler, M., Gil-Ad, I., Lomnitski, L., Korov, I., Baharav, E., Bar, M., et al. (2007). Immunomodulatory effect of selective serotonin reuptake inhibitors (SSRIs) on human T lymphocyte function and gene expression. Eur. Neuropsychopharmacol. 17, 774–780. doi: 10.1016/j.euroneuro.2007. 03.010

Tatebayashi, Y., Nihonmatsu-Kikuchi, N., Hayashi, Y., Yu, X., Soma, M., and Ikeda, K. (2012). Abnormal fatty acid composition in the frontopolar cortex of patients with affective disorders. Trans. Psychiatry 2:e204. doi: 10.1038/tp. 2012.132

Thomson, F., and Craighead, M. (2008). Innovative approaches for the treat- ment of depression: targeting the HPA axis. Neurochem. Res. 33, 691–707. doi: 10.1007/s11064-007-9518-3

Tonelli, L. H., Holmes, A., and Postolache, T. T. (2008). Intranasal immune challenge induces sex-dependent depressive-like behavior and cytokine expression in the brain. Neuropsychopharmacology 33, 1038–1048. doi: 10.1038/sj.npp.1301488

Touma, C., Fenzl, T., Ruschel, J., Palme, R., Holsboer, F., Kimura, M., et al. (2009). Rhythmicity in mice selected for extremes in stress reactivity: behavioural, endocrine and sleep changes resembling endophenotypes of major depression. PLoS ONE 4:e4325. doi: 10.1371/journal.pone.0004325

Triantafillidis, J. K., Merikas, E., and Gikas, A. (2013). Psychological factors and stress in inflammatory bowel disease. Expert Rev. Gastroenterol. Hepatol. 7, 225–238. doi: 10.1586/egh.13.4

Tynan, R. J., Naicker, S., Hinwood, M., Nalivaiko, E., Buller, K. M., Pow, D. V., et al. (2010). Chronic stress alters the density and morphology of microglia in a subset of stress-responsive brain regions. Brain Behav. Immun. 24, 1058–1068. doi: 10.1016/j.bbi.2010.02.001

Tyring, S., Gottlieb, A., Papp, K., Gordon, K., Leonardi, C., Wang, A., et al. (2006). Etanercept and clinical outcomes, fatigue, and depression in psoriasis: double- blind placebo-controlled randomised phase III trial. Lancet 367, 29–35. doi: 10.1016/S0140-6736(05)67763-X

Tyrka, A. R., Walters, O. C., Price, L. H., Anderson, G. M., and Carpenter, L. L. (2012). Altered response to neuroendocrine challenge linked to indices of the metabolic syndrome in healthy adults. Horm. Metab. Res. 44, 543–549. doi: 10.1055/s-0032-1306342

Udina, M., Castellvi, P., Moreno-Espana, J., Navines, R., Valdes, M., Forns, X., et al. (2012). Interferon-induced depression in chronic hepatitis C: a sys- tematic review and meta-analysis. J. Clin. Psychiatry 73, 1128–1138. doi: 10.4088/JCP.12r07694

Valkanova, V., and Ebmeier, K. P. (2013). Vascular risk factors and depression in later life: a systematic review and meta-analysis. Biol. Psychiatry 73, 406–413. doi: 10.1016/j.biopsych.2012.10.028

van Dartel, S. A. A., Fransen, J., Kievit, W., Flendrie, M., den Broeder, A. A., Visser, H., et al. (2013). Difference in the risk of serious infections in patients with rheumatoid arthritis treated with adalimumab, infliximab and etanercept: results from the Dutch Rheumatoid Arthritis Monitoring (DREAM) registry. Ann. Rheum. Dis. 72, 895–900. doi: 10.1136/annrheumdis-2012-201338

Van der Does, A. J. (2001). The effects of tryptophan depletion on mood and psychiatric symptoms. J. Affect. Disord. 64, 107–119. doi: 10.1016/S0165- 0327(00)00209-3

van Holten, T. C., Waanders, L. F., de Groot, P. G., Vissers, J., Hoefer, I. E., Pasterkamp, G., et al. (2013). Circulating biomarkers for predicting cardio- vascular disease risk; a systematic review and comprehensive overview of meta-analyses. PLoS ONE 8:e62080. doi: 10.1371/journal.pone.0062080

van Raalte, D. H., Ouwens, D. M., and Diamant, M. (2009). Novel insights into glucocorticoid-mediated diabetogenic effects: towards expansion of therapeutic options. Eur. J. Clin. Invest. 39, 81–93. doi: 10.1111/j.1365-2362.2008.02067.x van Reedt Dortland, A. K., Vreeburg, S. A., Giltay, E. J., Licht, C. M., Vogelzangs, N., van Veen, T., et al. (2013). The impact of stress systems and lifestyle on dys- lipidemia and obesity in anxiety and depression. Psychoneuroendocrinology 38, 209–218. doi: 10.1016/j.psyneuen.2012.05.017

van Rossum, E. F. C., Binder, E. B., Majer, M., Koper, J. W., Ising, M., Modell, S., et al. (2006). Polymorphisms of the glucocorticoid receptor gene and major depression. Biol. Psychiatry 59, 681–688. doi: 10.1016/j.biopsych.2006.02.007

van West, D., Van Den Eede, F., Del-Favero, J., Souery, D., Norrback, K.-F., Van Duijn, C., et al. (2005). Glucocorticoid receptor gene-based snp analy- sis in patients with recurrent major depression. Neuropsychopharmacology 31, 620–627. doi: 10.1038/sj.npp.1300898

Vignau, J., Costisella, O., Canva, V., Imbenotte, M., Duhamel, A., and Lhermitte, M. (2009). [Impact of interferon alpha immunotherapy on tryptophan metabolism in patients with chronic hepatitis, C. Results of a pilot studies on ten patients]. L'Encephale 35, 477–483. doi: 10.1016/j.encep.2007.09.007

Villeda, S. A., Luo, J., Mosher, K. I., Zou, B., Britschgi, M., Bieri, G., et al. (2011). The ageing systemic milieu negatively regulates neurogenesis and cognitive function. Nature 477, 90–94. doi: 10.1038/nature10357

Vogelzangs, N., Beekman, A. T., Dik, M. G., Bremmer, M. A., Comijs, H. C., Hoogendijk, W. J., et al. (2009). Late-life depression, cortisol, and the metabolic syndrome. Am. J. Geriatr. Psychiatry 17, 716–721. doi: 10.1097/JGP.0b013e3181aad5d7

Vreeburg, S. A., Hoogendijk, W. J., van Pelt, J., Derijk, R. H., Verhagen, J. C., van Dyck, R., et al. (2009). Major depressive disorder and hypothalamic-pituitary-adrenal axis activity: results from a large cohort study. Arch. Gen. Psychiatry 66, 617–626. doi: 10.1001/archgenpsychiatry.2009.50

Vreeburg, S. A., Zitman, F. G., van Pelt, J., Derijk, R. H., Verhagen, J. C., van Dyck, R., et al. (2010). Salivary cortisol levels in persons with and without different anxiety disorders. Psychosom. Med. 72, 340–347. doi: 10.1097/PSY.0b013e3181d2f0c8

Wake, H., Moorhouse, A. J., Jinno, S., Kohsaka, S., and Nabekura, J. (2009). Resting microglia directly monitor the functional state of synapses in vivo and determine the fate of ischemic terminals. J. Neurosci. 29, 3974–3980. doi: 10.1523/jneurosci.4363-08.2009

Walker, A. J., Burnett, S. A., Hasebe, K., McGillivray, J. A., Gray, L. J., McGee, S. L., et al. (2013). Chronic adrenocorticotrophic hormone treatment alters tri- cyclic antidepressant efficacy and prefrontal monoamine tissue levels. Behav. Brain Res. 242, 76–83. doi: 10.1016/j.bbr.2012.12.033

Wang, Y., Yang, F., Liu, Y. F., Gao, F., and Jiang, W. (2011). Acetylsalicylic acid as an augmentation agent in fluoxetine treatment resistant depressive rats. Neurosci. Lett. 499, 74–79. doi: 10.1016/j.neulet.2011.05.035

Warrington, T. P., and Bostwick, J. M. (2006). Psychiatric adverse effects of corticosteroids. Mayo Clin. Proc. 81, 1361–1367. doi: 10.4065/81. 10.1361

Watanabe, S., Kanada, S., Takenaka, M., and Hamazaki, T. (2004). Dietary n-3 fatty acids selectively attenuate LPS-induced behavioral depression in mice. Physiol. Behav. 81, 605–613. doi: 10.1016/j.physbeh.2004.02.021

Watson, S., Gallagher, P., Porter, R. J., Smith, M. S., Herron, L. J., Bulmer, S., et al. (2012). A randomized trial to examine the effect of mifepristone on neuropsy- chological performance and mood in patients with bipolar depression. Biol. Psychiatry 72, 943–949. doi: 10.1016/j.biopsych.2012.05.029

Wichers, M. C., Koek, G. H., Robaeys, G., Verkerk, R., Scharpe, S., and Maes, M. (2005). IDO and interferon-alpha-induced depressive symptoms: a shift in hypothesis from tryptophan depletion to neurotoxicity. Mol. Psychiatry 10, 538–544. doi: 10.1038/sj.mp.4001600

Wolfram, M., Bellingrath, S., Feuerhahn, N., and Kudielka, B. M. (2013). Emotional exhaustion and overcommitment to work are differentially asso- ciated with hypothalamus-pituitary-adrenal (HPA) axis responses to a low-dose ACTH1-24 (Synacthen) and dexamethasone-CRH test in healthy school teachers. Stress (Amst.) 16, 54–64. doi: 10.3109/10253890.2012. 683465

Young, A. H., Gallagher, P., Watson, S., Del-Estal, D., Owen, B. M., and Ferrier, I. N. (2004). Improvements in neurocognitive function and mood following adjunctive treatment with mifepristone (RU-486) in bipo- lar disorder. Neuropsychopharmacology 29, 1538–1545. doi: 10.1038/sj.npp.1300471

Zalachoras, I., Houtman, R., Atucha, E., Devos, R., Tijssen, A. M., Hu, P., et al. (2013). Differential targeting of brain stress circuits with a selective glucocor- ticoid receptor modulator. Proc. Natl. Acad. Sci. U.S.A. 110, 7910–7915. doi: 10.1073/pnas.1219411110

Zimmermann, P., Brückl, T., Nocon, A., Pfister, H., Binder, E. B., Uhr, M., et al. (2011). Interaction of FKBP5 gene variants and adverse life events in predicting depression onset: results from a 10-year prospective community study. Am. J. Psychiatry 168, 1107–1116. doi: 10.1176/appi.ajp.2011.10111577

Zorrilla, E. P., Luborsky, L., McKay, J. R., Rosenthal, R., Houldin, A., Tax, A., et al. (2001). The relationship of depression and stressors to immunolog- ical assays: a meta-analytic review. Brain Behav. Immun. 15, 199–226. doi: 10.1006/brbi.2000.0597

Zou, Y. F., Wang, F., Feng, X. L., Li, W. F., Tao, J. H., Pan, F. M., et al. (2010). Meta-analysis of FKBP5 gene polymorphisms association with treatment response in patients with mood disorders. Neurosci. Lett. 484, 56–61. doi: 10.1016/j.neulet.2010.08.019

15

Mechanisms of antidepressant resistance

Wissam El-Hage[1,2], Samuel Leman[1], Vincent Camus[1,2] and Catherine Belzung[1]*

[1] INSERM 930, Faculté de Sciences et Techniques, Université François Rabelais, Tours, France
[2] Centre Hospitalier Régional Universitaire de Tours, Centre Expert Dépression Résistante, Fondation FondaMental, Tours, France

Edited by:
Thibault Renoir, Florey Institute of Neuroscience and Mental Health, Australia

Reviewed by:
Jean-Philippe Guilloux, Université Paris Sud, France
Andre Carvalho, Federal University of Ceara, Brazil

***Correspondence:**
Catherine Belzung, INSERM 930, Faculté de Sciences et Techniques, Université François Rabelais, Parc Grandmont, F-37200 Tours, France
e-mail: catherine.belzung@univ-tours.fr

Depression is one of the most frequent and severe mental disorder. Since the discovery of antidepressant (AD) properties of the imipramine and then after of other tricyclic compounds, several classes of psychotropic drugs have shown be effective in treating major depressive disorder (MDD). However, there is a wide range of variability in response to ADs that might lead to non response or partial response or in increased rate of relapse or recurrence. The mechanisms of response to AD therapy are poorly understood, and few biomarkers are available than can predict response to pharmacotherapy. Here, we will first review markers that can be used to predict response to pharmacotherapy, such as markers of drug metabolism or blood-brain barrier (BBB) function, the activity of specific brain areas or neurotransmitter systems, hormonal dysregulations or plasticity, and related molecular targets. We will describe both clinical and preclinical studies and describe factors that might affect the expression of these markers, including environmental or genetic factors and comorbidities. This information will permit us to suggest practical recommendations and innovative treatment strategies to improve therapeutic outcomes.

Keywords: major depression, resistance, antidepressants, treatment-resistant depression, monoamine

INTRODUCTION

Major depressive disorder (MDD) is among the most frequent mental disorders, with an estimated lifetime prevalence of 1–16%, depending on the country (Andrade et al., 2003; Kessler and Ustun, 2004; Kessler et al., 2010). Recovering from MDD is a major challenge because the disease dramatically increases the risk of suicide (Cheng et al., 2000) and non-suicide mortality (Schulz et al., 2002). Practical guidelines recommend treating MDD with antidepressant (AD) therapy (NICE, 2004; Bauer et al., 2007; Ramasubbu et al., 2012). Since the initial serendipitous discovery of the AD effect of monoamine oxidase inhibitors (MAOIs) and tricyclics (TCAs), most ADs have been pharmacological agents that act on monoamine function, including serotonin (selective serotonin reuptake inhibitors, SSRIs), noradrenaline (noradrenaline reuptake inhibitors, NRIs), dopamine (such as bupropion), and melatonin (agomelatine). Some drugs act on several of these targets (serotonin and noradrenaline reuptake inhibitors, SNRIs) (Krishnan and Nestler, 2008). The main goals of treating MDD are to achieve remission and to maintain these therapeutic effects over time. In the absence of any reliable biomarker of MDD, the response to treatment is still based on clinical assessment as evidenced by changes on scores on standardized rating instruments, such as the Hamilton Depression Rating Scale (HDRS) (Hamilton, 1960) or the Montgomery Asberg Depression Rating Scale (Montgomery and Asberg, 1979). The response to ADs is typically characterized as "non-response" when only minimum improvement is achieved, "partial response" when the score on the standardized instrument decreases by 25–50%, "response" when a decrease of at least 50% is obtained, and "remission" when only residual clinical symptoms are reported, with a level of psychopathology under the typical threshold score currently correlated to MDD diagnosis (Nierenberg and DeCecco, 2001). Using these criteria, several studies, including the naturalistic STAR*D study, have shown that only one third of MDD patients receiving ADs achieve complete remission after a single AD trial (Trivedi et al., 2006). The remission rate reaches up to 60% after four trials, but the probability of remission drops significantly after the failure of two consecutive AD trials (Rush et al., 2006). Moreover, early improvement predicts sustained response and remission (Lam, 2012). Consequently, the concept of treatment-resistant depression (TRD) was proposed to describe depressive conditions that did not reach sufficient remission after treatment (Lehmann, 1974; Sartorius, 1974). Even several criteria have been proposed to define TRD-including non-response to one AD for at least 4 weeks or failure to respond to multiple trials of different classes of ADs-there is now an emerging consensus to consider any MDD patient that did not respond to two or more adequate (in terms of duration and dosage) AD trials of different classes as TRD (Berlim and Turecki, 2007). The characterization of TRD has been improved by considering the level of resistance (severity and duration) through staging classifications, such as the Antidepressant Treatment History Form (ATHF) (Sackeim et al., 1990), the Thase and Rush Model (Thase and Rush, 1997), the European Staging Model (Souery et al., 1999), the Massachusetts General Hospital Staging Model (MGH-s) (Fava, 2003), and the Maudsley Staging Model (MSM) (Fekadu et al., 2009) (for a review, see Ruhé et al., 2012).

Translational research enables to study the mechanisms of non response to ADs in animal models. Indeed, this involves invasive protocols, as particular proteins, brain areas or process have to be suppressed to elucidate their causal involvement in response to AD. Therefore, bioassays (forced swim test, tail suspension tests...) and more generally animal models have been designed that enable to induce a behavioral deficit after experimental manipulations (stressors during the developmental period, social defeat or unpredictable chronic stress during adulthood, chronic corticosterone). The induced modifications are then assessed via behavioral testing such as scoring of sucrose preference, of coat state, of grooming behavior, of anxiety-related behavior. It is usually observed that chronic ADs reverse the behavioral alterations that have been induced by the experimental manipulations and this enables to assess AD response (depending on the magnitude of the reversal that has been observed, and on the number of behavioral dimensions that have been counteracted). It is pivotal here to assess several different behaviors, as it can succeed that only a specific phenotype is reversed, and not the others as seen for example in David et al. (2009).

The main aim of this paper is to review the different potential predictors of response/non response to AD and discuss their clinical and practical implications. We will successively discuss the potential mechanisms and correlates of response to ADs with regard to some general clinical and pharmacological considerations and at the different levels of neurobiological understanding of AD mechanisms of action (Kupfer et al., 2012), with a particular consideration of the neuroanatomical, neurotransmission, molecular, and genetic levels, as well as to potential hormonal and neuroplasticity aspects (**Table 1**).

POOR RESPONSE TO ANTIDEPRESSANT THERAPY: CLINICAL CORRELATES

The efficacy of ADs has been strongly debated recently because of negative randomized controlled studies in which the response rates in the placebo control group were as high as 30–40% (Iovieno and Papakostas, 2012). Rather than arguing against the efficacy of ADs in MDD, these results indicated some methodological limitations of studies recently submitted to the European or US authorities (Khin et al., 2011). In particular, an inappropriately low baseline disease severity is likely the most problematic methodological flaw that eliminates the statistical significance of the difference in the response rate between the active and placebo groups (Kirsch et al., 2008; Fournier et al., 2010).

Another important methodological consideration is that even if the rating scales (such as the HDRS) on which the treatment response is assessed are robust and reliable, not all items of the scale (e.g., anxiety, somatic, early insomnia, hypochondriasis, and somatic symptoms) represent equal proportions of the observed change in the global score (Nelson et al., 2005). This could explain why a high level of anxiety symptoms could result in an underestimation of the response to treatment and why anxiety disorders are frequently associated with TRD (Souery et al., 2007). Other clinical characteristics are associated with a higher risk of low response to ADs. In particular, some MDD patients who meet the criteria for TRD are later revealed to suffer from bipolar disorder (Fekadu et al., 2012). Bipolar depression is less prone to respond to ADs than MDD (Gijsman et al., 2004), even though recent findings suggest that ADs may be as effective against bipolar depression as against MDD (Tondo et al., 2013; Vázquez et al., 2013).

Among clinical characteristics, older age has also been shown to be associated with a lower response rate to ADs. In a meta-analysis conducted on 15 late life MMD trials and 59 adult MDD trials, it was found that the response rate drops from 53.9% in

Table 1 | Mechanisms predicting response to antidepressants.

	Main predictors of poor response to antidepressant treatment
CLINICAL CORRELATES	
	• Bipolar depression • Older age in relation to age or somatic comorbidities (cardiac, cerebrovascular, neurodegenerative disorders) • Poor compliance to antidepressants in relation to low income, health insurance status, race/ethnicity
PHARMACOLOGICAL CORRELATES	
Drug metabolism	• Younger age, sex, smoking status, pregnancy, drug dose, diet, grapefruit, genetics, enzyme induction/inhibition • Ultra-rapid metabolizers in relation to hepatic metabolism: genetic differences in drug-metabolizing enzymes (cytochromes P450; e.g. CYP2D62, CYP2C19) • Alteration of hepatic, renal or cardiovascular functions • Polypharmacy enhances drug interactions, particularly fluvoxamine, fluoxetine, paroxetine, nefazodone
Blood-brain barrier	• Polymorphisms in genes coding for ABC transporter proteins, particularly the P-glycoprotein (P-gp) • Drugs that are substrates of P-gp have decreased penetration into the brain
NEUROBIOLOGICAL CORRELATES	
Brain structures	EEG (alpha and theta activities) • Lower alpha rhythmic activity in posterior regions (among amitriptyline non-responders) and in left hemisphere (SSRIs) • Higher theta rhythmic activity among imipramine non-responders • Decreased pre-treatment theta activity in the ACC Neuroimaging (fMRI, PET) • Lower baseline rostral ACC activity • Low ACC activity during functional tasks • Reduction in frontolimbic gray matter volumes (medial and orbital PFC) • Smaller baseline hippocampal volume • Abnormalities in corticolimbic connectivity • Higher right- over left hemisphere processing • Higher baseline metabolism in the amygdala and thalamus, and lower pretreatment metabolism in the medial PFC • Insula hypometabolism
Neurotransmission	Serotoninergic system • Alteration of the 5-HT_{1A} pre- and postsynaptic receptors dynamic • Polymorphism of the 5-HT transporter gene (short allele carriers) • SNPs of tryptophan hydroxylase genes (TPH1 and TPH2)

(Continued)

Table 1 | Continued

Main predictors of poor response to antidepressant treatment	
	• SNPs of the 5-HT1A receptor gene (1019C/G; 102T/C; 1438A/G) • Interaction between stressful life events and polymorphisms in 5-HT related genes Noradrenergic system • Alteration of the dopamine beta-hydroxylase enzyme/gene • Deficiency in organic cation transporter 2 • Polymorphisms of the noradrenaline transporter gene (-182T/C; 1287G/A) • Polymorphism of the catechol-O-methyltransferase gene (Val homozygous) • Early life stress events (via gene methylation or acetylation) Other systems • Decreased substance P in the cerebrospinal fluid • SNPs of the dystrobrevin-binding protein 1 gene (glutamatergic neurotransmission) • SNPs of the glutamate receptor ionotropic kainite 4 gene (rs1954787; rs12800734) • Deletion of the gene encoding the GABA transporter subtype 1 • Genetic variability in endocannabinoid receptors (CNR1; G allele of rs1049353 in females) • Deficit in the leptin system (decreased leptin serum levels, reduced leptin mRNA expression)
Neural plasticity	Molecular aspects • Polymorphism in the BDNF gene (Val allele carriers) • Alteration of BDNF in the dentate gyrus (hippocampus) • Alteration of protein p11, mediating the antidepressant activity of BDNF • Interaction between ongoing stress and the levels of BDNF • Zinc deficiency • Macrophage migration inhibitory factor deficiency Cellular targets • Alteration in adult hippocampal neurogenesis • Alteration of the generation of new functional neurons
Hormonal targets	HPA axis • Defect in the HPA axis regulation (defect in normalization of its overactivity) • No reduction of the cortisol response to a dexamethasone/CRH test after 2–3 weeks of treatment • Polymorphisms of genes coding for FKBP5, BclI, ER22/23EK, CRHR1 (rs242941), CRHR2 (rs2270007), CRH-BP, and hsp70 protein

(Continued)

Table 1 | Continued

Main predictors of poor response to antidepressant treatment	
	• Somatic condition: Cushing's disease • Interaction between stressors and genes (SERT, FKBP5, CRHR1) to predict response to treatment Thyrotropin releasing hormone • Hypothyroidism; Polymorphism of the deiodinase type 1 gene

ACC, Anterior cingulate cortex; BclI, ER22/23EK, Polymorphisms of glucocorticoid receptor gene; BDNF, Brain-derived neurotrophic factor; CRH, Corticotropin-releasing hormone; CRHR-BP, CRH binding protein; CRHR1, CRH receptor 1; CRHR2, CRH receptor 2; EEG, Electroencephalography; FKBP5, FK506 binding protein 5; fMRI, Functional magnetic resonance imaging; HPA, Hypothalamic-pituitary-adrenal; PET, Positron emission tomography; PFC, Prefrontal cortex; SERT, serotonin transporter; SNPs, Single-nucleotide polymorphisms; SSRIs, Selective serotonin reuptake inhibitors; 5-HT, Serotonin.

adults to 45.2% in older patients (Tedeschini et al., 2011). In adolescents, response rate has been shown to be much higher, several studies reporting response rate at week 36 from 65 (Tao et al., 2009) to 80% (March et al., 2006), with a mean remission rate of 67% (Cox et al., 2012). Whether age itself may explain the difference remains unclear because somatic comorbidities may have a role in increasing the risk of non-response or partial response to ADs in older patients, particularly cardiac (Scherrer et al., 2012), cerebrovascular (Miller et al., 2002), and neurodegenerative disorders (Price et al., 2011).

Sex also constitutes a clinical characteristic associated with difference in AD treatment response. Indeed, a study suggested that men respond more favorably to imipramine than women, and premenopausal women more frequently to fluvoxamine than men (Vermeiden et al., 2010). In animal studies, Goel et al. (2011) showed that acute citalopram induced higher neuronal activation in male brain than in females or gonadectomized males. This suggests a gonadal hormone influence on complex interactions between serotonin and neural circuits that mediate the stress axis (see section HPA Axis Regulation below) and could therefore explain some of the sex differences in the response to AD.

The lack of response to ADs may also be the consequence of non-adherence to the treatment as the rate of adherence to ADs has been estimated to be particularly low, varying over a period of six months from 12.4% for patients taking older MAOIs and TCAs to 29.3% for those taking SSRIs and 33.6% for those taking SNRIs (Sheehan et al., 2008). In a 9-week follow-up period, up to 20% of patients missed taking their treatment for at least four consecutive days (Demyttenaere et al., 2001). This poor compliance has been shown to alter the estimation of response and remission rates (Akerblad et al., 2006). According to Jin et al. (2008), various factors contribute to non-compliance. Jeon-Slaughter (2012) found that low income level, combined with health insurance status and race/ethnicity, predicted non-adherence to ADs. This was confirmed in a recent review (Rivero-Santana et al., 2013) that demonstrated that younger people were less compliant than older patients and minority ethnic patients were less compliant than white patients. Non-pharmacological interventions can improve the adherence to AD treatments. Vergouwen et al. (2003) found that collaborative interventions in primary care were associated with clinical benefit, particularly in patients suffering from MDD who were prescribed adequate dosages of ADs.

PREDICTORS OF POOR RESPONSE TO ANTIDEPRESSANT THERAPY: PHARMACOLOGICAL COMPONENT

DRUG METABOLISM

Availability of the drug to its brain targets is one of the first requisite conditions of its effect and clinical impact. However, various conditions affect drug delivery such as its metabolism. Drug metabolism is altered by a wide range of factors such as age, rate of expression of drug metabolism systems, comorbid disease, sex, pregnancy, environment, drug dose, enzyme induction/inhibition, diet, genetics... For instance, younger people metabolize drugs faster than elderly people, men faster than women, and smokers faster than non-smokers. AD medications are metabolized mainly in the liver into compounds that are typically pharmacologically active but with different properties than the parent drug. Drug metabolism may result in poor response. Hepatic metabolism mainly occurs via cytochrome P450 (CYP) enzymes, which comprise more than 200 isoenzymes (mainly CYP1A2, CYP2B6, CYP2D6, CYP2C9, CYP2C19, and CYP3A4/5): they account for 75% of drug metabolism (Guengerich, 2008), particularly oxidative metabolism.

Variations in CYP genes have been shown to be associated with modified pharmacokinetic clearance of ADs. In humans, CYP is encoded by 18 families and 43 subfamilies of genes, corresponding to 57 genes and more than 59 pseudogenes. Thus, many different genes may alter CYP, some patients being poor and others ultrarapid metabolizers. When ultrarapid metabolizers are treated with typical doses of ADs, they have low plasma concentrations and do not respond. Polymorphisms in genes for crucial CYP enzymes, such as CYP2D6 or CYP2C19, alter the metabolism of ADs and thus their plasma concentrations (Brosen, 2004). Carriers of the non-functional allele of CYP2C19 exhibit a 42% decrease in clearance of the SSRI citalopram compared to carriers of the functional allele (Yin et al., 2006). Bondolfi et al. (1996) investigated seven non-responders to citalopram; six were extensive CYP2D6 metabolizers, and all seven were extensive CYP2C19 metabolizers. Furthermore, when administered an inhibitor of these two enzymes, citalopram serum levels rose in all subjects, as well as the therapeutic response. However, Grasmäder et al. (2004) found that plasma concentrations of several ADs were altered depending on the CYP2D6 and CYP2C19 genotype, even if this genotype was unrelated to clinical response. Peters et al. (2008) using subjects from the STAR*D study found no association between 15 polymorphisms of four P450 genes (CYP2D6, CYP2C19, CYP3A4, and CYP3A5) and citalopram response. More recently, Mrazek et al. (2011) examined data from the white non-Hispanic subjects who were treated with citalopram in the same STAR*D sample. They found a modest association between CYP2C19 variation and remission following citalopram, particularly in a subset of patients able to tolerate the medication. Thus, evidence on the association between genetic variations in CYP and AD response is inconsistent and likely depends on the patients and drug used.

Among the environmental factors that influence pharmacokinetics, smoking, treatment adherence, and concurrent medications are particularly important. There are numerous drug interactions with cigarette smoking. Suzuki et al. (2011) found that smoking status significantly affected fluvoxamine concentration (only in the low 50 mg/d dose group). Together, CYP2D6 genotype and smoking status explained 23% of the variance in fluvoxamine concentration in this group.

Failure to respond to or tolerate a drug may be related to comorbid medical conditions (hepatic or renal insufficiency, cardiovascular disease) and/or to its related polypharmacy. Comorbid medical conditions that alter hepatic function are likely to decrease the rate of drug metabolism. In addition, co-prescriptions increase the risk of drug-drug interactions with ADs in the treatment of comorbid illness. Drug interactions are more likely to occur with high-risk drugs, such as fluvoxamine, fluoxetine, paroxetine, and nefazodone (Richelson, 1998). Coelho and Brum Cde (2009) investigated the interactions between ADs and antihypertensive and glucose-lowering drugs at two primary care units and found that 19 of 29 patients were exposed to 47 interactions involving pharmacokinetic and pharmacodynamic mechanisms. When initiating a new prescription, the physician should select an AD while considering comorbid medical conditions, including dosage adjustment, possible drug interactions, adverse effects, and tolerability issues. The physician should also inform the patient about the influence of co-administered drugs and simultaneous intake of beverages and food on the bioavailability of drugs. For instance, grapefruit juice consumption increases the mean peak plasma concentrations and the concentration-time curve of sertraline (Ueda et al., 2009) and fluvoxamine (Hori et al., 2003).

In case of TRD, therapeutic drug monitoring is a valuable tool for tailoring the dosage of the prescribed medication to the individual characteristics. Dose titration is strongly recommended to achieve therapeutic plasma concentrations that allow for the highest probability of response or remission. In addition to drug concentration measurements, symptom rating by the treating physician at baseline and at week 2 is recommended (Hiemke et al., 2011). In certain situations, AD monitoring could be combined with pharmacogenetic metabolism tests (Hiemke et al., 2011). For instance, when the concentrations are outside the reference range, pharmacogenetic tests could be recommended to detect polymorphisms that give rise to slow/rapid metabolizers. Winner et al. (2013) recently demonstrated that pharmacogenomic-directed prescribing reduced the incidence of adverse drug reactions and improved the efficacy of AD medication regimens. Thus, pharmacogenomic testing to determine metabolic capacity may be a valuable strategy to recognize individuals who will obtain a therapeutic benefit from a drug.

BLOOD-BRAIN BARRIER

Among the mechanisms of poor response to ADs, the drug efflux transporters that are expressed at the blood-brain barrier (BBB) and enable drugs to access the brain play a major role. The BBB is composed of brain capillary endothelial cells in association with pericytes and smooth muscle cells that delineate the circulating blood from glial cells and the neuronal terminals of the central nervous system. The BBB limits the traffic of substances to trans-cellular transport rather through the intercellular spaces because the tight junction system of the trans-membrane proteins acts as a physical barrier. Consequently, only lipophilic compounds of low molecular weight are able to cross the BBB. However, various transport systems ensure wider exchanges through the BBB, including the ATP-binding cassette (ABC transporters) system (for lipid-soluble molecules) (Benarroch, 2012). The human genome encodes 49 different ABC transporter proteins classified into seven subfamilies (ABCA to ABCG) (Dean et al., 2001). The P-glycoprotein (P-gp) encoded by the multi-drug resistance 1 (MDR1/ABCB1) gene, the breast cancer resistance protein encoded by the ABCG2 gene, and the multidrug resistance-associated proteins 4 and 5 are expressed by the brain endothelial cells and ensure active efflux of lipid-soluble molecules from the brain, reducing penetration of drugs into the brain. Compounds that interact with ABC transporters can be classified as substrates, modulators, or inhibitors. AD drugs interact mainly with P-gp. Thus, ADs that are substrates of P-gp are subject to greater efflux from brain endothelial cells and decreased penetration into the brain. Moreover, drug-drug interactions can also be the consequence of competing/synergic effects on P-gp. Several drugs, including cyclosporine, nifedipine, quinidine, and verapamil, are P-gp inhibitors (O'Brien et al., 2012). *In vivo* preclinical studies, particularly in P-gp knock-out mice, have demonstrated that not all ADs are subject to the same level of limitation to brain penetration by P-gp (Uhr et al., 2000, 2003; Uhr and Grauer, 2003; Karlsson et al., 2013). Moreover, metabolites of some ADs may not be substrates of P-gp, in contrast to their parent molecules (Weiss et al., 2003; Grauer and Uhr, 2004; Wang et al., 2008a). Clinical evidence of the role of P-gp in the response to ADs has been provided by studies of variants of the ABCB1 gene. Several single nucleotide polymorphisms (SNPs) of the ABCB1 gene have been identified and associated with a decreased clinical response to AD (Kato et al., 2008; Uhr et al., 2008; Sarginson et al., 2010; Lin et al., 2011; Singh et al., 2012) as well as a poorer tolerance profile (Roberts et al., 2002; Jensen et al., 2012; de Klerk et al., 2012), although several studies failed to replicate these results (Laika et al., 2006; Mihaljevic Peles et al., 2008; Menu et al., 2010). Furthermore, endogenous and synthetic glucocorticoids also act as P-gp substrates (Ueda et al., 1992; Schinkel et al., 1995; Uhr et al., 2002). Hyperactivity of the hypothalamus-pituitary-adrenal (HPA) axis is one of the most consistent biological hallmarks of MDD, and it has been suggested that increased penetration of glucocorticoids into the brain as a result of P-gp inhibition may contribute to normalization of HPA axis hyperactivity in MDD (O'Brien et al., 2012). These data suggest evaluation of P-gp inhibition as an augmentation strategy for improving response to AD therapy.

PREDICTORS OF POOR RESPONSE TO ANTIDEPRESSANT THERAPY: NEUROBIOLOGICAL COMPONENTS

Based on the understanding we have of the neurobiological mechanisms of action of ADs, the response to ADs can be explored at the following levels: brain structures, neurotransmission, and molecular targets. We will now describe each of these mechanisms (**Table 1**).

BRAIN STRUCTURES AND RESPONSE TO ANTIDEPRESSANTS

Various studies have explored brain changes associated with response to ADs by using electroencephalography (EEG) (alpha and theta activities) or neuroimaging (Functional magnetic resonance imaging: fMRI, Positron emission tomography: PET) that allow deducing potential mechanisms and markers of response to ADs.

Brain activity measurements by quantitative EEG in the resting state or during simple tasks have been used to predict response to ADs. Ulrich et al. (1986) observed increased alpha rhythmic activity (8–12 Hz) in the posterior regions of the head on both sides that was higher in amplitude on the dominant side in patients responding to amitriptyline. Subsequently, Knott et al. (1996) observed higher alpha and less theta rhythmic activity (4–7 Hz) among imipramine-responders than non-responders. Bruder et al. (2001) observed a difference in alpha asymmetry between fluoxetine responders and non-responders; non-responders displayed reduced alpha activity over the left hemisphere than the right, whereas responders tended to have the opposite asymmetry. Other studies focused on the brain regions associated with this altered alpha activity. Bruder et al. (2008) demonstrated that the difference between SSRI responders and non-responders involved occipital areas, where differences in alpha asymmetry were also observed. Theta activity was also investigated. EEG theta frequencies are generated in various brain areas, such as the medial prefrontal cortex (PFC), anterior cingulate cortex (ACC), hippocampus, amygdala, and ventral striatum. In the ACC, Pizzagalli et al. (2001) found an association between pre-treatment theta increases in rostral ACC and responses to nortriptyline. Mulert et al. (2007) reported similar findings with citalopram or reboxetine. This pre-treatment change in theta power in relationship to AD outcome has not been consistently observed (Cook et al., 2002). However, they demonstrated that the decrease in prefrontal cordance (i.e., the measure of quantitative EEG power that characterizes PFC function) that occurs after 1 week of treatment only in responders is also predictive of a better final outcome (Cook et al., 2002, 2009). In another study, Bares et al. (2008) found that reduction in the PFC theta quantitative EEG cordance value after the first week of treatment can predict the response to venlafaxine. Quantitative EEG measurements are now considered a promising clinical tool for predicting conventional AD treatment response (Leuchter et al., 2009, 2010). Interestingly, brain electrical activity has also been used to predict outcomes of non-conventional ADs, such as the NMDA receptor antagonist ketamine or non-pharmacological AD therapy, such as deep brain stimulation (DBS). For example, Duncan et al. (2013) recently demonstrated that measuring sleep slow wave activity (0.6–4 Hz) could predict ketamine response in individuals with TRD, whereas frontal theta quantitative EEG cordance has been shown to predict long-term AD response to subcallosal cingulate DBS in TRD patients (Broadway et al., 2012).

The involvement of the rostral ACC in TRD or treatment non-response is also supported by neuroimaging studies. Indeed, PET studies have observed increased baseline rostral ACC activity in MDD patients who subsequently responded to ADs (Mayberg et al., 1997; Saxena et al., 2003) while an fMRI study demonstrated that higher ACC activity during precise tasks, such as processing negative stimuli, was associated with the most robust treatment response (Davidson et al., 2003). Moreover, ACC activation during unsuccessful motor inhibition predicted response to escitalopram (Langenecker et al., 2007). Interestingly, a recent study showed that increased activity in the rostral ACC is a predictor not only of treatment outcome to conventional ADs but also to putative ADs, such as ketamine (Salvadore et al., 2009), or to non-pharmacological therapy, such as sleep deprivation (Wu et al., 1999). Non-response to ADs is correlated with low pre-treatment activity in the rostral ACC (Mayberg et al., 1997; Pizzagalli, 2011), which is one of the most reliable markers for predicting treatment outcome for conventional monoaminergic-acting ADs, intravenous ketamine treatment, and non-pharmacological treatments, such as electroconvulsive therapy (ECT) or repetitive transcranial magnetic stimulation (rTMS) (Pizzagalli, 2011). However, a low level of activity in the rostral ACC predicts a better outcome for cognitive behavioral therapy (CBT) (Fu et al., 2008; Pizzagalli, 2011; Roiser et al., 2012).

Gray matter brain volumes and, more recently, forebrain white matter integrity have also been measured in patients with MDD (first episode, remittent, or TRD). Frontolimbic gray matter areas (medial and orbital PFC) were reduced in the most severely depressed individuals (i.e., treatment-resistant/chronic group) (Serra-Blasco et al., 2013). Moreover, patients that did not respond to escitalopram exhibited microstructural abnormalities in fiber tracts connecting the cortex with limbic structures, such as the ACC (Alexopoulos et al., 2008). In addition, patients with TRD displayed abnormalities of both internal and external capsule integrity connecting cortical to subcortical nuclei and of the corpus callosum (Guo et al., 2012). Interestingly, these corticolimbic pathways are negatively impacted by adverse life events or by genetic polymorphism of the serotonin transporter (Alexopoulos et al., 2009; Choi et al., 2009), and corticolimbic connectivity increased as scores on the HDRS decreased during treatment (Anand et al., 2005). This suggests that assessing corticolimbic connectivity could be used to predict AD outcome. Further, the PFC region is one of the favorite targets for DBS in patients with TRD (Mayberg et al., 2005; Lozano et al., 2008; Malone et al., 2009). In addition, Dunkin et al. (2000) reported pre-treatment difference between fluoxetine responders and non-responders on PFC-related tasks reflecting executive dysfunction. Recently, Gupta et al. (2013) demonstrated that patients with TRD exhibited mildly reduced performance across all neurocognitive domains with a superimposed moderate impairment in verbal working memory. Finally, Bruder et al. (2004) investigated dichotic listening and demonstrated that patients who respond to SSRIs differed from non-responders in favoring left- over right-hemisphere processing of dichotic stimuli. Fluoxetine responders displayed greater left-hemisphere advantage for words and less right-hemisphere advantage for complex tones compared to non-responders. The cognitive, sensorial, or behavioral alterations shown in AD responders vs. non-responders are likely related to differences in the functioning of the brain areas underlying these functions, and thus, this suggests that brain alterations may also be valuable predictors of AD outcome.

The ACC is not the sole brain region whose activity can predict AD response. Indeed, improvement of MDD symptoms after AD has also been associated with lower pre-treatment metabolism (detected by PET) in the amygdala and thalamus and with higher pre-treatment metabolism in the medial PFC (Saxena et al., 2003). The hippocampus has also received some interest, and a recent study showed that MDD patients who met criteria for clinical remission at 8 weeks of AD treatment had larger pre-treatment hippocampal volumes than non-remitters, suggesting involvement of the hippocampus not only in the pathophysiology of MDD but also in treatment outcome (MacQueen et al., 2008; McKinnon et al., 2009). Larger hippocampal volume was also associated with a lower probability of relapse (Kronmüller et al., 2008). Microstructural abnormalities in the hippocampus have been suggested to indicate the vulnerability to treatment resistance (Ruhé et al., 2012). Further, a recent study pointed to a crucial role of the right insula: indeed, insula hypometabolism (detected via PET) was associated with poor response to escitalopram while the opposite was observed concerning cognitive behavior therapy, as insula hypometabolism was associated with good response to this cognitive therapeutic approach (McGrath et al., 2013). This indicates that neuroimaging can also help in selecting the appropriate treatment, and that brain activity does not predict poor response to treatment in a general way, but poor response to a particular therapeutic approach.

The crucial role of corticolimbic areas in the response to AD therapy has also been highlighted by recent impressive preclinical studies. These studies highlight the mechanisms underlying AD action in a given region. For example, Vialou et al. (2010) demonstrated that DeltaFosB induction in the nucleus accumbens was required for the effects of fluoxetine in the social defeat test, whereas Li et al. (2010) demonstrated that the effects of ketamine require synapse formation (particularly mTor-dependent synapse formation) in the PFC. Further, a recent paper showed that neural activity in the visual cortex during emotional processing predicts the response to scopolamine in depression (Furey et al., 2013).

Finally, TRD and/or treatment non-response can also be indirectly approached by studying the mechanism of non-pharmacological treatments, including vagus nerve stimulation therapy (VNS), ECT, and DBS. VNS is approved for the treatment of TRD. In VNS, a battery-powered generator is implanted in the chest wall and connected to a wire wrapped around the left vagus nerve in the neck. This wire sends intermittent electrical pulses through the vagal afferent connections to the brainstem, which may alter information processing in brain regions to which it projects, including the noradrenergic locus cœruleus and serotonergic nuclei as well as the thalamus, hypothalamus, central amygdala nucleus, bed nucleus of the stria terminalis, and nucleus accumbens, which are all disrupted during MDD. Functional imaging suggests that VNS leads to activity changes in the hypothalamus, orbitofrontal cortex, amygdala, hippocampus, insula, medial PFC, and cingulate (Bohning et al., 2001; Zobel et al., 2005), suggesting that VNS might aid in the recovery of MDD patients by reversing the pathophysiological alterations observed in MDD. ECT is based on the administration of brief electrical pulses to the scalp to induce depolarization of cortical neurons and thus brain seizures. It is among the most effective treatments for TRD and AD non-response. The mechanism of action of ECT remains a mystery, but the recent observation that electroconvulsive shock, the animal analogue of ECT, stimulates precursor cell proliferation in the subgranular zone of the dentate gyrus as well as hippocampal neurogenesis in the rat (Madsen et al., 2000) and monkey (Perera et al., 2007) suggests that pharmacological treatments and ECT may target a common endpoint, such as neuronal plasticity. Finally, because a number of clinical studies have demonstrated long-term effects of DBS in terms of improving symptoms of MDD (Bewernick et al., 2012; Lozano et al., 2012), the study of the neurobiological mechanisms underlying the beneficial effects of DBS will contribute to the understanding of TRD and of the mechanisms underlying poor response to AD. For example, a recent study by Schmuckermair et al. (2013) in a mouse model of TRD demonstrated that repeated nucleus accumbens DBS reversed depression-related behavior and coincided with changes in stress-induced neuronal activation of prelimbic, infralimbic, and cingulate areas in the lateral habenula and in the dentate gyrus of the hippocampus, where neurogenesis was also increased. In addition, Hamani et al. (2010) demonstrated that DBS in the rat ventromedial PFC induced a clear AD-like effect that was dependent on the integrity of the serotoninergic system.

NEUROTRANSMISSION AND RESPONSE TO ANTIDEPRESSANTS

Serotoninergic system

Because TCAs and SSRIs increase serotonin (5-HT: 5-hydroxytriptamine) availability in the synaptic cleft, the level of involvement of 5-HT in predicting AD response has been a focus of research. Consistent with predictions, tryptophan depletion (which is a precursor of the 5-HT synthesis) in subjects successfully treated with SSRI prevents AD effects (Delgado et al., 1999), indicating that 5-HT is essential for the action of SSRIs. More recently, the utilization of PET permitted the precise localization of this 5-HT action. SSRI treatment outcome was related to serotonin transporter (SERT) ratios between the raphe nuclei and serotonergic projection areas (habenula, amygdala, hippocampus, and subgenual cingulate cortex) before treatment (Lanzenberger et al., 2012). In animal models, depletion of 5-HT tissue content by para-chlorophenylalanine, an inhibitor of tryptophan hydroxylase (TPH), prevented the acute effects of SSRIs in a bioassay (O'Leary et al., 2007). Rodent studies also permitted the determination of the precise molecular target of AD action, particularly through the use of knockout mice for SERT and several 5-HT receptors. As expected, in a bioassay assessing effects of sub-acute injections of AD, the action of fluoxetine was abolished in SERT knockout mice, whereas the effect of a noradrenaline-preferring AD, desipramine, was conserved (Holmes et al., 2002). Once the blockade of the SERT has been achieved, the increased 5-HT in the synaptic cleft will bind to several 5-HT receptors. One of the most studied is the 5-HT_{1A} postsynaptic receptor. In initial studies, SSRIs failed to alter immobility in 5-HT_{1A} mutant mice, suggesting that 5HT_{1A} receptors are critical for the expression of AD-like responses to SSRIs (Mayorga et al., 2001; Santarelli et al., 2003). However, a more complex picture later emerged as other studies showed that the effects of SSRIs were still present in 5-HT_{1A} mutant mice (Guilloux et al., 2006; Holick et al., 2008). In fact, the use of 5-HT_{1A} mutants did not allow to distinguish the pre- and the post-synaptic 5-HT_{1A} receptors, and it is probable that the involvement of these receptors during chronic SSRIs is dynamic, as in the initial phase of the treatment the action of 5-HT on the 5-HT_{1A} somatodendritic receptors may oppose the action on the post-synaptic receptors, while during the second phase, the presynaptic receptors get desensitized (see below). It has also been shown that desipramine, a NRI, still exerts an AD-like effect in 5HT_{1A} receptor knockout mice despite reduced baseline immobility in the tail suspension test (Mayorga et al., 2001). However, the action on the postsynaptic 5-HT_{1A} receptors is compromised by a concomitant action on 5-HT_{1A} autoreceptors located in the raphe, which reduces the clinical efficacy of SSRIs and partly explains their delayed onset of action. Using conditional knockout mice for pre-synaptic 5-HT_{1A} receptors, it was observed that reduction of 5-HT_{1A}-autoreceptor expression with unchanged post-synaptic 5-HT_{1A} receptor expression induced AD-like behavior and augmented SSRI effects (Richardson-Jones et al., 2010). These observations were recently confirmed using another experimental strategy, intra-raphe infusion of small-interfering RNA (siRNA) sequences directed toward the 5-HT_{1A} autoreceptors. The siRNA decreased the expression of these receptors without affecting post-synaptic 5-HT_{1A} receptors, concomitant with a robust and rapid AD-like effect (Bortolozzi, Castañé, Semakova, Santana, Alvarado and Cortés, 2012).

The involvement of 5-HT_{1B} receptors is complex and depends upon the class of AD used, as well as on the methodology used to study their contribution (knockouts or pharmacological studies). Indeed, in 5HT_{1B} receptor knockout mice, desipramine still has AD-like effects (Mayorga et al., 2001) while pharmacological blockade of the 5-HT_{1B} receptors with GR 127935 or SB216641 (5-HT_{1B} receptor antagonists) potentiated the effects of the drug (Tatarczyñska et al., 2004). Concerning SSRIs, an increased sensitivity to these compounds has been observed in mutants (single mutants for the 5-HT_{1B} receptors) or after 5-HT_{1B} receptors antagonists (Mayorga et al., 2001), whereas other studies reported SSRI resistance in the mutants (Trillat et al., 1998). Finally, in double knockout for 5-HT_{1A} and the 5-HT_{1B} receptors the response to acute SSRI was impacted, but not the one to chronic SSRIs (Guilloux et al., 2011). Other 5-HT receptors are required for AD action, including the 5-HT_{2B} (Diaz et al., 2012), 5-HT_{2C} (Cryan and Lucki, 2000a) and 5-HT_4 receptors (Cryan and Lucki, 2000b; Lucas et al., 2007).

Genetic studies confirmed the involvement of 5-HT-related targets in the outcome of 5-HT therapy. For example, different studies indicated a polymorphism in the human gene encoding SERT (*SLC6A4*) as a predictor of response to AD. Heils et al. (1996) identified a functional polymorphism in the transcriptional region upstream of the *SLC6A4*-coding sequence (5-HTTLPR) that affects *SLC6A4* expression, in which the *l* allele yields twofold higher *SLC6A4* expression in the basal state than the *s* form. In a meta-analysis of the literature, Kato and Serretti (2010) demonstrated that the *l* variant is associated with a better response rate to AD than the *s* allele. Nakamura et al. (2000) further examined the polymorphic region and concluded that the alleles previously reported as *s* and *l* should be respectively divided into four (14A, 14B, 14C, and 14D) and six allelic variants (16A–16F). Smeraldi et al. (2006) demonstrated that among carriers of the *l* variant, 16F *l* carriers exhibited only a partial response to AD and 16D *l* carriers exhibited a marginally better response than 16A *l* allele carriers. Another polymorphism of *SLC6A4* has been associated with an increased response to ADs; carriers with the 12 allele displayed a greater response to ADs, particularly when this allele was also associated with the *l* variant of the SERT-linked polymorphic region (*5-HTTLPR*) gene (see (Kato and Serretti, 2010) for a review). However, these findings have not been consistently replicated.

Serotonin biosynthesis involves TPH. This enzyme has two isoforms encoded by TPH1 and TPH2 genes, and SNPs of both genes have been reported. A significant association of TPH1 218A/C with response to ADs has been reported (Serretti et al., 2001) but these findings were not replicated (Kato et al., 2007).

A total of 50 SNPs of the 5-HT_{1A} receptor gene have been described. Of particular interest is the 1019C/G (rs6295) SNP, which is related to the altered expression and function of 5-HT_{1A} receptors. Indeed, the G allele is associated with an increase in 5-HT_{1A} autoreceptors and thus a decrease in 5-HT neurotransmission. An association of this polymorphism with AD response was found only in Asian and not in Caucasian populations (Kato and Serretti, 2010). Two important common SNPs of the gene encoding the 5-HT_{2A} receptor, 102T/C and 1438A/G, have been described: the C variant of the 102T/C SNP is associated with lower 5-HT_{2A} receptor expression compared to the T variant, whereas the A variant of the 1438A/G SNP increases promoter activity compared to the G variant. Interestingly, the AD response was higher among the G/G genotype carriers than among the A/G or A/A carriers, although only in the Asian population (Kato and Serretti, 2010).

Polymorphisms combine with environmental factors in the etiology of MDD (El-Hage et al., 2009). For example, stressful life events predict a better response to escitalopram, but polymorphisms in 5-HT related genes, such as *5-HTTLPR*, alter these effects (Keers et al., 2011). Assessment of 5-HT-related polymorphisms or pre-treatment PET of 5-HT molecular targets would improve the prediction of treatment response. Specifically, targeting 5-HT_{1A} autoreceptors to eliminate their initial negative contribution during AD therapy would accelerate the onset of the beneficial effects of AD therapy.

Noradrenergic system

Drugs such as the TCA desipramine, and other TCAs that increase noradrenaline and serotonine neurotransmission, as well as the NRI reboxetine act by binding to the noradrenaline transporter which increases noradrenaline levels in the synaptic cleft, activating noradrenergic receptors. The enzyme dopamine beta-hydroxylase (*Dbh*) is responsible for the synthesis of epinephrine and noradrenaline. Mice unable to synthesize noradrenaline and epinephrine due to targeted disruption of the *Dbh* gene did not exhibit altered behavior in bioassays for depressive-like behavior, but ADs with a noradrenergic-preferring action such as desipramine or reboxetine failed to exert AD-like effects (Cryan et al., 2001). The same results were obtained with the MAOI pargyline and the atypical AD bupropion (Cryan et al., 2004). Surprisingly, the effects of the SSRIs fluoxetine, sertraline, and paroxetine were also absent or severely attenuated in *Dbh* knockout mice while the effects of another SSRI, citalopram, were not altered. Restoration of a normal noradrenergic level by L-*threo*-3,4-dihydroxyphenylserine restored the behavioral effects of both desipramine and paroxetine in the knockout mice, demonstrating that the AD non-response was due to altered noradrenergic function rather than developmental abnormalities resulting from chronic noradrenaline deficiency. Thus, noradrenaline may be involved in the effects of not only noradrenaline-acting AD drugs but also 5-HT-acting compounds. The beneficial action of noradrenergic-acting compounds in the treatment of MDD may be related to the α_2-adrenergic receptor because the AD-like effects of desipramine are reversed by α_2-adrenergic receptor antagonists, such as yohimbine or idazoxan (Yalcin et al., 2005; Zhang et al., 2009). Other adrenergic receptors are also involved: the cognitive effects of these treatments are mediated by post-synaptic α_1-adrenergic receptors in the mPFC (Bondi et al., 2010). However, β_2 or β_3 adrenergic receptors do not appear to play a pivotal role in AD effects (Zhang et al., 2009; Stemmelin et al., 2010).

Finally, the involvement of organic cation transporter 2 (OCT2) in non-response to AD is also of note. OCT2 is involved in monoamine clearance, and mice deficient in this protein exhibited an altered response to AD (Bacq et al., 2012).

The contribution of the noradrenergic system to AD effects is largely confirmed by genetic data. Several polymorphisms of the gene encoding the noradrenalin transporter (*SLC6A4*) have been associated with AD response, particularly the rs2242466 (–182T/C) and rs5569 (1287G/A) polymorphisms (Shiroma et al., 2010). Catechol-*O*-methyltransferase (COMT) plays a pivotal role in the degradation of noradrenalin and dopamine. Interestingly, the Val158Met (rs4680) polymorphism of the *COMT* gene is associated with AD response (Benedetti et al., 2009; Tsai et al., 2009). Baune et al. (2008) demonstrated a negative influence of the higher activity COMT 158Val/Val genotype on AD response during the first 6 weeks of treatment, possibly due to the consequent decrease in dopamine availability. MAOA is involved in the degradation of monoamines, and polymorphisms of MAOA have been associated with fluoxetine, paroxetine, or mirtazapine response (Yu et al., 2005; Tadić et al., 2007; Domschke et al., 2008b).

Xu et al. (2011) found that early life stress may interact with the *SLC6A2* polymorphism to alter AD response. Such effects might occur via epigenetic mechanisms, such as methylation or acetylation.

The assessment of polymorphisms of noradrenergic-related genes would improve the prediction of AD response. Combining ADs with α_2-adrenergic receptor agonists could also improve the response rate or accelerate the onset of therapeutic action.

Other neurotransmission systems

One reason for non-response to ADs targeting monoaminergic neurotransmission is that these drugs may be ineffective in patients with alterations of other neurotransmission systems. For example, psychomotor retardation, a symptom exhibited by a subgroup of patients with MDD, has been related to a deficit in dopaminergic neurotransmission, particularly in the dorsolateral PFC. Consequently, these patients may preferentially benefit from treatment directly targeting dopaminergic neurotransmission. This has been explored by Taylor et al. (2006), who demonstrated that MDD patients with reduced pre-treatment performance on neuropsychological tests had a poor outcome after 12 weeks of fluoxetine treatment.

Substance P has also been suggested to have a key role in AD response. For example, decreased substance P in the cerebrospinal fluid has been associated with poor response to ADs (Carpenter et al., 2008). This conclusion is supported by convincing genetic data because the D allele of the angiotensin-converting enzyme (ACE) gene, which is related to higher ACE plasma levels, is associated with higher substance P levels and a more rapid onset of AD response (Baghai et al., 2004; Bondy et al., 2005; Narasimhan and Lohoff, 2012).

There is increasing evidence for the involvement of glutamate neurotransmission in MDD, and glutamate receptors are now being explored as targets for the treatment of MDD. For example, a clinical effect was observed when riluzole, a glutamatergic-acting compound, was added to ongoing AD therapy in TRD patients (Sanacora et al., 2007, 2008). Ketamine has a rapid AD effect and improves symptoms in TRD patients or in patients not responding to ECT (Ibrahim et al., 2011).

This is confirmed by genetic studies. For example, studies have found an association between a SNP of the dystrobrevin-binding-protein 1 gene, which is involved in glutamatergic neurotransmission, and AD response (Pae et al., 2007b; Kim et al., 2008). Furthermore, according to the STAR*D study, a SNP (rs1954787) of the *GRIK4* (glutamate receptor ionotropic kainate 4) gene encoding kainate receptor subunit 1 is associated with response to citalopram (Mayer, 2007; Horstmann and Binder, 2009; Stawski et al., 2010; Narasimhan and Lohoff, 2012). This was confirmed in another cohort, the "Munich Antidepressant Response Signature" (MARS) project (Horstmann et al., 2008, 2010; Porcelli et al., 2011). Horstmann et al. (2010) identified another SNP (rs12800734) in the *GRIK4* gene that is more strongly associated with response to treatment.

Data to support the involvement of GABA (gamma-aminobutyric acid) in the response to ADs are sparse, and this neurotransmitter does not appear to have a pivotal role in AD effects. However, mice with a deletion of the gene encoding the GABA transporter subtype 1 (*GAT1*), which transports extracellular GABA into presynaptic neurons, exhibited non-response to fluoxetine and amitriptyline (Liu et al., 2007a).

The endocannabinoid system is a modulatory system with both central and peripheral actions. Two cannabinoid receptors have been characterized: CNR1 located predominantly in the brain, and CNR2 in peripheral immune tissue and in glial cells in the central nervous system. Interestingly, knockout mice for the CNR1 receptor displayed attenuated response to desipramine and paroxetine (Steiner et al., 2008). Mitjans et al. (2012, 2013) demonstrated that genetic variability in endocannabinoid receptors could play a role in clinical response. Specifically, molecular variations in the *CNR1* gene appear to differentiate the response to citalopram according to sex. In an analysis of SNP variability in the *CNR1* gene, Domschke et al. (2008a) reported that the G allele of rs1049353 leads to increased risk of non-response to in female patients. These results suggest a role of the *CNR1* gene in the etiology of MDD and clinical response to citalopram.

Leptin signaling may be involved in the pathophysiology of MDD. Kloiber et al. (2013) recently suggested an association of polymorphisms in the leptin gene with failure of AD to achieve remission. In this study, decreased leptin serum levels and reduced leptin mRNA expression were detected in patients with impaired treatment response, independently of their genotype configuration.

Endogenous opioids are involved in the regulation of mood and behavior. Three receptors (mu, delta, and kappa) interact with a family of endogenous opioid peptides (β-endorphin, enkephalins, and dynorphins). Studies in a mouse model of MDD have demonstrated that the combination of monoaminergic ADs and opioid receptor agonists can produce synergistic AD effects (Berrocoso and Mico, 2009). The mu receptor has been associated with citalopram response (Garriock et al., 2010). Haj-Mirzaian et al. (2013) demonstrated that elevated levels of endogenous opioids and nitric oxide due to bile-duct ligation in mice induced an AD-like effect. The effect was reversed by blockade of the nitrergic and opioid systems, suggesting an involvement of these systems in non-response. However, it is difficult to evaluate the risk-benefit balance of currently available mu opioid receptors agonists as ADs, partly because of their inherent abuse liability.

NEURAL PLASTICITY AND RESPONSE TO ANTIDEPRESSANTS

Molecular aspects

Once the AD has increased monoamines in the synaptic cleft or bound to post-synaptic serotoninergic or noradrenergic receptors, it activates second messengers, such as the cyclic adenosine monophosphate (cAMP) pathway, leading to the production of cAMP-dependent protein kinase (PKA). This activation may in turn stimulate nuclear transcription factors, such as cAMP response element binding protein (CREB), via phosphorylation. Activated CREB enhances the transcription of many target genes, including brain-derived neurotrophic factor (BDNF), which exerts its effects mainly by binding to its specific receptor: the tyrosine receptor kinase B (TrkB). Consequently, non-response to AD has been investigated in relationship to alterations of these targets, particularly when polymorphisms of the genes encoding these proteins have been reported.

BDNF secretion and intercellular trafficking are related to a SNP in the *BDNF* gene that causes a valine to methionine substitution (Val66Met). A meta-analysis by Kato and Serretti (2010) indicated a better response to ADs in Met allele carriers. Other neurotrophic/growth factors have also been implicated in TRD and/or in AD response, including vascular endothelial growth factor (VEGF), fibroblast growth factor 2, and insulin-like growth factor 1 (IGF-1).

In CREB mutant mice (CREBaD), the SSRI fluoxetine and NRI desipramine still induce AD-like effect in bioassays for depressive behavior (Conti et al., 2002). This effect is accompanied by a desipramine-induced attenuation of the stress-induced activation of the HPA axis in both CREBaD-deficient and control mice (Conti et al., 2002). Interestingly, the AD-induced increase in

BDNF in the cortex and hippocampus is absent in CREBaD-deficient mice (Conti et al., 2002), indicating that CREB may be a critical mediator of the transcriptional effects of AD.

Heterozygous *bdnf* $^{+/-}$ mice, in which the levels of BDNF in the brain are reduced by approximately half, and mice with an inducible deletion of *bdnf* in the forebrain exhibited blunted AD response in the forced swim test (Saarelainen et al., 2003; Monteggia et al., 2004). This result is related to the alteration of BDNF in the dentate gyrus of the hippocampus. Indeed, the selective deletion of BDNF in the dentate gyrus but not the CA1 region is sufficient to attenuate the effects of desipramine and citalopram in the forced swim test (Adachi et al., 2008). Further, in the BDNF$^{Met/Met}$ mice, chronic fluoxetine is no more able to reverse stress-related behavior (Chen et al., 2006; Yu et al., 2012), to increase hippocampal BDNF levels and to stimulate dentate gyrus synaptic plasticity (Bath et al., 2012). It is, however, to note that the action of desipramine is still present (Yu et al., 2012), which suggests a specific contribution of the 5-HT system in these effects. These findings are coherent with clinical findings as it was observed that serum levels of BDNF were low in MDD patients and this normalizes after remission (Molendijk et al., 2011). The molecular target of BDNF is TrkB, and mice with a conditional deletion of the TrkB gene restricted to the forebrain do not respond to ADs (Saarelainen et al., 2003). Similar results were observed in Aquaporin-4 (AQP4) knockout animals. AQP4 is a key molecule for maintaining water homeostasis in the CNS that is expressed in adult neural stem cells and astrocytes. AQP4 invalidation disrupts the chronic fluoxetine-induced enhancement of adult mouse hippocampal neurogenesis (which is also a process crucially involved in the AD response; see next section) as well as AD-evoked behavioral improvement under both basal conditions and a chronic, mild stress-evoked depressive state (Kong et al., 2009).

Stress induces changes in the brain that can persist for the lifespan. Variations in genes implicated in 5-HT neurotransmission may interact with environmental factors to influence AD response (El-Hage et al., 2009). One group of signaling pathways involved in the cellular stress response includes the family of mitogen-activated protein kinases (MAPKs). Bruchas et al. (2011), focusing on the dorsal raphe nucleus, a brain region in which corticotropin-releasing factor, kappa-opioid receptors, and 5-HT systems converge, demonstrated that social defeat stress causes an increase in the activity of the intracellular signaling molecule p38α MAPK. They demonstrated that p38α MAPK activation within the dorsal raphe nucleus is responsible for the ability of stress to trigger depressive-like states. They demonstrated that in 5-HT neurons, p38α MAPK acts to directly influence SERT trafficking and ultimately increase the rate of 5-HT reuptake.

Another key molecular player in the response to monoaminergic ADs is p11. Indeed, p11 is downregulated in several brain regions of MDD patients or in animal models of MDD (Svenningsson et al., 2006; Alexander et al., 2010), whereas ADs and ECT increase p11 in the frontal cortex and hippocampus (Svenningsson et al., 2006; Warner-Schmidt et al., 2010; Oh et al., 2013). This response appears to be related to BDNF because p11 is reduced in mice in which BDNF is downregulated and increased in mice in which BDNF is overexpressed (Warner-Schmidt et al., 2010). p11 is also regulated by glucocorticoids (Zhang et al., 2008) and pro-inflammatory cytokines (Warner-Schmidt et al., 2011). Mice that lack p11 throughout their body display a depressive-like phenotype (Svenningsson et al., 2006; Warner-Schmidt et al., 2009, 2010), and more interestingly, the response to AD drugs is reduced in these mice (Svenningsson et al., 2006; Egeland et al., 2011; Eriksson et al., 2013). Interestingly, the accumbens-restricted overexpression of p11 is sufficient to induce the depressive-like phenotype in mice but does not modify the response to ADs (Alexander et al., 2010), whereas ablation of p11 from pyramidal projection neurons in the cortical layer 5A does not alter depressive-like behavior but results in a diminished response to ADs (Schmidt et al., 2012a), indicating that the mechanisms underlying the pathophysiology of MDD might differ from the mechanisms underlying the response to ADs.

Recent studies have provided evidence for a *BDNF* gene × environment interaction. Stress and ADs have opposing actions on BDNF and neurogenesis. Stress decreases and ADs increase the expression of BDNF in the dentate gyrus granule cell layer. These changes contribute to the regulation of neurogenesis by stress and ADs (Duman and Li, 2012). Mutant mice with a heterozygous deletion of BDNF, which results in the expression of approximately half the normal levels of BDNF, display normal behavior under baseline conditions but exhibit a depressive phenotype upon exposure to stress and an altered response to ADs (Duman et al., 2007; Ibarguen-Vargas et al., 2009).

Other factors have been implicated in the response to AD (e.g., zinc and cytokines). Clinical evidence suggests that zinc deficiency induces depression- and anxiety-like behaviors. Zinc administration improves the efficacy of ADs in MDD patients and may be particularly relevant for TRD patients. Recent investigations on the molecular mechanisms responsible for these observations suggest a role for zinc in the regulation of neurotransmitters, antioxidant mechanisms, neurotrophic factors and neuronal precursor cells. The presynaptic release of zinc from axon terminals of glutamatergic neurons is prominent in the hippocampus, where zinc exerts complex pleiotropic effects on neuronal plasticity, neurogenesis, and neuronal viability, affecting learning, memory, and emotional regulation (Swardfager et al., 2013). The neuroprotective properties of zinc at physiological concentrations may be attributable to the blockade of excitotoxic Ca^{2+} in?ux and upregulation of cellular antioxidant systems. Chronic zinc administration can increase BDNF expression (Swardfager et al., 2013).

Conboy et al. (2011) explored the expression of macrophage migration inhibitory factor (MIF) in astrocytes and neurogenic cells in the subgranular zone of the rodent dentate gyrus and characterized its presence in stem cells, cells undergoing proliferation, and recently proliferated cells undergoing maturation. They found that MIF deficiency is associated with a phenotype characterized by increased anxiety- and depression-like behaviors. Furthermore, they determined that in the subgranular zone of the hippocampus, macrophage MIF expression is modulated in parallel with cell proliferation by stress, glucocorticoid levels, and fluoxetine. Both the genetic deletion of MIF and chronic treatment with the MIF antagonist Iso-1 resulted in reduced cell proliferation, and MIF deletion also abolished the enhanced proliferation induced by chronic fluoxetine.

Moon et al. (2012) provided evidence that macrophage MIF is regulated by long-term exercise and that it mediates induction of serotonin and neurotrophic factors, resulting in the amelioration of depressive behaviors in a rodent model. MIF was upregulated during both long-term voluntary exercise and repeated electroconvulsive seizure treatments. The authors demonstrated that MIF induced *TPH2* and *Bdnf* expression in the rat brain along with ERK1/2 activation, resulting in an increase in 5-HT levels by MIF. In addition, direct intra-brain administration of MIF induced an AD-like response in the forced swim test. These results demonstrate that MIF induces AD-like behavior and mediates the effect of exercise on mood improvement (Moon et al., 2012). Physical activity has neuroimmune effects that are likely involved in enhanced neuroplasticity, reduced oxidative stress, increases in 5-HT, dopamine, and noradrenaline, and enhanced glucocorticoid sensitivity (Eyre et al., 2013). Thus, physical activity should be recommended in addition to AD therapy to improve drug response.

Cellular targets

In the past 15 years, the process leading to the generation of new neurons in the adult hippocampus (adult neurogenesis) has been shown to be compromised in rodent models of MDD; this effect is prevented by administration of monoaminergic AD drugs (see Hanson et al., 2011; Eisch and Petrik, 2012; Petrik et al., 2012; Bambico and Belzung, 2013; Tanti and Belzung, 2013a,b for recent reviews). These data have been corroborated by clinical studies (Boldrini et al., 2009, 2012, 2013), although some contradictory findings have been initially reported (Reif et al., 2006). Furthermore, these data extend beyond pharmacotherapy, as increase in hippocampal neurogenesis has also been observed after ECT (Malberg et al., 2000) or VNS (Revesz et al., 2008). However, increase in adult hippocampal neurogenesis alone is insufficient to induce AD-like effects (Sahay et al., 2011). Interestingly, studies have established that the ability of AD treatments to stimulate neurogenesis applies to all phases of the generation of new cells (proliferation, maturation) and is observed in the ventral and dorsal hippocampus (Tanti and Belzung, 2013b). Furthermore, adult hippocampal neurogenesis is not only a correlate of the therapeutic action of monoaminergic drugs but appears to be essential to achieve recovery. Indeed, abolition of hippocampal neurogenesis by focal X-ray hippocampal irradiation suppresses some and/or all behavioral effects of fluoxetine and/or imipramine in animals (Santarelli et al., 2003; Airan et al., 2007; Surget et al., 2008, 2011; Wang et al., 2008b; David et al., 2009; Perera et al., 2011). Similar results are observed after genetic ablation of adult neurogenesis (Lehmann et al., 2013). However, the situation is more complicated if we consider the effects of newly developed putative ADs: indeed, whereas the effects of a CNR1 ligand are abolished by suppression of neurogenesis (Jiang et al., 2005) as observed with monoaminergic-acting compounds, most of the AD-like effects of MCHR1 (Melanin-concentrating hormone receptor 1), CRH1 (corticotrophin-releasing hormone), or V1b (Vasopressin V1b) antagonists are not prevented by ablation of neurogenesis (David et al., 2007; Surget et al., 2008). This result indicates that although the ability of the treatments used in the clinic (which all target monoaminergic systems) to elicit remission relies on neurogenesis, the therapeutic effects of a drug can also be achieved via neurogenesis-independent mechanisms. For example, the dual orexine receptor almorexant induces AD-like effects but can decrease neurogenesis in some cases (Nollet et al., 2012), and rTMS suppresses the survival rate of proliferating cells (Czéh et al., 2002). The ability of new cells to contribute to recovery requires the incorporation of the new neurons into a functional network, which occurs when these cells are 4–8 weeks old. Thus, the use of an anti-mitotic agent to suppress neurogenesis revealed that the ablation of 2-week-old cells did not modify the effects of ADs (Bessa et al., 2009), whereas the 4-week-old cells are recruited after successful AD therapy to facilitate the regulation of the HPA axis after disruption by chronic stress (Surget et al., 2011). Therefore, it appears that hippocampal neurogenesis can be considered a process underlying AD non-response, related to the generation of new functional neurons.

The essential role of adult hippocampal neurogenesis in achieving remission is further supported by the observation that environmental factors that contribute to remission also act on adult hippocampal neurogenesis. Indeed, environmental enrichment and running both enable recovery and stimulate neurogenesis. Furthermore, the AD-like effects of environmental enrichment are suppressed by genetic abolition of neurogenesis (Schloesser et al., 2010). Factors associated with higher AD non-response, such as aging, are also related to lower hippocampal neurogenesis (Couillard-Despres et al., 2009).

Several hypotheses have been formulated regarding the function of adult hippocampal neurogenesis. According to some authors, this process might be crucial for pattern separation (Clelland er al., 2009; Sahay et al., 2011; Nakashiba et al., 2012; Tronel et al., 2012), a process that enables the differentiation of two closely overlapping stimuli. Thus, a deficit in pattern separation might lead to overgeneralization and cognitive bias. A restoration of such a deficit could contribute to remission. Others claim that hippocampal neurogenesis is required for contextual memory (Shors et al., 2001; Dupret et al., 2008; Deng et al., 2009; Trouche et al., 2009). Hippocampal neurogenesis is essential for regulation of the HPA axis (Schloesser et al., 2009; Snyder et al., 2011; Surget et al., 2011), and an increase in neurogenesis might facilitate recovery via normalization of HPA axis function. Finally, hippocampal neurogenesis have also been proposed to be crucial for anxiety behavior (Revest et al., 2009; Fuss et al., 2010; Mateus-Pinheiro et al., 2013) or executive functions (Burghardt et al., 2012); if restored, these functions would enable the subject to react more accurately to the environment. Interestingly, all of the above-mentioned processes are disturbed in MDD and could be essential to achieving remission (see Tanti and Belzung, 2013a,b, for reviews).

If hippocampal neurogenesis is crucial in achieving remission, any strategy that leads to an increase in the number of new neurons in this structure could facilitate recovery or accelerate the onset of therapeutic outcome when combined with ADs. Several processes have been shown to increase neurogenesis, including environment enrichment, physical exercise, and learning. Thus, one can speculate that combining any of these activities with AD treatment could increase the therapeutic outcome of pharmacotherapy.

HORMONAL TARGETS AND RESPONSE TO ANTIDEPRESSANTS

HPA axis regulation

It has been repeatedly demonstrated that ~50% of patients with MDD exhibit a dysfunction of the tuning of the HPA axis (Young et al., 1991; Holsboer, 2000; Pariante and Miller, 2001; Pariante, 2003), which can be measured using the dexamethasone-suppression test or combined dexamethasone/CRH test. Indeed, these patients exhibit dexamethasone non-suppression, indicating a defect in the negative feedback that enables the suppression of the secretion of glucocorticoids in healthy subjects. This dysregulation is restored after effective AD therapy, and interestingly, the therapeutic action of the treatment only occurs once normal feedback of the HPA axis has been restored (see Belzung and Billette De Villemeur, 2010, for a review), indicating that restoration of the HPA axis regulation is mandatory to enable recovery. Interestingly, normalization of HPA axis overactivity also occurs after successful ECT (Kling et al., 1994), indicating that this property goes beyond classical pharmacotherapy. Thus, the tuning of the HPA axis may be related to the ability to achieve a therapeutic outcome after treatment. If this outcome cannot be achieved, a resistance and/or non-response to treatment should be observed (Ising et al., 2007; Binder et al., 2009; Hennings et al., 2009; Schüle et al., 2009; Horstmann et al., 2010). This relationship has been demonstrated: a defect in HPA axis regulation is not only a signature of MDD or of remission but also a predictor of treatment non-response. Indeed, using the combined dexamethasone/CRH test, Brouwer et al. (2006) demonstrated that the AD response rate in high-ACTH patients was significantly lower than that in intermediate-ACTH patients. Similar results have been reported by Ising et al. (2007), who demonstrated that patients who do not exhibit a reduction of the cortisol response to a dexamethasone/CRH test after 2–3 weeks of treatment are not likely to respond to the current treatment. However, this has not been confirmed in two other studies (Paslakis et al., 2010; Carpenter et al., 2011). For example, Carpenter et al. (2011) rather found an increased pre-treatment cortisol after DEX/CRH to be associated with sertraline response. Possibly, rapid initial improvement of the cortisol response following DEX/CRH would be a more effective predictor of response outcome.

At the molecular level, the negative feedback on the HPA axis mainly occurs via the binding of glucocorticoids, such as cortisol or corticosterone, on specific receptors, such as the glucocorticoid receptors (GRs), which have low affinity for glucocorticoids and are thus only activated when a high level of stress hormones is present. The mode of action of GRs is very complex: in the absence of glucocorticoids, GRs are packaged into a large molecular complex consisting of chaperone heat-shock proteins, such as *hsp90* and *hsp70*, and co-chaperones, such as *FKBP51*, which bind to the receptor and keep it inactive, thus decreasing the affinity of GRs for glucocorticoids. High *FKBP51* induces inhibition of glucocorticoid-related GR activation, and thus, *FKBP51* can be considered a negative feedback loop regulating GRs (Schmidt et al., 2012b). Interestingly, in MDD subjects, peripheral *FKBP51* reduction is a marker for successful AD therapeutic outcome because FKBP51 levels are diminished in AD responders but not non-responders(Cattaneo et al., 2013).

The contribution of HPA regulation to treatment outcome after AD has been confirmed by studies investigating the contribution of genes involved in the tuning of the stress axis after treatment. Most findings concern the *FKBP5* gene. Several reports have investigated the association of *FKBP5* polymorphisms with the response to AD drugs. In 2004, a strong association between polymorphisms of the *FKBP5* gene and the response to AD was observed in 280 depressed patients of the MARS sample (Binder et al., 2004). These results were subsequently replicated in the STAR*D sample (Lekman et al., 2008) as well as in another German sample (Kirchheiner et al., 2008). Interestingly, this relationship appears to be independent of the class of AD drug because it was observed in patients treated with TCAs, SSRIs, or mirtazapine. However, two smaller studies of Spanish and Korean subjects reported negative associations in small samples (Papiol et al., 2007; Tsai et al., 2007). In fact, in the patients carrying the genotypes associated with faster response to AD, pre-treatment HPA-axis dysregulation was low compared to other patients (Binder et al., 2004), which might have facilitated the normalization of the HPA-axis and thus recovery.

Polymorphisms of the *GR* gene have also been studied in association with treatment outcome. Studies have demonstrated that the BclI and ER22/23EK polymorphisms are associated with the response to ADs (Brouwer et al., 2006; van Rossum et al., 2006). Other association studies have focused on the influence of polymorphisms in the *CRHR1*, *CRHR2*, and *CRH-BP* genes. Allele G carriers at the rs2270007 site of the *CRHR2* gene exhibited a worse response to the SSRI citalopram (Papiol et al., 2007) when compared to other alleles. Similarly, in a Chinese population, polymorphism at the rs242941 site of the *CRH1* gene has been associated with fluoxetine response (Liu et al., 2007b). Finally, polymorphisms of genes related to hsp70 protein have also been associated with poor response to AD (Pae et al., 2007a). Taken together, these genetic studies strengthen the view that a pre-treatment defect in HPA axis regulation may predict poor treatment outcome.

Environmental studies further corroborate this assertion. Hyperactivity of the HPA axis is related to chronic stress. Interestingly, two recent publications reported that elevated stress prior to treatment was associated with a good response to SSRIs (Keers et al., 2010; Horacek et al., 2011). However, other studies have shown the opposite (Monroe et al., 1992) or no association (Bock et al., 2009). These discrepancies could be related to gene × environment interactions because the effects of stress on treatment outcome may vary according to genotype. For example, in patients carrying more than one *s* allele of the *SERT* gene (which is associated with increased vulnerability to stress), the occurrence of a stressor predicted a poor response to ADs (Mandelli et al., 2009; Keers et al., 2011). Similar findings were obtained using a large sample of patients treated with escitalopram; in patients carrying polymorphisms inducing vulnerability to stress, such as polymorphism at the rs1360780 site of the *FKBP5* gene and at the rs110402 site of the *CRHR1* gene, stressors were predictive of response to treatment (Keers and Uher, 2012).

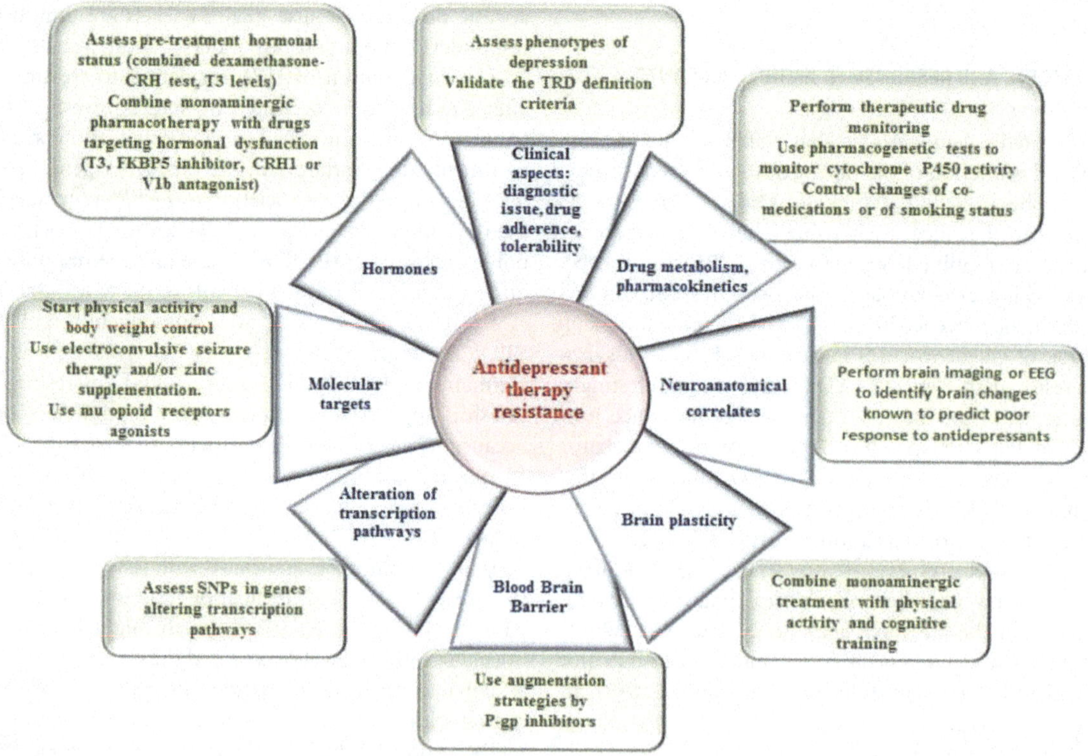

FIGURE 1 | Mechanisms (in blue) associated with antidepressant therapy resistance and recommendations for clinical practice (in green).

Finally, evidence for the involvement of HPA axis feedback dysregulation in AD non-response is also provided by data from patients with diseases that are highly comorbid with MDD, such as Cushing's disease. Cushing's disease is a syndrome related to chronic glucocorticoid excess, due either to an overproduction of ACTH caused by a pituitary adenoma (66% of patients), to an adrenal adenoma or carcinoma (24% of patients), or to ectopic causes (10% of patients). Approximately half of the patients display MDD (Sonino and Fava, 2002; Pereira et al., 2010). Interestingly, MDD patients with Cushing's disease are poor responder to treatment with classical AD therapy (Sonino et al., 1986, 1993), whereas a good therapeutic outcome can be achieved by treatments that normalize the HPA overactivity (Sonino and Fava, 2002; Pereira et al., 2010). These results confirm that excessive function of the HPA axis is associated with AD non-response.

To improve drug response, pre-treatment HPA dysfunction should be assessed with the dexamethasone suppression test or, preferably, the combined dexamethasone/CRH, as this latter test appears to be more specific (Ising et al., 2007). Polymorphisms of HPA-related genes, such as the *FKBP5*, *CRHR1*, or GR genes, would also be highly relevant, even if they are not yet currently used in clinical practice. If these markers predict poor HPA function, one could predict that treatments targeting the HPA axis (CRF1 antagonists, V1b receptor antagonists, GR antagonists, FRBP51 inhibitors) could be useful therapeutic strategies to improve drug response as well as the onset of response when combined with more conventional ADs.

Thyrotropin releasing hormone (TRH)

The relationship between thyroid function and MDD is well-known. Indeed, hypothyroidism is associated with MDD, and TRH levels correlate with symptom severity (Bauer et al., 2009). Furthermore, MDD patients exhibit alterations in several markers of thyroid function, particularly of the thyroid hormone triiodothyronine (T3) (see Hage and Azar, 2012 for a review). Interestingly, T3 is widely used to improve the therapeutic outcome of AD drugs in patients who exhibit poor response to treatment (Aronson et al., 1996; Nierenberg et al., 2006), particularly in those treated with TCAs. Successful treatment with T3 alone has also been reported in some older studies (Feldmesser-Reiss, 1958; Flach et al., 1958; Wilson et al., 1974). These findings are further supported by preclinical evidence. Indeed, T3 alone elicited an AD-like effect in a bio-assay for AD response (Lifschytz et al., 2006, 2011), whereas the combination of T3 with chronic fluoxetine increased the effects of the SSRI (Brochet et al., 1987; Eitan et al., 2010). This effect appears to be related to thyroid function because it has also been shown that the effects of TCAs are reduced in rats in which hypothyroidism has been provoked by the addition of propylthiouracil to their drinking water (Martin et al., 1987). The effects of T3 occur via an interaction with nuclear thyroid hormone receptors (TRs). Four such receptors have been described: α-1, α-2, β-1, and β-2. It would be of interest to determine which of these receptors might mediate the effects of T3. A recent study demonstrated that administration of dronedarone, a specific TRα antagonist, prevented the AD-like effects of T3, suggesting that the TRα receptor is responsible for the effects of T3 (Lifschytz et al., 2011). This observation is consistent with the finding that TRα receptors are the most highly expressed TRs in the brain (Williams, 2008) as well as with the observation that mice in which this receptor is mutated display depressive-like behavior (Pilhatsch et al., 2010).

Few studies have investigated the association of polymorphisms of thyroid function-related genes with MDD and AD response. However, the relationship of a polymorphism of the deiodinase type I (*D1*) gene (D1 converts inactive T4 to active T3) with the ability of T3 to augment the effects of AD has been investigated (Papakostas et al., 2009).

Interestingly, the effects of T3 in patients undergoing AD therapy are particularly remarkable in some subcategories of patients, particularly in women (Altshuler et al., 2001; Agid and Lerer, 2003) and in patients with atypical MDD.

Further progress could certainly be achieved in improving AD response by (a) dosing pre-treatment T3 hormones in patients and (b) studying polymorphisms of thyroid function related genes. Such studies would enable the segregation of patients according to their thyroid hormone status and the initiation of co-therapy with T3 at the beginning of AD therapy in those patients with the highest thyroid dysfunction.

DISCUSSION

To summarize, we know from various evidence from the litterature that response to ADs can be driven but also altered at various levels (**Table 1**). Derived from these data, several peripheral or central biomarkers can now enable predicting an increased risk of non-response to AD treatment. They include markers genetic testing (polymorphisms of *P450, ABCB1, SERT, NERT, COMT, MAOA, leptin, FKBP5, hsp70, GR, BclI, CRHR1, CRHR2, BDBF, D1, TRα* genes, etc), plasmatic dosage (BDNF, cortisol, FKBP51, etc.) or brain imaging. Predictors of treatment response can easily be uncovered by deduction from predictors of treatment non-response: for example, if a poor response to ADs is met in Val allele carriers of the BDNF gene, this also indicates that good response might be achieved in the Met carriers. If poor response is shown in patients having low rostral cingulate activity, high response is observed in patients exhibiting elevated pretreatment rostral cingulate activity.

Based on the potential mechanisms of response to AD, several practical implications may be deducted (see **Figure 1**). Some of these conclusions have entered clinical routine and are now part of practical recommendations, such as augmentation therapy by thyroid hormones, and are sustained by strong clinical evidence (Shelton et al., 2010). However, other innovative strategies may enter further clinical investigation through randomized controlled studies. Among these new strategies, controlling co-medications, smoking status, or weight, assessing pre-treatment hormonal status combined with dexamethasone/CRH tests and T3 levels, investigating SNPs of specific genes known to be implicated in AD non-response, and the use of brain imaging or EEG to identify brain changes known to predict poor response to ADs are among the most promising. A more systematic referral to therapeutic drug monitoring (plasma concentration quantification) would also be useful as it appears to be largely insufficiently used given the considerable inter-individual variability in the pharmacokinetic characteristics of drugs. It enables the adaptation of the dosage of ADs to achieve the plasma drug concentration that ensures the highest probability of response (Hiemke et al., 2011). New augmentation strategies could also be developed based on the evidence reported in the present review, such as combining monoaminergic treatment with physical activity, cognitive training, stress reduction, P-gp inhibitors, mu opioid receptors agonists, zinc, and drugs targeting hormonal dysfunction (T3, FKBP5 inhibitor, or CRH1 or V1b antagonists). Switching ADs from one ineffective AD to a similar or different class of ADs and from SSRI/SNRIs to TCAs, MAOIs, and non-conventional antidepressant drugs, such as NMDA antagonists, may be other valuable strategies, as well as switching to somatic therapies, such as ECT, rTMS, VNS, or DBS.

One of the main obstacles to improving care strategies is the wide heterogeneity of patients labeled as suffering from TRD and/or showing insufficient response to conventional AD. This heterogeneity is the consequence of the relatively poor specificity of the criteria for diagnosis, which are still based on clinical evaluation; even the rating scales typically used to assess clinical response exhibit relatively good inter-rater and test-retest validity. Moving toward a more systematic use of biomarkers may improve the characterization of clinical phenotypes of MDD and their biological, imaging or genetic, proteomic and metabolomic correlates (Leuchter et al., 2010). As we have extensively reviewed, although TRD and/or treatment non-response is a considerable challenge to improving patient outcome and preventing severe complications of prolonged depressive states, it represents a unique opportunity to better understand mechanism of action of ADs and thus to better understand the pathophysiology of MDD and improve its clinical characterization. This potential makes research on TRD and/or treatment non-response a high priority for new research developments at both the preclinical and clinical levels.

REFERENCES

Adachi, M., Barrot, M., Autry, A. E., Theobald, D., and Monteggia, L. M. (2008). Selective loss of brain-derived neurotrophic factor in the dentate gyrus attenuates antidepressant efficacy. Biol. Psychiatry 63, 642–649. doi: 10.1016/j.biopsych.2007.09.019

Agid, O., and Lerer, B. (2003). Algorithm-based treatment of major depression in an outpatient clinic: clinical correlates of response to a specific serotonin reuptake inhibitor and to triiodothyronine augmentation. Int. J. Neuropsychopharmacol. 6, 41–49. doi: 10.1017/S14611457 0200322X

Airan, R. D., Meltzer, L. A., Roy, M., Gong, Y., Chen, H., and Deisseroth, K. (2007). High-speed imaging reveals neurophysiological links to behavior in an animal model of depression. Science 317, 819–823. doi: 10.1126/science.1144400

Akerblad, A. C., Bengtsson, F., von Knorring, L., and Ekselius, L. (2006). Response, remission and relapse in relation to adherence in primary care treatment of depression: a 2-year outcome study. Int. Clin. Psychopharmacol. 21, 117–124. doi: 10.1097/01.yic.0000199452.16682.b8

Alexander, B., Warner-Schmidt, J.,

Eriksson, T., Tamminga, C., Arango-Lievano, M., Ghose, S., et al. (2010). Reversal of depressed behaviors in mice by p11 gene therapy in the nucleus accumbens. Science Transl. Med. 2, 54ra76. doi: 10.1126/scitranslmed.3001079

Alexopoulos, G. S., Murphy, C. F., Gunning-Dixon, F. M., Glatt, C. E., Latoussakis, V., Kelly, et al. (2009). Serotonin transporter polymorphisms, microstructural white matter abnormalities and remission of geriatric depression. J. Affect. Disord. 119, 132–141. doi: 10.1016/j.jad.2009.03.004

Alexopoulos, G. S., Murphy, C. F., Gunning-Dixon, F. M., Latoussakis, V., Kanellopoulos, D., Klimstra, S., et al. (2008). Microstructural white matter abnormalities and remission of geriatric depression. Am. J. Psychiatry 165, 238–244. doi: 10.1176/appi.ajp.2007.07050744

Altshuler, L. L., Bauer, M., Frye, M. A., Gitlin, M. J., Mintz, J., Szuba, M. P., et al. (2001). Does thyroid supplementation accelerate tricyclic antidepressant response. A review and meta-analysis of the literature. Am. J. Psychiatry 158, 1617–1622. doi: 10.1176/appi.ajp.158.10.1617

Anand, A., Li, Y., Wang, Y., Wu, J., Gao, S., Bukhari, L., et al. (2005). Antidepressant effect on connectivity of the mood-regulating circuit: an FMRI study. Neuropsychopharmacology 30, 1334–1344. doi: 10.1038/sj.npp. 1300725

Andrade, L., Caraveo-Anduaga, J. J., Berglund, P., Bijl, R. V., de Graaf, R., Vollebergh, W., et al. (2003). The epidemiology of major depressive episodes: results from the International Consortium of Psychiatric Epidemiology (ICPE) Surveys. Int. J. Methods Psychiatr. Res. 12, 3–21. doi: 10.1002/mpr.138

Aronson, R., Offman, H., Joffe, R., and Naylor, C. (1996). Triiodothyronine augmentation in treatment of refractory depression. Arch. Gen. Psychiatry 53, 842–848. doi: 10.1001/archpsyc.1996.01830090090013

Bacq, A., Balasse, L., Biala, G., Guiard, B., Gardier, A. M., Schinkel, A., et al. (2012). Organic cation transporter 2 controls brain norepinephrine and sero-tonin clearance and antidepressant response. Mol. Psychiatry 17, 926–939. doi: 10.1038/mp.2011.87

Baghai, T., Schule, C., Zill, P., Deiml, T., Eser, D., Zwanzger, P., et al. (2004). The angiotensin I converting enzyme insertion/deletion polymorphism influences therapeutic outcome in major depressed women, but not in men. Neurosci. Lett. 363, 38–42. doi: 10.1016/j.neulet.2004.03.052

Bambico, F. R., and Belzung, C. (2013). "Novel Insights into depression and antidepressants: a synergy between synaptogenesis and neurogenesis," in Neurogenesis and Neural Plasticity, Vol. 15. eds C. Belzung and P. Wigmore (Berlin; Heidelberg: Springer-Verlag), 243–291. doi: 10.1007/7854_2012_234

Bares, M., Brunovsky, M., Kopecek, M., Novak, T., Stopkova, P., Kozeny, J., et al. (2008). Early reduction in prefrontal theta QEEG cordance value predicts response to venlafaxine treatment in patients with resistant depressive disorder. Eur. Psychiatry 23, 350–355. doi: 10.1016/j.eurpsy.2008.03.001

Bath, K. G., Jing, D. Q., Dincheva, I., Neeb, C. C., Pattwell, S. S., Chao, M. V., et al. (2012). BDNF Val66Met impairs fluoxetine-induced enhancement of adult hippocampus plasticity. Neuropsychopharmacology 37, 1297–1304. doi: 10.1038/npp.2011.318

Bauer, M., Bschor, T., Pfennig, A., Whybrow, P. C., Angst, J., Versiani, M., et al. (2007). World Federation of Societies of Biological Psychiatry (WFSBP) guide-lines for biological treatment of unipolar depressive disorders in primary care. World J. Biol. Psychiatry 8, 67–104. doi: 10.1080/15622970701227829

Bauer, M., Silverman, D. H. S., Schlagenhauf, F., London, E. D., Geist, C. L., van Herle, K., et al. (2009). Brain glucose metabolism in hypothyroidism: a positron emission tomography study before and after thyroid hormone replacement therapy. J. Clin. Endocrinol. Metab. 94, 2922–2929. doi: 10.1210/jc.2008-2235

Baune, B. T., Hohoff, C., Berger, K., Neumann, A., Mortensen, S., Roehrs, T., et al. (2008). Association of the COMT val158met variant with antidepressant treatment response in major depression. Neuropsychopharmacology 33, 924–932. doi: 10.1038/sj.npp.1301462

Belzung, C., and Billette De Villemeur, E. (2010). The design of new antidepres-sants: can formal models help. A first attempt using a model of the hippocampal control over the HPA axis based on a review from the literature. Behav. Pharmacol. 21, 677–689. doi: 10.1097/FBP.0b013e328340d630

Benarroch, E. E. (2012). Blood-brain barrier: recent developments and clinical correlations. Neurology 78, 1268–1276. doi: 10.1212/WNL.0b013e318250d8bc

Benedetti, F., Colombo, C., Pirovano, A., Marino, E., and Smeraldi, E. (2009). The catechol-O-methyltransferase Val(108/158)Met polymorphism affects antidepressant response to paroxetine in a naturalistic setting. Psychopharmacology 203, 155–160. doi: 10.1007/s00213-008-1381-7

Berlim, M. T., and Turecki, G. (2007). What is the meaning of treatment resistant/refractory major depression (TRD). A systematic review of current randomized trials. Eur. Neuropsychopharmacol. 17, 696–707. doi: 10.1016/j.euroneuro.2007.03.009

Berrocoso, E., and Mico, J. A. (2009). Cooperative opioid and serotonergic mechanisms generate superior antidepressant-like effects in a mice model of depression. Int. J. Neuropsychopharmacol. 12, 1033–1044. doi: 10.1017/S1461145709000236

Bessa, J. M., Ferreira, D., Melo, I., Marques, F., Cerqueira, J. J., Palha, J. A., et al. (2009). The mood-improving actions of antidepressants do not depend on neurogenesis but are associated with neuronal remodeling. Mol. Psychiatry 14, 764–773. doi: 10.1038/mp.2008.119

Bewernick, B. H., Kayser, S., Sturm, V., and Schlaepfer, T. E. (2012). Longterm effects of nucleus accumbens deep brain stimulation in treatment-resistant depression: evidence for sustained efficacy. Neuropsychopharmacology 37, 1975–1985. doi: 10.1038/npp.2012.44

Binder, E. B., Künzel, H. E., Nickel, T., Kern, N., Pfennig, A., Majer, M., et al. (2009). HPA-axis regulation at in-patient admission is associated with antidepressant therapy outcome in male but not in female depressed patients. Psychoneuroendocrinology 34, 99–109. doi: 10.1016/j.psyneuen.2008. 08.018

Binder, E. B., Salyakina, D., Lichtner, P., Wochnik, G. M., Ising, M., Putz, B., et al. (2004). Polymorphisms in FKBP5 are associated with increased recurrence of depressive episodes and rapid response to antidepressant treatment. Nat. Genet. 36, 1319–1325. doi: 10.1038/ng1479

Bock, C., Bukh, J. D., Vinberg, M., Gether, U., and Kessing, L. V. (2009). Do stressful life events predict medical treatment outcome in first episode of depression. Soc. Psychiatry Psychiatr. Epidemiol. 44, 752–760. doi: 10.1007/s00127-008-0491-1

Bohning, D. E., Lomarev, M. P., Denslow, S., Nahas, Z., Shastri, A., and George, M. S. (2001). Feasibility of vagus nerve stimulation-synchronized blood oxygenation level-dependent functional MRI. Invest. Radiol. 36, 470–479. doi: 10.1097/00004424-200108000-00006

Boldrini, M., Hen, R., Underwood, M. D., Rosoklija, G. B., Dwork, A. J., Mann, J. J., et al. (2012). Hippocampal angiogenesis and progenitor cell proliferation are increased with antidepressant use in major depression. Biol. Psychiatry 72, 562–571. doi: 10.1016/j.biopsych.2012.04.024

Boldrini, M., Santiago, A. N., Hen, R., Dwork, A. J., Rosoklija, G. B., Tamir, H., et al. (2013). Hippocampal granule neuron number and dentate gyrus volume in antidepressant-treated and untreated major depression. Neuropsychopharmacology 38, 1068–1077. doi: 10.1038/npp. 2013.5

Boldrini, M., Underwood, M. D., Hen, R., Rosoklija, G. B., Dwork, A. J., John Mann, J., et al. (2009). Antidepressants increase neural progenitor cells in the human hippocampus. Neuropsychopharmacology 34, 2376–2389. doi: 10.1038/npp.2009.75

Bondi, C. O., Jett, J. D., and Morilak, D. A. (2010). Beneficial effects of desipramine on cognitive function of chronically stressed rats are mediated byalpha1-adrenergic receptors in medial prefrontal cortex. Prog. Neuropsychopharmacol. Biol. Psychiatry 34, 913–923. doi: 10.1016/j.pnpbp.2010.04.016

Bondolfi, G., Chautems, C., Rochat, B., Bertschy, G., and Baumann, P. (1996). Non-response to citalopram in depressive patients: pharmacokinetic and clinical consequences of a fluvoxamine augmentation. Psychopharmacology (Berl.) 128, 421–425. doi: 10.1007/s002130050152

Bondy, B., Baghai, T. C., Zill, P., Schule, C., Eser, D., Deiml, T., et al. (2005). Genetic variants in the angiotensin I-converting-enzyme (ACE) and angiotensin II receptor (AT1) gene and clinical outcome in depression. Prog. Neuropsychopharmacol. Biol. Psychiatry 29, 1094–1099. doi: 10.1016/j.pnpbp.2005.03.015

Bortolozzi, A., Castañé, A., Semakova, J., Santana, N., Alvarado, G., Cortés, R., et al. (2012). Selective siRNA-mediated suppression of 5-HT1A autoreceptors evokes strong anti-depressant-like effects. Mol. Psychiatry 17, 612–623. doi: 10.1038/mp.2011.92

Broadway, J. M., Holtzheimer, P. E., Hilimire, M. R., Parks, N. A., Devylder, J. E., Mayberg, H. S., et al. (2012). Frontal theta cordance predicts 6-month antidepressant response to subcallosal cingulate deep brain stimulation for treatment-resistant depression: a pilot study. Neuropsychopharmacology 37, 1764–1772. doi: 10.1038/npp.2012.23

Brochet, D. M., Martin, P., Soubrié, P., and Simon, P. (1987). Triiodothyronine potentiation of antidepressant-induced reversal of learned helplessness in rats. Psychiatry Res. 21, 267–275. doi: 10.1016/0165-1781(87)90031-X

Brosen, K. (2004). Some aspects of genetic polymorphism in the biotransformation of antidepressants. Therapie 59, 5–12. doi: 10.2515/therapie:2004003

Brouwer, J. P., Appelhof, B. C., van Rossum, E. F., Koper, J. W., Fliers, E., Huyser, J., et al. (2006). Prediction of treatment response by HPA-axis and glucocor-ticoid receptor polymorphisms in major depression. Psychoneuroendocrinology 31, 1154–1163. doi: 10.1016/j.psyneuen.2006.08.001

Bruchas, M. R., Schindler, A. G., Shankar, H., Messinger, D. I., Miyatake, M., Land, B. B., et al. (2011). Selective p38α MAPK deletion in serotonergic neurons produces stress resilience in models of depression and addiction. Neuron 71, 498–511. doi: 10.1016/j.neuron.2011.06.011

Bruder, G. E., Sedoruk, J. P., Stewart, J. W., McGrath, P. J., Quitkin, F. M., and Tenke, C. E. (2008). Electroencephalographic alpha measures predict therapeutic response to a selective serotonin reuptake inhibitor antidepres-sant: pre- and post-treatment findings. Biol. Psychiatry 63, 1171–1177. doi: 10.1016/j.biopsych.2007.10.009

Bruder, G. E., Stewart, J. W., McGrath, P. J., Deliyannides, D., and Quitkin, F. M. (2004). Dichotic listening tests of functional brain asymmetry predict response to fluoxetine in depressed women and men. Neuropsychopharmacology 29, 1752–1761. doi: 10.1038/sj.npp.1300519

Bruder, G. E., Stewart, J. W., Tenke, C. E., McGrath, P. J., Leite, P., Bhattacharya, N., et al. (2001). Electroencephalographic and perceptual asymmetry differences between responders and nonresponders to an SSRI antidepressant. Biol. Psychiatry 48, 416–425. doi: 10.1016/S0006-3223(00)01016-7

Burghardt, N. S., Park, E. H., Hen, R., and Fenton, A. A. (2012). Adult-born hippocampal neurons promote cognitive flexibility in mice. Hippocampus 22, 1795–1808. doi: 10.1002/hipo.22013

Carpenter, L. L., Bayat, L., Moreno, F., Kling, M. A., Price, L. H., Tyrka, A. R., et al. (2008). Decreased cerebrospinal fluid concentrations of substance P in treatment-resistant depression and lack of alteration after acute adjunct vagus nerve stimulation therapy. Psychiatry Res. 157, 123–129. doi: 10.1016/j.psychres.2007.04.016

Carpenter, L. L., Tyrka, A. R., Lee, J. K., Tracy, A. P., Wilkinson, C. W., and Price, L. H. (2011). A placebo-controlled study of sertraline's effect on cortisol response to the dexamethasone/corticotropin-releasing hormone test in healthy adults. Psychopharmacology (Berl.) 218, 371–379. doi: 10.1007/s00213-011-2336-y

Cattaneo, A., Gennarelli, M., Uher, R., Breen, G., Farmer, A., Aitchison, K. J., et al. (2013). Candidate genes expression profile associated with antidepres-sants response in the GENDEP study: differentiating between baseline 'predictors' and longitudinal 'targets'. Neuropsychopharmacology 38, 377–385. doi: 10.1038/npp.2012.191

Cheng, A. T., Chen, T. H., Chen, C. C., and Jenkins, R. (2000). Psychosocial and psychiatric risk factors for suicide. Case-control psychological autopsy study. Br. J. Psychiatry 177, 360–365. doi: 10.1192/bjp.177.4.360

Chen, Z. Y., Jing, D., Bath, K. G., Ieraci, A., Khan, T., Siao, C. J., et al. (2006). Genetic variant BDNF (Val66Met) polymorphism alters anxiety-related behav-ior. Science 314, 140–143. doi: 10.1126/science.1129663

Choi, J., Jeong, B., Rohan, M. L., Polcari, A. M., and Teicher, M. H. (2009). Preliminary evidence for white matter tract abnormalities in young adults exposed to parental verbal abuse. Biol. Psychiatry 65, 227–234. doi: 10.1016/j.biopsych.2008.06.022

Clelland, C. D., Choi, M., Romberg, C., Clemenson, G. D. Jr., Fragniere, A., Tyers, P., et al. (2009). A functional role for adult hippocampal neurogenesis in spatial pattern separation. Science. 325, 210–213. doi: 10.1126/science.1173215

Coelho, P. V., and Brum Cde, A. (2009). Interactions between antidepressants and antihypertensive and glucose lowering drugs among patients in the HIPERDIA Program, Coronel Fabriciano, Minas Gerais State, Brazil. Cad. Saude Publica. 25, 2229–2236. doi: 10.1590/S0102-311X2009001000013

Conboy, L., Varea, E., Castro, J. E., Sakouhi-Ouertatani, H., Calandra, T., Lashuel, H. A., et al. (2011). Macrophage migration inhibitory factor is critically involved in basal and fluoxetine-stimulated adult hippocampal cell proliferation and in anxiety, depression, and memory-related behaviors. Mol. Psychiatry 16, 533–547. doi: 10.1038/mp.2010.15

Conti, A. C., Cryan, J. F., Dalvi, A., Lucki, I., and Blendy, J. A. (2002). cAMP response element-binding protein is essential for the upregulation of brain-derived neurotrophic factor transcription, but not the behavioral or endocrine responses to antidepressant drugs. J. Neurosci. 22, 3262–3268.

Cook, I. A., Hunter, A. M., Abrams, M., Siegman, B., and Leuchter, A. F. (2009). Midline and right frontal brain function as a physiologic biomarker of remission in major depression. Psychiatry Res. 174, 152–157. doi: 10.1016/j.pscychresns.2009.04.011

Cook, I. A., Leuchter, A. F., Morgan, M., Witte, E., Stubbeman, W. F., Abrams, M., et al. (2002). Early changes in prefrontal activity characterize clinical responders to antidepressants. Neuropsychopharmacology 27, 120–131. doi: 10.1016/S0893-133X(02)00294-4

Couillard-Despres, S., Wuertinger, C., Kandasamy, M., Caioni, M., Stadler, K., Aigner, R., et al. (2009). Ageing abolishes the effects of fluox-etine on neurogenesis. Mol. Psychiatry 14, 856–864. doi: 10.1038/mp. 2008.147

Cox, G. R., Callahan, P., Churchill, R., Hunot, V., Merry, S. N., Parker, A. G., et al. (2012). Psychological therapies versus antidepressant medication, alone and in combination for depression in children and adolescents. Cochrane Database Syst. Rev. 11:CD008324. doi: 10.1002/14651858.CD008324.pub2

Cryan, J. F., Dalvi, A., Jin, S. H., Hirsch, B. R., Lucki, I., and Thomas, S. A. (2001). Use of dopamine-beta-hydroxylase-deficient mice to determine the role of nore-pinephrine in the mechanism of action of antidepressant drugs. J. Pharmacol. Exp. Ther. 298, 651–657.

Cryan, J. F., and Lucki, I. (2000a). Antidepressant-like behavioral effects mediated by 5-Hydroxytryptamine2C receptors. J. Pharmacol. Exp. Ther. 295, 1120–1126.

Cryan, J. F., and Lucki, I. (2000b). 5-HT4 receptors do not mediate the antidepressant-like behavioral effects of fluoxetine in a modified forced swim test. Eur. J. Pharmacol. 409, 295–299. doi: 10.1016/S0014-2999(00) 00858-X

Cryan, J. F., O'Leary, O. F., Jin, S. H., Friedland, J. C., Ouyang, M., Hirsch, B. R., et al. (2004). Norepinephrine-deficient mice lack responses to antidepressant drugs, including selective serotonin-reuptake inhibitors. Proc. Natl. Acad. Sci. U.S.A. 101, 8186–8191. doi: 10.1073/pnas.0401080101

Czéh, B., Welt, T., Fischer, A. K., Erhardt, A., Schmitt, W., Müller, M. B., et al. (2002). Chronic psychosocial stress and concomitant repetitive tran-scranial magnetic stimulation: effects on stress hormone levels and adult hippocampal neurogenesis. Biol. Psychiatry 52, 1057–1065. doi: 10.1016/S0006-3223(02)01457-9

David, D. J., Klemenhagen, K. C., Holick, K. A., Saxe, M. D., Mendez, I., Santarelli, L., et al. (2007). Efficacy of the MCHR1 antagonist N-[3-(1-{[4-(3, 4-difluorophenoxy)phenyl]methyl}(4-piperidyl))-4-methylphenyl]-2-methylpropanamide (SNAP 94847) in mouse models of anxiety and depression following acute and chronic administration is independent of hippocampal neurogenesis. J. Pharmacol. Exp. Ther. 321, 237–248. doi: 10.1124/jpet.106.109678

David, D. J., Samuels, B. A., Rainer, Q., Wang, J.-W., Marsteller, D., Mendez, I., et al. (2009). Neurogenesis-dependent and -independent effects of fluox-etine in an animal model of anxiety/depression. Neuron 62, 479–493. doi: 10.1016/j.neuron.2009.04.017

Davidson, R. J., Irwin, W., Anderle, M. J., and Kalin, N. H. (2003). The neural substrates of affective processing in depressed patients treated with venlafaxine. Am. J. Psychiatry 160, 64–75. doi: 10.1176/appi.ajp.160.1.64

Dean, M., Rzhetsky, A., and Allikmets, R. (2001). The human ATP-binding cassette (ABC) transporter superfamily. Genome Res. 11, 1156–1166. doi: 10.1101/gr.GR-1649R de Klerk, O. L., Nolte, I. M., Bet, P. M., Bosker, F. J., Snieder, H., den Boer, J. A., et al. (2012). ABCB1 gene variants influence tolerance to selective serotonin reup-take inhibitors in a large sample of Dutch cases with major depressive disorder. Pharmacogenomics J. 13, 349–353. doi: 10.1038/tpj.2012.16

Delgado, P. L., Miller, H. L., Salomon, R. M., Licinio, J., Krystal, J. H., Moreno, F. A., et al. (1999). Tryptophan-depletion challenge in depressed patients treated with desipramine or fluoxetine: implications for the role of serotonin in the mechanism of antidepressant action. Biol. Psychiatry 46, 212–220. doi: 10.1016/S0006-3223(99)00014-1

Demyttenaere, K., Mesters, P., Boulanger, B., Dewe, W., Delsemme,

M. H., Gregoire, J., et al. (2001). Adherence to treatment regimen in depressed patients treated with amitriptyline or fluoxetine. J. Affect. Disord. 65, 243–252. doi: 10.1016/S0165-0327(00)00225-1

Deng, W., Saxe, M. D., Gallina, I. S., and Gage, F. H. (2009). Adult-born hippocampal dentate granule cells undergoing maturation modulate learning and memory in the brain. J. Neurosci. 29, 13532–13542. doi: 10.1523/JNEUROSCI.3362-09.2009

Diaz, S. L., Doly, S., Narboux-Nême, N., Fernández, S., Mazot, P., Banas, S. M., et al. (2012). 5-HT(2B) receptors are required for serotonin-selective antidepressant actions. Mol. Psychiatry 17, 154–163. doi: 10.1038/mp. 2011.159

Domschke, K., Dannlowski, U., Ohrmann, P., Lawford, B., Bauer, J., Kugel, H., et al. (2008a). Cannabinoid receptor 1 (CNR1) gene: impact on antidepressant treatment response and emotion processing in major depression. Eur. Neuropsychopharmacol. 18, 751–759. doi: 10.1016/j.euroneuro.2008.05.003

Domschke, K., Hohoff, C., Mortensen, L. S., Roehrs, T., Deckert, J., Arolt, V., et al. (2008b). Monoamine oxidase A variant influences antidepressant treatment response in female patients with Major Depression. Prog. Neuropsychopharmacol. Biol. Psychiatry 32, 224–228. doi: 10.1016/j.pnpbp.2007.08.011

Duman, C. H., Schlesinger, L., Kodama, M., Russell, D. S., and Duman, R. S. (2007). A role for MAP kinase signaling in behavioral models of depression and antidepressant treatment. Biol. Psychiatry 61, 661–670. doi: 10.1016/j.biopsych.2006.05.047

Duman, R. S., and Li, N. (2012). A neurotrophic hypothesis of depression: role of synaptogenesis in the actions of NMDA receptor antagonists. Philos. Transl. R. Soc. Lond. B Biol. Sci. 367, 2475–2484. doi: 10.1098/rstb.2011.0357

Duncan, W. C. Jr., Selter, J., Brutsche, N., Sarasso, S., and Zarate, C. A. Jr. (2013). Baseline delta sleep ratio predicts acute ketamine mood response in major depressive disorder. J. Affect. Disord. 145, 115–119. doi: 10.1016/j.jad.2012.05.042

Dunkin, J. J., Leuchter, A. F., Cook, I. A., Kasl-Godley, J. E., Abrams, M., and Rosenberg-Thompson, S. (2000). Executive dysfunction predicts nonresponse to fluoxetine in major depression. J. Affect. Disord. 60, 13–23. doi: 10.1016/S0165-0327(99)00157-3

Dupret, D., Revest, J.-M., Koehl, M., Ichas, F., De Giorgi, F., Costet, P., et al. (2008). Spatial relational memory requires hippocampal adult neurogenesis. PLoS ONE 3:e1959. doi: 10.1371/journal.pone.0001959

Egeland, M., Warner-Schmidt, J., Greengard, P., and Svenningsson, P. (2011). Co-expression of serotonin 5-HT(1B) and 5-HT(4) receptors in p11 containing cells in cerebral cortex, hippocampus, caudate-putamen and cerebellum. Neuropharmacology 61, 442–450. doi: 10.1016/j.neuropharm.2011.01.046

Eisch, A. J., and Petrik, D. (2012). Depression and hippocampal neurogenesis: a road to remission. Science 338, 72–75. doi: 10.1126/science. 1222941

Eitan, R., Landshut, G., Lifschytz, T., Einstein, O., Ben-Hur, T., and Lerer, B. (2010). The thyroid hormone, triiodothyronine, enhances fluoxetine-induced neurogenesis in rats: possible role in antidepressant-augmenting properties. Int. J. Neuropsychopharmacol. 13, 553–561. doi: 10.1017/S1461145709990769

El-Hage, W., Powell, J. F., and Surguladze, S. A. (2009). Vulnerability to depression: what is the role of stress genes in gene x environment interaction. Psychol. Med. 39, 1407–1411. doi: 10.1017/S0033291709005236

Eriksson, T. M., Alvarsson, A., Stan, T. L., Zhang, X., Hascup, K. N., Hascup, E. R., et al. (2013). Bidirectional regulation of emotional memory by 5-HT(1B) receptors involves hippocampal p11. Mol. Psychiatry. 18, 1096–1105. doi: 10.1038/mp.2012.130

Eyre, H. A., Papps, E., and Baune, B. T. (2013). Treating depression and depression-like behavior with physical activity: an immune perspective. Front. Psychiatry 4:3. doi: 10.3389/fpsyt.2013.00003

Fava, M. (2003). Diagnosis and definition of treatment-resistant depression. Biol. Psychiatry 53, 649–659. doi: 10.1016/S0006-3223(03)00231-2

Fekadu, A., Rane, L. J., Wooderson, S. C., Markopoulou, K., Poon, L., and Cleare, A. J. (2012). Prediction of longer-term outcome of treatment-resistant depression in tertiary care. Br. J. Psychiatry 201, 369–375. doi: 10.1192/bjp.bp.111.102665

Fekadu, A., Wooderson, S. C., Markopoulou, K., and Cleare, A. J. (2009). The Maudsley Staging Method for treatment-resistant depression: prediction of longer-term outcome and persistence of symptoms. J. Clin. Psychiatry 70, 952–957. doi: 10.4088/JCP.08m04728

Feldmesser-Reiss, E. E. (1958). The application of triiodothyronine in the treatment of mental disorders. J. Nerv. Ment. Dis. 127, 540–545. doi: 10.1097/00005053-195812000-00007

Flach, F. F., Celian, C. I., and Rawson, R. W. (1958). Treatment of psychiatric disorders with triiodothyronine. Am. J. Psychiatry 114, 841–842.

Fournier, J. C., DeRubeis, R. J., Hollon, S. D., Dimidjian, S., Amsterdam, J. D., Shelton, R. C., et al. (2010). Antidepressant drug effects and depression severity: a patient-level meta-analysis. JAMA 303, 47–53. doi: 10.1001/jama.2009.1943

Fu, C. H., Williams, S. C., Cleare, A. J., Scott, J., Mitterschiffthaler, M. T., Walsh, N. D., et al. (2008). Neural responses to sad facial expressions in major depression following cognitive behavioral therapy. Biol. Psychiatry 64, 505–512. doi: 10.1016/j.biopsych.2008.04.033

Furey, M. L., Drevets, W. C., Hoffman, E. M., Frankel, E., Speer, A. M., and Zarate, C. A. Jr. (2013). Potential of pretreatment neural activity in the visual cortex during emotional processing to predict treatment response to scopolamine in major depressive disorder. JAMA Psychiatry 70, 280–290. doi: 10.1001/2013.jamapsychiatry.60

Fuss, J., Ben Abdallah, N. M. B., Hensley, F. W., Weber, K.-J., Hellweg, R., and Gass, P. (2010). Deletion of running-induced hippocampal neurogenesis by irradiation prevents development of an anxious phenotype in mice. PLoS ONE 5:e12769. doi: 10.1371/journal.pone.0012769

Garriock, H. A., Tanowitz, M., Kraft, J. B., Dang, V. C., Peters, E. J., Jenkins, G. D., et al. (2010). Association of mu-opioid receptor variants and response to citalopram treatment in major depressive disorder. Am. J. Psychiatry 167, 565–573. doi: 10.1176/appi.ajp.2009.08081167

Gijsman, H. J., Geddes, J. R., Rendell, J. M., Nolen, W. A., and Goodwin, G. M. (2004). Antidepressants for bipolar depression: a systematic review of randomized, controlled trials. Am. J. Psychiatry 161, 1537–1547. doi: 10.1176/appi.ajp.161.9.1537

Goel, N., Plyler, K. S., Daniels, D., and Bale, T. L. (2011). Androgenic influence on serotonergic activation of the HPA stress axis. Endocrinology 152, 2001–2010. doi: 10.1210/en.2010-0964

Grasmäder, K., Verwohlt, P. L., Rietschel, M., Dragicevic, A., Müller, M., Hiemke, C., et al. (2004). Impact of polymorphisms of cytochrome-P450 isoenzymes 2C9, 2C19 and 2D6 on plasma concentrations and clinical effects of antidepressants in a naturalistic clinical setting. Eur. J. Clin. Pharmacol. 60, 329–336. doi: 10.1007/s00228-004-0766-8

Grauer, M. T., and Uhr, M. (2004). P-glycoprotein reduces the ability of amitriptyline metabolites to cross the blood brain barrier in mice after a 10-day administration of amitriptyline. J. Psychopharmacol. 18, 66–74. doi: 10.1177/0269881104042831

Guengerich, F. P. (2008). Cytochrome P450 and chemical toxicology. Chem. Res. Toxicol. 21, 70–83. doi: 10.1021/tx700079z

Guilloux, J. P., David, D. J., Guiard, B. P., Chenu, F., Repérant, C., Toth, M., et al. (2006). Blockade of 5-HT1A receptors by (+/-)-pindolol potentiates cortical 5-HT outflow, but not antidepressant-like activity of paroxetine: microdialysis and behavioral approaches in 5-HT1A receptor knockout mice. Neuropsychopharmacology 31, 2162–2172. doi: 10.1038/sj.npp.1301019

Guilloux, J. P., David, D. J., Xia, L., Nguyen, H. T., Rainer, Q., Guiard, B. P., et al. (2011). Characterization of 5-HT(1A/1B)-/-mice: an animal model sensitive to anxiolytic treatments. Neuropharmacology 61, 478–488. doi: 10.1016/j.neuropharm.2011.02.009

Guo, W. B., Liu, F., Chen, J. D., Xu, X. J., Wu, R. R., Ma, C. Q., et al. (2012). Altered white matter integrity of forebrain in treatment-resistant depression: a diffusion tensor imaging study with tract-based spatial statistics. Prog. Neuropsychopharmacol. Biol. Psychiatry 38, 201–206. doi: 10.1016/j.pnpbp.2012.03.012

Gupta, M., Holshausen, K., Best, M. W., Jokic, R., Milev, R., Bernard, T., et al. (2013). Relationships among neurocognition, symptoms, and functioning in treatment-resistant depression. Arch. Clin. Neuropsychol. 28, 272–281. doi: 10.1093/arclin/act002

Hage, M. P., and Azar, S. T. (2012). The link between thyroid function and depression. J. Thyroid Res. 2012:8. doi: 10.1155/2012/590648

Haj-Mirzaian, A., Hamzeh, N., Javadi-Paydar, M., Abdollahzadeh Estakhri, M. R., and Dehpour, A. R. (2013). Resistance to depression through interference of opioid and nitrergic systems in bile-duct ligated mice. Eur. J. Pharmacol. 708, 38–43. doi: 10.1016/j.ejphar.2013.03.013

Hamani, C., Diwan, M., Macedo, C. E., Brandão, M. L., Shumake, J.,

Gonzalez-Lima, F., et al. (2010). Antidepressant-like effects of medial prefrontal cortex deep brain stimulation in rats. Biol. Psychiatry 67, 117–124. doi: 10.1016/j.biopsych.2009.08.025

Hamilton, M. (1960). A rating scale for depression. J. Neurol. Neurosurg. Psychiatry 23, 56–62. doi: 10.1136/jnnp.23.1.56

Hanson, N. D., Owens, M. J., and Nemeroff, C. B. (2011). Depression, antidepressants, and neurogenesis: a critical reappraisal. Neuropsychopharmacology 36, 2589–2602. doi: 10.1038/npp.2011.220

Heils, A., Teufel, A., Petri, S., Stöber, G., Riederer, P., Bengel, D., et al. (1996). Allelic variation of human serotonin transporter gene expression. J. Neurochem. 66, 2621–2624. doi: 10.1046/j.1471-4159.1996.66062621.x

Hennings, J. M., Owashi, T., Binder, E. B., Horstmann, S., Menke, A., Kloiber, S., et al. (2009). Clinical characteristics and treatment outcome in a representative sample of depressed inpatients—findings from the Munich Antidepressant Response Signature (MARS) project. J. Psychiatr. Res. 43, 215–229. doi: 10.1016/j.jpsychires.2008.05.002

Hiemke, C., Baumann, P., Bergemann, N., Conca, A., Dietmaier, O., Egberts, K., et al. (2011). AGNP consensus guidelines for therapeutic drug monitoring in psychiatry: update 2011. Pharmacopsychiatry 44, 195–235. doi: 10.1055/s-0031-1286287

Holick, K. A., Lee, D. C., Hen, R., and Dulawa, S. C. (2008). Behavioral effects of chronic fluoxetine in BALB/cJ mice do not require adult hippocampal neurogenesis or the serotonin 1A receptor. Neuropsychopharmacology 33, 406–417. doi: 10.1038/sj.npp.1301399

Holmes, A., Yang, R. J., Murphy, D. L., and Crawley, J. N. (2002). Evaluation of antidepressant-related behavioral responses in mice lacking the serotonin transporter. Neuropsychopharmacology 27, 914–923. doi: 10.1016/S0893-133X(02)00374-3

Holsboer, F. (2000). The corticosteroid receptor hypothesis of depression. Neuropsychopharmacology 23, 477–501. doi: 10.1016/S0893-133X(00)00159-7

Horacek, J., Rozehnalova, E., Rosslerova, H., and Dvorak, A. (2011). The influence of stressful life events on development of depression and treatment response in the population of patients in higher age. Ceska Slov. Psychiatr. 106, 311–317.

Hori, H., Yoshimura, R., Ueda, N., Eto, S., Shinkai, K., Sakata, S., et al. (2003). Grapefruit juice-fluvoxamine interaction -is it risky or not. J. Clin. Psychopharmacol. 23, 422–424. doi: 10.1097/01.jcp.0000085423.74359.f2

Horstmann, S., Binder, E. B. (2009). Pharmacogenomics of antidepressant drugs. Pharmacol. Ther. 124, 57–73. doi: 10.1016/j.pharmthera.2009.06.007

Horstmann, S., Lucae, S., Menke, A., Hennings, J. M., Ising, M., Roeske, D., et al. (2010). Polymorphisms in GRIK4, HTR2A, and FKBP5 show interactive effects in predicting remission to antidepressant treatment. Neuropsychopharmacology 35, 727–740. doi: 10.1038/npp.2009.180

Horstmann, S., Lucae, S., Menke, A., Ising, M., Muller-Myhsok, B., Holsboer, F., et al. (2008). Association of GRIK4 and HTR2A genes with antidepressant treatment in the MARS cohort of depressed inpatients. Eur. Neuropsychopharm. 18, S214–S215. doi: 10.1016/S0924-977X(08)70255-4

Ibarguen-Vargas, Y., Surget, A., Vourc'h, P., Leman, S., Andres, C. R., Gardier, A. M., et al. (2009). Deficit in BDNF does not increase vulnerability to stress but dampens antidepressant-like effects in the unpredictable chronic mild stress. Behav. Brain Res. 202, 245–251. doi: 10.1016/j.bbr.2009.03.040

Ibrahim, L., Diazgranados, N., Luckenbaugh, D. A., Machado-Vieira, R., Baumann, J., Mallinger, A. G., et al. (2011). Rapid decrease in depressive symptoms with an N-methyl-d-aspartate antagonist in ECT-resistant major depression. Prog. Neuropsychopharmacol. Biol. Psychiatry 35, 1155–1159. doi: 10.1016/j.pnpbp.2011.03.019

Iovieno, N., and Papakostas, G. I. (2012). Correlation between different levels of placebo response rate and clinical trial outcome in major depressive disorder: a meta-analysis. J. Clin. Psychiatry 73, 1300–1306. doi: 10.4088/JCP.11r07485

Ising, M., Horstmann, S., Kloiber, S., Lucae, S., Binder, E. B., Kern, N., et al. (2007). Combined dexamethasone/corticotropin releasing hormone test predicts treat-ment response in major depression—a potential biomarker. Biol. Psychiatry 62, 47–54. doi: 10.1016/j.biopsych.2006.07.039

Jensen, B. P., Roberts, R. L., Vyas, R., Bonke, G., Jardine, D. L., and Begg, E. J. (2012). Influence of ABCB1 (P-glycoprotein) haplotypes on nortriptyline pharmacoki-netics and nortriptyline-induced postural hypotension in healthy volunteers. Br. J. Clin. Pharmacol. 73, 619–628. doi: 10.1111/j.1365-2125.2011.04126.x

Jeon-Slaughter, H. (2012). Economic factors in of patients' nonadherence to antide-pressant treatment. Soc. Psychiatry Psychiatr. Epidemiol. 47, 1985–1998. doi: 10.1007/s00127-012-0497-6

Jiang, W., Zhang, Y., Xiao, L., Van Cleemput, J., Ji, S.-P., Bai, G., et al. (2005). Cannabinoids promote embryonic and adult hippocampus neurogenesis and produce anxiolytic-and antidepressant-like effects. J. Clin. Investig. 115, 3104–3116. doi: 10.1172/JCI25509

Jin, J., Sklar, G. E., Min Sen Oh, V., and Chuen Li, S. (2008). Factors affecting therapeutic compliance: a review from the patient's perspective. Ther. Clin. Risk Manag. 4, 269–286.

Karlsson, L., Carlsson, B., Hiemke, C., Ahlner, J., Bengtsson, F., Schmitt, U., et al. (2013). Altered brain concentrations of citalopram and escitalopram in P-glycoprotein deficient mice after acute and chronic treatment. Eur. Neuropsychopharmacol. 23, 1636–1644. doi: 10.1016/j.euroneuro.2013.01.003

Kato, M., Fukuda, T., Serretti, A., Wakeno, M., Okugawa, G., Ikenaga, Y., et al. (2008). ABCB1 (MDR1) gene polymorphisms are associated with the clinical response to paroxetine in patients with major depressive disorder. Prog. Neuropsychopharmacol. Biol. Psychiatry 32, 398–404. doi: 10.1016/j.pnpbp.2007.09.003

Kato, M., and Serretti, A. (2010). Review and meta-analysis of antidepressant pharmacogenetic findings in major depressive disorder. Mol. Psychiatry 15, 473–500. doi: 10.1038/mp.2008.116

Kato, M., Wakeno, M., Okugawa, G., Fukuda, T., Azuma, J., Kinoshita, T., et al. (2007). No association of TPH1 218A/C polymorphism with treatment response and intolerance to SSRIs in Japanese patients with major depression. Neuropsychobiology 56, 167–171. doi: 10.1159/000119734

Keers, R., and Uher, R. (2012). Gene-environment interaction in major depression and antidepressant treatment response. Curr. Psychiatry Rep. 14, 129–137. doi: 10.1007/s11920-011-0251-x

Keers, R., Uher, R., Gupta, B., Rietschel, M., Schulze, T. G., Hauser, J., et al. (2010). Stressful life events, cognitive symptoms of depression and response to antidepressants in GENDEP. J. Affect. Disord. 127, 337–342. doi: 10.1016/j.jad.2010.06.011

Keers, R., Uher, R., Huezo-Diaz, P., Smith, R., Jaffee, S., Rietschel, M., et al. (2011). Interaction between serotonin transporter gene variants and life events predicts response to antidepressants in the GENDEP project. Pharmacogenomics J. 11, 138–145. doi: 10.1038/tpj.2010.14

Kessler, R. C., Birnbaum, H. G., Shahly, V., Bromet, E., Hwang, I., McLaughlin, K. A., et al. (2010). Age differences in the prevalence and co-morbidity of DSM-IV major depressive episodes: results from the WHO world mental health survey initiative. Depress. Anxiety. 27, 351–364. doi: 10.1002/da.20634

Kessler, R. C., and Ustun, T. B. (2004). The World Mental Health (WMH) Survey Initiative Version of the World Health Organization (WHO) Composite International Diagnostic Interview (CIDI). Int. J. Methods Psychiatr. Res. 13, 93–121. doi: 10.1002/mpr.168

Khin, N. A., Chen, Y. F., Yang, Y., Yang, P., and Laughren, T. P. (2011). Exploratory analyses of efficacy data from major depressive disorder trials submitted to the US Food and Drug Administration in support of new drug applications. J. Clin. Psychiatry 72, 464–472. doi: 10.4088/JCP.10m06191

Kim, J. J., Mandelli, L., Pae, C. U., De Ronchi, D., Jun, T. Y., Lee, C., et al. (2008). Is there protective haplotype of dysbindin gene (DTNBP1) 3 polymorphisms for major depressive disorder. Prog. Neuropsychopharmacol. Biol. Psychiatry 32, 375–379. doi: 10.1016/j.pnpbp.2007.09.002

Kirchheiner, J., Lorch, R., Lebedeva, E., Seeringer, A., Roots, I., Sasse, J., et al. (2008). Genetic variants in FKBP5 affecting response to antidepressant drug treatment. Pharmacogenomics 9, 841–846. doi: 10.2217/14622416. 9.7.841

Kirsch, I., Deacon, B. J., Huedo-Medina, T. B., Scoboria, A., Moore, T. J., and Johnson, B. T. (2008). Initial severity and antidepressant benefits: a meta-analysis of data submitted to the Food and Drug Administration. PLoS Med. 5:e45. doi: 10.1371/journal.pmed.0050045

Kling, M. A., Geracioti, T. T., Licinio, J., Michelson, D., Oldfield, E. H., and Gold, P. W. (1994). Effects of electroconvulsive therapy on the CRH–ACTH– cortisol system in melancholic depression. Psychopharmacol. Bull. 30, 489–494.

Kloiber, S., Ripke, S., Kohli, M. A., Reppermund, S., Salyakina, D., Uher, et al. (2013). Resistance to antidepressant treatment is associated with polymorphisms in the leptin gene, decreased leptin mRNA expression, and decreased leptin serum levels. Eur. Neuropsychopharmacol. 23, 653–662. doi: 10.1016/j.euroneuro.2012.08.010

Knott, V. J., Telner, J. I., Lapierre, Y. D., Browne, M., and Horn, E. R. (1996). Quantitative EEG in the prediction of antidepressant response to imipramine. J. Affect. Disord. 39, 175–184. doi: 10.1016/0165-0327(96)00003-1

Kong, H., Sha, L. L., Fan, Y., Xiao, M., Ding, J. H., Wu, J., et al. (2009). Requirement of AQP4 for antidepressive efficiency of fluoxetine: implication in adult hippocampal neurogenesis. Neuropsychopharmacology. 34, 1263–1276. doi: 10.1038/npp.2008.185

Krishnan, V., and Nestler, E. J. (2008). The molecular neurobiology of depression. Nature 455, 894–902. doi: 10.1038/nature07455

Kronmüller, K. T., Pantel, J., Köhler, S., Victor, D., Giesel, F., Magnotta, V. A., et al. (2008). Hippocampal volume and 2-year outcome in depression. Br. J. Psychiatry 192, 472–473. doi: 10.1192/bjp.bp.107.040378

Kupfer, D. J., Frank, E., and Phillips, M. L. (2012). Major depressive disorder: new clinical, neurobiological, and treatment perspectives. Lancet 379, 1045–1055. doi: 10.1016/S0140-6736(11)60602-8

Laika, B., Leucht, S., and Steimer, W. (2006). ABCB1 (P-glycoprotein/MDR1) gene G2677T/a sequence variation (polymorphism): lack of association with side effects and therapeutic response in depressed inpatients treated with amitripty-line. Clin. Chem. 52, 893–895. doi: 10.1373/clinchem.2006.066605

Lam, R. W. (2012). Onset, time course and trajectories of improvement with antidepressants. Eur. Neuropsychopharmacol. 22(Suppl. 3), S492–S498. doi: 10.1016/j.euroneuro.2012.07.005

Langenecker, S. A., Kennedy, S. E., Guidotti, L. M., Briceno, E. M., Own, L. S., Hooven, T., et al. (2007). Frontal and limbic activation during inhibitory control predicts treatment response in major depressive disorder. Biol. Psychiatry 62, 1272–1280. doi: 10.1016/j.biopsych.2007.02.019

Lanzenberger, R., Kranz, G. S., Haeusler, D., Akimova, E., Savli, M., Hahn, A., et al. (2012). Prediction of SSRI treatment response in major depression based on serotonin transporter interplay between median raphe nucleus and projection areas. Neuroimage 63, 874–881. doi: 10.1016/j.neuroimage.2012. 07.023

Lehmann, H. E. (1974). Therapy-resistant depressions -a clinical classification. Pharmakopsychiatr. Neuropsychopharmakol. 7, 156–163. doi: 10.1055/s-0028-1094425

Lehmann, M. L., Brachman, R. A., Martinowich, K., Schloesser, R. J., and Herkenham, M. (2013). Glucocorticoids orchestrate divergent effects on mood through adult neurogenesis. J. Neuroscience. 33, 2961–2972. doi: 10.1523/JNEUROSCI.3878-12.2013

Lekman, M., Laje, G., Charney, D., Rush, A. J., Wilson, A. F., Sorant, A. J., et al. (2008). The FKBP5-gene in depression and treatment response—an association study in the Sequenced Treatment Alternatives to Relieve Depression (STAR*D) cohort. Biol. Psychiatry 63, 1103–1110. doi: 10.1016/j.biopsych.2007. 10.026

Leuchter, A. F., Cook, I. A., Gilmer, W. S., Marangell, L. B., Burgoyne, K. S., Howland, R. H., et al. (2009). Effectiveness of a quantitative electroencephalo-graphic biomarker for predicting differential response or remission with escitalopram and bupropion in major depressive disorder. Psychiatry Res. 169, 132–138. doi: 10.1016/j.psychres.2009.04.004

Leuchter, A. F., Cook, I. A., Hamilton, S. P., Narr, K. L., Toga, A., Hunter, A. M., et al. (2010). Biomarkers to predict antidepressant response. Curr. Psychiatry Rep. 12, 553–562. doi: 10.1007/s11920-010-0160-4

Li, N., Lee, B., Liu, R. J., Banasr, M., Dwyer, J. M., Iwata, M., et al. (2010). mTOR-dependent synapse formation underlies the rapid antidepressant effects of NMDA antagonists. Science 329, 959–964. doi: 10.1126/science.1190287

Lifschytz, T., Segman, R., Shalom, G., Lerer, B., Gur, E., Golzer, T., et al. (2006). Basic mechanisms of augmentation of antidepressant effects with thy-roid hormone. Curr. Drug Targets 7, 203–210. doi: 10.2174/138945006775515482

Lifschytz, T., Zozulinsky, P., Eitan, R., Landshut, G., Ohayon, S., and Lerer, B. (2011). Effect of triiodothyronine on antidepressant screening tests in mice and on presynaptic 5-HT1A receptors: mediation by thyroid hormone α receptors. J. Pharmacol. Exp. Ther. 337, 494–502. doi: 10.1124/jpet.111.179564

Lin, K. M., Chiu, Y. F., Tsai, I. J., Chen, C. H., Shen, W. W., Liu, S. C., et al. (2011). ABCB1 gene polymorphisms are associated with the severity of major depressive disorder and its response to escitalopram treatment. Pharmacogenet. Genomics. 21, 163–170. doi: 10.1097/FPC.0b013e32833db216

Liu, G. X., Cai, G. Q., Cai, Y. Q., Sheng, Z. J., Jiang, J., Mei, Z., et al. (2007a). Reduced anxiety and depression-like behaviors in mice lacking GABA transporter subtype 1. Neuropsychopharmacology 32, 1531–1539. doi: 10.1038/sj.npp.1301281

Liu, Z., Zhu, F., Wang, G., Xiao, Z., Tang, J., Liu, W., et al. (2007b). Association study of corticotropin-releasing hormone receptor1 gene polymorphisms and antide-pressant response in major depressive disorders. Neurosci. Lett. 414, 155–158. doi: 10.1016/j.neulet.2006.12.013

Lozano, A. M., Giacobbe, P., Hamani, C., Rizvi, S. J., Kennedy, S. H., Kolivakis, T. T., et al. (2012). A multicenter pilot study of subcallosal cingulate area deep brain stimulation for treatment-resistant depression. J. Neurosurg. 116, 315–322. doi: 10.3171/2011.10.JNS102122

Lozano, A. M., Mayberg, H. S., Giacobbe, P., Hamani, C., Craddock, R. C., and Kennedy, S. H. (2008). Subcallosal cingulate gyrus deep brain stimulation for treatment-resistant depression. Biol. Psychiatry 64, 461–467. doi: 10.1016/j.biopsych.2008.05.034

Lucas, G., Rymar, V. V., Du, J., Mnie-Filali, O., Bisgaard, C., Manta, S., et al. (2007). Serotonin(4) (5-HT(4)) receptor agonists are putative antidepressants with a rapid onset of action. Neuron 55, 712–725. doi: 10.1016/j.neuron.2007.07.041

MacQueen, G. M., Yucel, K., Taylor, V. H., Macdonald, K., and Joffe, R. (2008). Posterior hippocampal volumes are associated with remission rates in patients with major depressive disorder. Biol. Psychiatry 64, 880–883. doi: 10.1016/j.biopsych.2008.06.027

Madsen, T. M., Treschow, A., Bengzon, J., Bolwig, T. G., Lindvall, O., and Tingström, A. (2000). Increased neurogenesis in a model of electroconvul-sive therapy. Biol. Psychiatry 47, 1043–1049. doi: 10.1016/S0006-3223(00)00228-6

Malberg, J. E., Eisch, A. J., Nestler, E. J., and Duman, R. S. (2000). Chronic antide-pressant treatment increases neurogenesis in adult rat hippocampus. J. Neurosci. 20, 9104–9110.

Malone, D. A. Jr., Dougherty, D. D., Rezai, A. R., Carpenter, L. L., Friehs, G. M., et al. (2009). Deep brain stimulation of the ventral capsule/ventral striatum for treatment-resistant depression. Biol. Psychiatry 65, 267–275. doi: 10.1016/j.biopsych.2008.08.029

Mandelli, L., Marino, E., Pirovano, A., Calati, R., Zanardi, R., Colombo, C., et al. (2009). Interaction between SERTPR and stressful life events on response to antidepressant treatment. Eur. Neuropsychopharmacol. 19, 64–67. doi: 10.1016/j.euroneuro.2008.08.005

March, J., Silva, S., Vitiello, B., and TADS Team. (2006). The Treatment for Adolescents with Depression Study (TADS): methods and message at 12 weeks. J. Am. Acad. Child Adolesc. Psychiatry 45, 1393–1403. doi: 10.1097/01.chi.0000237709.35637.c0

Martin, P., Massol, J., Belon, J. P., Gaudel, G., and Soubrié, P. (1987). Thyroid function and reversal by antidepressant drugs of depressive-like behavior (escape deficits) in rats. Neuropsychobiology 18, 21–26. doi: 10.1159/000118388

Mateus-Pinheiro, A., Pinto, L., Bessa, J. M., Morais, M., Alves, N. D., Monteiro, et al. (2013). Sustained remission from depressive-like behavior depends on hippocampal neurogenesis. Transl. Psychiatry 3, e210. doi: 10.1038/tp.2012.141 Mayberg, H. S., Brannan, S. K., Mahurin, R. K., Jerabek, P. A., Brickman, J. S., Tekell, J. L., et al. (1997). Cingulate function in depression: a potential predic-tor of treatment response. Neuroreport 8, 1057–1061. doi: 10.1097/00001756-199703030-00048

Mayberg, H. S., Lozano, A. M., Voon, V., McNeely, H. E., Seminowicz, D., Hamani, C., et al. (2005). Deep brain stimulation for treatment-resistant depression. Neuron 45, 651–660. doi: 10.1016/j.neuron.2005.02.014

Mayer, M. L. (2007). GRIK4 and the kainate receptor. Am. J. Psychiatry 164, 1148. doi: 10.1176/appi.ajp.2007.07060996

Mayorga, A. J., Dalvi, A., Page, M. E., Zimov-Levinson, S., Hen, R., and Lucki, I. (2001). Antidepressant-like behavioral effects in 5-hydroxytryptamine(1A) and 5-hydroxytryptamine(1B) receptor mutant mice. J. Pharmacol. Exp. Ther. 298, 1101–1107.

McGrath, C. L., Kelley, M. E., Holtzheimer, P. E., Dunlop, B. W., Craighead, W. E., Franco, A. R., et al. (2013). Toward a neuroimaging treatment selection biomarker for major depressive disorder. JAMA Psychiatry 12, 1–9. doi: 10.1001/jamapsychiatry.2013.143

Menu, P., Gressier, F., Verstuyft, C., Hardy, P., Becquemont, L., and Corruble, E. (2010). Antidepressants and ABCB1 gene C3435T functional polymor-phism: a naturalistic study. Neuropsychobiology 62, 193–197. doi: 10.1159/000319361

Mihaljevic Peles, A., Bozina, N., Sagud, M., Rojnic Kuzman, M., and Lovric, M. (2008). MDR1 gene polymorphism: therapeutic response to paroxetine among patients with major depression. Prog. Neuropsychopharmacol. Biol. Psychiatry 32, 1439–1444. doi: 10.1016/j.pnpbp.2008.03.018

Miller, M. D., Lenze, E. J., Dew, M. A., Whyte, E., Weber, E., Begley, A. E., et al. (2002). Effect of cerebrovascular risk factors on depression treatment outcome in later life. Am. J. Geriatr. Psychiatry 10, 592–598. doi: 10.1176/appi.ajgp.10.5.592

Mitjans, M., Gastó, C., Catalán, R., Fañanás, L., and Arias, B. (2012). Genetic variability in the endocannabinoid system and 12-week clinical response to citalopram treatment: the role of the CNR1, CNR2 and FAAH genes. J. Psychopharmacol. 26, 1391–1398. doi: 10.1177/0269881112454229

Mitjans, M., Serretti, A., Fabbri, C., Gastó, C., Catalán, R., Fañanás, L., et al. (2013). Screening genetic variability at the CNR1 gene in both major depression etiology and clinical response to citalopram treatment. Psychopharmacology (Berl.) 227, 509–519. doi: 10.1007/s00213-013-2995-y

Molendijk, M. L., Bus, B. A., Spinhoven, P., Penninx, B. W., Kenis, G., Prickaerts, J., et al. (2011). Serum levels of brain-derived neurotrophic factor in major depressive disorder: state-trait issues, clinical features and pharmacological treatment. Mol. Psychiatry 16, 1088–1095. doi: 10.1038/mp.2010.98

Monroe, S. M., Thase, M. E., and Simons, A. D. (1992). Social factors and the psychobiology of depression: relations between life stress and rapid eye movement sleep latency. J. Abnorm. Psychol. 101, 528–537. doi: 10.1037/0021-843X.101.3.528

Monteggia, L. M., Barrot, M., Powell, C. M., Berton, O., Galanis, V., Gemelli, T., et al. (2004). Essential role of brain-derived neurotrophic factor in adult hippocampal function. Proc. Natl. Acad. Sci. U.S.A. 101, 10827–10832. doi: 10.1073/pnas.0402141101

Montgomery, S. A., and Asberg, M. (1979). A new depression scale designed to be sensitive to change. Br. J. Psychiatry 134, 382–389. doi: 10.1192/bjp.134.4.382 Moon, H. Y., Kim, S. H., Yang, Y. R., Song, P., Yu, H. S., Park, H. G., et al. (2012). Macrophage migration inhibitory factor mediates the antidepressant actions of voluntary exercise. Proc. Natl. Acad. Sci. U.S.A. 109, 13094–13099. doi: 10.1073/pnas.1205535109

Mrazek, D. A., Biernacka, J. M., O'Kane, D. J., Black, J. L., Cunningham, J. M., Drews, M. S., et al. (2011). CYP2C19 variation and citalopram response. Pharmacogenet. Genomics. 21, 1–9. doi: 10.1097/FPC.0b013e328340bc5a

Mulert, C., Juckel, G., Brunnmeier, M., Karch, S., Leicht, G., Mergl, R., et al. (2007). Prediction of treatment response in major depression: integration of concepts. J. Affect. Disord. 98, 215–225. doi: 10.1016/j.jad.2006.07.021

McKinnon, M., Yucel, K., Nazarov, A., and MacQueen, G. (2009). A meta-analysis examining clinical predictors of hippocampal volume in patients with major depressive disorder. J. Psychiatry Neurosci. 34, 41–54.

Nakamura, M., Ueno, S., Sano, A., and Tanabe, H. (2000). The human serotonin transporter gene linked polymorphism (5-HTTLPR) shows ten novel allelic variants. Mol. Psychiatry 5, 32–38. doi: 10.1038/sj.mp.4000698

Nakashiba, T., Cushman, J. D., Pelkey, K. A., Renaudineau, S., Buhl, D. L., McHugh, T. J., et al. (2012). Young dentate granule cells mediate pattern separation, whereas old granule cells facilitate pattern completion. Cell 149, 188–201. doi: 10.1016/j.cell.2012.01.046

Narasimhan, S., and Lohoff, F. W. (2012). Pharmacogenetics of antidepressant drugs: current clinical practice and future directions. Pharmacogenomics 13, 441–464. doi: 10.2217/pgs.12.1

Nelson, J. C., Clary, C. M., Leon, A. C., and Schneider, L. S. (2005). Symptoms of late-life depression: frequency and change during treatment. Am. J. Geriatr. Psychiatry 13, 520–526. doi: 10.1176/appi.ajgp.13.6.520

NICE. (2004). Depression: Management of Depression in Primary and Secondary Care. London: Clinical guidelines, CG23, National Institute for Clinical Excellence.

Nierenberg, A. A., and DeCecco, L. M. (2001). Definitions of antidepressant treat-ment response, remission, nonresponse, partial response, and other relevant outcomes: a focus on treatment-resistant depression. J. Clin. Psychiatry 62 (Suppl. 16), 5–9.

Nierenberg, A. A., Fava, M., Trivedi, M. H., Wisniewski, S. R., Thase, M. R., McGrath, P. J., et al. (2006). A comparison of lithium and T(3) augmentation following two failed medication treatments for depression: a STAR*D report. Am. J. Psychiatry 163, 1519–1530. doi: 10.1176/appi.ajp.163.9.1519

Nollet, M., Gaillard, P., Tanti, A., Girault, V., Belzung, C., and Leman, S. (2012). Neurogenesis-independent antidepressant-like effects on behavior and stress axis response of a dual orexin receptor antagonist in a rodent model of depression. Neuropsychopharmacology 37, 2210–2221. doi: 10.1038/npp.2012.70

O'Brien, F. E., Dinan, T. G., Griffin, B. T., and Cryan, J. F. (2012). Interactions between antidepressants and P-glycoprotein at the blood-brain barrier: clini-cal significance of in vitro and in vivo findings. Br. J. Pharmacol. 165, 289–312. doi: 10.1111/j.1476-5381.2011.01557.x

Oh, Y. S., Gao, P., Lee, K. W., Ceglia, I., Seo, J. S., Zhang, X., et al. (2013). SMARCA3, a chromatin remodeling factor, is required for p11-dependent antidepressant action. Cell 152, 831–843. doi: 10.1016/j.cell.2013.01.014

O'Leary, O. F., Bechtholt, A. J., Crowley, J. J., Hill, T. E., Page, M. E., and Lucki, I. (2007). Depletion of serotonin and catecholamines block the acute behavioral response to different classes of antidepressant drugs in the mouse tail suspension test. Psychopharmacology (Berl.). 192, 357–371. doi: 10.1007/s00213-007-0728-9

Pae, C. U., Mandelli, L., Serretti, A., Patkar, A. A., Kim, J. J., Lee, C. U., et al. (2007a). Heat-shock protein-70 genes and response to antidepressants in major depression. Prog. Neuropsychopharmacol. Biol. Psychiatry 31, 1006–1011. doi: 10.1016/j.pnpbp.2007.02.011

Pae, C. U., Serretti, A., Mandelli, L., De Ronchi, D., Patkar, A. A., Jun, T. Y., et al. (2007b). Dysbindin associated with selective serotonin reuptake inhibitor antidepressant efficacy. Pharmacogenet. Genomics. 17, 69–75. doi: 10.1097/01.fpc.0000236330.03681.6d

Papakostas, G. I., Cooper-Kazaz, R., Appelhof, B. C., Posternak, M. A., Johnson, D. P., Klibanski, A., et al. (2009). Simultaneous initiation (coinitiation) of pharma-cotherapy with triiodothyronine and a selective serotonin reuptake inhibitor for major depressive disorder: a quantitative synthesis of double-blind studies. Int. Clin. Psychopharmacol. 24, 19–25. doi: 10.1097/YIC.0b013e328314dfaf

Papiol, S., Arias, B., Gastó, C., Gutiérrez, B., Catalán, R., and Fañanás, L. (2007). Genetic variability at HPA axis in major depression and clinical response to antidepressant treatment. J. Affect. Disord. 104, 83–90. doi: 10.1016/j.jad.2007.02.017

Pariante, C. M. (2003). Depression, stress and the adrenal axis. J. Neuroendocrinol. 15, 811–812. doi: 10.1046/j.1365-2826.2003.01058.x

Pariante, C. M., and Miller, A. H. (2001). Glucocorticoid receptors in major depres-sion: relevance to pathophysiology and treatment. Biol. Psychiatry 49, 391–404. doi: 10.1016/S0006-3223(00)01088-X

Paslakis, G., Heuser, I., Schweiger, U., and Deuschle, M. (2010). A single DEX/CRH test in male drug-free depressed patients is associated with the clinical response to treatment with fluoxetine. J. Psychiatr. Res. 44, 1154–1157. doi: 10.1016/j.jpsychires.2010.04.010

Pereira, A. M., Tiemensma, J., and Romijn, J. A. (2010). Neuropsychiatric disorders in cushing's syndrome. Neuroendocrinology 92(Suppl. 1), 65–70. doi: 10.1159/000314317

Perera, T. D., Coplan, J. D., Lisanby, S. H., Lipira, C. M., Arif, M., Carpio, C., et al. (2007). Antidepressant-induced neurogenesis in the hippocampus of adult non-human primates. J. Neurosci. 27, 4894–4901. doi: 10.1523/JNEUROSCI.0237-07.2007

Perera, T. D., Dwork, A. J., Keegan, K. A., Thirumangalakudi, L., Lipira, C. M., Joyce, N., et al. (2011). Necessity of hippocampal neurogenesis for the therapeu-tic action of antidepressants in adult nonhuman primates. PLoS ONE 6:e17600. doi: 10.1371/journal.pone.0017600

Peters, E. J., Slager, S. L., Kraft, J. B., Jenkins, G. D., Reinalda, M. S., McGrath, P. J., et al. (2008). Pharmacokinetic genes do not influence response or tolerance to citalopram in the STAR*D sample. PLoS ONE 3:e1872. doi: 10.1371/jour-nal.pone.0001872

Petrik, D., Lagace, D. C., and Eisch, A. J. (2012). The neurogenesis hypothesis of affective and anxiety disorders: are we mistaking the scaffolding for the building. Neuropharmacology 62, 21–34. doi: 10.1016/j.neuropharm.2011.09.003

Pilhatsch, M., Winter, C., Nordström, K., Vennström, B., Bauer, M., and Juckel, G. (2010). Increased depressive behaviour in mice harboring the mutant thyroid hormone receptor alpha 1. Behav. Brain Res. 214, 187–192. doi: 10.1016/j.bbr.2010.05.016

Pizzagalli, D. A. (2011). Frontocingulate dysfunction in depression: toward biomarkers of treatment response. Neuropsychopharmacology 36, 183–206. doi: 10.1038/npp.2010.166

Pizzagalli, D., Pascual-Marqui, R. D.,

Nitschke, J. B., Oakes, T. R., Larson, C. L., Abercrombie, H. C., et al. (2001). Anterior cingulate activity as a predictor of degree of treatment response in major depression: evidence from brain electrical tomography analysis. Am. J. Psychiatry 158, 405–415. doi: 10.1176/appi.ajp.158.3.405

Porcelli, S., Fabbri, C., Drago, A., Gibiino, S., De Ronchi, D., and Serretti, A. (2011). Genetics and antidepressants: where we are. Clin Neuropsychiatry 8, 99–150.

Price, A., Rayner, L., Okon-Rocha, E., Evans, A., Valsraj, K., Higginson, I. J., et al. (2011). Antidepressants for the treatment of depression in neurological disorders: a systematic review and meta-analysis of randomised controlled trials. J. Neurol. Neurosurg. Psychiatry 82, 914–923. doi: 10.1136/jnnp.2010.230862

Ramasubbu, R., Beaulieu, S., Taylor, V. H., Schaffer, A., and McIntyre, R. S. (2012). The CANMAT task force recommendations for the management of patients with mood disorders and comorbid medical conditions: diagnostic, assessment, and treatment principles. Ann. Clin. Psychiatry 24, 82–90.

Reif, A., Fritzen, S., Finger, M., Strobel, A., Lauer, M., Schmitt, A., et al. (2006). Neural stem cell proliferation is decreased in schizophrenia, but not in depression. Mol. Psychiatry 11, 514–522. doi: 10.1038/sj.mp.4001791

Revest, J. M., Dupret, D., Koehl, M., Funk-Reiter, C., Grosjean, N., Piazza, P. V., et al. (2009). Adult hippocampal neurogenesis is involved in anxiety-related behaviors. Mol. Psychiatry 14, 959–967. doi: 10.1038/mp.2009.15

Revesz, D., Tjernstrom, M., Ben-Menachem, E., and Thorlin, T. (2008). Effects of vagus nerve stimulation on rat hippocampal progenitor proliferation. Exp. Neurol. 214, 259–265. doi: 10.1016/j.expneurol.2008.08.012

Richardson-Jones, J. W., Craige, C. P., Guiard, B. P., Stephen, A., Metzger, K. L., Kung, H. F., et al. (2010). 5-HT1A autoreceptor levels determine vul-nerability to stress and response to antidepressants. Neuron 65, 40–52. doi: 10.1016/j.neuron.2009.12.003

Richelson, E. (1998). Pharmacokinetic interactions of antidepressants. J. Clin. Psychiatry 59(Suppl. 10), 22–26. doi: 10.4065/72.9.835

Rivero-Santana, A., Perestelo-Perez, L., Pérez-Ramos, J., Serrano-Aguilar, P., and De Las Cuevas, C. (2013). Sociodemographic and clinical predictors of compliance with antidepressants for depressive disorders: systematic review of observational studies. Patient Prefer. Adherence 7, 151–169. doi: 10.2147/PPA.S39382

Roberts, R. L., Joyce, P. R., Mulder, R. T., Begg, E. J., and Kennedy, M. A. (2002). A common P-glycoprotein polymorphism is associated with nortriptyline-induced postural hypotension in patients treated for major depression. Pharmacogenomics J. 2, 191–196. doi: 10.1038/sj.tpj.6500099

Roiser, J. P., Elliott, R., and Sahakian, B. J. (2012). Cognitive mechanisms of treatment in depression. Neuropsychopharmacology 37, 117–136. doi: 10.1038/npp.2011.183

Ruhé, H. G., van Rooijen, G., Spijker, J., Peeters, F. P., and Schene, A. H. (2012). Staging methods for treatment resistant depression. A systematic review. J. Affect. Disord. 137, 35–45. doi: 10.1016/j.jad.2011.02.020

Rush, A. J., Trivedi, M. H., Wisniewski, S. R., Nierenberg, A. A., Stewart, J. W., Warden, D., et al. (2006). Acute and longer-term outcomes in depressed out-patients requiring one or several treatment steps: a STAR*D report. Am. J. Psychiatry 163, 1905–1917. doi: 10.1176/appi.ajp.163.11.1905

Saarelainen, T., Hendolin, P., Lucas, G., Koponen, E., Sairanen, M., MacDonald, E., et al. (2003). Activation of the TrkB neurotrophin receptor is induced by antide-pressant drugs and is required for antidepressant-induced behavioral effects. J. Neurosci. 23, 349–357.

Sackeim, H. A., Prudic, J., Devanand, D. P., Decina, P., Kerr, B., and Malitz, S. (1990). The impact of medication resistance and continuation pharmacother-apy on relapse following response to electroconvulsive therapy in major depression. J. Clin. Psychopharmacol. 10, 96–104. doi: 10.1097/00004714-199004000-00004

Sahay, A., Scobie, K. N., Hill, A. S., O'Carroll, C. M., Kheirbek, M. A., Burghardt, N. S., et al. (2011). Increasing adult hippocampal neurogenesis is sufficient to improve pattern separation. Nature 472, 466–470. doi: 10.1038/nature09817

Salvadore, G., Cornwell, B. R., Colon-Rosario, V., Coppola, R., Grillon, C., Zarate, et al. (2009). Increased anterior cingulate cortical activity in response to fearful faces: a neurophysiological biomarker that predicts rapid antidepressant response to ketamine. Biol. Psychiatry 65, 289–295. doi: 10.1016/j.biopsych.2008.08.014

Sanacora, G., Kendell, S. F., Levin, Y., Simen, A. A., Fenton, L. R., Coric, V., et al. (2007). Preliminary evidence of riluzole efficacy in antidepressant-treated patients with residual depressive symptoms. Biol. Psychiatry 61, 822–825. doi: 10.1016/j.biopsych.2006.08.037

Sanacora, G., Zarate, C. A., Krystal, J. H., and Manji, H. K. (2008). Targeting the glutamatergic system to develop novel, improved therapeutics for mood disorders. Nat. Rev. Drug. Discov. 7, 426–437. doi: 10.1038/nrd2462

Santarelli, L., Saxe, M., Gross, C., Surget, A., Battaglia, F., Dulawa, S., et al. (2003). Requirement of hippocampal neurogenesis for the behavioral effects of antidepressants. Science 301, 805–809. doi: 10.1126/science.1083328

Sarginson, J. E., Lazzeroni, L. C., Ryan, H. S., Ershoff, B. D., Schatzberg, A. F., and Murphy, G. M. Jr. (2010). ABCB1 (MDR1) polymorphisms and antidepressant response in geriatric depression. Pharmacogenet. Genomics. 20, 467–475. doi: 10.1097/FPC.0b013e32833b593a

Sartorius, N. (1974). Description and classification of depressive disorders. Contributions for the definition of the therapy-resistance and of therapy resistant depressions. Pharmakopsychiatr. Neuropsychopharmakol. 7, 76–79. doi: 10.1055/s-0028-1094404

Saxena, S., Brody, A. L., Ho, M. L., Zohrabi, N., Maidment, K. M., and Baxter, L. R. Jr. (2003). Differential brain metabolic predictors of response to paroxetine in obsessive-compulsive disorder versus major depression. Am. J. Psychiatry 160, 522–532. doi: 10.1176/appi.ajp.160.3.522

Scherrer, J. F., Chrusciel, T., Garfield, L. D., Freedland, K. E., Carney, R. M., Hauptman, P. J., et al. (2012). Treatment-resistant and insufficiently treated depression and all-cause mortality following myocardial infarction. Br. J. Psychiatry 200, 137–142. doi: 10.1192/bjp.bp.111.096479

Schinkel, A. H., Wagenaar, E., van Deemter, L., Mol, C. A., and Borst, P. (1995). Absence of the mdr1a P-Glycoprotein in mice affects tissue distribution and pharmacokinetics of dexamethasone, digoxin, and cyclosporin A. J. Clin. Invest. 96, 1698–1705. doi: 10.1172/JCI118214

Schloesser, R. J., Lehmann, M., Martinowich, K., Manji, H. K., and Herkenham, M. (2010). Environmental enrichment requires adult neurogenesis to facili-tate the recovery from psychosocial stress. Mol. Psychiatry 15, 1152–1163. doi: 10.1038/mp.2010.34

Schloesser, R. J., Manji, H. K., and Martinowich, K. (2009). Suppression of adult neurogenesis leads to an increased hypothalamo-pituitary-adrenal axis response. Neuroreport 20, 553–557. doi: 10.1097/WNR.0b013e3283293e59

Schmidt, E. F., Warner-Schmidt, J. L., Otopalik, B. G., Pickett, S. B., Greengard, P., and Heintz, N. (2012a). Identification of the cortical neurons that mediate antidepressant responses. Cell 149, 1152–1163. doi: 10.1016/j.cell.2012.03.038

Schmidt, M. V., Paez-Pereda, M., Holsboer, F., and Hausch, F. (2012b). The prospect of FKBP51 as a drug target. Chem. Med. Chem. 7, 1351–1359. doi: 10.1002/cmdc.201200137

Schmuckermair, C., Gaburro, S., Sah, A., Landgraf, R., Sartori, S. B., and Singewald, N. (2013). Behavioral and neurobiological effects of deep brain stimulation in a mouse model of high anxiety-and depression-like behavior. Neuropsychopharmacology 38, 1234–1244. doi: 10.1038/npp.2013.21

Schüle, C., Baghai, T. C., Eser, D., Häfner, S., Born, C., Herrmann, S., et al. (2009). The combined dexamethasone/CRH Test (DEX/CRH test) and prediction of acute treatment response in major depression. PLoS ONE 4:e4324. doi: 10.1371/journal.pone.0004324

Schulz, R., Drayer, R. A., and Rollman, B. L. (2002). Depression as a risk factor for non-suicide mortality in the elderly. Biol. Psychiatry 52, 205–225. doi: 10.1016/S0006-3223(02)01423-3

Serra-Blasco, M., Portella, M. J., Gómez-Ansón, B., de Diego-Adeliño, J., Vives-Gilabert, Y., Puigdemont, D., et al. (2013). Effects of illness duration and treatment resistance on grey matter abnormalities in major depression. Br. J. Psychiatry. 202, 434–440. doi: 10.1192/bjp.bp.112.116228

Serretti, A., Zanardi, R., Rossini, D., Cusin, C., Lilli, R., and Smeraldi, E. (2001). Influence of tryptophan hydroxylase and serotonin transporter genes on fluvoxamine antidepressant activity. Mol. Psychiatry 6, 586–592. doi: 10.1038/sj.mp.4000876

Sheehan, D. V., Keene, M. S., Eaddy, M., Krulewicz, S., Kraus, J. E., and Carpenter, D. J. (2008). Differences in medication adherence and health-care resource utilization patterns: older versus newer antidepressant agents in patients with depression and/or anxiety disorders. CNS Drugs 22, 963–973. doi: 10.2165/00023210-200822110-00005

Shelton, R. C., Osuntokun, O., Heinloth, A. N., and Corya, S. A.

(2010). Therapeutic options for treatment-resistant depression. CNS Drugs 24, 131–161. doi: 10.2165/11530280-000000000-00000

Shiroma, P. R., Geda, Y. E., and Mrazek, D. A. (2010). Pharmacogenomic implications of variants of monoaminergic-related genes in geriatric psychiatry. Pharmacogenomics 11, 1305–1330. doi: 10.2217/pgs.10.118

Shors, T. J., Miesegaes, G., Beylin, A., Zhao, M., Rydel, T., and Gould, E. (2001). Neurogenesis in the adult is involved in the formation of trace memories. Nature 410, 372–376. doi: 10.1038/35066584

Singh, A. B., Bousman, C. A., Ng, C. H., Byron, K., and Berk, M. (2012). ABCB1 polymorphism predicts escitalopram dose needed for remission in major depression. Transl. Psychiatry 2, e198. doi: 10.1038/tp.2012.115

Smeraldi, E., Serretti, A., Artioli, P., Lorenzi, C., and Catalano, M. (2006). Serotonin transporter gene-linked polymorphic region: possible pharmaco-genetic implications of rare variants. Psychiatr. Genet. 16, 153–158. doi: 10.1097/01.ypg.0000218611.53064.a0

Snyder, J. S., Soumier, A., Brewer, M., Pickel, J., and Cameron, H. A. (2011). Adult hippocampal neurogenesis buffers stress responses and depressive behaviour. Nature 476, 458–461. doi: 10.1038/nature10287

Sonino, N., Boscaro, M., Ambroso, G., Merola, G., and Mantero, F. (1986). Prolonged treatment of Cushing's disease with metyrapone and aminog-lutethimide. IRCS Med. Sci. 14, 485–486.

Sonino, N., and Fava, G. A. (2002). Residual symptoms in depression. An emerging therapeutic concept. Prog. NeuroPsychopharmacol. Biol. Psychiatry 26, 763–770. doi: 10.1016/S0278-5846(02)00200-2

Sonino, N., Fava, G. A., Belluardo, P., Girelli, M. E., and Boscaro, M. (1993). Course of depression in Cushing's syndrome: response to treatment and comparison with Graves' disease. Horm. Res. 39, 202–206. doi: 10.1159/000182736

Souery, D., Amsterdam, J., de Montigny, C., Lecrubier, Y., Montgomery, S., Lipp, O., et al. (1999). Treatment resistant depression: methodological overview and operational criteria. Eur. Neuropsychopharmacol. 9, 83–91. doi: 10.1016/S0924-977X(98)00004-2

Souery, D., Oswald, P., Massat, I., Bailer, U., Bollen, J., Demyttenaere, K., et al. (2007). Group for the study of resistant depression. clinical factors associated with treatment resistance in major depressive disorder: results from a European multicenter study. J. Clin. Psychiatry 68, 1062–1070. doi: 10.4088/JCP.v68n0713

Stawski, P., Janovjak, H., and Trauner, D. (2010). Pharmacology of ionotropic glutamate receptors: a structural perspective. Bioorg. Med. Chem. 18, 7759–7772. doi: 10.1016/j.bmc.2010.09.012

Steiner, M. A., Wanisch, K., Monory, K., Marsicano, G., Borroni, E., Bächli, H., et al. (2008). Impaired cannabinoid receptor type 1 signaling interferes with stress-coping behavior in mice. Pharmacogenomics J. 8, 196–208. doi: 10.1038/sj.tpj.6500466

Stemmelin, J., Cohen, C., Yalcin, I., Keane, P., and Griebel, G. (2010). Implication of beta3-adrenoceptors in the antidepressant-like effects of amibegron using Adrb3 knockout mice in the chronic mild stress. Behav. Brain Res. 206, 310–312. doi: 10.1016/j.bbr.2009.09.003

Surget, A., Saxe, M., Leman, S., Ibarguen-Vargas, Y., Chalon, S., Griebel, G., et al. (2008). Drug-dependent requirement of hippocampal neurogenesis in a model of depression and of antidepressant reversal. Biol. Psychiatry 64, 293–301. doi: 10.1016/j.biopsych.2008.02.022

Surget, A., Tanti, A., Leonardo, E. D., Laugeray, A., Rainer, Q., Touma, C., et al. (2011). Antidepressants recruit new neurons to improve stress response regula-tion. Mol. Psychiatry 16, 1177–1188. doi: 10.1038/mp.2011.48

Suzuki, Y., Sugai, T., Fukui, N., Watanabe, J., Ono, S., Inoue, Y., et al. (2011). CYP2D6 genotype and smoking influence fluvoxamine steady-state concentra-tion in Japanese psychiatric patients: lessons for genotype-phenotype association study design in translational pharmacogenetics. J. Psychopharmacol. 25, 908–914. doi: 10.1177/0269881110370504

Svenningsson, P., Chergui, K., Rachleff, I., Flajolet, M., Zhang, X., El Yacoubi, M., et al. (2006). Alterations in 5-HT1B receptor function by p11 in depression-like states. Science 311, 77–80. doi: 10.1126/science.1117571

Swardfager, W., Herrmann, N., McIntyre, R. S., Mazereeuw, G., Goldberger, K., Cha, D. S., et al. (2013). Potential roles of zinc in the pathophysiology and treatment of major depressive disorder. Neurosci. Biobehav. Rev. 37, 911–929. doi: 10.1016/j.neubiorev.2013.03.018

Tadic′, A., Müller, M. J., Rujescu, D., Kohnen, R., Stassen, H. H., Dahmen, N., et al. (2007). The MAOA T941G polymorphism and short-term treatment response to mirtazapine and paroxetine in major depression. Am. J. Med. Genet. B. Neuropsychiatr. Genet. 144B, 325–331. doi: 10.1002/ajmg.b.30462

Tanti, A., and Belzung, C. (2013a). Hippocampal neurogenesis: a biomarker for

depression or antidepressant effects. Methodological considerations and per-spectives for future research. Cell Tissue Res. 354, 203–219. doi: 10.1007/s00441-013-1612-z

Tanti, A., and Belzung, C. (2013b). Neurogenesis along the septo-temporal axis of the hippocampus: are depression and the action of antidepressants region-specific. Neuroscience. 252, 234–252. doi: 10.1016/j.neuroscience.2013.08.017

Tao, R., Emslie, G., Mayes, T., Nakonezny, P., Kennard, B., and Hughes, C. (2009). Early prediction of acute antidepressant treatment response and remission in pediatric major depressive disorder. J. Am. Acad. Child Adolesc. Psychiatry 48, 71–78. doi: 10.1097/CHI.0b013e318190043e

Tatarczyńska, E., Kłodzin′ ska, A., Stachowicz, K., and Chojnacka-Wójcik, E. (2004). Effect of combined administration of 5-HT1A or 5-HT1B/1D receptor antago-nists and antidepressants in the forced swimming test. Eur. J. Pharmacol. 487, 133–142. doi: 10.1016/j.ejphar.2004.01.008

Taylor, B. P., Bruder, G. E., Stewart, J. W., McGrath, P. J., Halperin, J., Ehrlichman, H., et al. (2006). Psychomotor slowing as a predictor of fluoxetine nonresponse in depressed outpatients. Am. J. Psychiatry 163, 73–78. doi: 10.1176/appi.ajp.163.1.73

Tedeschini, E., Levkovitz, Y., Iovieno, N., Ameral, V. E., Nelson, J. C., and Papakostas, G. I. (2011). Efficacy of antidepressants for late-life depression: a meta-analysis and meta-regression of placebo-controlled randomized trials. J. Clin. Psychiatry 72, 1660–1668. doi: 10.4088/JCP.10r06531

Thase, M. E., and Rush, A. J. (1997). When at first you don't succeed: sequential strategies for antidepressant nonresponders. J. Clin. Psychiatry 58(Suppl. 13), 23–29.

Tondo, L., Baldessarini, R. J., Vázquez, G., Lepri, B., and Visioli, C. (2013). Clinical responses to antidepressants among 1036 acutely depressed patients with bipolar or unipolar major affective disorders. Acta Psychiatr. Scand. 127, 355–364. doi: 10.1111/acps.12023

Trillat, A. C., Malagié, I., Bourin, M., Jacquot, C., Hen, R., and Gardier, A. M. (1998). Homozygote mice deficient in serotonin 5-HT1B receptor and antide-pressant effect of selective serotonin reuptake inhibitors. C. R. Seances Soc. Biol. Fil. 192, 1139–1147.

Trivedi, M. H., Rush, A. J., Wisniewski, S. R., Nierenberg, A. A., Warden, D., Ritz, L., et al. (2006). Evaluation of outcomes with citalopram for depression using measurement-based care in STAR*D: implications for clinical practice. Am. J. Psychiatry 163, 28–40. doi: 10.1176/appi.ajp.163.1.28

Tronel, S., Belnoue, L., Grosjean, N., Revest, J. M., Piazza, P. V., Koehl, M., and Abrous, D. N. (2012). Adult-born neurons are necessary for extended contextual discrimination. Hippocampus 22, 292–298. doi: 10.1002/hipo. 20895

Trouche, S., Bontempi, B., Roullet, P., and Rampon, C. (2009). Recruitment of adult-generated neurons into functional hippocampal networks contributes to updating and strengthening of spatial memory. Proc. Natl. Acad. Sci. U.S.A. 106, 5919–5924. doi: 10.1073/pnas.0811054106

Tsai, S. J., Gau, Y. T., Hong, C. J., Liou, Y. J., Yu, Y. W., and Chen, T. J. (2009). Sexually dimorphic effect of catechol-O-methyltransferase val158met polymor-phism on clinical response to fluoxetine in major depressive patients. J. Affect. Disord. 113, 183–187. doi: 10.1016/j.jad.2008.04.017

Tsai, S. J., Hong, C. J., Chen, T. J., and Yu, Y. W. (2007). Lack of supporting evidence for a genetic association of the FKBP5 polymorphism and response to antidepressant treatment. Am. J. Med. Genet. B. Neuropsychiatr. Genet. 144B, 1097–1098. doi: 10.1002/ajmg.b.30246

Ueda, K., Okamura, N., Hirai, M., Tanigawara, Y., Saeki, T., Kioka, N., et al. (1992). Human P-glycoprotein transports cortisol, aldosterone, and dexamethasone, but not progesterone. J. Biol. Chem. 267, 24248–24252.

Ueda, N., Yoshimura, R., Umene-Nakano, W., Ikenouchi-Sugita, A., Hori, H., Hayashi, K., et al. (2009). Grapefruit juice alters plasma sertraline levels after single ingestion of sertraline in healthy volunteers. World J. Biol. Psychiatry 10(4 Pt 3), 832–835. doi: 10.1080/15622970802688069

Uhr, M., and Grauer, M. T. (2003). abcb1ab P-glycoprotein is involved in the uptake of citalopram and trimipramine into the brain of mice. J. Psychiatr. Res.

37, 179–185. doi: 10.1016/S0022-3956(03)00022-0

Uhr, M., Grauer, M. T., and Holsboer, F. (2003). Differential enhancement of antidepressant penetration into the brain in mice with abcb1ab (mdr1ab) P-glycoprotein gene disruption. Biol. Psychiatry 54, 840–846. doi: 10.1016/S0006-3223(03)00074-X

Uhr, M., Holsboer, F., and Müller, M. B. (2002). Penetration of endogenous steroid hormones corticosterone, cortisol, aldosterone and progesterone into the brain is enhanced in mice deficient for both mdr1a and mdr1b P-glycoproteins. J. Neuroendocrinol. 14, 753–759. doi: 10.1046/j.1365-2826.2002.00836.x

Uhr, M., Steckler, T., Yassouridis, A., and Holsboer, F. (2000). Penetration of amitriptyline, but not of fluoxetine, into brain is enhanced in mice with blood-brain barrier deficiency due to mdr1a P-glycoprotein gene disruption. Neuropsychopharmacology 22, 380–387. doi: 10.1016/S0893-133X(99)00095-0

Uhr, M., Tontsch, A., Namendorf, C., Ripke, S., Lucae, S., Ising, M., et al. (2008). Polymorphisms in the drug transporter gene ABCB1 predict antide-pressant treatment response in depression. Neuron 57, 203–209. doi: 10.1016/j.neuron.2007.11.017

Ulrich, G., Renfordt, E., and Frick, K. (1986). The topographical distribution of alpha-activity in the resting EEG of endogenous-depressive inpatients with and without clinical-response to pharmacotherapy. Pharmacopsychiatry 19, 272–273. doi: 10.1055/s-2007-1017230

Van Rossum, E. F., Binder, E. B., Majer, M., Koper, J. W., Ising, M., Modell, S., et al. (2006). Polymorphisms of the glucocorticoid receptor gene and major depression. Biol. Psychiatry 59, 681–688. doi: 10.1016/j.biopsych.2006.02.007

Vázquez, G. H., Tondo, L., Undurraga, J., and Baldessarini, R. J. (2013). Overview of antidepressant treatment of bipolar depression. Int. J. Neuropsychopharmacol. 22, 1–13. doi: 10.1017/S1461145713000023

Vergouwen, A. C., Bakker, A., Katon, W. J., Verheij, T. J., and Koerselman, F. (2003). Improving adherence to antidepressants: a systematic review of interventions. J. Clin. Psychiatry 64, 1415–1420. doi: 10.4088/JCP.v64n1203

Vermeiden, M., van den Broek, W. W., Mulder, P. G., and Birkenhäger, T. K. (2010). Influence of gender and menopausal status on antidepressant treat-ment response in depressed inpatients. J. Psychopharmacol. 24, 497–502. doi: 10.1177/0269881109105137

Vialou, V., Robison, A. J., Laplant, Q. C., Covington, H. E. 3rd, Dietz, D. M., et al. (2010). DeltaFosB in brain reward circuits mediates resilience to stress and antidepressant responses. Nat. Neurosci. 13, 745–752. doi: 10.1038/ nn.2551

Wang, J. S., Zhu, H. J., Gibson, B. B., Markowitz, J. S., Donovan, J. L., and DeVane, C. L. (2008a). Sertraline and its metabolite desmethylsertraline, but not bupropion or its three major metabolites, have high affinity for P-glycoprotein. Biol. Pharm. Bull. 31, 231–234. doi: 10.1248/bpb.31.231

Wang, J. W., David, D. J., Monckton, J. E., Battaglia, F., and Hen, R. (2008b). Chronic fluoxetine stimulates maturation and synaptic plasticity of adult-born hippocampal granule cells. J. Neuroscience 28, 1374–1384. doi: 10.1523/JNEUROSCI.3632-07.2008

Warner-Schmidt, J. L., Chen, E. Y., Zhang, X., Marshall, J. J., Morozov, A., Svenningsson, P., et al. (2010). A role for p11 in the antidepressant action of brainderived neurotrophic factor. Biol. Psychiatry 68, 528–535. doi: 10.1016/j.biopsych.2010.04.029

Warner-Schmidt, J. L., Flajolet, M., Maller, A., Chen, E. Y., Qi, H., Svenningsson, P., et al. (2009). Role of p11 in cellular and behavioral effects of 5-HT4 recep-tor stimulation. J. Neurosci. 29, 1937–1946. doi: 10.1523/JNEUROSCI.5343-08.2009

Warner-Schmidt, J. L., Vanover, K. E., Chen, E. Y., Marshall, J. J., and Greengard, P. (2011). Antidepressant effects of selective serotonin reuptake inhibitors (SSRIs) are attenuated by antiinflammatory drugs in mice and humans. Proc. Natl. Acad. Sci. U.S.A. 108, 9262–9267. doi: 10.1073/pnas.1104836108

Weiss, J., Dormann, S. M., Martin-Facklam, M., Kerpen, C. J., Ketabi-Kiyanvash, N., and Haefeli, W. E. (2003). Inhibition of P-glycoprotein by newer antide-pressants. J. Pharmacol. Exp. Ther. 305, 197–204. doi: 10.1124/jpet.102. 046532

Williams, G. R. (2008). Neurodevelopmental and neurophysiological actions of thyroid hormone. J. Neuroendocrinol. 20, 784–794. doi: 10.1111/j.1365-2826.2008.01733.x

Wilson, I. C., Prange, A. J. Jr., and Lara, P. P. (1974). "Triiodothyronine alone and with imipramine in the treatment of depressed women," in The Thyroid Axis, Drugs and Behavior, ed A. J. Prange (New York, NY: Raven Press), 49–61.

Winner, J., Allen, J. D., Altar, C. A., and Spahic-Mihajlovic, A. (2013). Psychiatric pharmacogenomics predicts health resource utilization of outpatients with anxiety and depression. Transl. Psychiatry 3, e242. doi: 10.1038/tp.2013.2

Wu, J., Buchsbaum, M. S., Gillin, J. C., Tang, C., Cadwell, S., Wiegand, M., et al. (1999). Prediction of antidepressant effects of sleep deprivation by metabolic rates in the ventral anterior cingulate and medial prefrontal cortex. Am. J. Psychiatry 156, 1149–1158.

Xu, Z., Zhang, Z., Shi, Y., Pu, M., Yuan, Y., Zhang, X., et al. (2011). Influence and interaction of genetic polymorphisms in catecholamine neurotransmitter sys-tems and early life stress on antidepressant drug response. J. Affect. Disord. 133, 165–173. doi: 10.1016/j.jad.2011.04.011

Yalcin, I., Aksu, F., and Belzung, C. (2005). Effects of desipramine and tramadol in a chronic mild stress model in mice are altered by yohimbine but not by pindolol. Eur. J. Pharmacol. 514, 165–174. doi: 10.1016/j.ejphar.2005.03.029

Yin, O. Q., Wing, Y. K., Cheung, Y., Wang, Z. J., Lam, S. L., Chiu, H. F., et al. (2006). Phenotype-genotype relationship and clinical effects of citalopram in Chinese patients. J. Clin. Psychopharmacol. 26, 367–372. doi: 10.1097/01.jcp.0000227355.54074.14

Young, E. A., Haskett, R. F., Murphy-Weinberg, V., Watson, S. J., and Akil, H. (1991). Loss of glucocorticoid fast feedback in depression. Arch. Gen. Psychiatry 48, 693–699. doi: 10.1001/archpsyc.1991.01810320017003

Yu, H., Wang, D. D., Wang, Y., Liu, T., Lee, F. S., and Chen, Z. Y. (2012). Variant brain-derived neurotrophic factor Val66Met polymorphism alters vulnerability to stress and response to antide-pressants. J. Neurosci. 32, 4092–4101. doi: 10.1523/JNEUROSCI. 5048-11.2012

Yu, Y. W., Tsai, S. J., Hong, C. J., Chen, T. J., Chen, M. C., and Yang, C. W. (2005). Association study of a monoamine oxidase a gene promoter polymorphism with major depressive disorder and antidepressant response. Neuropsychopharmacology 30, 1719–1723. doi: 10.1038/sj.npp.1300785

Zhang, H. T., Whisler, L. R., Huang, Y., Xiang, Y., and O'Donnell, J. M. (2009). Postsynaptic alpha-2 adrenergic receptors are critical for the antidepressant-like effects of desipramine on behavior. Neuropsychopharmacology 34, 1067–1077. doi: 10.1038/npp.2008.184

Zhang, L., Li, H., Su, T. P., Barker, J. L., Maric, D., Fullerton, C. S., et al. (2008). p11 is up-regulated in the forebrain of stressed rats by gluco-corticoid acting via two specific glucocorticoid response elements in the p11 promoter. Neuroscience 153, 1126–1134. doi: 10.1016/j.neuroscience.2008.03.022

Zobel, A., Joe, A., Freymann, N., Clusmann, H., Schramm, J., Reinhardt, M., et al. (2005). Changes in regional cerebral blood flow by therapeutic vagus nerve stimulation in depression: an exploratory approach. Psychiatry Res. 139, 165–179. doi: 10.1016/j.pscychresns.2005.02.010

16

Relaxin-3/RXFP3 networks: an emerging target for the treatment of depression and other neuropsychiatric diseases

Craig M. Smith[1,2] *, Andrew W. Walker[1,2], Ihaia T. Hosken[1,2], Berenice E. Chua[1], Cary Zhang[1,2], Mouna Haidar[1,2] and Andrew L. Gundlach[1,2,3] *

[1] Peptide Neurobiology Laboratory, Neuropeptides Division, The Florey Institute of Neuroscience and Mental Health, The University of Melbourne, VIC, Australia
[2] Florey Department of Neuroscience and Mental Health, The University of Melbourne, VIC, Australia
[3] Department of Anatomy and Neuroscience, The University of Melbourne, VIC, Australia

Edited by:
Laurence Lanfumey, Institut National de la Santé et de la Recherche Médicale, France

Reviewed by:
Sara Morley-Fletcher, Centre National de la Recherche Scientifique-University Lille, France
Pascal Bonaventure, Janssen Research & Development, LLC, USA

***Correspondence:**
Craig M. Smith and Andrew L. Gundlach, Peptide Neurobiology Laboratory, Neuropeptides Division, The Florey Institute of Neuroscience and Mental Health, The University of Melbourne, 30 Royal Parade, Parkville, VIC 3052, Australia
e-mail: craig.smith@florey.edu.au; andrew.gundlach@florey.edu.au

Animal and clinical studies of gene-environment interactions have helped elucidate the mechanisms involved in the pathophysiology of several mental illnesses including anxiety, depression, and schizophrenia; and have led to the discovery of improved treatments. The study of neuropeptides and their receptors is a parallel frontier of neuropsychopharmacology research and has revealed the involvement of several peptide systems in mental illnesses and identified novel targets for their treatment. Relaxin-3 is a newly discovered neuropeptide that binds, and activates the G-protein coupled receptor, RXFP3. Existing anatomical and functional evidence suggests relaxin-3 is an arousal transmitter which is highly responsive to environmental stimuli, particularly neurogenic stressors, and in turn modulates behavioral responses to these stressors and alters key neural processes, including hippocampal theta rhythm and associated learning and memory. Here, we review published experimental data on relaxin-3/RXFP3 systems in rodents, and attempt to highlight aspects that are relevant and/or potentially translatable to the etiology and treatment of major depression and anxiety. Evidence pertinent to autism spectrum and metabolism/eating disorders, or related psychiatric conditions, is also discussed. We also nominate some key experimental studies required to better establish the therapeutic potential of this intriguing neuromodulatory signaling system, including an examination of the impact of RXFP3 agonists and antagonists on the overall activity of distinct or common neural substrates and circuitry that are identified as dysfunctional in these debilitating brain diseases.

Keywords: relaxin-3, RXFP3, neuropeptide, arousal, stress, mood and depression, autism spectrum disorders, eating disorders

INTRODUCTION

It has now become widely accepted by neuroscientists and the clinical community that mental illness can arise from multiple sources and causes, including genetic mutations or epigenetic effects, and key environmental impacts during early development, and adolescence. A need for an ongoing reappraisal of how best to study and classify mental illness is also acknowledged, including the development of circuit-level frameworks for understanding different modality deficits in depression (e.g., Nestler, 1998; Willner et al., 2013), autism spectrum disorders (ASD; e.g., Haznedar et al., 2000; Markram and Markram, 2010; Yizhar et al., 2011b; Fan et al., 2012), and schizophrenia (e.g., Spencer et al., 2003; O'Donnell, 2011; Millan et al., 2012; Jiang et al., 2013).

Similarly, novel structural and molecular targets in brain that might underpin better treatments for the debilitating conditions encompassed by the clinical spectrum of anxiety, major depression, and related psychiatric illnesses need to be identified and explored. In this regard, it is clear that neuromodulatory systems that utilize monoamine and peptide transmitters play a key role in the neurophysiology of circuits associated with affective behavior and cognition (Hoyer and Bartfai, 2012; Marder, 2012; van den Pol, 2012), and they can be both aberrant in psychiatric pathology and targets for novel treatments (e.g., Domschke et al., 2011; Hoyer and Bartfai, 2012; Lin and Sibille, 2013).

Relaxin-3 is a highly conserved neuropeptide that is abundantly expressed in four small groups of largely γ-aminobutyric acid (GABA) projection neurons in mammalian brain (Bathgate et al., 2002; Burazin et al., 2002; Tanaka et al., 2005), and is involved in regulating aspects of physiological and behavioral stress responses and the integration of sensory inputs (see Smith et al., 2011). Recent reviews have highlighted the putative role of relaxin-3 in the control of feeding and the neuroendocrine axis (Tanaka, 2010; Ganella et al., 2012, 2013b). However, existing neuroanatomical and functional evidence also suggests the GABA/relaxin-3 system acts as a broad "arousal" network which is highly responsive to environmental stimuli (neurogenic stressors) and modulates stress responses and other key behaviors/neural processes. These effects are mediated via a variety of mechanisms, such as influencing hippocampal theta rhythm and associated learning and memory, and via putative actions throughout the limbic system (Tanaka et al., 2005; Ma et al., 2009a, 2013; Banerjee et al., 2010). Here, in the broader context of the potential for neuropeptide-receptor systems as therapeutic drug targets (Hoyer and Bartfai, 2012), we review existing experimental data on relaxin-3 and modulation of its receptor, relaxin family peptide 3 receptor (RXFP3), in rodents and highlight its relevance to the etiology of various neuropsychiatric disorders.

NEUROPEPTIDE-RECEPTOR SYSTEMS AS TARGETS FOR TREATMENT OF NEUROPSYCHIATRIC DISORDERS

Since the early discovery of "substance P" (von Euler and Gaddum, 1931), a plethora of neuropeptide-receptor systems have been identified and characterized (see Hoyer and Bartfai, 2012). Neuropeptides are commonly co-released with GABA/glutamate and monoamine transmitters, and generally signal through G-protein coupled receptors to modulate a broad range of neural processes and behaviors. The potential attractiveness of neuropeptide-receptor systems as therapeutic drug targets is enhanced by their high level of signaling specificity. For example, expression of neuropeptides is often restricted to small populations of neurons within a small number of brain nuclei (e.g., orexin, MCH, and neuropeptide S; Xu et al., 2004; Sakurai, 2007; Saito and Nagasaki, 2008), and neuropeptides frequently bind to their receptors with high affinity and specificity due to their generally large allosteric binding sites (Hoyer and Bartfai, 2012). Neuropeptides are also often preferentially released under states of high neuronal firing frequency in response to the nervous system being challenged, as can occur during acute or chronic environmental stress and/or in association with neuropsychiatric disorders (Hökfelt et al., 2000, 2003; Holmes et al., 2003).

These characteristics suggest that therapeutic drugs which target neuropeptide systems may be less prone to unwanted "non-specific" side-effects compared to current drug treatments. For example, although tricyclic antidepressants are relatively effective at increasing 5-hydroxytrypamine (5-HT) and noradrenaline signaling to reduce the symptoms of major depression, they are hampered by cross-reactivity with other transmitter systems and reduce histamine and cholinergic signaling, which contributes to unwanted side effects (Westenberg, 1999). Even their "replacement" drugs (selective serotonin reuptake inhibitors, SSRIs) are associated with shortcomings such as slow onset of action and patient resistance, and side effects including sexual dysfunction, and weight gain (Nestler, 1998). Similar problems have been encountered in the development of antipsychotics to treat schizophrenia (Tandon, 2011), suggesting that more selective drugs that target relevant peptide receptors could have broad therapeutic applications (Hökfelt et al., 2003; Holmes et al., 2003; Hoyer and Bartfai, 2012).

Interest in the therapeutic potential of neuropeptide-receptor systems has further increased following a number of studies which implicate their dysregulation as contributing to disease susceptibility. For example, narcolepsy is strongly associated with reduced orexin signaling (Burgess and Scammell, 2012); post-traumatic stress syndrome (PTSD) susceptibility and panic has been linked to pituitary adenylate cyclase-activating polypeptide (PACAP) receptor-1 and corticotrophin-releasing factor (CRF) receptor-2 signaling (Ressler et al., 2011; Lebow et al., 2012; see also Dore et al., 2013); and neuropeptide Y (NPY) and CRF appear to play a role not only in the underlying pathophysiology of schizophrenia and depression, but as likely downstream mediators of the therapeutic effects following treatment with monoamine-targeting drugs (Arborelius et al., 1999; Ishida et al., 2007; Zorrilla and Koob, 2010; Nikisch et al., 2011). Not surprisingly, the antidepressant potential of drugs which directly target NPY and CRF signaling is currently under investigation (Paez-Pereda et al., 2011), while drugs that target receptors for neurotrophic factors and other neuropeptides, such as brain-derived neurotrophic factor (BDNF; Vithlani et al., 2013) and neuropeptide S (NPS; Pape et al., 2010), offer considerable promise as antidepressants and anxiolytics (Schmidt and Duman, 2010; McGonigle, 2011), in light of the effects of the native peptides in relevant animal models of neurogenesis, and neural structure and activity (Rotzinger et al., 2010; Pulga et al., 2012).

However, from a translational viewpoint, over the last two decades pharmaceutical and biotechnology groups have been attempting to target neuropeptide systems to treat various CNS disorders and despite encouraging pre-clinical data, clinical studies investigating the antidepressant potential of neuropeptide receptor-targeting drugs have yielded mixed findings. For example, the neurokinin 1 (NK_1) antagonist "aprepitant," which is effective at treating nausea during chemotherapy (de Wit et al., 2004), was unsuccessful in the treatment of major depression (Keller et al., 2006). CRF receptor-1 antagonists are also yet to demonstrate clear antidepressant properties (Binneman et al., 2008), although anxiolytic effects are promising (Bailey et al., 2011); and trials of these compounds against alcohol abuse and relapse are being undertaken (Zorrilla et al., 2013). NPY agonists were initially observed to inhibit circulating stress hormones during sleep in healthy controls (Antonijevic et al., 2000), while subsequent testing in depressed patients failed to confer therapeutic effects (Held et al., 2006). Although frustrating for industry *and* clinical and basic researchers, in regard to depression, these findings are more likely to reflect the complex underlying nature of the targeted disorder and its symptoms, rather than inherent flaws with neuropeptide-receptor systems as drug targets. Indeed, more recently, drugs that target orexin receptors have demonstrated promise in the treatment of sleep disorders (Hoyer and Jacobson, 2013; Winrow and Renger, 2014).

THE NEUROPEPTIDE RELAXIN-3 AND ITS RECEPTOR, RXFP3

Relaxin-3 is a two chain, 51 amino acid neuropeptide discovered by our laboratory in 2001 (Bathgate et al., 2002; Burazin et al., 2002; Rosengren et al., 2006). Relaxin-3 is the ancestral gene of the relaxin family of peptides (Wilkinson et al., 2005), which includes the namesake peptide "relaxin" (H2 relaxin or relaxin-2 in humans) that was observed to relax the pelvic ligament in guinea pigs almost a century ago (Hisaw, 1926). In contrast to the many and varied peripheral actions of relaxin (Sherwood, 2004; Bathgate et al., 2013a), relaxin-3 is abundantly expressed within the mammalian brain (Bathgate et al., 2002; Burazin et al., 2002) and acts as a neurotransmitter by activating its cognate G-protein coupled receptor, RXFP3 [also known as GPCR135, SALPR, and GPR100; Matsumoto et al., 2000; Liu et al., 2003; Boels et al., 2004; see Bathgate et al., 2006, 2013a]. Although research in this area is still in its relative infancy (Smith et al., 2011), several key features have highlighted relaxin-3/RXFP3 systems as an attractive putative target for the treatment of cognitive deficits, and neuropsychiatric disorders, including depression.

Neuroanatomical studies conducted in the rat (Burazin et al., 2002; Tanaka et al., 2005; Ma et al., 2007), mouse (Smith et al., 2010) and macaque (Ma et al., 2009b,c) have revealed that relaxin-3 is mainly expressed within neurons of the pontine *nucleus incertus* (NI; Goto et al., 2001; Olucha-Bordonau et al., 2003; Ryan et al., 2011), while smaller populations are present in the pontine raphé, periaqueductal gray, and a region dorsal to the substantia nigra (see **Figure 1**). Relaxin-3 containing neurons in these areas innervate a broad range of target forebrain regions rich in RXFP3. NI relaxin-3 neurons are predominately GABAergic (Ma et al., 2007; Cervera-Ferri et al., 2012), and it is likely relaxin-3 signaling confers complimentary inhibitory effects to the primary transmitter, as in cell-based studies RXFP3 activation is linked to $G_{i/o}$ and reduces cAMP accumulation (van der Westhuizen et al., 2007). In recent electrophysiological experiments, however, RXFP3 activation was able to hyperpolarize *or* depolarize presumed RXFP3-positive neurons within the rat intergeniculate leaflet (Blasiak et al., 2013), suggesting the effect of receptor activation or inhibition may vary with the neurochemical phenotype and connectivity of the target neuron, as described for other peptides. RXFP3 activation also stimulates ERK1/2 MAP kinase and other pathways *in vitro* (van der Westhuizen et al., 2010), although related changes in gene expression or precise roles of RXFP3 signaling within distinct neuronal populations *in vivo* remain unknown.

The distribution of relaxin-3-positive axons and RXFP3 mRNA/binding sites within key midbrain, hypothalamic, limbic, and septohippocampal circuits of the rodent and primate brain (Ma et al., 2007, 2009b; Smith et al., 2010) suggests relaxin-3/RXFP3 neural networks represent an "arousal" system that modulates behavioral outputs such as feeding and the responses to stress; and associated neuronal processes including spatial and emotional memory and hippocampal theta rhythm (see **Figure 1**). These actions have been investigated in a number of functional studies in rodents (see Ma et al., 2009a; Smith et al., 2011; Ganella et al., 2012 for review). As numerous neuropsychiatric disorders are either associated with alterations in these processes and behaviors, and/or can be therapeutically treated by drugs which modulate these processes and behaviors (Mazure, 1998; Anand et al., 2005; McGonigle, 2011; Tandon, 2011; Millan et al., 2012), the relaxin-3/RXFP3 system has considerable potential as a novel therapeutic target and warrants further investigation.

RELAXIN-3/RXFP3 SIGNALING: A NOVEL TARGET FOR THE TREATMENT OF DEPRESSION?

IS RELAXIN-3 IS AN "AROUSAL" TRANSMITTER?

Wakefulness, along with highly aroused behavioral states such as when an animal is alert, attentive, active, or engaged in exploratory behavior, are mediated by the interactive signaling of a range of "arousal" neurotransmitters (Saper et al., 2005). Several arousal transmitters and their associated neural networks and single or multiple target receptors have been identified, including the monoamines 5-HT, acetylcholine, noradrenaline, and dopamine (Nestler, 1998; Saper et al., 2005; Berridge et al., 2012), and the peptides orexin, melanin-concentrating hormone (MCH) NPY, CRF, and NPS (Hökfelt et al., 2003; Xu et al., 2004; Ishida et al., 2007; Sakurai, 2007; Zee and Manthena, 2007; Bittencourt, 2011). Indeed, it is now widely thought, based particularly on studies using optogenetic control of neural pathways, that selective spatiotemporal recruitment and coordinated activity of various cell type-specific brain circuits may underlie the neural integration of reward, learning, arousal, and feeding.

As mentioned, considerable neuroanatomical evidence suggests relaxin-3 should be thought of as an arousal neurotransmitter. For example, relaxin-3 neurons project to several areas that regulate arousal, such as the midbrain, cortex, thalamus, and limbic and septohippocampal regions, in a similar way as the monoamine and other peptide arousal systems (Ma et al., 2007; Smith et al., 2010, 2011). In fact, the "restricted" localization of relaxin-3 (GABA) neurons and the broadly distributed relaxin-3 projections throughout the brain are remarkably similar to those of the raphé/5-HT (Steinbusch, 1981; Monti and Jantos, 2008; Lesch and Waider, 2012) and locus coeruleus/noradrenaline (Jones et al., 1977; Takagi et al., 1980; Berridge et al., 2012) pathways/networks.

Arousal neurotransmitter systems are extensively interconnected, and relaxin-3 fibers, and RXFP3 are enriched within the pedunculopontine/laterodorsal tegmentum and basal forebrain, periaqueductal gray and lateral hypothalamus; which contain interconnected populations of neurons which produce acetylcholine, dopamine and orexin/MCH, respectively (Saper et al., 2005). Furthermore, along with 5-HT and orexin fibers and receptors (Meyer-Bernstein and Morin, 1996; Marchant et al., 1997; Peyron et al., 1998; Thankachan and Rusak, 2005; Pekala et al., 2011), relaxin-3 fibers/RXFP3 are enriched within the sensory and photic integrative thalamic center, known as the intergeniculate leaflet (Harrington, 1997; Morin, 2013), and application of an RXFP3 agonist can excite (depolarize) NPY neurons within this region (Blasiak et al., 2013), which project to the suprachiasmatic nucleus and promote wakefulness (Shinohara et al., 1993; Thankachan and Rusak, 2005; Zee and Manthena, 2007). Furthermore, rat NI relaxin-3 neurons express the 5-HT_{1A} receptor (and possibly other 5-HT receptors), and chronic 5-HT depletion increased relaxin-3 mRNA in the NI (Miyamoto et al., 2008); while in preliminary electrophysiological studies, bath application of orexin activated rat NI relaxin-3 neurons in a brain slice preparation (Blasiak et al., 2010).

Indeed, arousal and stress transmitter systems, including CRF and orexin peptides and their receptors, have long been implicated in reward and drug seeking behavior (Koob, 2010; Kim et al., 2012) and we recently demonstrated that antagonism of RXFP3 in brain – specifically within the bed nucleus of the stria terminalis – reduced self-administration of alcohol and cue- and stress (yohimbine)-induced relapse in alcohol-preferring iP rats (Ryan

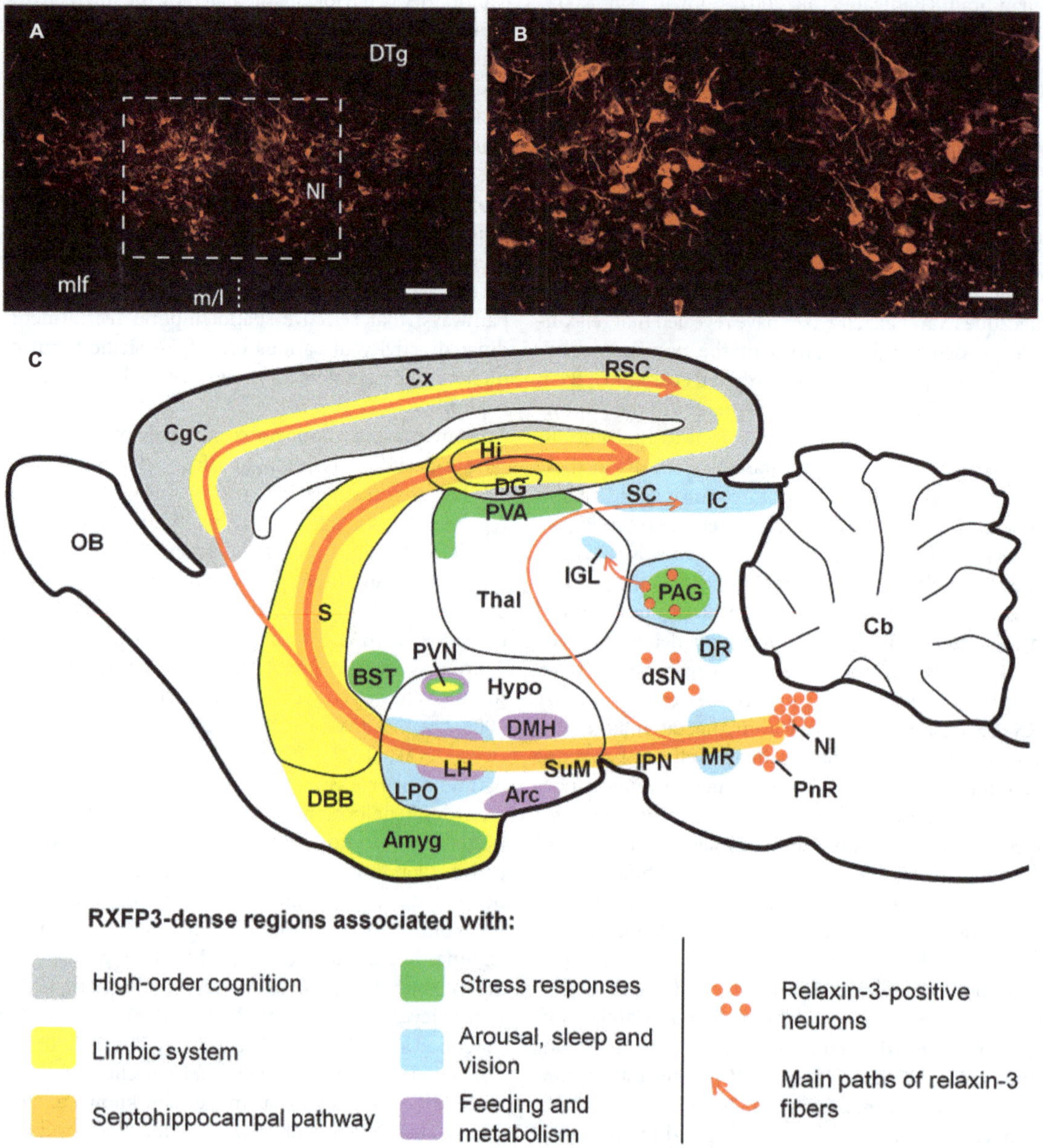

FIGURE 1 | (A,B) Low and high magnification micrographs of a coronal section through the mouse NI, displaying neurons positive for relaxin-3-like fluorescent immunoreactivity. The region displayed in **(B)** is outlined in **(A)**. The location of the midline (m/l) is indicated with a dotted line. Anterior-posterior coordinates from bregma, −5.38 mm. Scale bars **A**, 100 μm; **B**, 250 μm. **(C)** Schematic parasagittal representation of the rodent brain, illustrating the ascending relaxin-3 system and the distribution of RXFP3 in regions grouped by function. Amyg, amygdala; Arc, arcuate nucleus; BST, bed nucleus of stria terminalis; Cb, cerebellum; CgC, cingulate cortex; Cx, cerebral cortex; DBB, diagonal band of Broca; DG, dentate gyrus; DMH, dorsomedial nucleus of hypothalamus; DR, dorsal raphé nucleus; dSN, region dorsal to the substantia nigra; DTg, dorsal tegmental nucleus; Hi, hippocampus; Hypo, hypothalamus; IC, inferior colliculus; IGL, intergeniculate leaflet; IPN, interpeduncular nucleus; LH, lateral hypothalamus; LPO, lateral preoptic area; MLF, medial longitudinal fasciculus; MR, median raphé; NI, nucleus incertus; OB, olfactory bulb; PAG, periaqueductal gray; PnR, pontine raphé; PVA, paraventricular thalamic area; PVN, paraventricular hypothalamic nucleus; RSC, retrosplenial cortex; S, septum; SC, super colliculus; SuM, supramammillary nucleus; Thal, thalamus.

et al., 2013b). As monoamines (Nutt et al., 1999; Berridge et al., 2012) and peptides (Nemeroff, 1992; Brundin et al., 2007; McGonigle, 2011) are established or putative targets for the development of antidepressant drugs (Willner et al., 2013), the status of relaxin-3/RXFP3 as a similar and likely interconnected arousal system suggests a similar therapeutic potential.

Abnormal sleep and the disruption of circadian rhythm are common symptoms of the major neurodegenerative diseases (Hastings and Goedert, 2013) and neurological disorders such as depression (Berger et al., 2003), schizophrenia (Van Cauter et al., 1991), and anxiety (Monti and Monti, 2000), and the success of current pharmacological treatments for these diseases appears to be mediated in part through normalizing these symptoms (McClung, 2007). In line with neuroanatomical features, a number of functional studies suggest that relaxin-3 signaling promotes wakefulness. In rats, relaxin-3 mRNA displays a circadian pattern of expression which peaks during the dark/active phase (Banerjee et al., 2005), and intracerebroventricular (icv) infusion of an RXFP3 agonist during the light/inactive phase has been reported to increase locomotor activity (Sutton et al., 2009). These data were partly replicated in mice, in which chronic virally mediated delivery of an RXFP3 agonist into the cerebroventricular system slowed the decline in locomotor activity associated with habituation to a novel environment (Smith et al., 2013a). Mixed background (129S5:B6) relaxin-3 knockout (KO) mice were also hypoactive compared to wildtype littermate controls when placed in novel environments (Smith et al., 2009), and although this phenotype was not reproduced in C57BL/6J backcrossed colonies; during the dark/active phase backcrossed relaxin-3 KO mice traveled less distance on voluntary home-cage running wheels and appeared to spend more time sleeping than wildtype controls (Smith et al., 2012). These data are consistent with a possible regulation of circadian activity by relaxin-3/RXFP3 signaling in the IGL and network-induced changes in SCN activity (Blasiak et al., 2013), a possibility that is currently being explored in both wildtype and gene deletion mouse strains (Hosken et al., 2013).

RELAXIN-3 NEURONS ARE INVOLVED IN THE RESPONSE TO STRESS

A current view of the stress response is the behavioral and physiological changes generated in the face of, or in anticipation of, a perceived threat. The stress response involves activation of the sympathetic nervous system and recruitment of the hypothalamic-pituitary-adrenal (HPA) axis. When an animal encounters a social, physical or other stressor, these endogenous systems are stimulated and generate a "fight-or-flight" response to manage the "stressful" situation. Acutely, these changes are considered advantageous, but when an organism is subjected to prolonged or chronic stressors, the continuous irregularity in homeostasis is considered detrimental and leads to metabolic and behavioral disturbances (McEwen, 2007). Chronic stress is a well-known trigger for depression in humans, which often involves prolonged over-activation of the HPA axis, resulting in increased circulating glucocorticoids (Mazure, 1998; McEwen, 2007). Since its discovery in 1982 by the late Wylie Vale and others (Bittencourt, 2013), CRF has been shown to play a key role in the stress response *and* in major depression (Nemeroff, 1992; Arborelius et al., 1999; Paez-Pereda et al., 2011). A major source of CRF expression is the parvocellular neurons of the paraventricular hypothalamic nucleus (PVN) that project to the portal circulatory system. In response to stress, CRF is released which triggers the HPA axis by stimulating the release of adrenocorticotropic hormone (ACTH) by the pituitary gland. ACTH binds to receptors in the adrenal gland, which responds by secreting cortisol (corticosterone in rodents). CRF is also expressed within a number of other brain regions including the extended amygdala and the raphé nuclei (Cummings et al., 1983; Morin et al., 1999) and produces a range of extra-pituitary effects via CRF_1 and CRF_2 receptors that are broadly expressed throughout the brain (Chalmers et al., 1995; Van Pett et al., 2000).

Relaxin-3 neurons within the rat NI express high levels of CRF_1 receptor (Bittencourt and Sawchenko, 2000; Tanaka et al., 2005; Ma et al., 2013), and the majority of these neurons are activated (i.e., display increased relaxin-3 mRNA, Fos immunoreactivity and/or depolarization) following a restraint stress or icv injection of CRF (Tanaka et al., 2005; Lenglos et al., 2013; Ma et al., 2013). Relaxin-3 expression in the NI was also increased following a repeated swim stress, and this effect was blocked via pre-administration of the CRF_1 antagonist, antalarmin (Banerjee et al., 2010). NI neurons are also activated by a range of other stressors, including foot shock, treadmill running, and food deprivation (Ryan et al., 2011), although their impact on relaxin-3 expression has not been assessed. Similarly, the responsiveness of the other relaxin-3 neuron populations has not yet been investigated. The stress-responsiveness of relaxin-3 neurons appears highly conserved, as gene microarray analysis of three-spine stickleback fish revealed that exposure to a predator markedly increased relaxin-3 expression in the brain compared to controls (Sanogo et al., 2011).

Although the precise location and identity of the CRF neurons that innervate relaxin-3 neurons is unknown, the NI receives strong afferent inputs from the CRF-rich lateral and medial preoptic area (Lenglos et al., 2013; Ma et al., 2013), while the close proximity of the NI to the fourth ventricle suggests that volume transfer is also possible (Bittencourt and Sawchenko, 2000). Current data (Lenglos et al., 2013; Ma et al., 2013) and the plasticity of CRF *and* CRF receptor expression (see Dabrowska et al., 2013) suggest the level of CRF innervation and activation of the NI/(relaxin-3) cells may be altered under different physiological and pathological conditions, along with other aspects of their overall phenotype.

In addition to responding to stress, relaxin-3/RXFP3 signaling is able to modulate a variety of stress-related responses. In a recent report, C57B/6J backcrossed relaxin-3 KO mice were reported to display a "subtle decrease" in anxiety-like behavior compared to WT controls (Watanabe et al., 2011b), although a similar phenotype was not observed in a largely parallel study (Smith et al., 2012). In a more relevant set of experiments which highlight the anti-depressant potential of relaxin-3/RXFP3 signaling, icv infusion of a specific RXFP3 agonist reduced anxiety- and depressive-like behavior in rats (Ryan et al., 2013a). These findings have been partly corroborated by an independent study, which observed similar reductions in anxiety-like behavior following icv infusion of relaxin-3 in rats (Nakazawa et al., 2013). These pharmacological effects might be mediated, at least in part, by actions in the amygdala, which is largely responsible for conferring anxiety-related symptoms that are commonly experienced during depression (Holmes et al., 2012). The central and medial amygdala displays some of the highest densities of RXFP3 expression within the rodent brain (Ma et al., 2007; Smith et al., 2010), and injection of a specific RXFP3 agonist into the central amygdala reduced the characteristic freezing fear response displayed by rats when anticipating a foot shock following conventional auditory fear conditioning (Ma et al., 2010).

Relaxin family peptide 3 receptor expression is also highly enriched within the PVN (Ma et al., 2007; Smith et al., 2010), and icv injection of relaxin-3 in rats increased CRF and *c-fos* mRNA within the PVN and increased plasma ACTH, indicative of HPA axis activation (Watanabe et al., 2011a). These findings suggest that although the net sum of behavioral responses following "global" (or intra-amygdala) RXFP3 activation appears to be anxiolytic/antidepressant in nature (Nakazawa et al., 2013; Ryan et al., 2013a), RXFP3 signaling can in fact either promote or attenuate different aspects of the stress response, depending on the brain region modulated. This feature is shared with several other neuropeptides. For example, rodent studies have demonstrated that orexin and galanin signaling can either increase or decrease anxiety-like behavior, depending on the brain region(s) targeted (Bing et al., 1993; Möller et al., 1999; Lungwitz et al., 2012), while icv administration of NPS has been shown to decrease anxiety while increasing HPA axis activity (Xu et al., 2004; Smith et al., 2006). NPY (possibly from the arcuate nucleus) can activate the HPA axis via NPY Y1 receptors expressed on PVN CRF neurons (Albers et al., 1990; Dimitrov et al., 2007); but icv administration of NPY and a specific Y1 agonist inhibits fear behavior during contextual fear conditioning (Lach and de Lima, 2013).

High densities of relaxin-3-positive fibers and RXFP3 mRNA/binding sites are also present within several other brain structures that contribute to the central stress response and have been implicated in the etiology of anxiety and depression (Ma et al., 2007; Smith et al., 2010), including the: (i) *dorsal raphé*, which contains stress-responsive 5-HT neurons that are critical for determining depression susceptibility and recovery (Zhang et al., 2012; Challis et al., 2013); (ii) *hippocampus*, which expresses high densities of glucocorticoid receptors and often displays reduced volume and neurogenesis and impaired function in depressed patients (Manji et al., 2003; Videbech and Ravnkilde, 2004; Willner et al., 2013); (iii) *periaqueductal gray*, which is involved in fear behavior and associated autonomic responses (Vianna et al., 2001), and which contains relaxin-3 neurons positive for $CRF_{1/2}$ immunoreactivity (Blasiak et al., 2013); (iv) *bed nucleus of the stria terminalis*, which constitutes a stress integration center that contains CRF-expressing and other peptide containing GABA/glutamate neurons, which strongly influence the PVN and are reportedly dysfunctional in several psychiatric disorders, including depression, anxiety-disorders, and addiction (Dunn, 1987; Walker et al., 2009; Koob, 2010; Lebow et al., 2012; Crestani et al., 2013; Zheng and Rinaman, 2013); (v) *medial preoptic area*, in which neurons also express high levels of CRF and strongly project to and influence the PVN (Marson and Foley, 2004; Lenglos et al., 2013); (vi) *lateral habenula*, a key structure mediating the response to emotionally negative states (Willner et al., 2013), in which neuron activity was shown recently to be regulated by levels of β-CaMK II expression and to be sufficient to either induce or alleviate depressive-like symptoms in rodents, depending on whether these neurons were activated or inhibited, respectively (Li et al., 2013); (vii) *anterior cingulate cortex*, which acts to stabilize emotional responses via inhibitory projections to the amygdala that are often reduced in depressed patients (Anand et al., 2005; Willner et al., 2013) and; (viii) *medial prefrontal cortex*, which is dysfunctional in depressed patients and strongly projects to the PVN and amygdala to suppress behavioral responses to stress (Espejo and Minano, 1999). The medial prefrontal cortex is of additional interest, as it forms a main source of afferent input into the NI (Goto et al., 2001). A recent study has also demonstrated that stimulation of CRF_1 positive NI neurons that project to the medial prefrontal cortex (either electrophysiologically or via administration of CRF) act to inhibit this region, while electrical or CRF-mediated stimulation of the whole NI impaired long term potentiation within the hippocampo-prelimbic medial prefrontal cortical pathway (Farooq et al., 2013).

RELAXIN-3 NEURONS MODULATE HIPPOCAMPAL ACTIVITY

A key feature of hippocampal function is a state of synchronous neuronal firing at theta rhythm (4–10 Hz in humans), which is required for the hippocampus to mediate its important roles in memory formation and retrieval, spatial navigation, and rapid eye movement (REM) sleep (Vertes and Kocsis, 1997). Hippocampal function is disrupted by elevated circulating glucocorticoids during chronic stress, which can contribute to the cognitive deficits seen in depression (Murphy et al., 2001; Clark et al., 2009). Furthermore, a common hallmark of depression is stress-related increases in REM sleep (Kimura et al., 2010), which is robustly reduced to normal levels following antidepressant treatment (Argyropoulos and Wilson, 2005), an effect partly mediated by 5-HT signaling (Adrien, 2002). In light of the critical role that hippocampal theta rhythm plays in normal neurological function and its propensity for disruption in disease states, it is not surprising that almost all currently available anxiolytic and pro-cognitive drugs alter hippocampal theta rhythm (McNaughton and Gray, 2000). It has in fact been suggested that this feature can be used as an "output" for screening the potential effectiveness of new psychoactive drugs (McNaughton et al., 2007).

The ability of ascending brainstem nuclei such as the *reticularis pontis oralis* (RPO) and median raphé to modulate hippocampal theta rhythm is well established. These functions are mediated not only by projections to the hippocampus, but also via innervation of several "nodes" of the septohippocampal system such as the interpeduncular nucleus (IPN), supramammillary nucleus, posterior hypothalamus, and medial septum (Vertes and Kocsis, 1997). In particular, the medial septum has been termed the hippocampal theta rhythm "pace-maker" and contains populations of cholinergic and GABAergic neurons which provide alternating synchronous excitatory/inhibitory input to reciprocally connected hippocampal neurons (Vertes and Kocsis, 1997; Wang, 2002; Hangya et al., 2009). The NI sits adjacent to, and is strongly interconnected with, the RPO, median raphé and IPN, and efferent relaxin-3-positive projections innervate the hippocampus and the major nodes of the septohippocampal pathway (Ma et al., 2007; Teruel-Marti et al., 2008; Smith et al., 2010; Cervera-Ferri et al., 2012), including the medial septum which displays a high density of relaxin-3 immunoreactive fibers and terminals which make synaptic contacts with hippocampal-projecting cholinergic and GABAergic neurons in the rat (Olucha-Bordonau et al., 2012).

Functional studies have confirmed the regulation of hippocampal theta rhythm by the NI. In anesthetized rats, electrical stimulation of the NI induced hippocampal theta rhythm, whereas electrolytic lesion of the NI blocked the ability of the RPO to generate hippocampal theta rhythm (Nunez et al., 2006; Teruel-Marti et al., 2008). In conscious rats with electrolytic lesions of the NI, theta-dependent behaviors are impaired such as the acquisition of fear extinction in a contextual auditory conditioned fear paradigm (Pereira et al., 2013). Simultaneous recording of hippocampal and NI field potentials (Cervera-Ferri et al., 2011) and electrophysiological recording of NI neurons (Ma et al., 2013) have also revealed that these two structures are "theta-synchronized" and individual neurons display coherent firing. Although it is likely that these actions are primarily conferred by GABA (or to a much lesser extent, glutamate) transmission of these septohippocampal-projecting NI neurons (Ma et al., 2007; Cervera-Ferri et al., 2012), relaxin-3/RXFP3 signaling nonetheless appears capable of contributing to this functional effect. Our laboratory has shown that local infusion of an RXFP3 agonist into the medial septum of anesthetized rats promotes hippocampal theta rhythm, while medial septum infusion of an RXFP3 antagonist in conscious rats inhibits hippocampal theta and theta-dependent spatial memory measured in a spontaneous alternation task (Ma et al., 2009a).

RELEVANCE OF RELAXIN-3/RXFP3 SIGNALING TO SOCIAL BEHAVIOR AND AUTISM?

In rodents, social behavior is highly dependent upon three aspects of brain function: (i) *arousal*, which is required for motivation to engage in social contact, and mediates appropriate mood responses (Crawley et al., 1981); (ii) *stress responses*, which regulate levels of social withdrawal/anxiety (File and Seth, 2003) and; (iii) *exploration and social recognition*, which is associated with hippocampal theta rhythm activity (Maaswinkel et al., 1997). Notably, relaxin-3 has been demonstrated to modulate all of these behavioral aspects.

Abnormal social behavior is associated with depression and is a key symptom of ASD (Millan et al., 2012; Bishop-Fitzpatrick et al., 2013). Human imaging studies indicate that autism is often characterized by structural abnormalities in limbic structures such as the hippocampus (Haznedar et al., 2000; Ohnishi et al., 2000), which according to post-mortem studies consists of principal neurons that are smaller in size and are more densely packed (Bauman and Kemper, 2005). The amygdala is another major limbic structure that has been the focus of many human (van Elst et al., 2000) and animal (Amaral et al., 2003) studies of social aggression, and in rodent models of autism, hyperexcitability and enhanced long term potentiation in lateral amygdala neurons has been reported (Lin et al., 2013). Reduced activity of the anterior cingulate cortex has been observed in human autistic patients, which is correlated with deficits in attention and executive control (Fan et al., 2012). The PVN is another major limbic structure relevant to autism partly due to the presence of oxytocin neurons, which are crucial for mother-infant bonding (Mogi et al., 2010) and promote social interaction (Lukas et al., 2011). Autism is associated with loss of PVN oxytocin neurons (McNamara et al., 2008), and oxytocin is displaying considerable promise in clinical treatment of this disorder (Yamasue et al., 2012). The PVN also contains neurons that express vasopressin, which reciprocally interact with oxytocin neurons and strongly influence social behaviors such as aggression (Caldwell et al., 2008), suggesting similar therapeutic potential (Ring, 2011; Lukas and Neumann, 2013).

Relaxin-3/RXFP3 systems are well placed to modulate social behavior and other symptoms of ASD due to their presence throughout the limbic hippocampus, amygdala, anterior cingulate cortex, and PVN. Particularly intriguing, however, is the strong link between relaxin-3 and oxytocin. Oxytocin receptors are expressed within the rat and mouse NI (Vaccari et al., 1998; Yoshida et al., 2009), and microarray/peptidomics analysis revealed that the most striking neurochemical change that occurred within the rat hypothalamus following acute icv infusion of relaxin-3 and resultant activation of RXFP3 (and RXFP1) was a large (>10-fold) upregulation of oxytocin (Nakazawa et al., 2013). In contrast, chronic hypothalamic RXFP3 signaling resulted in an opposite effect, as viral-mediated hypothalamic delivery of an RXFP3 agonist for 3 months reduced hypothalamic oxytocin mRNA by ~50% (Ganella et al., 2013a). Whether some or all oxytocin neurons express RXFP3 or whether these effects are mediated in part or in full by indirect actions, remains to be determined experimentally. Similarly, vasopressin neurons may also be targeted by RXFP3 signaling (Ganella et al., 2013a).

Despite the potential for a role of relaxin-3/RXFP3 signaling in aspects of social behavior, only a single functional study has thus far been reported, which observed that compared to wildtype littermate controls, female 129S5:B6 mixed background relaxin-3 KO mice engaged in fewer encounters with a novel mouse in a social interaction test (Smith et al., 2009). Therefore, further studies including those that test the therapeutic potential of RXFP3 agonists in validated rodent models of major ASD symptoms are required. These might also include assessment of aggressive behavior, with the presence of RXFP3 in brain "defensive centers" such as the amygdala, PAG, and ventromedial hypothalamus (see Future Studies of Relaxin-3/RXFP3 System).

RELAXIN-3/RXFP3 CONTROL OF FEEDING AND RELEVANCE FOR EATING DISORDERS?

It is generally accepted that obesity has rapidly reached epidemic proportions, but is also one of the leading preventable causes of death worldwide. Notably, there is evidence that obesity associated metabolic signals markedly increase the odds of developing depression; and depressed mood not only impairs motivation, quality of life and overall functioning, but also further increases the risks of complications associated with obesity (Hryhorczuk et al., 2013). Therefore, curbing the global growth in obesity and associated health problems, and demands on public healthcare, is a major challenge which offers huge economic reward for agencies that develop effective treatments (Kopelman, 2000; Carter et al., 2012; Roux and Donaldson, 2012; Adan, 2013). Conversely, a smaller but important niche exists for the development of orexigenic agents to treat symptoms of decreased appetite and/or cachexia associated with cancer and its treatment, immune deficiency, and anorexia nervosa (Sodersten et al., 2006).

RXFP3 is present in several hypothalamic feeding centers in rat brain (Kishi and Elmquist, 2005) including the PVN (Liu et al., 2003), lateral hypothalamus, arcuate, and dorsomedial nuclei (Sutton et al., 2004; Ma et al., 2007). These data prompted a series of pharmacological studies which consistently demonstrated that relaxin-3 and selective RXFP3 agonist peptides are potently orexigenic in rats following acute delivery into the lateral cerebral ventricle (Liu et al., 2005, 2009; McGowan et al., 2005; Sutton et al., 2009; Shabanpoor et al., 2012; Hossain et al., 2013) or various hypothalamic regions (McGowan et al., 2007). Chronic delivery of RXFP3 agonists via repeated intra-PVN injection (McGowan et al., 2006), osmotic minipump (icv) infusion (Hida et al., 2006; Sutton et al., 2009), or viral constructs injected into the PVN (Ganella et al., 2013a) also reliably increase food consumption and bodyweight, and result in metabolic changes such as increased plasma levels of leptin, insulin, and adiponectin, and decreased plasma levels of growth hormone and thyroid stimulating hormone. Co-administration of RXFP3 antagonists are able to prevent the increases in feeding induced by acute RXFP3 agonist injections (Kuei et al., 2007; Haugaard-Jonsson et al., 2008), but a significant reduction in feeding behavior produced by acute blockade of endogenous relaxin-3/RXFP3 signaling in satiated *and* food restricted rats is yet to be reported; suggesting a graded impact on this heavily regulated homeostatic behavior. Furthermore, relaxin-3 KO mice (C57BL/6J background) do not display any overt differences in feeding or bodyweight under normal housing and dietary conditions (Watanabe et al., 2011b; Smith et al., 2012), despite an earlier report that mixed (129S5:B6) background relaxin-3 KO mice fed on a diet with higher than normal (moderate) fat content were largely resistant to the obesity observed in WT controls (Sutton et al., 2009). Clearly this is an important area for further research in normal and other suitable transgenic mice. A recent study suggested that relaxin-3/RXFP3 signaling may be more important under specific physiological conditions, as in stressed female rats with intermittent access to palatable liquid food, relaxin-3 expression in the NI was increased in food restricted versus *ad libitum* fed animals (Lenglos et al., 2013).

Increased feeding is a common side effect of antipsychotic medications (Theisen et al., 2003), and acute atypical (clozapine) and typical (chlorpromazine and fluphenazine) antipsychotic treatments increased the number of Fos-positive cells in the rat NI (Rajkumar et al., 2013). On this basis, it was hypothesized that increased NI activation may be partly responsible for the antipsychotic drug induced increase in feeding behavior, which if correct, would suggest that relaxin-3/RXFP3 signaling might also play a role. Further evidence supporting this theory comes from a gene association study, in which >400 schizophrenia patients undergoing treatment with antipsychotic medications were assessed, many of whom displayed co-morbid metabolic syndromes (Munro et al., 2012). Interestingly, a polymorphism within the RXFP3 gene was significantly associated with obesity, while one polymorphism in the relaxin-3 gene and two in the RXFP3 gene were significantly associated with hypercholesterolemia.

In another gene association study, members of a Puerto Rican family with schizophrenia had a mutation within a chromosome 5p locus, which had earlier been identified in similar studies of familial schizophrenia-like symptoms (Bespalova et al., 2005). This locus contains the RXFP3 gene, and although sequencing of the coding region and proximal promoter did not reveal functionally significant variants, further upstream or downstream promoter regions were not assessed. Antipsychotics block dopamine D2 receptors and are the primary therapy for psychotic, *positive* symptoms (hallucinations/delusions) of schizophrenia (Tandon, 2011; Castle et al., 2013). It is possible, however, that modulation of endogenous relaxin-3/RXFP3 signaling might reduce the severity of the *negative* affective symptoms and cognitive deficits displayed in schizophrenic patients. These putative roles might be mediated via actions within limbic structures to modulate relevant neural circuits that regulate theta and other frequency brain oscillations, to enhance attention, working, and episodic memory (Ma et al., 2009a; Millan et al., 2012). However, experimental evidence in support of this speculation is yet to be gathered.

Overall, given the enormity of the obesity epidemic and associated health problems and the lack of understanding of, and effective pharmacological therapies for, eating disorders such as anorexia nervosa, there is a strong justification for further studies that involve chronic manipulation of RXFP3 signaling to assess feeding, metabolism, and body weight.

FUTURE STUDIES OF THE RELAXIN-3/RXFP3 SYSTEM

Considerable experimental evidence obtained over the last decade suggests that endogenous relaxin-3/RXFP3 signaling promotes arousal and contributes to the central response to stress, and the highly conserved nature of this peptide/receptor system suggests it plays important biological roles. Current data suggest that drugs which act to increase relaxin-3/RXFP3 signaling are likely to have therapeutic/beneficial effects in a range of clinical conditions. Like many other complex neuromodulatory (peptide) systems, however, receptor modulation in different brain regions may confer differential effects; and in a therapeutic context, increased brain RXFP3 activation may produce both beneficial *and* "undesirable" effects. With RXFP3 agonists, in some disorders these may include increased HPA axis activity (Watanabe et al., 2011a) and bodyweight gain (McGowan et al., 2005; Ganella et al., 2012; Lenglos et al., 2013); while with RXFP3 antagonists these may include decreased arousal and motivation. Therefore, characterizing precise direct and indirect actions of relaxin-3/RXFP3 signaling within the major RXFP3-rich regions of the rodent brain remains an important long term goal. Similarly, neurons in the relaxin-3 rich NI express a large array of receptors for transmitters, and monoamine and peptide modulators (Blasiak et al., 2010; Ryan et al., 2011; Ma et al., 2013), and it will be important to carefully assess how these signals are integrated by the NI relaxin-3 system.

Studies which have centrally administered RXFP3 agonists have mainly employed the icv route, and although it is often assumed that peptides are able to access receptors throughout the whole brain (Bittencourt and Sawchenko, 2000), recent studies in our laboratory using fluorophore-conjugated relaxin family peptides suggest that periventricular regions such as the PVN may be exposed to higher concentrations of peptide (Chan et al., 2013). Although RXFP3 agonists or antagonists have been locally infused into the bed nucleus of the stria terminalis (Ryan et al., 2013b), central amygdala (Ma et al., 2010), medial septum (Ma et al., 2009a), and hypothalamic nuclei (McGowan et al., 2007) of rodents, in connection with actions on reward, fear, spatial memory, and feeding, respectively; many other RXFP3-rich brain regions including those distal to the ventricular system remain to be targeted, including the median raphé, superior and inferior colliculus, intergeniculate leaflet, IPN, supramammillary nucleus, diagonal band of Broca, fields within the dorsal and ventral hippocampus, and the retrosplenial and cingulate cortices (see **Figure 1**). Intranasal delivery may be a viable alternate route of peptide administration based on recent studies with insulin, oxytocin/vasopressin and NPS (e.g., Ionescu et al., 2012), but ultimately, characterization of the net effects of activating RXFP3 throughout the brain is required, using highly stable peptides or small synthetic molecules that cross the blood–brain barrier (Bathgate et al., 2013b) and can be administered systemically.

In addition to characterizing the function of relaxin-3/RXFP3 at a regional level, it is crucial to characterize the populations of neurons that express RXFP3 within each nucleus/region, and whether they are stimulated or inhibited following RXFP3 activation. Such functional data will provide valuable insights into the mechanisms of relaxin-3 action, but to date, this has only been partially achieved in the intergeniculate leaflet (Blasiak et al., 2013). Based on equivalent studies of similar systems such as the orexins, such features may be complicated, despite the relative simplicity of the one ligand/one receptor, relaxin-3/RXFP3 system.

In the context of arousal, an RXFP3-rich area of particular interest is the lateral hypothalamus (Ma et al., 2007; Smith et al., 2010). If it is assumed that RXFP3 activation *inhibits* receptor-positive neurons, then it is possible that relaxin-3/RXFP3 may promote arousal by directly inhibiting neurons which express MCH, which act to inhibit arousal (Saito and Nagasaki, 2008). Alternatively, activation of RXFP3 expressed on GABAergic interneurons which project to and inhibit orexin/dynorphin/(neurotensin) neurons in the area (Alam et al., 2005; Burt et al., 2011; Furutani et al., 2013), may indirectly disinhibit these neurons, increasing the activity of these arousal-promoting networks. If, however, RXFP3 signaling directly *stimulates* specific target neurons, these scenarios could be reversed. Similar hypothetical circuits can be conceived involving sleep active neurons that express galanin in the ventrolateral preoptic area (Gaus et al., 2002), 5-HT and non 5-HT neurons in the dorsal and median raphé (Morin and Meyer-Bernstein, 1999; Kirby et al., 2000; Kocsis et al., 2006), and a host of other systems throughout the brain (Smith et al., 2013b). Traditional immunohistochemical approaches to achieving this goal have been hampered, however, as sufficiently sensitive and specific antisera for RXFP3 are currently unavailable. An alternative approach has observed relaxin-3-positive fibers in the rat medial septum terminating on neurons expressing choline acetyltransferase, parvalbumin, and glutamate decarboxylase (Olucha-Bordonau et al., 2012); but this "indirect" method is labor intensive and future studies would benefit from the development of an RXFP3 antibody, or transgenic mice which express a reporter gene under the control of the RXFP3 promoter (e.g., Chee et al., 2013).

Acute icv infusion of an RXFP3 agonist decreased the time rats spent immobile in the Porsolt forced swim test (Ryan et al., 2013a), which is used to test for putative antidepressant drug action. However, more recently this measure of "depressive-like" behavior has been described as having poor predictive, face, and construct validity (Nestler and Hyman, 2010), particularly as such changes in behavior are evident in rodents following acute administration of SSRIs, while these drugs require chronic administration over weeks in humans before therapeutic effects are observed. It is also possible that the Porsolt paradigm, which was developed to test drugs that target monoamine systems, may not be optimal for assessing drugs that target neuropeptide receptors. Therefore, it will be important to test the antidepressant potential of acute and chronic delivery of RXFP3 agonists against behavioral measures such as anhedonia and aberrant reward-associated perception, and memory in additional validated rodent models of depression, such as the chronic unpredictable mild stress, chronic social defeat, and chronic methamphetamine withdrawal models (Nestler and Hyman, 2010; Russo and Nestler, 2013) and/or assess effects on brain activity patterns (McNaughton and Gray, 2000).

Similarly, it will be of interest to assess whether RXFP3 agonists (or antagonists) can improve social behavior in one or more of the rodent models of ASD, such as the commonly used BTBR (Silverman et al., 2010) and transgenic mouse strains (Peca et al., 2011). Determining whether RXFP3 antagonists are protective against the obesity and metabolic syndromes induced by high fat diets in rodents is also a logical and important goal (Panchal and Brown, 2011; Ganella et al., 2012).

These studies would benefit greatly from the development of small molecule RXFP3 agonists and antagonists with a stable *in vivo* half-life that can cross the blood–brain barrier, and hence could be administered peripherally. Such compounds would penetrate the brain more evenly and in a manner more closely resembling the method that would eventually be adopted in humans, rather than preferentially accessing regions near the ventricular system, which occurs following icv infusions. Peripheral delivery methods also circumvent the need for surgical implantation of indwelling guide cannulae in experimental studies. The development of such compounds has not been reported, however, despite initial efforts by some groups (e.g., Alvarez-Jaimes et al., 2012).

In the meantime, further experimental studies are likely to benefit from recently developed and novel methods to manipulate the relaxin-3/RXFP3 system. For example, the RXFP3 agonist "R3/I5" has been successfully delivered chronically into the PVN of rats using an adeno-associated viral construct (Ganella et al., 2013a), which improves upon previous studies which relied on repeated injections (McGowan et al., 2006) or osmotic minipump infusions of exogenous peptide (Hida et al., 2006; Sutton et al., 2009), which are stressful and invasive techniques that can potentially alter behavior. The development and study of conditional rxfp3 KO mice in which RXFP3 protein could be deleted either globally or within specific brain regions in adult mice would not only help characterize the regional role of endogenous relaxin-3/RXFP3 signaling, but should also prevent the "masking" of phenotypes which may occur due to developmental compensation in life-long relaxin-3 KO mice (Smith et al., 2012).

The clustered/restricted distribution of relaxin-3 neurons within the NI readily enables targeting of these neurons with injected viral constructs (Callander et al., 2012), which could be used to drive the expression of virally encoded genes of interest under the control of the relaxin-3 promoter (Tanaka et al., 2009). Cell type-specific expression of light-gated ion channels has become a powerful resource for the anatomical and functional deconstruction of neuronal networks and allows the structural dynamics and electrical activity of genetically defined neurons to be manipulated and analyzed on the millisecond timescale (Zhang et al., 2010; Yizhar et al., 2011a; Kalmbach et al., 2012). The overall function of relaxin-3 NI neurons could be similarly assessed via targeted expression of channelrhodopsins and related functional measures. Similarly, the expression in NI GABA/relaxin-3 expressing neurons of excitatory and inhibitory "Designer Receptors Exclusively Activated by Designer Drugs" (DREADDs; Nawaratne et al., 2008; Sasaki et al., 2011; Farrella and Roth, 2013; Wess et al., 2013) will allow the effects of acute and chronic activation/inhibition of these neurons on brain circuit activity and behavior to be conveniently studied in freely moving animals. These studies will be important in delineating whether in the NI, it is relaxin-3 or GABA signaling or GABA signaling specifically associated with the relaxin-3-expressing neurons that is primarily linked to effects on brain network activity and changes in behavior (see e.g., GABA/AgRP neurons in the arcuate nucleus in control of feeding (Atasoy et al., 2012; Liu et al., 2013).

For effective drug development in the future, the definition and characterization of depression and antidepressant drug treatment effects, currently based heavily on symptomatic criteria, needs to be improved, so that greater emphasis is placed on the underlying dysfunction at the circuit, neuron, and transmitter level (see Millan et al., 2012; Willner et al., 2013). In this regard, characterizing the potential involvement of novel transmitter systems such as relaxin-3 in the etiology of depression will be of interest. Although relaxin-3 and RXFP3 are genetically highly conserved between rodents and humans, more experiments are needed to demonstrate conserved functions of these signaling networks. The anatomical distribution of relaxin-3 and RXFP3 in non-human primate brain is very similar to that observed in rat and mouse (Ma et al., 2009b,c); and so "select" studies in non-human primates should be informative (Willard and Shively, 2012). Further studies of any potential involvement of relaxin-3 in the etiology of neurological or psychiatric diseases are also warranted (*c.f.* Lin and Sibille, 2013). For example, in addition to comprehensive searches for polymorphisms in the relaxin-3 or RXFP3 genes that might result in altered neurotransmission and affective behavior; once suitably validated assays for human relaxin-3 peptide and/or RXFP3 protein levels are available, studies to determine whether these are altered in patients who suffer from depression and other mental disorders could be completed, as potential markers for dysregulation of relaxin-3/RXFP3 related signaling. Any such findings would, based on prior experience with other peptide-receptor systems such as NPS and PACAP (Pape et al., 2010; Ressler et al., 2011), provide a significant stimulus to this relatively new area of research.

Finally, there are clear signs in the academic literature and emerging from government agencies and Pharma that the field of psychiatric disease research is entering a new era in relation to better understanding and improved drug and environmental-based treatments. This involves an emphasis on analyzing the neural circuitry that causes these brain diseases, rather than a reliance on more "isolated" conventional neurotransmitter and receptor based studies or isolated gene-based studies (Millan et al., 2012; Abbott, 2013; Insel et al., 2013a,b). Thus, newly identified signaling systems like relaxin-3/RXFP3 will need to be studied in the context of regulatory impacts on key neural circuits under physiological and pathological conditions in human (patient-relevant) and industry-validated experimental models, and demonstrate genuine efficacy to restore the required balance of excitatory/inhibitory transmission in one or more diseases.

However, given the relative paucity of new therapeutic drug discoveries in the field over the last several decades using "older style" techniques, this recent realization and redirection in psychiatric disease research in some way removes any disadvantage a "new, little investigated" system such as this might have over other more exhaustively explored systems. Certainly, based on what is known regarding the anatomical distribution of relaxin-3/RXFP3 networks and the prominent effects they can demonstrate on fundamental processes (such as coherent neural firing in the "septohippocampal system" and associated limbic circuits (Farooq et al., 2013; Ma et al., 2013) and effects on circadian activity related circuits (Smith et al., 2012; Blasiak et al., 2013), there is reason for optimism regarding its ability to be relevant therapeutically and to attract the attention of major Pharma.

CONCLUSION

The study of neuropeptide-receptor systems is a key area of neuropsychopharmacology research and has revealed the involvement of several peptide systems in mental illnesses, in addition to identifying novel targets for their treatment. Relaxin-3 is a highly conserved neuropeptide in mammalian brain. Relaxin-3 neurons located in the midbrain and pons, innervate a broad range of RXFP3-rich circuits (hypothalamic, septohippocampal, and limbic) to modify stress, arousal, and other modalities that are often dysfunctional in neuropsychiatric diseases. Therefore, further elucidating the full array of relaxin-3/RXFP3 network effects under normal and pathological conditions represents an important and promising research goal, which may eventually help meet the challenges and opportunities for improving the symptomatic treatment of sufferers of conditions such as anxiety and major depression, and the social and cognitive deficits in neurodevelopmental, and degenerative disorders, by restoring the required balance of excitatory/inhibitory transmission within the appropriate neural circuits.

ACKNOWLEDGMENTS

The research in the authors' laboratory reviewed here was supported by grants from the National Health and Medical Research Council (NHMRC) of Australia (509246, 1005988, and 1024885) and the Pratt and Besen Foundations, and by the Victorian Government Strategic Investment. Andrew L. Gundlach is an NHMRC (Australia) Senior Research Fellow and a Brain & Behavior Research Foundation (USA) NARSAD Independent Investigator. The authors acknowledge the contribution of their current and former colleagues to the relaxin-3 related research reviewed.

REFERENCES

Abbott, A. (2013). Novartis reboots brain division. Nature 502, 153–154. doi: 10.1038/502153a

Adan, R. A. H. (2013). Mechanisms underlying current and future anti-obesity drugs. Trends Neurosci. 36, 133–140. doi: 10.1016/j.tins.2012.12.001

Adrien, J. (2002). Neurobiological basis for the relation between sleep and depression. Sleep Med. Rev. 6, 341–351.

Alam, M. N., Kumar, S., Bashir, T., Suntsova, N., Methippara, M. M., Szymusiak, R., et al. (2005). GABA-mediated control of hypocretin-but not melanin-concentrating hormone-immunoreactive neurones during sleep in rats. J. Physiol. (Lond.) 563, 569–582. doi: 10.1113/jphysiol.2004.076927

Albers, H. E., Ottenweller, J. E., Liou, S. Y., Lumpkin, M. D., and Anderson, E. R. (1990). Neuropeptide Y in the hypothalamus: effect on corticosterone and single-unit activity. Am. J. Physiol. 258, R376–R382.

Alvarez-Jaimes, L., Sutton, S. W., Nepomuceno, D., Motley, S. T., Cik, M., Stocking, E., et al. (2012). In vitro pharmacological characterization of RXFP3 allosterism: an example of probe dependency. PLoS ONE 7:e30792. doi: 10.1371/journal.pone.0030792

Amaral, D. G., Bauman, M. D., Capitanio, J. P., Lavenex, P., Mason, W. A., Mauldin-Jourdain, M. L., et al. (2003). The amygdala: is it an essential component of the neural network for social cognition? Neuropsychologia 41, 517–522. doi: 10.1016/S0028-3932(02)00310-X

Anand, A., Li, Y., Wang, Y., Wu, J., Gao, S., Bukhari, L., et al. (2005). Activity and connectivity of brain mood regulating circuit in depression: a functional magnetic resonance study. Biol. Psychiatry 57, 1079–1088. doi: 10.1016/j.biopsych.2005.02.021

Antonijevic, I. A., Murck, H., Bohlhalter, S., Frieboes, R. M., Holsboer, F., and Steiger, A. (2000). Neuropeptide Y promotes sleep and inhibits ACTH and cortisol release in young men. Neuropharmacology 39, 1474–1481. doi: 10.1016/S0028-3908(00)00057-5

Arborelius, L., Owens, M. J., Plotsky, P. M., and Nemeroff, C. B. (1999). The role of corticotropin-releasing factor in depression and anxiety disorders. J. Endocrinol. 160, 1–12. doi: 10.1677/joe.0.1600001

Argyropoulos, S. V., and Wilson, S. J. (2005). Sleep disturbances in depression and the effects of antidepressants. Int. Rev. Psychiatry 17, 237–245. doi: 10.1080/09540260500104458

Atasoy, D., Betley, J. N., Su, H. H., and Sternson, S. M. (2012). Deconstruc-tion of a neural circuit for hunger. Nature 488, 172–177. doi: 10.1038/nature 11270

Bailey, J. E., Papadopoulos, A., Diaper, A., Phillips, S., Schmidt, M., van der Ark, P., et al. (2011). Preliminary evidence of anxiolytic effects of the CRF1 receptor antagonist R317573 in the 7.5% CO2 proof-of-concept exper-imental model of human anxiety. J. Psychopharmacol. 25, 1199–1206. doi: 10.1177/0269881111400650

Banerjee, A., Ma, S., Ortinau, S., Smith, C. M., Layfield, S., Burazin, T. C. D., et al. (2005). Relaxin-3 neurons in the nucleus incertus – projection patterns, response to swim stress and relaxin-3 neuronal signalling. Soc. Neurosci. Abstr. 35, 59.57.

Banerjee, A., Shen, P.-J., Ma, S., Bathgate, R. A. D., and Gundlach, A. L. (2010). Swim stress excitation of nucleus incertus and rapid induction of relaxin-3 expression via CRF1 activation. Neuropharmacology 58, 145–155. doi: 10.1016/j.neuropharm.2009.06.019

Bathgate, R. A. D., Halls, M. L., van der Westhuizen, E. T., Callander, G. E., Kocan, M., and Summers, R. J. (2013a). Relaxin family peptides and their receptors. Physiol. Rev. 93, 405–480. doi: 10.1152/physrev.00001.2012

Bathgate, R. A. D., Oh, M. H., Ling, W. J., Kaas, Q., Hossain, M. A., Gooley, P. R., et al. (2013b). Elucidation of relaxin-3 binding interactions in the extracellular loops of RXFP3. Front. Endocrinol. (Lausanne) 4:13. doi: 10.3389/fendo.2013. 00013

Bathgate, R. A. D., Ivell, R., Sanborn, B. M., Sherwood, O. D., and Summers, R. J. (2006). International Union of Pharmacology LVII: recommendations for the nomenclature of receptors for relaxin family peptides. Pharmacol. Rev. 58, 7–31. doi: 10.1124/pr.58.1.9

Bathgate, R. A. D., Samuel, C. S., Burazin, T. C. D., Layfield, S., Claasz, A. A., Reytomas, I. G., et al. (2002). Human relaxin gene 3 (H3) and the equivalent mouse relaxin (M3) gene. Novel members of the relaxin peptide family. J. Biol. Chem. 277, 1148–1157. doi: 10.1074/jbc.M1078 82200

Bauman, M. L., and Kemper, T. L. (2005). Neuroanatomic observations of the brain in autism: a review and future directions. Int. J. Dev. Neurosci. 23, 183–187. doi: 10.1016/j.ijdevneu.2004.09.006

Berger, M., Van Calker, D., and Riemann, D. (2003). Sleep and manipulations of the sleep-wake rhythm in depression. Acta Psychiatr. Scand. 108, 83–91. doi: 10.1034/j.1600-0447.108.s418.17.x

Berridge, C. W., Schmeichel, B. E., and España, R. A. (2012). Noradrener-gic modulation of wakefulness/arousal. Sleep Med. Rev. 16, 187–197. doi: 10.1016/j.smrv.2011.12.003

Bespalova, I. N., Angelo, G. W., Durner, M., Smith, C. J., Siever, L. J., Buxbaum, J. D., et al. (2005). Fine mapping of the 5p13 locus linked to schizophrenia and schizotypal personality disorder in a Puerto Rican family. Psychiatry Genet. 15, 205–210. doi: 10.1097/00041444-200509000-00012

Bing, O., Möller, C., Engel, J. A., Soderpalm, B., and Heilig, M. (1993). Anxiolytic-like action of centrally administered galanin. Neurosci. Lett. 164, 17–20. doi: 10.1016/0304-3940(93)90846-D

Binneman, B., Feltner, D., Kolluri, S., Shi, Y., Qiu, R., and Stiger, T. (2008). A 6-week randomized, placebo-controlled trial of CP-316,311 (a selective CRH1 antagonist) in the treatment of major depression. Am. J. Psychiatry 165, 617–620. doi: 10.1176/appi.ajp.2008.07071199

Bishop-Fitzpatrick, L., Minshew, N. J., and Eack, S. M. (2013). A systematic review of psychosocial interventions for adults with autism spectrum disorders. J. Autism Dev. Disord. 43, 687–694. doi: 10.1007/s10803-012-1615-8

Bittencourt, J. C. (2011). Anatomical organization of the melanin-concentrating hormone peptide family in the mammalian brain. Gen. Comp. Endocrinol. 172, 185–197. doi: 10.1016/j.ygcen.2011.03.028

Bittencourt, J. C. (2013). The tale of a person and a peptide: Wylie W. Vale Jr. and the role of corticotropin-releasing factor in the stress response. J. Chem. Neuroanat. 54, 1–4. doi: 10.1016/j.jchemneu.2013.04.005

Bittencourt, J. C., and Sawchenko, P. E. (2000). Do centrally administered neuropep-tides access cognate receptors?: an analysis in the central corticotropin-releasing factor system. J. Neurosci. 20, 1142–1156.

Blasiak, A., Blasiak, T., Lewandowski, M. H., Hossain, M. A., Wade, J. D., and Gundlach, A. L. (2013). Relaxin-3 innervation of the intergeniculate leaflet of the rat thalamus – neuronal tract-tracing and in vitro electrophysiological studies. Eur. J. Neurosci. 37, 1284–1294. doi: 10.1111/ejn.12155

Blasiak, A., Gundlach, A. L., and Lewandowski, M. H. (2010). Orexins increase nucleus incertus neuronal activity: implications for a possible reinforcing arousal drive. FENS Abstr. 5, 104.2.

Boels, K., Hermans-Borgmeyer, I., and Schaller, H. C. (2004). Identification of a mouse orthologue of the G-protein-coupled receptor SALPR and its expression in adult mouse brain and during development. Dev. Brain Res. 152, 265–268. doi: 10.1016/j.devbrainres.2004.06.002

Brundin, L., Bjorkqvist, M., Petersen, A., and Traskman-Bendz, L. (2007). Reduced orexin levels in the cerebrospinal fluid of suicidal patients with major depressive disorder. Eur. Neuropsychopharmacol. 17, 573–579. doi: 10.1016/j.euroneuro.2007.01.005

Burazin, T. C. D., Bathgate, R. A. D., Macris, M., Layfield, S., Gundlach, A. L., and Tregear, G. W. (2002). Restricted, but abundant, expression of the novel rat gene-3 (R3) relaxin in the dorsal tegmental region of brain. J. Neurochem. 82, 1553–1557. doi: 10.1046/j.1471-4159.2002.01114.x

Burgess, C. R., and Scammell, T. E. (2012). Narcolepsy: neural mechanisms of sleepi-ness and cataplexy. J. Neurosci. 32, 12305–12311. doi: 10.1523/JNEUROSCI.2630-12.2012

Burt, J., Alberto, C. O., Parsons, M. P., and Hirasawa, M. (2011). Local network regulation of orexin neurons in the lateral hypothalamus. Am. J. Phys-iol. Regul. Integr. Comp. Physiol. 301, R572–R580. doi: 10.1152/ajpregu.006 74.2010

Caldwell, H. K., Lee, H. J., Macbeth, A. H., and Young, W. S. III. (2008). Vasopressin: behavioral roles of an "original" neuropeptide. Prog. Neurobiol. 84, 1–24. doi: 10.1016/j.pneurobio.2007.10.007

Callander, G. E., Ma, S., Ganella, D. E., Wimmer, V. C., Gundlach, A. L., Thomas, W. G., et al. (2012). Silencing relaxin-3 in nucleus incertus of adult rodents: a viral vector-based approach to investigate neuropeptide function. PLoS ONE 7:e42300. doi: 10.1371/journal.pone.0042300

Carter, R., Mouralidarane, A., Ray, S., Soeda, J., and Oben, J. (2012). Recent advancements in drug treatment of obesity. Clin. Med. 12, 456–460. doi: 10.7861/clinmedicine.12-5-456

Castle, D., Keks, N., Newton, R., Schweitzer, I., Copolov, D., Paoletti, N., et al. (2013). Pharmacological approaches to the management of schizophrenia: 10 years on. Australas Psychiatry 21, 329–334. doi: 10.1177/1039856213486211

Cervera-Ferri, A., Guerrero-Martinez, J., Bataller-Mompean,

M., Taberner-Cortes, A., Martinez-Ricos, J., Ruiz-Torner, A., et al. (2011). Theta synchronization between the hippocampus and the nucleus incertus in urethane-anesthetized rats. Exp. Brain Res. 211, 177–192. doi: 10.1007/s00221-011-2666-3

Cervera-Ferri, A., Rahmani, Y., Martinez-Bellver, S., Teruel-Marti, V., and Martinez-Ricos, J. (2012). Glutamatergic projection from the nucleus incertus to the septohippocampal system. Neurosci. Lett. 517, 71–76. doi: 10.1016/j.neulet.2012.04.014

Challis, C., Boulden, J., Veerakumar, A., Espallergues, J., Vassoler, F. M., Pierce, R. C., et al. (2013). Raphe GABAergic neurons mediate the acquisition of avoidance after social defeat. J. Neurosci. 33, 13978–13988. doi: 10.1523/JNEUROSCI.2383-13.2013

Chalmers, D. T., Lovenberg, T. W., and De Souza, E. B. (1995). Localization of novel corticotropin-releasing factor receptor (CRF2) mRNA expression to specific subcortical nuclei in rat brain: comparison with CRF1 receptor mRNA expression. J. Neurosci. 15, 6340–6350.

Chan, L. J., Smith, C. M., Chua, B. E., Lin, F., Bathgate, R. A. D., Separovic, F., et al. (2013). Synthesis of fluorescent analogues of relaxin family peptides and their preliminary in vitro and in vivo characterization. Front. Chem. 1:30. doi: 10.3389/fchem.2013.00030

Chee, M. J. S., Pissios, P., and Maratos-Flier, E. (2013). Neurochemical characterization of neurons expressing melanin-concentrating hormone receptor 1 in the mouse hypothalamus. J. Comp. Neurol. 521, 2208–2234. doi: 10.1002/cne.23273

Clark, L., Chamberlain, S. R., and Sahakian, B. J. (2009). Neurocognitive mechanisms in depression: implications for treatment. Ann. Rev. Neurosci. 32, 57–74. doi: 10.1146/annurev.neuro.31.060407.125618

Crawley, J. N., Hays, S. E., O'Donohue, T. L., Paul, S. M., and Goodwin, F. K. (1981). Neuropeptide modulation of social and exploratory behaviors in laboratory rodents. Peptides 2(Suppl. 1), 123–129. doi: 10.1016/0196-9781(81)90066-8

Crestani, C. C., Alves, F. H. F., Gomes, F. V., Resstel, L. B. M., Correa, F. M. A., nd Herman, J. P. (2013). Mechanisms in the bed nucleus of the stria terminalis involved in control of autonomic and neuroendocrine functions: a review. Curr. Neuropharmacol. 11, 141–159. doi: 10.2174/1570159X11311020002

Cummings, S., Elde, R., Ells, J., and Lindall, A. (1983). Corticotropin-releasing factor immunoreactivity is widely distributed within the central nervous system of the rat: an immunohistochemical study. J. Neurosci. 3, 1355–1368.

Dabrowska, J., Hazra, R., Guo, J.-D., Witt, S. D., and Rainnie, D. G. (2013). Central CRF neurons are not created equal: phenotypic differences in CRF-containing neurons of the rat paraventricular hypothalamus and the bed nucleus of the stria terminalis. Front. Neurosci. 7:156. doi: 10.3389/fnins.2013.00156

de Wit, R., Herrstedt, J., Rapoport, B., Carides, A. D., Guoguang-Ma, J., Elmer, M., et al. (2004). The oral NK(1) antagonist, aprepitant, given with standard antiemetics provides protection against nausea and vomiting over multiple cycles of cisplatin-based chemotherapy: a combined analysis of two randomised, placebo-controlled phase III clinical trials. Eur. J. Cancer 40, 403–410. doi: 10.1016/S0959-8049(03)00931-6

Dimitrov, E. L., DeJoseph, M. R., Brownfield, M. S., and Urban, J. H. (2007). Involvement of neuropeptide Y Y1 receptors in the regulation of neuroen-docrine corticotropin-releasing hormone neuronal activity. Endocrinology 148, 3666–3673. doi: 10.1210/en.2006-1730

Domschke, K., Reif, A., Weber, H., Richter, J., Hohoff, C., Ohrmann, P., et al. (2011). Neuropeptide S receptor gene – converging evidence for a role in panic disorder. Mol. Psychiatry 16, 938–948. doi: 10.1038/mp.2010.81

Dore, R., Iemolo, A., Smith, K. L., Wang, X., Cottone, P., and Sabino, V. (2013). CRF mediates the anxiogenic and anti-rewarding, but not the anorectic effects of PACAP. Neuropsychopharmacology 38, 2160–2169. doi: 10.1038/npp.2013.113

Dunn, J. D. (1987). Plasma corticosterone responses to electrical stimulation of the bed nucleus of the stria terminalis. Brain Res. 407, 327–331. doi: 10.1016/0006-8993(87)91111-5

Espejo, E. F., and Minano, F. J. (1999). Prefrontocortical dopamine depletion induces antidepressant-like effects in rats and alters the profile of desipramine during Porsolt's test. Neuroscience 88, 609–615. doi: 10.1016/S0306-4522(98)00258-9

Fan, J., Bernardi, S., Dam, N. T., Anagnostou, E., Gu, X., Martin, L., et al. (2012). Functional deficits of the attentional networks in autism. Brain Behav. 2, 647–660. doi: 10.1002/brb3.90

Farooq, U., Rajkumar, R., Sukumaran, S., Wu, Y., Tan, W. H., and Dawe, G. S. (2013). Corticotropin-releasing factor infusion into nucleus incertus suppresses medial prefrontal cortical activity and hippocampo-medial prefrontal cortical long-term potentiation. Eur. J. Neurosci. 38, 2516–2525. doi: 10.1111/ejn.12242

Farrella, M. S., and Roth, B. L. (2013). Pharmacosynthetics: reimagining the pharmacogenetic approach. Brain Res. 1511, 6–20. doi: 10.1016/j.brainres.2012.09.043

File, S. E., and Seth, P. (2003). A review of 25 years of the social interaction test. Eur. J. Pharmacol. 463, 35–53. doi: 10.1016/S0014-2999(03)01273-1

Furutani, N., Hondo, M., Kageyama, H., Tsujino, N., Mieda, M., Yanagisawa, M., et al. (2013). Neurotensin co-expressed in orexin-producing neurons in the lateral hypothalamus plays an important role in regulation of sleep/wakefulness states. PLoS ONE 8:e62391. doi: 10.1371/journal.pone.0062391

Ganella, D. E., Callander, G. E., Ma, S., Bye, C. R., Gundlach, A. L., and Bath-gate, R. A. D. (2013a). Modulation of feeding by chronic rAAV expression of a relaxin-3 peptide agonist in rat hypothalamus. Gene Ther. 20, 703–716. doi: 10.1038/gt.2012.83

Ganella, D. E., Ma, S., and Gundlach, A. L. (2013b). Relaxin-3/RXFP3 signaling and neuroendocrine function–a perspective on extrinsic hypothalamic control. Front. Endocrinol. (Lausanne) 4:128. doi: 10.3389/fendo.2013.00128

Ganella, D. E., Ryan, P. J., Bathgate, R. A. D., and Gundlach, A. L. (2012). Increased feeding and body weight gain after acute/chronic hypothalamic activation of RXFP3 by relaxin-3 and receptor-selective synthetic and rAAV-driven agonist peptides: functional and therapeutic implications. Behav. Pharmacol. 23, 516–525. doi: 10.1097/FBP.0b013e3283576999

Gaus, S. E., Strecker, R. E., Tate, B. A., Parker, R. A., and Saper, C. B. (2002). Ventrolateral preoptic nucleus contains sleep-active, galaninergic neurons in multiple mammalian species. Neuroscience 115, 285–294. doi: 10.1016/S0306-4522(02)00308-1

Goto, M., Swanson, L. W., and Canteras, N. S. (2001). Connections of the nucleus incertus. J. Comp. Neurol. 438, 86–122. doi: 10.1002/cne.1303

Hangya, B., Borhegyi, Z., Szilágyi, N., Freund, T. F., and Varga, V. (2009). GABAergic neurons of the medial septum lead the hippocampal network during theta activity. J. Neurosci. 29, 8094–8102. doi: 10.1523/JNEUROSCI.5665-08.2009

Harrington, M. E. (1997). The ventral lateral geniculate nucleus and the intergenic-ulate leaflet: interrelated structures in the visual and circadian systems. Neurosci. Biobehav. Rev. 21, 705–727. doi: 10.1016/S0149-7634(96)00019-X

Hastings, M. H., and Goedert, M. (2013). Circadian clocks and neurodegen-erative diseases: time to aggregate? Curr. Opin. Neurobiol. 23, 1–8. doi: 10.1016/j.conb.2013.05.004

Haugaard-Jonsson, L. M., Hossain, M. A., Daly, N. L., Bathgate, R. A. D., Wade, J. D., Craik, D. J., et al. (2008). Structure of the R3/I5 chimeric relaxin peptide, a selective GPCR135 and GPCR142 agonist. J. Biol. Chem. 283, 23811–23818. doi: 10.1074/jbc.M800489200

Haznedar, M. M., Buchsbaum, M. S., Wei, T. C., Hof, P. R., Cartwright, C., Bienstock, C. A., et al. (2000). Limbic circuitry in patients with autism spectrum disorders studied with positron emission tomography and magnetic resonance imaging. Am. J. Psychiatry 157, 1994–2001. doi: 10.1176/appi.ajp.157. 12.1994

Held, K., Antonijevic, I., Murck, H., Kuenzel, H., and Steiger, A. (2006). Neuropep-tide Y (NPY) shortens sleep latency but does not suppress ACTH and cortisol in depressed patients and normal controls. Psychoneuroendocrinology 31, 100–107. doi: 10.1016/j.psyneuen.2005.05.015

Hida, T., Takahashi, E., Shikata, K., Hirohashi, T., Sawai, T., Seiki, T., et al. (2006). Chronic intracerebroventricular administration of relaxin-3 increases body weight in rats. J. Recept. Signal Transduct. Res. 26, 147–158. doi: 10.1080/10799890600623373

Hisaw, F. L. (1926). Experimental relaxation of the pubic ligament of the guinea pig. Proc. Soc. Exp. Biol. Med. 23, 661–663. doi: 10.3181/00379727-23-3107

Hökfelt, T., Bartfai, T., and Bloom, F. (2003). Neuropeptides: opportunities for drug discovery. Lancet Neurol. 2, 463–472. doi: 10.1016/S1474-4422(03) 00482-4

Hökfelt, T., Broberger, C., Xu, Z.-Q. D., Sergeyev, V., Ubink, R., and Diez, M. (2000). Neuropeptides– an overview. Neuropharmacology 39, 1337–1356. doi: 10.1016/S0028-3908(00)00010-1

Holmes, A., Heilig, M., Rupniak, N. M., Steckler, T., and Griebel, G. (2003). Neuropeptide systems as novel therapeutic targets for depression and anxiety disorders. Trends Pharmacol. Sci. 24, 580–588. doi: 10.1016/j.tips.2003.09.011

Holmes, A. J., Lee, P. H., Hollinshead, M. O., Bakst, L., Roffman, J. L., Smoller, J. W., et al. (2012). Individual differences in amygdala-medial prefrontal anatomy link negative affect, impaired social functioning, and polygenic depression risk. J. Neurosci. 32, 18087–18100. doi: 10.1523/JNEUROSCI.2531-12.2012

Hosken, I. T., Smith, C. M., Chua, B. E., and Gundlach, A. L. (2013). "Consequences of relaxin-3 null mutation in mice on food-entrainable arousal," in Proceedings of Sixth International Conference on Relaxin and Related Peptides, Florence.

Hossain, M. A., Smith, C. M., Ryan, P. J., Buchler, E., Bathgate, R. A. D., Gundlach, A. L., et al. (2013). Chemical synthesis and orexigenic activity of rat/mouse relaxin-3. Amino Acids 44, 1529–1536. doi: 10.1007/s00726-013-1478-0

Hoyer, D., and Bartfai, T. (2012). Neuropeptides and neuropeptide receptors: drug targets, and peptide and non-peptide ligands: a tribute to Prof Dieter Seebach. Chem. Biodiv. 9, 2367–2387. doi: 10.1002/cbdv.201200288

Hoyer, D., and Jacobson, L. H. (2013). Orexin in sleep, addiction and more: is the perfect insomnia drug at hand? Neuropeptides 47, 477–488. doi: 10.1016/j.npep.2013.10.009

Hryhorczuk, C., Sharma, S., and Fulton, S. E. (2013). Metabolic distur-bances connecting obesity and depression. Front. Neurosci. 7:177. doi: 10.3389/fnins.2013.00177

Insel, T., Krystal, J., and Ehlers, M. (2013a). New drug development for cognitive enhancement in mental health: challenges and opportunities. Neuropharmacology 64, 2–7. doi: 10.1016/j.neuropharm.2012.07.041

Insel, T. R., Voon, V., Nye, J. S., Brown, V. J., Altevogt, B. M., Bullmore, E. T., et al. (2013b). Innovative solutions to novel drug development in mental health. Neu-rosci. Biobehav. Rev. 37, 2438–2444. doi.org/10.1016/j.neubiorev.2013.1003.1022

Ionescu, I. A., Dine, J., Yen, Y. C., Buell, D. R., Herrmann, L., Holsboer, F., et al. (2012). Intranasally administered neuropeptide S (NPS) exerts anx-iolytic effects following internalization into NPS receptor-expressing neurons. Neuropsychopharmacology 37, 1323–1337. doi: 10.1038/npp.2011.317

Ishida, H., Shirayama, Y., Iwata, M., Katayama, S., Yamamoto, A., Kawahara, R., et al. (2007). Infusion of neuropeptide Y into CA3 region of hippocampus pro-duces antidepressant-like effect via Y1 receptor. Hippocampus 17, 271–280. doi: 10.1002/hipo.20264

Jiang, Z., Cowell, R. M., and Nakazawa, K. (2013). Convergence of genetic and environmental factors on parvalbumin-positive interneurons in schizophrenia. Front. Behav. Neurosci. 7:116. doi: 10.3389/fnbeh.2013.00116

Jones, B. E., Halaris, A. E., McIlhany, M., and Moore, R. Y. (1977). Ascending projections of the locus coeruleus in the rat. I. Axonal transport in central noradrenaline neurons. Brain Res. 127, 1–21. doi: 10.1016/0006-8993(77)90377-8

Kalmbach, A., Hedrick, T., and Waters, J. (2012). Selective optogenetic stimulation of cholinergic axons in neocortex. J. Neurophysiol. 107, 2008–2019. doi: 10.1152/jn.00870.2011

Keller, M., Montgomery, S., Ball, W., Morrison, M., Snavely, D., Liu, G., et al. (2006). Lack of efficacy of the substance P (neurokinin1 receptor) antagonist Aprepitant in the treatment of major depressive disorder. Biol. Psychiatry 59, 216–223. doi: 10.1016/j.biopsych.2005.07.013

Kim, A. K., Brown, R. M., and Lawrence, A. J. (2012). The role of orexins/hypocretins in alcohol use and abuse: an appetitive-reward relationship. Front. Behav. Neurosci. 6:78. doi: 10.3389/fnbeh.2012.00078

Kimura, M., Müller-Preuss, P., Lu, A., Wiesner, E., Flachskamm, C., Wurst, W., et al. (2010). Conditional corticotropin-releasing hormone overexpression in the mouse forebrain enhances rapid eye movement sleep. Mol. Psychiatry 15, 154–165. doi: 10.1038/mp.2009.46

Kirby, L. G., Rice, K. C., and Valentino, R. J. (2000). Effects of corticotropin-releasing factor on neuronal activity in the serotonergic dorsal raphe nucleus. Neuropsychopharmacology 22, 148–162. doi: 10.1016/S0893-133X(99)00093-7

Kishi, T., and Elmquist, J. K. (2005). Body weight is regulated by the brain: a link between feeding and emotion. Mol. Psychiatry 10, 132–146. doi: 10.1038/sj.mp.4001638

Kocsis, B., Varga, V., Dahan, L., and Sik, A. (2006). Serotonergic neuron diversity: identification of raphe neurons with discharges time-locked to the hippocampal theta rhythm. Proc. Natl. Acad. Sci. U.S.A. 103, 1059–1064. doi: 10.1073/pnas.0508360103

Koob, G. F. (2010). The role of CRF and CRF-related peptides in the dark side of addiction. Brain Res. 1314, 3–14. doi: 10.1016/j.brainres.2009.11.008

Kopelman, P. G. (2000). Obesity as a medical problem. Nature 404, 635–643.

Kuei, C., Sutton, S., Bonaventure, P., Pudiak, C., Shelton, J., Zhu, J., et al. (2007). R3 (BΔ23-27) R/I5 chimeric peptide, a selective antagonist for GPCR135 and GPCR142 over relaxin receptor LGR7. J. Biol. Chem. 282, 25425. doi: 10.1074/jbc.M701416200

Lach, G., and de Lima, T. C. (2013). Role of NPY Y1 receptor on acquisition, con-solidation and extinction on contextual fear conditioning: dissociation between anxiety, locomotion and non-emotional memory behavior. Neurobiol. Learn. Mem. 103, 26–33. doi: 10.1016/j.nlm.2013.04.005

Lebow, M., Neufeld-Cohen, A., Kuperman, Y., Tsoory, M., Gil, S., and Chen, A. (2012). Susceptibility to PTSD-like behavior is mediated by corticotropin-releasing factor receptor type 2 levels in the bed nucleus of the stria terminalis. J. Neurosci. 32, 6906–6916. doi: 10.1523/JNEUROSCI.4012-11.2012

Lenglos, C., Mitra, A., Guevremont, G., and Timofeeva, E. (2013). Sex differences in the effects of chronic stress and food restriction on body weight gain and brain expression of CRF and relaxin-3 in rats. Genes Brain Behav. 12, 370–387. doi: 10.1111/gbb.12028

Lesch, K. P., and Waider, J. (2012). Serotonin in the modulation of neural plasticity and networks: implications for neurodevelopmental disorders. Neuron 76, 175–191. doi: 10.1016/j.neuron.2012.09.013

Li, K., Zhou, T., Liao, L., Yang, Z., Wong, C., Henn, F., et al. (2013). βCaMKII in lateral habenula mediates core symptoms of depression. Science 341, 1016–1020. doi: 10.1126/science.1240729

Lin, H. C., Gean, P. W., Wang, C. C., Chan, Y. H., and Chen, P. S. (2013). The amygdala excitatory/inhibitory balance in a valproate-induced rat autism model. PLoS ONE 8:e55248. doi: 10.1371/journal.pone.0055248

Lin, L. C., and Sibille, E. (2013). Reduced brain somatostatin in mood disorders: a common pathophysiological substrate and drug target? Front. Pharmacol. 4:110. doi: 10.3389/fphar.2013.00110

Liu, C., Chen, J., Kuei, C., Sutton, S., Nepomuceno, D., Bonaventure, P., et al. (2005). Relaxin-3/insulin-like peptide 5 chimeric peptide, a selective ligand for G protein-coupled receptor (GPCR)135 and GPCR142 over leucine-rich repeat-containing G protein-coupled receptor 7. Mol. Pharmacol. 67, 231–240. doi: 10.1124/mol.104.006700

Liu, C., Eriste, E., Sutton, S., Chen, J., Roland, B., Kuei, C., et al. (2003). Identification of relaxin-3/INSL7 as an endogenous ligand for the orphan G-protein-coupled receptor GPCR135. J. Biol. Chem. 278, 50754–50764. doi: 10.1074/jbc.M308995200

Liu, C., Kuei, C., Sutton, S., Shelton, J., Zhu, J., Nepomuceno, D., et al. (2009). Prob-ing the functional domains of relaxin-3 and the creation of a selective antagonist for RXFP3/GPCR135 over relaxin receptor RXFP1/LGR7. Ann. N. Y. Acad. Sci. 1160, 31–37. doi: 10.1111/j.1749-6632.2008.03790.x

Liu, T., Wang, Q., Berglund, E. D., and Tong, Q. (2013). Action of neurotransmitter: a key to unlock the AgRP neuron feeding circuit. Front. Neurosci. 6:200. doi: 10.3389/fnins.2012.00200

Lukas, M., and Neumann, I. D. (2013). Oxytocin and vasopressin in rodent behaviors related to social dysfunctions in autism spectrum disorders. Behav. Brain Res. 251, 85–94. doi: 10.1016/j.bbr.2012.08.011

Lukas, M., Toth, I., Reber, S. O., Slattery, D. A., Veenema, A. H., and Neumann, I. D. (2011). The neuropeptide oxytocin facilitates pro-social behavior and prevents social avoidance in rats and mice. Neuropsychopharmacology 36, 2159–2168. doi: 10.1038/npp.2011.95

Lungwitz, E. A., Molosh, A., Johnson, P. L., Harvey, B. P., Dirks, R. C., Dietrich, A., et al. (2012). Orexin-A induces anxiety-like behavior through interactions with glutamatergic receptors in the bed nucleus of the stria terminalis of rats. Physiol. Behav. 107, 726–732. doi: 10.1016/j.physbeh.2012.05.019

Ma, S., Blasiak, A., Olucha-Bordonau, F. E., Verberne, A. J., and Gundlach, A. L. (2013). Heterogeneous responses of nucleus incertus neurons to corticotropin-releasing factor and coherent activity with hippocampal theta rhythm in the rat. J. Physiol. (Lond.) 591, 3981–4001. doi: 10.1113/jphysiol.2013. 254300

Ma, S., Bonaventure, P., Ferraro, T., Shen, P. J., Burazin, T. C. D., Bathgate, R. A. D., et al. (2007). Relaxin-3 in GABA projection neurons of nucleus incertus suggests widespread influence on forebrain circuits via G-protein-coupled receptor-135 in the rat. Neuroscience 144, 165–190. doi: 10.1016/j.neuroscience.2006. 08.072

Ma, S., Kastman, H., Olucha-Bordonau, F. E., Capogna, M., Hossain, A., Wade, J. D., et al. (2010). Relaxin-3 receptor activation in the central amygdala enhances fear extinction in the rat: implications for relaxin-3 control of emotion. Soc. Neurosci. Abstr. 809.24.

Ma, S., Olucha-Bordonau, F. E., Hossain, M. A., Lin, F., Kuei, C., Liu, C., et al. (2009a). Modulation of hippocampal theta oscillations and spatial memory by relaxin-3 neurons of the nucleus incertus. Learn. Mem. 16, 730–742. doi: 10.1101/lm.1438109

Ma, S., Sang, Q., Lanciego, J. L., and Gundlach, A. L. (2009b). Localization of relaxin-3 in brain of Macaca fascicularis -Identification of nucleus incertus in primate. J. Comp. Neurol. 517, 700–712. doi: 10.1002/cne.22197

Ma, S., Shen, P. J., Sang, Q., Lanciego, J. L., and Gundlach, A. L. (2009c). Distribution of relaxin-3 mRNA and immunoreactivity and RXFP3-binding sites in the brain of the macaque, Macaca fascicularis. Ann. N. Y. Acad. Sci. 1160, 256–258. doi: 10.1111/j.1749-6632.2009.03954.x

Maaswinkel, H., Gispen, W. H., and Spruijt, B. M. (1997). Executive function of the hippocampus in social behavior in the rat. Behav. Neurosci. 111, 777–784. doi: 10.1037/0735-7044.111.4.777

Manji, H. K., Quiroz, J. A., Sporn, J., Payne, J. L., Denicoff, K., Gray, A. N., et al. (2003). Enhancing neuronal plasticity and cellular resilience to develop novel, improved therapeutics for difficult-to-treat depression. Biol. Psychiatry 53, 707– 742. doi: 10.1016/S0006-3223(03)00117-3

Marchant, E. G., Watson, N. V., and Mistlberger, R. E. (1997). Both neuropeptide Y and serotonin are necessary for entrainment of circadian rhythms in mice by daily treadmill running schedules. J. Neurosci. 17, 7974 –7987.

Marder, E. (2012). Neuromodulation of neuronal circuits: back to the future. Neuron 76, 1–11. doi: 10.1016/j.neuron.2012.09.010

Markram, K., and Markram, H. (2010). The intense world theory – a unify-ing theory of the neurobiology of autism. Front. Hum. Neurosci. 4:224. doi: 10.3389/fnhum.2010.00224

Marson, L., and Foley, K. A. (2004). Identification of neural pathways involved in genital reflexes in the female: a combined anterograde and retrograde tracing study. Neuroscience 127, 723–736. doi: 10.1016/j.neuroscience.2004. 04.063

Matsumoto, M., Kamohara, M., Sugimoto, T., Hidaka, K., Takasaki, J., Saito, T., et al. (2000). The novel G-protein coupled receptor SALPR shares sequence sim-ilarity with somatostatin and angiotensin receptors. Gene 248, 183–189. doi: 10.1016/S0378-1119(00)00123-2

Mazure, C. M. (1998). Life stressors as risk factors in depression. Clin. Psychol. Sci. Pract. 5, 291–313. doi: 10.1111/j.1468-2850.1998. tb00151.x

McClung, C. A. (2007). Circadian genes, rhythms and the biology of mood disorders. Pharmacol. Ther. 114, 222–232. doi: 10.1016/j.pharmthera.2007.02.003

McEwen, B. S. (2007). Physiology and neurobiology of stress and adaptation: central role of the brain. Physiol. Rev. 87, 873–904. doi: 10.1152/physrev.000 41.2006

McGonigle, P. (2011). Peptide therapeutics for CNS indications. Biochem. Pharma-col. 83, 559–566. doi: 10.1016/j.bcp.2011.10.014

McGowan, B. M., Stanley, S. A., Smith, K. L., Minnion, J. S., Donovan, J., Thompson, E. L., et al. (2006). Effects of acute and chronic relaxin-3 on food intake and energy expenditure in rats. Regul. Peptides 136, 72–77. doi: 10.1016/j.regpep.2006. 04.009

McGowan, B. M., Stanley, S. A., Smith, K. L., White, N. E., Connolly, M. M., Thompson, E. L., et al. (2005). Central relaxin-3 administration causes hyper-phagia in male Wistar rats. Endocrinology 146, 3295–3300. doi: 10.1210/en. 2004-1532

McGowan, B. M., Stanley, S. A., White, N. E., Spangeus, A., Patterson, M., Thompson, E. L., et al. (2007). Hypothalamic mapping of orexigenic action and Fos-like immunoreactivity following relaxin-3 administration in male Wistar rats. Am. J. Physiol. Endocrinol. Metab. 292, E913–E919. doi: 10.1152/ajpendo.003 46.2006

McNamara, I. M., Borella, A. W., Bialowas, L. A., and Whitaker-Azmitia, P. M. (2008). Further studies in the developmental hyperserotonemia model (DHS) of autism: social, behavioral and peptide changes. Brain Res. 1189, 203–214. doi: 10.1016/j.brainres.2007.10.063

McNaughton, N., and Gray, J. A. (2000). Anxiolytic action on the behavioural inhibition system implies multiple types of arousal contribute to anxiety. J. Affect. Disord. 61, 161–176. doi: 10.1016/S0165-0327(00) 00344-X

McNaughton, N., Kocsis, B., and Hajos, M. (2007). Elicited hippocampal theta rhythm: a screen for anxiolytic and procognitive drugs through changes in hippocampal function? Behav. Pharmacol. 18, 329–346. doi: 10.1097/FBP.0b013e3282ee82e3

Meyer-Bernstein, E. L., and Morin, L. P. (1996). Differential serotonergic innervation of the suprachiasmatic nucleus and the intergeniculate leaflet and its role in circadian rhythm modulation. J. Neurosci. 16, 2097–2111.

Millan, M. J., Agid, Y., Brüne, M., Bullmore, E. T., Carter, C. S., Clayton, N. S., et al. (2012). Cognitive dysfunction in psychiatric disorders: characteristics, causes and the quest for improved therapy. Nat. Rev. Drug Discov. 11, 141–168. doi: 10.1038/nrd3628

Miyamoto, Y., Watanabe, Y., and Tanaka, M. (2008). Developmental expression and serotonergic regulation of relaxin 3/INSL7 in the nucleus incertus of rat brain. Regul. Peptides 145, 54–59. doi: 10.1016/j.regpep.2007.08.010

Mogi, K., Nagasawa, M., and Kikusui, T. (2010). Developmental consequences and biological significance of mother-infant bonding. Prog. Neuropsychopharmacol. Biol. Psychiatry 35, 1232–1241. doi: 10.1016/j.pnpbp.2010.08.024

Möller, C., Sommer, W., Thorsell, A., and Heilig, M. (1999). Anxiogenic-like action of galanin after intra-amygdala administration in the rat. Neuropsychopharma-cology 21, 507–512. doi: 10.1016/S0893-133X(98)00102-X

Monti, J. M., and Jantos, H. (2008). The roles of dopamine and serotonin, and of their receptors, in regulating sleep and waking. Prog. Brain Res. 172, 625–646. doi: 10.1016/S0079-6123(08)00929-1

Monti, J. M., and Monti, D. (2000). Sleep disturbance in generalized anxiety disorder and its treatment. Sleep Med. Rev. 4, 263–276. doi: 10.1053/smrv.19 99.0096

Morin, L. P. (2013). Neuroanatomy of the extended circadian rhythm system. Exp. Neurol. 243, 4–20. doi: 10.1016/j.expneurol.2012.06.026

Morin, L. P., and Meyer-Bernstein, E. L. (1999). The ascending serotoner-gic system in the hamster: comparison with projections of the dorsal and median raphe nuclei. Neuroscience 91, 81–105. doi: 10.1016/S0306-4522(98) 00585-5

Morin, S. M., Ling, N., Liu, X. J., Kahl, S. D., and Gehlert, D. R. (1999). Differential distribution of urocortin-and corticotropin-releasing factor-like immunore-activities in the rat brain. Neuroscience 92, 281–291. doi: 10.1016/S0306-4522(98)00732-5

Munro, J., Skrobot, O., Sanyoura, M., Kay, V., Susce, M. T., Glaser, P. E., et al. (2012). Relaxin polymorphisms associated with metabolic disturbance in patients treated with antipsychotics. J. Psychopharmacol. 26, 374–379. doi: 10.1177/0269881111408965

Murphy, F. C., Rubinsztein, J. S., Michael, A., Rogers, R. D., Robbins, T. W., Paykel, E. S., et al. (2001). Decision-making cognition in mania and depression. Psychol. Med. 31, 679–693. doi: 10.1017/S0033291701003804

Nakazawa, C. M., Shikata, K., Uesugi, M., Katayama, H., Aoshima, K., Tahara, K., et al. (2013). Prediction of relaxin-3-induced downstream pathway resulting in anxiolytic-like behaviors in rats based on a microarray and peptidome analy-sis. J. Recept. Signal Transduct. Res. 33, 224–233. doi: 10.3109/10799893.2012. 756895

Nawaratne, V., Leach, K., Suratman, N., Loiacono, R. E., Felder, C. C., Armbruster, B. N., et al. (2008). New insights into the function of M4 muscarinic acetylcholine receptors gained using a novel allosteric modulator and a DREADD (designer receptor exclusively activated by a designer drug). Mol. Pharmacol. 74, 1119–1131. doi: 10.1124/mol.108.049353

Nemeroff, C. B. (1992). New vistas in neuropeptide research in neuropsychiatry: focus on corticotropin-releasing factor. Neuropsychopharmacology 6, 69–75.

Nestler, E. J. (1998). Antidepressant treatments in the 21st century. Biol. Psychiatry 44, 526–533. doi: 10.1016/S0006-3223(98)00095-X

Nestler, E. J., and Hyman, S. E. (2010). Animal models of neuropsychiatric disorders. Nat. Neurosci. 13, 1161–1169. doi: 10.1038/nn.2647

Nikisch, G., Baumann, P., Liu, T., and Mathe, A. A. (2011). Quetiapine affects neuropeptide Y and corticotropin-releasing hormone in cerebrospinal fluid from schizophrenia patients: relationship to depression and anxiety symptoms and to treatment response. Int. J. Neuropsychopharmacol. 15, 1051–1061. doi: 10.1017/S1461145711001556

Nunez, A., Cervera-Ferri, A., Olucha-Bordonau, F., Ruiz-Torner, A., and Teruel, V. (2006). Nucleus incertus contribution to hippocampal theta rhythm generation. Eur. J. Neurosci. 23, 2731–2738. doi: 10.1111/j.1460-9568.2006. 04797.x

Nutt, D. J., Forshall, S., Bell, C., Rich,

A., Sandford, J., Nash, J., et al. (1999). Mechanisms of action of selective serotonin reuptake inhibitors in the treatment of psychiatric disorders. Eur. Neuropsychopharmacol. 9 S81–S86. doi: 10.1016/S0924-977X(99)00030-9

O'Donnell, P. (2011). Adolescent onset of cortical disinhibition in schizophre-nia: insights from animal models. Schizophr. Bull. 37, 484–492. doi: 10.1093/schbul/sbr028

Ohnishi, T., Matsuda, H., Hashimoto, T., Kunihiro, T., Nishikawa, M., Uema, T., et al. (2000). Abnormal regional cerebral blood flow in childhood autism. Brain 123 1838–1844. doi: 10.1093/brain/123.9.1838

Olucha-Bordonau, F. E., Otero-Garcia, M., Sanchez-Perez, A. M., Nunez, A., Ma, S., and Gundlach, A. L. (2012). Distribution and targets of the relaxin-3 inner-vation of the septal area in the rat. J. Comp. Neurol. 520, 1903–1939. doi: 10.1002/cne.23018

Olucha-Bordonau, F. E., Teruel, V., Barcia-Gonzalez, J., Ruiz-Torner, A., Valverde-Navarro, A. A., and Martinez-Soriano, F. (2003). Cytoarchitecture and efferent projections of the nucleus incertus of the rat. J. Comp. Neurol. 464, 62–97. doi: 10.1002/cne.10774

Paez-Pereda, M., Hausch, F., and Holsboer, F. (2011). Corticotropin releasing factor receptor antagonists for major depressive disorder. Expert Opin. Investig. Drugs 20, 519–535. doi: 10.1517/13543784.2011.565330

Panchal, S. K., and Brown, L. (2011). Rodent models for metabolic syndrome research. J. Biomed. Biotechnol. 35, 1982.

Pape, H.-C., Jüngling, K., Seidenbecher, T., Lesting, J., and Reinscheid, R. K. (2010). Neuropeptide S: a transmitter system in the brain regulating fear and anxiety. Neuropharmacology 58, 29–34. doi: 10.1016/j.neuropharm.2009.06.001

Peca, J., Feliciano, C., Ting, J. T., Wang, W., Wells, M. F., Venkatraman, T. N., et al. (2011). Shank3 mutant mice display autistic-like behaviours and striatal dysfunction. Nature 472, 437–442. doi: 10.1038/nature09965

Pekala, D., Blasiak, T., Raastad, M., and Lewandowski, M. H. (2011). The influence of orexins on the firing rate and pattern of rat intergeniculate leaflet neurons -electrophysiological and immunohistological studies. Eur. J. Neurosci. 34, 1406– 1418. doi: 10.1111/j.1460-9568.2011.07868.x

Pereira, C. W., Santos, F. N., Sanchez-Perez, A. M., Otero-Garcia, M., Marchioro, M., Ma, S., et al. (2013). Electrolytic lesion of the nucleus incertus retards extinction of auditory conditioned fear. Behav. Brain Res. 247, 201–210. doi: 10.1016/j.bbr.2013.03.025

Peyron, C., Tighe, D. K., van den Pol, A. N., de Lecea, L., Heller, H. C., Sutcliffe, J. G., et al. (1998). Neurons containing hypocretin (orexin) project to multiple neuronal systems. J. Neurosci. 18, 9996–10015.

Pulga, A., Ruzza, C., Rizzi, A., Guerrini, R., and Calo, G. (2012). Anxiolytic-and panicolytic-like effects of neuropeptide S in the mouse elevated T-maze. Eur. J. Neurosci. 36, 3531–3537. doi: 10.1111/j.1460-9568.2012.08265.x

Rajkumar, R., See, L. K., and Dawe, G. S. (2013). Acute antipsychotic treatments induce distinct c-Fos expression patterns in appetite-related neuronal structures of the rat brain. Brain Res. 1508, 34–43. doi: 10.1016/j.brainres.2013. 02.050

Ressler, K. J., Mercer, K. B., Bradley, B., Jovanovic, T., Mahan, A., Kerley, K., et al. (2011). Post-traumatic stress disorder is associated with PACAP and the PAC1 receptor. Nature 470, 492–497. doi: 10.1038/nature09856

Ring, R. H. (2011). A complicated picture of oxytocin action in the central nervous system revealed. Biol. Psychiatry 69, 818–819. doi: 10.1016/j.biopsych.2011.03.020

Rosengren, K. J., Lin, F., Bathgate, R. A. D., Tregear, G. W., Daly, N. L., Wade, J. D., et al. (2006). Solution structure and novel insights into the determinants of the receptor specificity of human relaxin-3. J. Biol. Chem. 281, 5845–5851. doi: 10.1074/jbc.M511210200

Rotzinger, S., Lovejoy, D. A., and Tan, L. A. (2010). Behavioral effects of neuropeptides in rodent models of depression and anxiety. Peptides 31, 736–756. doi: 10.1016/j.peptides.2009.12.015

Roux, L., and Donaldson, C. (2012). Economics and obesity: costing the problem or evaluating solutions? Obes. Res. 12, 173–179. doi: 10.1038/oby.2004.23

Russo, S. J., and Nestler, E. J. (2013). The brain reward circuitry in mood disorders. Nat. Rev. Neurosci. 14, 609–625. doi: 10.1038/nrn3381

Ryan, P. J., Buchler, E., Shabanpoor, F., Hossain, M. A., Wade, J. D., Lawrence, A. J., et al. (2013a). Central relaxin-3 receptor (RXFP3) activation decreases anxiety-and depressive-like behaviours in the rat. Behav. Brain Res. 244, 142–151. doi: 10.1016/j.bbr.2013.01.034

Ryan, P. J., Kastman, H. E., Krstrew, E. V., Chirlov, L., Rosengren, K. J., Hossain, M. A., et al. (2013b). Relaxin-3/RXFP3 system regulates alcohol-seeking. Proc. Natl. Acad. Sci. U.S.A. 110, 20789–20794. doi: 10.1073/pnas.1317 807110

Ryan, P. J., Ma, S., Olucha-Bordonau, F. E., and Gundlach, A. L. (2011). Nucleus incertus – an emerging modulatory role in arousal, stress and memory. Neurosci. Biobehav. Rev. 35, 1326–1341. doi: 10.1016/j.neubiorev.2011.02.004

Saito, Y., and Nagasaki, H. (2008). The melanin-concentrating hormone system and its physiological functions. Results Probl. Cell Differ. 46, 159–179. doi: 10.1007/400_2007_052

Sakurai, T. (2007). The neural circuit of orexin (hypocretin): maintaining sleep and wakefulness. Nat. Rev. Neurosci. 8, 171–181. doi: 10.1038/nrn2092

Sanogo, Y. O., Hankison, S., Band, M., Obregon, A., and Bell, A. M. (2011). Brain transcriptomic response of threespine sticklebacks to cues of a predator. Brain Behav. Evol. 77, 270–285. doi: 10.1159/000328221

Saper, C. B., Scammell, T. E., and Lu, J. (2005). Hypothalamic regulation of sleep and circadian rhythms. Nature 437, 1257–1263. doi: 10.1038/nature04284

Sasaki, K., Suzuki, M., Mieda, M., Tsujino, N., Roth, B., and Sakurai, T. (2011). Pharmacogenetic modulation of orexin neurons alters sleep/wakefulness states in mice. PLoS ONE 6:e20360. doi: 10.1371/journal.pone.0020360

Schmidt, H. D., and Duman, R. S. (2010). Peripheral BDNF produces antidepressant-like effects in cellular and behavioral models. Neuropsychophar-macology 35, 2378–2391. doi: 10.1038/npp.2010.114

Shabanpoor, F., Akhter Hossain, M., Ryan, P. J., Belgi, A., Layfield, S., Kocan, M., et al. (2012). Minimization of human relaxin-3 leading to high-affinity analogues with increased selectivity for relaxin-family peptide 3 receptor (RXFP3) over RXFP1. J. Med. Chem. 55, 1671–1681. doi: 10.1021/jm201505p

Sherwood, O. D. (2004). Relaxin's physiological roles and other diverse actions. Endocr. Rev. 25, 205–234. doi: 10.1210/er.2003-0013

Shinohara, K., Tominaga, K., Isobe, Y., and lnouye, S.-I. T. (1993). Photic regulation of peptides located in the ventrolateral subdivision of the suprachiasmatic nucleus of the rat: daily variations of vasoactive intestinal polypeptide, gastrin-releasing peptide, and neuropeptide Y. J. Neurosci. 13, 793–800.

Silverman, J. L., Tolu, S. S., Barkan, C. L., and Crawley, J. N. (2010). Repetitive self-grooming behavior in the BTBR mouse model of autism is blocked by the mGluR5 antagonist MPEP. Neuropsychopharmacology 35, 976–989. doi: 10.1038/npp.2009.201

Smith, C. M., Blasiak, A., Ganella, D. E., Chua, B. E., Layfield, S. L., Bathgate, R. A. D., et al. (2013a). "Viral-mediated delivery of an RXFP3 agonist into brain promotes arousal in mice," in Proceedings of Sixth International Conference on Relaxin and Related Peptides, Florence.

Smith, C. M., Chua, B. E., Walker, A. W., and Gundlach, A. L. (2013b). "Potential hypothalamic targets of relaxin-3 innervation: a perspective," in Proceedings of Sixth International Conference on Relaxin and Related Peptides, Florence.

Smith, C. M., Hosken, I. T., Sutton, S. W., Lawrence, A. J., and Gundlach, A. L. (2012). Relaxin-3 null mutation mice display a circadian hypoactivity phenotype. Genes Brain Behav. 11, 94–104. doi: 10.1111/j.1601-183X.2011.00730.x

Smith, C. M., Lawrence, A. J., Sutton, S. W., and Gundlach, A. L. (2009). Behavioral phenotyping of mixed-background (129S5:B6) relaxin-3 knockout mice. Ann. N. Y. Acad. Sci. 1160, 236–241. doi: 10.1111/j.1749-6632.2009.03953.x

Smith, C. M., Ryan, P. J., Hosken, I. T., Ma, S., and Gundlach, A. L. (2011). Relaxin-3 systems in the brain – the first 10 years. J. Chem. Neuroanat. 42, 262–275. doi: 10.1016/j.jchemneu.2011.05.013

Smith, C. M., Shen, P. J., Banerjee, A., Bonaventure, P., Ma, S., Bathgate, R. A. D., et al. (2010). Distribution of relaxin 3 and RXFP3 within arousal, stress, affective, and cognitive circuits of mouse brain. J. Comp. Neurol. 518, 4016–4045. doi: 10.1002/cne.22442

Smith, K. L., Patterson, M., Dhillo, W. S., Patel, S. R., Semjonous, N. M., Gardiner, J. V., et al. (2006). Neuropeptide S stimulates the hypothalamo-pituitary-adrenal axis and inhibits food intake. Endocrinology 147, 3510–3518. doi: 10.1210/en.2005-1280

Sodersten, P., Bergh, C., and Zandian, M. (2006). Understanding eating disorders. Horm. Behav. 50, 572–578. doi: 10.1016/j.yhbeh.2006.06.030

Spencer, K. M., Nestor, P. G., Niznikiewicz, M. A., Salisbury, D. F., Shenton, M. E., and McCarley, R. W. (2003). Abnormal neural synchrony in schizophrenia. J. Neurosci. 23, 7407–7411.

Steinbusch, H. W. (1981). Distribution of serotonin-immunoreactivity in the central nervous system of the rat-cell bodies and terminals. Neuroscience 6, 557–618. doi: 10.1016/0306-4522(81)90146-9

Sutton, S. W., Bonaventure, P., Kuei, C., Roland, B., Chen, J., Nepomuceno, D., et al. (2004). Distribution of G-protein-coupled receptor (GPCR)135 binding sites and receptor mRNA in the rat brain suggests a role for relaxin-3 in neuroendocrine and sensory processing. Neuroendocrinology 80, 298–307. doi: 10.1159/0000 83656

Sutton, S. W., Shelton, J., Smith, C., Williams, J., Yun, S., Motley, T., et al. (2009). Metabolic and neuroendocrine responses to RXFP3 modulation in the central nervous system. Ann. N. Y. Acad. Sci. 1160, 242–249. doi: 10.1111/j.1749-6632.2008.03812.x

Takagi, H., Shiosaka, S., Tohyama, M., Senba, E., and Sakanaka, M. (1980). Ascending components of the medial forebrain bundle from the lower brain stem in the rat, with special reference to raphe and catecholamine cell groups. A study by the HRP method. Brain Res. 193, 315–337. doi: 10.1016/0006-8993(80)90168-7

Tanaka, M. (2010). Relaxin-3/insulin-like peptide 7, a neuropeptide involved in the stress response and food intake. FEBS J. 277, 4990–4997. doi: 10.1111/j.1742-4658.2010.07931.x

Tanaka, M., Iijima, N., Miyamoto, Y., Fukusumi, S., Itoh, Y., Ozawa, H., et al. (2005). Neurons expressing relaxin 3/INSL 7 in the nucleus incertus respond to stress. Eur. J. Neurosci. 21, 1659–1670. doi: 10.1111/j.1460-9568.2005. 03980.x

Tanaka, M., Watanabe, Y., and Yoshimoto, K. (2009). Regulation of relaxin 3 gene expression via cAMP-PKA in a neuroblastoma cell line. J. Neurosci. Res. 87, 820–829. doi: 10.1002/jnr.21895

Tandon, R. (2011). Antipsychotics in the treatment of schizophrenia: an overview. J. Clin. Psychiatry 72(Suppl. 1), 4–8. doi: 10.4088/JCP.10075su1.01

Teruel-Marti, V., Cervera-Ferri, A., Nunez, A., Valverde-Navarro, A. A., Olucha-Bordonau, F. E., and Ruiz-Torner, A. (2008). Anatomical evidence for a ponto-septal pathway via the nucleus incertus in the rat. Brain Res. 1218, 87–96. doi: 10.1016/j.brainres.2008.04.022

Thankachan, S., and Rusak, B. (2005). Juxtacellular recording/labeling anal-ysis of physiological and anatomical characteristics of rat intergeniculate leaflet neurons. J. Neurosci. 25, 9195–9204. doi: 10.1523/JNEUROSCI.2672-05.2005

Theisen, F. M., Linden, A., Konig, I. R., Martin, M., Remschmidt, H., and Hebebrand, J. (2003). Spectrum of binge eating symptomatology in patients treated with clozapine and olanzapine. J. Neural Transm. 110, 111–121.

Vaccari, C., Lolait, S. J., and Ostrowski, N. L. (1998). Comparative distribution of vasopressin V1b and oxytocin receptor messenger ribonucleic acids in brain. Endocrinology 139, 5015–5033.

Van Cauter, E., Linkowski, P., Kerkhofs, M., Hubain, P., L'Hermite-Baleriaux, M., Leclercq, R., et al. (1991). Circadian and sleep-related endocrine rhythms in schizophrenia. Arch. Gen. Psychiatry 48, 348. doi: 10.1001/archpsyc.1991.01810280064009

van den Pol, A. N. (2012). Neuropeptide transmission in brain circuits. Neuron 76, 98–115. doi: 10.1016/j.neuron.2012.09.014

van der Westhuizen, E. T., Christopoulos, A., Sexton, P. M., Wade, J. D., and Summers, R. J. (2010). H2 relaxin is a biased ligand relative to H3 relaxin at the relaxin family peptide receptor 3 (RXFP3). Mol. Pharmacol. 77, 759–772. doi: 10.1124/mol.109.061432

van der Westhuizen, E. T., Werry, T. D., Sexton, P. M., and Summers, R. J. (2007). The relaxin family peptide receptor 3 activates extracellular signal-regulated kinase 1/2 through a protein kinase C-dependent mechanism. Mol. Pharmacol. 71, 1618– 1629. doi: 10.1124/mol.106.032763

van Elst, L. T., Woermann, F. G., Lemieux, L., Thompson, P. J., and Trimble, M. R. (2000). Affective aggression in patients with temporal lobe epilepsy: a quantitative MRI study of the amygdala. Brain 123, 234–243. doi: 10.1093/brain/123. 2.234

Van Pett, K., Viau, V., Bittencourt, J. C., Chan, R. K., Li, H. Y., Arias, C., et al. (2000). Distribution of mRNAs encoding CRF receptors in brain and pituitary of rat and mouse. J. Comp. Neurol. 428, 191–212. doi:10.1002/1096-9861(20001211)428:2<191::AID-CNE1>3.0.CO;2-U

Vertes, R. P., and Kocsis, B. (1997). Brainstem-diencephalo-septohippocampal systems controlling the theta rhythm of the hippocampus. Neuroscience 81, 893–926.

Vianna, D. M., Graeff, F. G., Landeira-Fernandez, J., and Brandao, M. L. (2001). Lesion of the ventral periaqueductal gray reduces conditioned fear but does not change freezing induced by stimulation of the dorsal periaqueductal gray. Learn. Mem. 8, 164–169. doi: 10.1101/lm.36101

Videbech, P., and Ravnkilde, B. (2004). Hippocampal volume and depres-sion: a meta-analysis of MRI studies. Am. J. Psychiatry 161, 1957–1966. doi: 10.1176/appi.ajp.161.11.1957

Vithlani, M., Hines, R. M., Zhong, P., Terunuma, M., Hines, D. J., Revilla-Sanchez, R., et al. (2013). The ability of BDNF to modify neurogenesis and depressive-like behaviors is dependent upon phosphorylation of tyrosine residues 365/367 in the GABAA-receptor γ2 subunit. J. Neurosci. 33, 15567–15577. doi: 10.1523/JNEUROSCI.1845-13.2013

von Euler, U. S., and Gaddum, J. H. (1931). An unidentified depressor substance in certain tissue extracts. J. Physiol. 72, 74.

Walker, D. L., Miles, L. A., and Davis, M. (2009). Selective participation of the bed nucleus of the stria terminalis and CRF in sustained anxiety-like vs. phasic fear-like responses. Prog. Neuropsychopharmacol. Biol. Psychiatry 33, 1291–1308. doi: 10.1016/j.pnpbp.2009.06.022

Wang, X. J. (2002). Pacemaker neurons for the theta rhythm and their syn-chronization in the septohippocampal reciprocal loop. J. Neurophysiol. 87, 889–900.

Watanabe, Y., Miyamoto, Y., Matsuda, T., and Tanaka, M. (2011a). Relaxin-3/INSL7 regulates the stress-response system in the rat hypothalamus. J. Mol. Neurosci. 43, 169–174. doi: 10.1007/s12031-010-9468-0

Watanabe, Y., Tsujimura, A., Takao, K., Nishi, K., Ito, Y., Yasuhara, Y., et al. (2011b). Relaxin-3-deficient mice showed slight alteration in anxiety-related behavior. Front. Behav. Neurosci. 5:50. doi: 10.3389/fnbeh.2011.00050

Wess, J., Nakajima, K., and Jain, S. (2013). Novel designer receptors to probe GPCR signaling and physiology. Trends Pharmacol. Sci. 34, 385–392. doi: 10.1016/j.tips.2013.04.006

Westenberg, H. G. (1999). Pharmacology of antidepressants: selectivity or multiplicity? J. Clin. Psychiatry 60(Suppl. 17), 4–8.

Wilkinson, T. N., Speed, T. P., Tregear, G. W., and Bathgate, R. A. D. (2005). Evolution of the relaxin-like peptide family. BMC Evol. Biol. 5:14. doi: 10.1186/1471-2148-5-14

Willard, S. L., and Shively, C. A. (2012). Modeling depression in adult female cynomolgus monkeys (Macaca fascicularis). Am. J. Primatol. 74, 528–542. doi: 10.1002/ajp.21013

Willner, P., Scheel-Krüger, J., and Belzung, C. (2013). The neurobiology of depres-sion and antidepressant action. Neurosci. Biobehav. Rev. 37, 2331–2371. doi: 10.1016/j.neubiorev.2012.12.007

Winrow, C. J., and Renger, J. J. (2014). Discovery and development of orexin receptor antagonists as therapeutics for insomnia. Br. J. Pharmacol. 171, 283–293. doi: 10.1111/bph.12261

Xu, Y. L., Reinscheid, R. K., Huitron-Resendiz, S., Clark, S. D., Wang, Z., Lin, S. H., et al. (2004). Neuropeptide S: a neuropeptide promoting arousal and anxiolytic-like effects. Neuron 43, 487–497. doi: 10.1016/j.neuron.2004.08.005

Yamasue, H., Yee, J. R., Hurlemann, R., Rilling, J. K., Chen, F. S., Meyer-Lindenberg, A., et al. (2012). Integrative approaches utilizing oxytocin to enhance prosocial behavior: from animal and human social behavior to autistic social dysfunction. J. Neurosci. 32, 14109–14117. doi: 10.1523/JNEUROSCI.3327-12.2012

Yizhar, O., Fenno, L. E., Davidson, T. J., Mogri, M., and Deisseroth, K. (2011a). Optogenetics in neural systems. Neuron 71, 9–34. doi: 10.1016/j.neuron.2011. 06.004

Yizhar, O., Fenno, L. E., Prigge, M., Schneider, F., Davidson, T. J., O'Shea, D. J., et al. (2011b). Neocortical excitation/inhibition balance in information processing and social dysfunction. Nature 477, 171–178. doi: 10.1038/nature10360

Yoshida, M., Takayanagi, Y., Inoue, K., Kimura, T., Young, L. J., Onaka, T., et al. (2009). Evidence that oxytocin exerts anxiolytic effects via oxytocin receptor expressed in serotonergic neurons in mice. J. Neurosci. 29, 2259–2271. doi: 10.1523/JNEUROSCI.5593-08.2009

Zee, P. C., and Manthena, P. (2007). The brain's master circadian clock: implications and opportunities for therapy of sleep disorders. Sleep Med. Rev. 11, 59–70. doi: 10.1016/j.smrv.2006.06.001

Zhang, F., Gradinaru, V., Adamantidis, A. R., Durand, R., Airan, R. D., de Lecea, L., et al. (2010). Optogenetic interrogation of neural circuits: technol-ogy for probing mammalian brain structures. Nat. Protoc. 5, 439–456. doi: 10.1038/nprot.2009.226

Zhang, J., Fan, Y., Li, Y., Zhu, H.,

Wang, L., and Zhu, M. Y. (2012). Chronic social defeat up-regulates expression of the serotonin transporter in rat dorsal raphe nucleus and projection regions in a glucocorticoid-dependent manner. J. Neurochem. 123, 1054–1068. doi: 10.1111/jnc. 12055

Zheng, H., and Rinaman, L. (2013). Yohimbine anxiogenesis in the elevated plus maze requires hindbrain noradrenergic neurons that target the anterior ventro-lateral bed nucleus of the stria terminalis. Eur. J. Neurosci. 37, 1340–1349. doi: 10.1111/ejn.12123

Zorrilla, E. P., Heilig, M., de Wit, H., and Shaham, Y. (2013). Behav-ioral, biological, and chemical perspectives on targeting CRF(1) receptor antagonists to treat alcoholism. Drug Alcohol Depend. 128, 175–186. doi: 10.1016/j.drugalcdep.2012.12.017

Zorrilla, E. P., and Koob, G. F. (2010). Progress in corticotropin-releasing factor-1 antagonist development. Drug Discov. Today 15, 371–383. doi: 10.1016/j.drudis.2010.02.011

17

Antidepressant effects of ketamine: mechanisms underlying fast-acting novel antidepressants

Caroline A. Browne*[1] *and Irwin Lucki*[1,2]

[1] *Department of Psychiatry, University of Pennsylvania, Philadelphia, PA, USA*
[2] *Department of Pharmacology, University of Pennsylvania, Philadelphia, PA, USA*

Edited by:
Maarten Van Den Buuse, Mental Health Research Institute, Australia

Reviewed by:
Charles H. Large, Autifony Therapeutics Limited, Italy
Kenji Hashimoto, Chiba University Center for Forensic Mental Health, Japan

***Correspondence:**
Irwin Lucki, Department of Psychiatry, University of Pennsylvania, 125 South 31st Street, Room 2204, Philadelphia, PA 19104-3404, USA
e-mail: lucki@mail.med.upenn.edu

Newer antidepressants are needed for the many individuals with major depressive disorder (MDD) that do not respond adequately to treatment and because of a delay of weeks before the emergence of therapeutic effects. Recent evidence from clinical trials shows that the NMDA antagonist ketamine is a revolutionary novel antidepressant because it acts rapidly and is effective for treatment-resistant patients. A single infusion of ketamine alleviates depressive symptoms in treatment-resistant depressed patients within hours and these effects may be sustained for up to 2 weeks. Although the discovery of ketamine's effects has reshaped drug discovery for antidepressants, the psychotomimetic properties of this compound limit the use of this therapy to the most severely ill patients. In order to develop additional antidepressants like ketamine, adequate preclinical behavioral screening paradigms for fast-acting antidepressants need to be established and used to identify the underlying neural mechanisms. This review examines the preclinical literature attempting to model the antidepressant-like effects of ketamine. Acute administration of ketamine has produced effects in behavioral screens for antidepressants like the forced swim test, novelty suppression of feeding and in rodent models for depression. Protracted behavioral effects of ketamine have been reported to appear after a single treatment that last for days. This temporal pattern is similar to its clinical effects and may serve as a new animal paradigm for rapid antidepressant effects in humans. In addition, protracted changes in molecules mediating synaptic plasticity have been implicated in mediating the antidepressant-like behavioral effects of ketamine. Current preclinical studies are examining compounds with more specific pharmacological effects at glutamate receptors and synapses in order to develop additional rapidly acting antidepressants without the hallucinogenic side effects or abuse potential of ketamine.

Keywords: ketamine, antidepressants, depression, animal models, BDNF

INTRODUCTION

Major depressive disorder (MDD) is a serious public health problem and one of the most common psychiatric disorders, with a lifetime prevalence of 17% in the United States (Kessler et al., 2005). Although the currently available antidepressants provide a measurable degree of therapy, approximately 50% of individuals diagnosed with MDD do not respond adequately to first–line treatment with conventional antidepressants (Trivedi et al., 2006; Fava et al., 2008). Moreover, the 3–4 week delay in the onset of therapeutic efficacy is particularly difficult for patients with persistent suicidal ideation. Patients that emerge as treatment resistant, defined as failing two or more trials of medication, are more severely ill with comorbid anxiety disorders and are at increased risk of suicide for an extended period of time (Joffe et al., 1993; Souery et al., 2007; Schosser et al., 2012). Therefore, there is a pressing medical need to develop rapidly acting therapeutics that are capable of immediately relieving the depressive symptomology, and persisting in their action as an antidepressant, for patients unable to respond to conventional therapies.

Recently it has been demonstrated that the NMDA receptor antagonist ketamine has rapid-acting and transient antidepressant effects in patients that are treatment resistant (Mathew et al., 2012). However, the discovery of ketamine is no panacea. The psychotomimetic properties and abuse potential of ketamine necessitate caution in promoting this particular compound as a general treatment for MDD. Understanding the underlying mechanism of action of ketamine linked to behavioral improvement is of significant importance for the development of novel, more improved antidepressants beyond the use of ketamine. This review will focus on the molecular alterations and animal behavior studies that have been used to measure potential correlates of the antidepressant effects of ketamine. As ketamine produces clinical antidepressant effects with a different time course and apparently different neurochemical mechanism than conventional antidepressants, the results of these studies have revealed new paradigms that can be used to identify novel compounds which may have a similar therapeutic potential and time course as ketamine in targeting treatment resistant depression (TRD).

KETAMINE—CLINICAL TRIALS

The initial clinical trials were double blind crossover studies that utilized a single infusion of ketamine (0.5 mg/kg) administered intravenously over a 40 min period (Berman et al., 2000; Zarate et al., 2006). Berman et al reported decreases in depressive symptomology, which emerged progressively over the first 3 days in all of the eight patients that were treated; one patient continued to show antidepressant-like effects 2 weeks post-infusion. Similarly, Zarate and colleagues reported a significant and rapid alleviation of depressive symptoms in 12 individuals on the first day, with six subjects exhibiting symptom alleviation for a least 1 week; two of these subjects continued to show antidepressant effects 2 weeks post-single ketamine infusion. Subsequent studies reported significant efficacy of ketamine in reducing suicidal ideation in individuals exhibiting TRD (Diazgranados et al., 2010). Moreover, a proof of concept trial conducted in treatment-resistant bipolar patients revealed a more rapid onset of antidepressant effects following ketamine infusion concomitant to their valproate and lithium treatment compared to previous studies conducted in MDD patients. However, the alleviation of depressive symptoms in the bipolar study persisted for only 3 days compared to the 7 days reported in earlier trials. In addition, ketamine had significant efficacy in patients resistant to electroconvulsive therapy (ECT) and produced more rapid antidepressant effects compared to ECT (Ibrahim et al., 2011). Unlike the almost immediate alleviation of depressive symptomology associated with ketamine infusion, similar reductions in symptoms were observed approximately 1–2 weeks following the first of the thrice-weekly ECT exposures. Furthermore, the use of ketamine as the anesthetic prior to ECT has been suggested to improve outcome and response to ECT (Hoyer et al., 2013). Indeed, the administration of ketamine/propofol (ketofol) improved the severity of seizure duration, induced an earlier onset of the antidepressant effect and significantly improved cognitive performances compared to propofol (Wang et al., 2012). Recently, it was reported that subanesthetic doses of S-ketamine with propofol actually worsened the post-treatment disorientation in some patients (Jarventausta et al., 2013). Further research is ongoing to determine the benefit of the S-enantiomer over the commonly used racemic mixture of ketamine. One group suggested that S-ketamine did not induce the transient psychotomimetic effects evident in the initial phase of infusion (Segmiller et al., 2013).

An extensive clinical trial involving 67 patients at two sites with documented TRD established the most definitive antidepressant efficacy of ketamine, in comparison with the benzodiazepine, midazolam, used as an active placebo control (Murrough et al., 2013). The response rates to ketamine vs. midazolam were 64 and 28%, respectively, with ketamine significantly reducing scores in the MADRS by 7.95 points. Ketamine-treated patients continued to exhibit improved scores over the 7-day period post-infusion compared to midazolam, however, the reduction of depressive scores on day 7 was no longer significant. Although most studies of ketamine have involved only a small number of patients, this is the best-designed and most extensive clinical trial to confirm the efficacy of ketamine in rapidly and persistently alleviating depressive symptomology.

Because the clinical effects of ketamine are transient, studies have assessed the efficacy of ketamine administration when given chronically. Significant improvement of symptoms persisted following six infusions of ketamine over 11 days, although the 9 patients treated in this trial eventually relapsed 19 days after the final infusion (aan het Rot et al., 2010). In addition, the effects of oral administration of ketamine given over a long-term period yielded positive findings, with patients exhibiting improved mood over the 28-day treatment period. Interestingly, although the level of symptom alleviation was the same as that achieved by I.V. infusion of ketamine, oral ketamine did not elicit a significant effect on depressive symptoms until day 14 of treatment but fortunately did relieve anxiety symptoms within 3 days of treatment (Irwin et al., 2013). Psychotomimetic effects were not observed in these patients; however, there were some reports of sleep disturbances and diarrhea. Moreover, another study conducted in bipolar patients using sublingual ketamine indicated significant (70%) numbers of individuals exhibiting improved mood with limited side effects with rapid onset of action. These data indicate that further evaluation of the administration route of ketamine and their side effect profiles may be beneficial.

Although there is a clear consensus on the rapidity of the antidepressant effect of ketamine in TRD, with most patients experiencing elevated mood starting approximately 120 min post-infusion, not all patients respond to ketamine treatment. Response rates across studies have ranged between 25 and 85% at 24 h and 14–70% at 72 h (Aan Het Rot et al., 2012). In addition, the duration of the antidepressant effect has varied across studies. In most of the trials conducted so far, only approximately half of the patients exhibited relief of depressive symptoms from ketamine lasting past 72 h. The reasons underlying variability in the response to ketamine are unknown. Given the heterogeneous nature of depression, a number of genetic, environmental and patient characteristics may be associated with treatment response. For example, patients with a family history of alcohol use disorder (AUD) exhibit better outcomes in response to ketamine administration, reporting less psychotomimetic disturbances and greater reductions of depression symptoms, compared to MDD patients without a history of AUD (Phelps et al., 2009). In addition, potential biomarkers or genetic variants will likely be found to augment or prevent responsiveness to ketamine.

Some clinical studies have tried to identify the critical pharmacological characteristics of ketamine associated with treatment response. Modification of the NMDA receptor subunit NR2B may confer an increased treatment response; indeed, NR2B antagonists, CP-1016060 and MK-0657 have shown good efficacy in treating TRD patients (Preskorn et al., 2008; Ibrahim et al., 2012a). AZD6765, a NMDA channel blocker, was assessed for its antidepressant-like qualities in a double blind crossover study involving 22 subjects. Although no psychotomimetic effects of this compound were reported, depressive symptoms were alleviated only for the first 2 h following infusion (Zarate et al., 2013). Similarly, administration of riluzole, (a sodium channel blocker, which indirectly inhibits glutamate release) for 4 weeks following ketamine infusion did not potentiate symptom improvement compared to placebo (Ibrahim et al., 2012b). These reports and a growing literature indicate that the mechanisms of action mediating ketamine's antidepressant effects have not yet been identified and are not elicited simply by the blockade of NMDA receptors.

ANTIDEPRESSANT-LIKE BEHAVIORAL EFFECTS OF KETAMINE IN RODENTS

The ability of ketamine to affect depressive-like behavior in a number of preclinical behavioral paradigms and models of depression has been widely studied in the past few years. Many reports indicate that acute administration of ketamine produces antidepressant-like effects in rodents (**Table 1**). However, some of the findings have not been replicated consistently by other laboratories. The literature concerning the antidepressant-like effects of ketamine is reviewed here, focusing on the effects of varying test conditions on behavioral outcomes. In addition, many studies have now reported that the effects of a single dose of ketamine can be measured over a protracted period of time lasting between days to weeks (**Table 2**). The time course of these protracted effects resembles the time course for ketamine's clinical effects (Yilmaz et al., 2002; Maeng et al., 2008), and may represent a new animal behavioral paradigm that correlates with the clinical effects of rapidly acting antidepressants.

FORCED SWIM TEST (FST)

The FST is the most frequently used behavioral test for measuring depressive-like behavior in rodents. It has also been a frequently used test within the preclinical ketamine literature. Mice and rats placed in cylinders containing water rapidly become immobile, demonstrated by floating passively or making only movements necessary to remain afloat. Based on an immobility response induced by inescapable exposure to stress, the FST also has strong predictive validity because short-term administration of antidepressant compounds from a variety of pharmacological classes reduces immobility time in the FST. These drugs include tricyclic compounds, MAO inhibitors, atypical antidepressants, and SSRIs (Cryan et al., 2005). Furthermore, the behavioral effects of tricyclics and SSRIs do not last beyond a few hours following their acute administration (Hoshaw et al., 2008).

Several groups have reported that a single administration of ketamine produced acute reductions of immobility in the FST shortly after injection (**Table 1**). Although the majority of these studies utilized a 10 mg/kg dose administered intraperitoneally (i.p.), subanesthetic doses of ketamine ranging from 10–50 mg/kg have produced antidepressant-like effects in the FST. However, some studies failed to detect acute effects of ketamine using the FST in mice (Bechtholt-Gompf et al., 2011) or in rats (Popik et al., 2008).

A feature of ketamine's pharmacology distinct from conventional antidepressants is that it produces protracted behavioral effects persisting between one to several days after administration (**Table 2**). The majority of studies indicate that the FST remains sensitive to the protracted effects of ketamine up to 1 week after a single injection (**Table 1**). These protracted effects were reported to persist for 8 days (Ma et al., 2013), 10 days (Yilmaz et al., 2002), 12 days (Garcia et al., 2008a), and 2 weeks (Maeng et al., 2008). Interestingly, antidepressant-like effects of ketamine were observed in the FST 2 months following the cessation of a 15-day treatment of rats during adolescence (Parise et al., 2013). This result is in line with other studies that have used a 10 or 12-day dosing regimen to establish longer-lasting effects of chronic ketamine on depressive-like activity in the FST (Tizabi et al., 2012; Akinfiresoye and Tizabi, 2013). Only one study examining the protracted effects of ketamine failed to report this finding (Lindholm et al., 2012).

The presence of chronic stress has been shown to facilitate the detection of antidepressant-like effects of ketamine in the FST (Koike et al., 2013a). There are also significant strain differences in the sensitivity to ketamine. For example, Wistar rats are insensitive to the antidepressant-like effects of low dose ketamine (2.5 and 5 mg/kg) following chronic treatment. In contrast, WKY rats were extremely sensitive to ketamine-induced reductions in FST immobility (Tizabi et al., 2012). WKY rats have a high baseline immobility level in the FST, which may allow for a greater sensitivity to compounds. Moreover, WKY rats are a genetic model of pathological depression and anxiety (Will et al., 2003; Solberg et al., 2004), which could provide them greater sensitivity to the effects of ketamine. Finally, the WKY strain is insensitive to SSRIs (Lopez-Rubalcava and Lucki, 2000; Tejani-Butt et al., 2003; Will et al., 2003) showing that ketamine is active under conditions where current antidepressants are ineffective. This feature makes WKY rats a useful strain in which to assess novel compounds resembling ketamine, which may be screened for efficacy in TRD.

TAIL SUSPENSION TEST (TST)

The TST is widely used in the preclinical ketamine literature as a less stressful test of behavioral despair when mice are suspended from their tail (Steru et al., 1985; Cryan et al., 2005). TST has predictive validity because it measures antidepressant-like responses from various classes of drugs. Ketamine reduces immobility levels in mice acutely, with studies reporting reductions in immobility time at 30 min (Mantovani et al., 2003; Rosa et al., 2003; Cruz et al., 2009; Koike et al., 2011a) and 24 h (Koike et al., 2011b) following a single injection of ketamine.

The most effective dose in the TST was 30 mg/kg. ICR mice were particularly sensitive to ketamine and continued to exhibit decreased immobility 72 h after treatment (Koike et al., 2011b). Furthermore, a lower dose of ketamine (10 mg/kg) was effective in reducing TST immobility increased by chronic mild stress (CMS) 48 h after ketamine injection (Ma et al., 2013). In contrast, two studies indicated that the acute reduction in immobility by high dose ketamine (50 and 160 mg/kg) was not maintained 1 week following treatment in mice (Popik et al., 2008; Bechtholt-Gompf et al., 2011). These data suggest that the TST is most valuable in the assessment of the more immediate antidepressant effects of ketamine. However, exposure to stress could increase the sensitivity to ketamine in the TST. To date there are no studies that have investigated whether the TST is sensitive to a chronic dosing regimen of ketamine.

NOVELTY SUPPRESSED FEEDING (NSF)

Exposure to a novel environment produces an anxiety-like phenotype in rodents known as hyponeophagia. In the NSF and novelty-induced hypophagia (NIH) tests, the latency to feed is increased and the amount of food consumption is reduced in a

Table 1 | Acute effects of ketamine.

References	Species and strain	Ketamine—supplier and dose	Behavioral alterations	Molecular alterations
ACUTE EFFECTS OF KETAMINE				
Burgdorf et al., 2013	Male adult (2–3 months) Sprague-Dawley rats	Fort Dodge (Butler, USA), I.V., I.P., and S.C. 10 mg/kg	Reduced immobility in FST 20–60 min and 24 h post i.p. Injection (10 mg/kg). Reduced latency to feed in the NIH 1 h post 10 mg/kg i.v.	Increased NR2B and GluR1 expression in the mPFC and HC 24 h post-injection
Carrier and Kabbaj, 2013	Male (250–270 g) and female (200–225 g) Sprague-Dawley rats	Fort Dodge (Butler Schein), Inc. 2.5–0 mg/kg	Latency to feed was reduced in the NSF 24 h post-injection (5 and 10 mg/kg). Increased sucrose consumption of males 48 h post-injection in the SPT. Reduced immobility in FST in males & females 30 min post-injection	Increased mTOR phosphorylation in males and females, reduced eEF2 phosphorylation in males (5 mg/kg)
Gigliucci et al., 2013	Male (280–320 g) Sprague- Dawley rats	Vetoquinol Ltd., UK (1.0 mg/ml). 10–25 mg/kg i.p.	Rats exhibited antidepressant-like effects in the FST at 1 or 24 h after a single injection of ketamine. Ketamine was ineffective following 3 injections (24, 5 and 1 h prior to testing). Ketamine (25 mg/kg) reversed stress-induced immobility; this was prevented by *p*CPA treatment at 24 h but not at 1 h post-injection	Depletion of cortical serotonin levels by *p*CPA (1.0 mg/kg once daily for 3 days) attenuated the antidepressant-like effect of ketamine in the FST
Koike et al., 2013a	Male Sprague-Dawley rats (185–325 g at testing)	Ketalar® Sankyo Yell Pharmaceutical Co., Ltd., 1–10 mg/kg i.p.	Ketamine (10 mg/kg) decreased immobility 30 min post-treatment in rats exposed to 21 days of corticosterone administration	N/A
Koike et al., 2013b	Male ICR (5 weeks) and male C57BL/6j (9 weeks)	Ketalar® Sankyo Yell Pharmaceutical Co., Ltd. 30 mg/kg i.p.	Ketamine decreased immobility in the FST & latency to feed in the NSF at 30 min and 24 h post-injection. K252a prevented ketamine's effects at 24 h.	N/A
Muller et al., 2013	Male Sprague Dawley rats (330–400 g)	Fort-Dodge (Pfizer CT), USA. 15 mg/kg (i.p.)	Reduced immobility in FST 2 h post-injection	Increased p-αCamKII and decreased SNARE complex expression 1– 4 h post-injection. No effect on GSK-3 activity. Protracted increased in synapsin expression1 h to 7 days post-injection
Walker et al., 2013	CD-1 mice (6 wks. old) and C57BL/6J mice (12 weeks old)	Fort Dodge Animal Health 6 mg/kg (i.p.)	Ketamine co-administered with LPS but not pretreatment 24 h prior blocked LPS-induced immobility in FST and anhedonia in the SPT. 10 h post LPS, ketamine administration reversed the anhedonia in SPT, this was blocked by NBQX	Ketamine did not block the LPS-induced increases in kynurenine metabolites, cytokines or BDNF expression at 6–28 h
Iijima et al., 2012	C57Bl/6J mice (9 weeks)	Sigma-Aldrich 30 mg/kg (i.p.)	Latency to feed in the NSF was reduced at 30 min and 24 h post-injection. Rapamycin reversed the 24 h reduction in NSF latency	N/A

(Continued)

Table 1 | Continued

References	Species and strain	Ketamine—supplier and dose	Behavioral alterations	Molecular alterations
Liu et al., 2012	BDNF knockin mice, (Val66Met SNP) Val/Met, Met/Met and Val/Val (WT) 6–8 months	Hospira Inc. 10 mg/kg (i.p.)	24 h post-injection the AD effects of ketamine in the FST were blocked in Met/Met mice	Met/Met knockin mice are insensitive to the molecular effects of ketamine on spine head diameter and spine length modulated in WT mice
Yang et al., 2012	Male Wistar rats (180–220 g)	Gutian Pharmaceutical CO. Ltd., Fuijan, China 10 mg/kg (i.p.)	Reduced immobility in FST 30 min post-injection	Increased mTOR phosphorylation in HC and PFC
Yang et al., 2013b	Male Wistar rats (200–300 g)	Gutian Pharmaceutical CO. Ltd., Fuijan, China 5–15 mg/kg (i.p.)	Dose-dependent reduction in immobility in the FST 30 min post-injection	Increased BDNF levels in the HC following 10 and 15 mg/kg. Dose dependent increase in phosphorylated mTOR levels in HC
Wang et al., 2011	Male Wistar rats (60 days old)	Sigma-Aldrich 15 mg/kg (i.p.)	Decreased immobility in the FST 60 min post-injection	Increased BDNF expression and decreased phosphorylation of GluR1 (Ser845) in HC 60 min post-injection
Beurel et al., 2011	WT and GSK-3 Knock in mice	10 mg/kg (i.p.)	AD effects in LH in WT but not GSK-3 knock-in mice	Increased pGSK-3β (CTX and HC) 30 and 60 min post-injection
Koike et al., 2011a	Male ICR mice (25–35 g)	Sigma-Aldrich 3–30 mg/kg (i.p.)	Ketamine reduced immobility in the TST 24 h post 30 mg/kg injection. Rapamycin reversed the ketamine-induced reduction in TST immobility	N/A
Reus et al., 2011	Male Wistar rats (60 days old)	Fort Dodge Animal Health—0.1 g/ml injectable solution, 5–10 mg/kg	Immobility in the FST was reduced at 60 min postinjection by 10 mg/kg only	Ketamine 5 mg/kg increased the expression of BDNF, CREB, and PKC phosphorylation in the PFC. 5mg/kg increased BDNF in the HC and Amg. 10 mg/kg decreased BDNF in the PFC, HC, and Amg. 10 mg/kg increased CREB expression and PKC phosphorylation in the PFC
Li et al., 2010	Male Sprague Dawley rats (150–250 g)	Sigma-Aldrich 10 mg/kg (i.p.)	Ketamine produced AD effects in the FST, LH and NSF test 24 h post-injection, blocked by rapamycin	Ketamine 10 mg/kg activated mTOR, ERK, and PKB/Akt signaling, blocked by NBQX, Ketamine 10 mg/kg increased expression of certain synaptic proteins at 2, 6, and 72 h post-injection, blocked by rapamycin
Ghasemi et al., 2010	Male NMRI mice (23–30 g)	Sigma-Aldrich 0.5–5 mg/kg (i.p)	Ketamine reduced immobility in the FST 45 min post-injection (2 and 5 mg/kg)	N/A
Cruz et al., 2009	Male Swiss mice (25–35 g)	Sigma-Aldrich 6.35–50 mg/kg (i.p.)	12.5, 25, and 50 mg/kg ketamine reduced immobility in the FST 30 min	N/A

(Continued)

Table 1 | Continued

References	Species and strain	Ketamine—supplier and dose	Behavioral alterations	Molecular alterations
			post-injection. Only 50 mg/kg ketamine reduced immobility in the TST	
Engin et al., 2009	Male Sprague-Dawley rats (180–360 g)	10–50 mg/kg (i.p.)	Ketamine (50 mg/kg) increased the % of open arm entries in the EPM. Both doses decreased immobility in the FST 30 min post-injection	N/A
Rezin et al., 2009	Male Wistar rats (300 g)	Fort Dodge Animal Health 15 mg/kg (i.p.)	Ketamine did not reverse the CMS-induced reduction in consumption of sweet food	Ketamine reversed the CMS-induced reductions in mitochondrial respiratory chain enzymes
Garcia et al., 2008a	Male Wistar rats (60 days old)	Fort Dodge (Brazil) 5, 10, and 15 mg/kg (i.p.)	1 h post-injection ketamine (5 & 10 mg/kg) significantly reduced immobility in the FST	BDNF increased in the HC following ketamine injection (15 mg/kg)
Hayase et al., 2006	Male ICR mice (60–90 days old)	Sankyo Co., Ltd. Tokyo, Japan 30–1.0 mg/kg (i.p.)	Ketamine increased the latency to immobility in the FST and was anxiolytic in the EPM at both doses 60 and 120 min post-injection	N/A
Rosa et al., 2003	Swiss mice male and female (30–40 g)	Sigma-Aldrich 5 mg/kg (i.p.)	Ketamine reduced immobility in the TST 30 min post-injection	N/A
Mantovani et al., 2003	Male Swiss mice 35–45 g)	0.1 mg/kg (i.p.)	Ketamine reduced immobility in the TST 30 min post-injection	N/A

This table outlines studies that have assessed the antidepressant-like effects of ketamine at 30 min to 24 h post-administration in commonly used behavioral tests. Molecular alterations of relevance to ketamine's molecular mechanism of action are also reported. FST, forced swim test; TST, tail suspension test; LH, learned helplessness; NSF, novelty suppressed feeding; SPT, sucrose preference test; EPM, elevated plus maze; AD, antidepressant; CMS, chronic mild stress; LPS, lipopolysaccharide; HC, hippocampus; CTX, cortex; Amg, amygdala; mPFC, medial prefrontal cortex; WT, wild type.

novel environment. These tests, based on a similar principle, differ in methodology; NSF requires acute food deprivation 24 h prior to testing whereas the NIH utilizes an 8–10-day training period without deprivation. These tests have considerable face validity, although interpretation of results with the NSF may be limited by the use of food deprivation. Hyponeophagia is one of the few anxiety-related tests that are reliably attenuated following chronic, but not acute, administration of antidepressant drugs (Bodnoff et al., 1988; Dulawa and Hen, 2005). In contrast, ketamine reduced the latency to eat within hours of treatment. The effective dose range for ketamine in this task varied across studies: 30 min and 24 h following 5–10 mg/kg (Li et al., 2010; Carrier and Kabbaj, 2013) and 30 mg/kg (Iijima et al., 2012), but all tests resulted in a significant reduction in the latency to feed in the novel environment. Moreover, ketamine (10 mg/kg) successfully reduced the latency to eat in the NIH 1 h post-injection (Burgdorf et al., 2013). More protracted effects of acute ketamine treatment (3 mg/kg) were observed 48 h following treatment in mice exposed to chronic stress, although ketamine did not reduce feeding latency in stress naïve mice in this study (Autry et al., 2011).

Overall, these data suggest that hyponeophagia is highly sensitive to a single dose of ketamine, although additional parameters of these tests remain to be examined more systematically. The fact that ketamine produced anxiolytic effects rapidly whereas conventional antidepressants require chronic treatment for weeks agrees with a more rapid onset of clinical effects. As TRD patients exhibit increased comorbid anxiety compared to treatment responsive MDD patients, the usefulness of assessing ketamine in anxiety tests should not be overlooked.

SUCROSE PREFERENCE TEST (SPT)

Sucrose consumption is widely accepted as a measure of anhedonia in rodents and has significant face validity in terms of its sensitivity to chronic stress and antidepressant treatment. Repeated administration of ketamine (7 days) reversed the decrease in sucrose consumption in rats exposed to chronic stress. Although it should be noted that this dosing regimen with ketamine also increased sweet food consumption in both stressed and non-stressed rats (Garcia et al., 2009). Furthermore, administration of a low dose of ketamine (0.5 mg/kg) for 10 days significantly increased sucrose consumption in WKY rats (Akinfiresoye and Tizabi, 2013). Marked increases in sucrose consumption in rats persisted at 1, 3, 5, and 7 days after a single treatment with ketamine (10 mg/kg) (Li et al., 2011), indicating significant protracted effects of ketamine on this behavior.

Table 2 | Protracted effects of ketamine.

References	Species and strain	Ketamine—supplier and dose	Behavioral alterations	Molecular alterations
PROTRACTED EFFECTS OF KETAMINE				
Akinfiresoye and Tizabi, 2013	Male WKY rats	Fort-Dodge (Henry Schien), 0.25 and 0.5 mg/kg (i.p.), administered daily for 10 days	Only chronic administration of 0.5 mg/kg reduced immobility in the FST and increased sucrose intake in the SPT	0.25 mg/kg ketamine did not alter mTOR phosphorylation or synapsin 1 and BDNF expression
Liu et al., 2013	Male Sprague-Dawley rats (150–250 g)	Hospira Inc., 1 and 10 mg/kg (i.p.)	Ketamine reduced immobility in the FST 24 h and 1 week following a single 10 mg/kg injection. This effect was not observed 2 weeks post-injection	Ketamine increased p- S6K, p-ERK, p-Akt but not p-mTOR or GSK-3b 1 h post-injection (10 mg/kg). These changes were not detected 24 h post-injection. 5-HT and hypocretin induced EPSCs were increased 24 h following ketamine treatment (10 mg/kg). Ketamine 1 and 10 mg/kg increased spine head diameter and spine density
Ma et al., 2013	C57Bl/6J mice (7 wks. old 20 g)	Gutian Pharmaceutical CO. Ltd., Fuijan, China. 10 mg/kg (i.p.)	Ketamine reversed CMS-induced increases in immobility in the FST and TST 48 h post-treatment. Ketamine reversed CMS-induced reductions in sucrose intake in the SPT, 24 h, 4, 6, and 8 days post-treatment. In non-stressed animals ketamine reduced immobility in the TST and FST at 3 and 24 h post-injection	N/A
Parise et al., 2013	Male adolescent Sprague-Dawley rats (post-natal day 35–49)	Fort-Dodge (Schein), 5, 10, and 20 mg/kg (i.p.). Administered twice a day for either 1 or 15 days	Ketamine (10 and 20 mg/kg) reduced immobility in the FST 24 h after the 2nd injection. CMS-induced immobility was reversed by ketamine (20 mg/kg). No effect of ketamine on SPT was observed. Two months after chronic ketamine treatment rats exhibited an anxiolytic phenotype on the EPM and AD effects in the FST	N/A
Lindholm et al., 2012	Adult male C57Bl/6J and WT & BDNF ± mice	Sigma-Aldrich 20 and 50 mg/kg (i.p.)	Decreased immobility in FST in WT mice at 45 min but not 7 days post-injection	No alterations in TrkB phosphorylation at 60 min or 7 days post-injection
Tizabi et al., 2012	Male and Female WKY and Wistar rats	Fort-Dodge (Schein), 0.25–5 mg/kg (i.p.), administered once or daily for 10 days	No acute/chronic effect of ketamine on Wistar immobility levels in the FST. 2.5 and 5 mg/kg reduced immobility of WKY rats in the FST; the 5 mg/kg dose had protracted effects 1 week post-injection. Chronic administration of 2.5 and	Ketamine (chronic 0.5 mg/kg paradigm) increased AMPA receptor binding & the AMPA/NMDA ration in WKY rats

(Continued)

Table 2 | Continued

References	Species and strain	Ketamine—supplier and dose	Behavioral alterations	Molecular alterations
			5 mg/kg reduced immobility of WKY but not Wistar. The effect of the 2.5 mg.kg dose were evident 1 week following the cessation of treatment	
Autry et al., 2011	Adult male C57BL/6 WT and inducible BDNF KO mutants	Fort Dodge Animal Health 3 mg/kg (i.p.)	No effect in EPM or fear conditioning 24 h post-injection. Reduced FST immobility at 30 min, 3 h, 24 h, and 1 week, blocked by NBQX. Reduced latency to feed in NSF, increased sucrose intake & decreased immobility in CMS mice 30 min post-injection. Rapamycin did not block ketamine-induced reductions in FST immobility 30 min post-injection. Anisomycin prevented the effects of ketamine in the NSF & FST. TrkB KO mice did not response to ketamine	Increased TrkB activation. Increased BDNF protein but not mRNA at 30 min and 1 h post-injection. Decreased phosphorylation of eEF2 in HC. Blocked spontaneous activity of NMDARs in HC cultures
Bechtholt-Gompf et al., 2011	CD-1 and BALB/c mice	Sigma-Aldrich, dose range 0.5–3.0 mg/kg	Reduced immobility in TST 1 h post-injection (1.0 mg/kg), not observed at day 7. No effect on FST immobility at any dose, or time point	N/A
Koike et al., 2011b	Male ICR mice (25–35 g) and male Sprague-Dawley rats (230–350 g)	Sigma-Aldrich 3–30 mg/kg (i.p.)	Ketamine reduced the number of failures to escape in the LH test 30 min post 10 mg/kg injection. Reduced immobility in the TST 30 min & 72 h post 30 mg/kg injection	N/A
Li et al., 2011	Male Sprague Dawley rats (150–250 g)	Sigma-Aldrich 10 mg/kg (i.p.)	Ketamine reversed CMS-induced anhedonia in the NSF test 2 days post-injection. Sucrose consumption was increased 1, 3, 5, and 7 days following the single ketamine injection	Ketamine reversed CMS-induced deficits in synaptic EPSCs, spine density and synaptic protein expression. At 7 days post-treatment these effects were still apparent
Yilmaz et al., 2002)	Male Wistar rats (280–310 g)	Parke-Davis 50 mg/ml stock 1.0 mg/kg (i.p.)	Ketamine reduced FST at 3, 7, and 10 days post-injection, (this was only in the second test of each day).	N/A
Garcia et al., 2009	Wistar rats (300–350 g)	Fort Dodge Animal Health 15 mg/kg once on day 7 or daily for 7 days	CMS-induced reductions in sucrose intake, weight loss, adrenal hypertrophy, and	No differences in HC BDNF concentrations

(Continued)

Table 2 | Continued

References	Species and strain	Ketamine—supplier and dose	Behavioral alterations	Molecular alterations
			increased ACTH and corticosterone levels were reversed by acute and chronic ketamine administration. Chronic ketamine increased sucrose intake in controls	
Garcia et al., 2008b	Wistar rats (300–350 g)	Fort Dodge Animal Health, 5, 10, and 15 mg/kg—daily i.p. injections for 12 days	All doses reduced immobility in the FST	HC BDNF concentrations were not altered
Popik et al., 2008	Male Wistar rats (270 g) and male Sprague Dawley rats (275 g), C57/Bl/Han male mice (24 g) and Male Swiss mice (28 g)	Biowet, Pulawy, Poland, FST rats, 1.0 mg/kg. TST mice, 50–1.0 mg/kg. FST mice, 1.25–10 mg/kg	Reduction of immobility in the FST in mice but not in rats at 30 min post-injection only (50 mg/kg). Ketamine reduced immobility in the TST at 40 min but not at 1 week post-injection	N/A
Maeng et al., 2008	Mice	Sigma-Aldrich 0.5–10 mg/kg (i.p.)	Ketamine reduced the number of escape failures in LH 24 h post-injection. Ketamine (2.5 mg/kg) reduced immobility in the FST at 30 min and 2 weeks post-injection	Ketamine reduced phosphorylation of HC GluR1 (S845), rescued by NBQX

This table outlines studies that have assessed the antidepressant-like effects of ketamine from day 2, or, 48 h post-administration onwards in commonly used behavioral tests. In some of these studies earlier time points have been assessed, the results are also included in this table. Molecular alterations of relevance to ketamine's molecular mechanism of action are also reported. FST, forced swim test; TST, tail suspension test; LH, learned helplessness; NSF, novelty suppressed feeding; SPT, sucrose preference test; EPM, elevated plus maze; AD, antidepressant; CMS, chronic mild stress; LPS, lipopolysaccharide; HC, hippocampus; CTX, cortex; Amg, amygdala; mPFC, medial prefrontal cortex; WTm, wild type.

Decreases in sucrose consumption induced by exposure to LPS (Walker et al., 2013) and CMS (Ma et al., 2013) were reversed following a single ketamine treatment. Protracted effects of acute ketamine treatment were evident in CMS exposed mice tested at 4, 6, and 8 days after a single ketamine treatment (Ma et al., 2013). In contrast, the consumption of sugar pellets in CMS exposed rats was not altered by ketamine treatment (Rezin et al., 2009), although this particular test is not directly comparable to the traditional SPT. It should be noted that there is a lack of consensus on the most appropriate SPT protocol to model an anhedonic state in rats. Nevertheless, these data support the use of the SPT as a sensitive screening test for rapid-acting antidepressant-like drugs such as ketamine.

ELEVATED PLUS MAZE (EPM)

The EPM is frequently used to measure anxiety behavior in rodents (Bourin, 1997; Rodgers et al., 1997) and has strong predictive validity for screening anxiolytics. However, it is generally not sensitive to antidepressant treatments. Ketamine induced an anxiolytic phenotype in rats during exposure to the EPM 30 min after a single ketamine injection (Engin et al., 2009). A similar effect was observed in mice 1 and 2 h following treatment (Hayase et al., 2006). These studies indicate that the EPM was not sensitive to low doses of ketamine; only higher doses (30 mg/kg) induced a significant anxiolytic effect. Moreover, lower doses of ketamine did not induce an anxiolytic response in the EPM in stress naïve mice (Autry et al., 2011). The lack of effect of low doses of ketamine is also characteristic of the TST. Parise and colleagues described significant anxiolytic effects in the EPM in rats 2 months after the completion of a 15-day dosing regimen of 20 mg/kg per day during adolescence (Parise et al., 2013). Although the presence of drug effects after such a long interval could indicate sensitivity to the protracted effects of ketamine, developmental factors may have played a greater role. At present the EPM can only be proposed as a tool for assessing the more immediate anxiolytic effects of ketamine.

LOCOMOTOR ACTIVITY

Antidepressant-like effects of ketamine are usually evaluated in conjunction with spontaneous activity, because increased motor activity can produce false positive effects in the aforementioned behavioral tasks. Ketamine produces significant hyperactivity immediately following injection; 10 min post i.p. injection of low dose ketamine (5–15 mg/kg), rats displayed hyperactivity in spontaneous activity (da Silva et al., 2010). In addition, repeated administration of ketamine (50 mg/kg) sensitized rats to its hyperactive effects (Popik et al., 2008).

However, most studies have reported either no change or a reduction of locomotor activity after ketamine. A reduction of open field behavior was produced by ketamine in rats at 30 min post 50 mg/kg (Engin et al., 2009) and 1 h post 10 and 25 mg/kg (Gigliucci et al., 2013). In addition, a single injection of ketamine did not alter locomotor activity beyond 30 min post-injection in rats (Reus et al., 2011; Tizabi et al., 2012; Yang et al., 2012; Akinfiresoye and Tizabi, 2013) or in mice (Lindholm et al., 2012). At 24 h post-injection, there was no effect on locomotor activity in mice by ketamine or by the NMDA antagonists CPP and MK-801 (Autry et al., 2011).

Furthermore, chronic administration of low dose ketamine did not affect spontaneous activity in adult rats (Garcia et al., 2008b; Ma et al., 2013). Interestingly, it was shown recently that hyperactivity was displayed in adolescent but not adult rats following chronic ketamine administration (Parise et al., 2013). Many of the experiments assessed in this review did not measure the effects of ketamine on locomotor activity at the dose and time point used. However, taken together, the data suggest it is important practice to assess changes in activity measures post-treatment to identify and eliminate the involvement of any potential locomotor effect in the behavioral responses to ketamine.

LEARNED HELPLESSNESS (LH)

The LH model of depression produces escape deficits in rodents exposed to unpredictable and uncontrollable stress (Seligman et al., 1980). LH is a popular model of depression as it has good face validity and induces a number of endophenotypes that can be measured in other behavioral tasks, including the FST and NSF. Repeated treatment with antidepressants reversed the coping behavior deficits in rats and mice (Shanks and Anisman, 1988; Caldarone et al., 2000). A single administration of ketamine (10 mg/kg) has been reported to reverse the deficits in coping behavior induced by learned helplessness 30–60 min (Beurel et al., 2011; Koike et al., 2011a) and 24 h after treatment (Maeng et al., 2008; Li et al., 2010). Furthermore, ketamine is effective in producing antidepressant-like effects in the LH in CMS-treated mice at even a lower dose (3 mg/kg) (Autry et al., 2011). Currently, there is no information regarding the protracted effects of ketamine in LH.

CHRONIC MILD STRESS (CMS)

Exposure to the CMS model induces depressive behavior in rodents following the presentation of a series of stressors in an unpredictable sequence over a prolonged period of time. CMS produces a number of behavioral changes in rodents thought to resemble features of depressed patients, such as anhedonia or loss of grooming (Willner, 1997, 2005). CMS satisfies most of the criteria of validity for an animal model of depression; it is etiologically relevant with good design, resulting in similar pathological alterations observed in humans that are sensitive to chronic antidepressant treatment. The behavioral and molecular changes induced by CMS are reversed by treatment with antidepressant drugs, but only after administration for several weeks. In contrast, ketamine reversed the behavioral and physiological alterations induced by CMS in rats following acute administration and the effects were maintained following chronic treatment. Acute and chronic treatment with ketamine reversed the increase in adrenal gland weight, promoted regain of body weight, and normalized circulating corticosterone and ACTH levels (Garcia et al., 2009). Physiological alterations induced by CMS were reversed by acute ketamine treatment in a similar study but failed to reverse CMS-induced anhedonia in the SPT (Rezin et al., 2009). In addition, CMS-exposed adolescent rats exhibited decreased immobility, increased sucrose consumption and latency to feed immediately following acute ketamine treatment (Parise et al., 2013).

Because the CMS is accepted as a rodent model of depression, CMS is an ideal paradigm with which to screen the antidepressant-like effects of novel therapeutics like ketamine. Reversal of CMS-induced depressive-like phenotypes measured using the mouse FST, NSF, and SPT has been reported by ketamine in the absence of any drug effect in stress naïve mice (Autry et al., 2011). Furthermore, the effect of ketamine in the NSF test was observed to persist in CMS mice 48 h post-injection. In line with these findings, two similar studies have indicated an increased sensitivity of CMS-exposed mice to ketamine (Li et al., 2011; Ma et al., 2013). Taken together, the CMS data is the most consistent and possibly the most valid method of examining the antidepressant-like effects of ketamine in preclinical studies.

KETAMINE—MOLECULAR MECHANISMS OF ACTION

In order to develop novel and more effective antidepressants, the molecular mechanisms underlying the protracted behavioral improvement associated with ketamine treatment need to be understood fully. The majority of this information has been garnered from preclinical animal studies and the principle findings are detailed in the following section.

NMDA AND AMPA RECEPTORS

Currently the hypothesis for ketamine's mechanism of action focuses on a cascade of neurochemical events that are initiated shortly after administration of ketamine. The events then persist in a protracted manner for days following its metabolism and elimination.

Reductions in neurogenesis and synaptic plasticity play a key role in the pathophysiology of MDD. Synaptic plasticity refers to the dynamic capability of synapses to form and retract processes, thereby modifying synaptic strength and communication. The most well studied mechanisms mediating changes in plasticity are long-term potentiation (LTP) and long-term depression (LTD). These processes involve significant alterations in pre and post-synaptic scaffolding proteins and glutamate receptors, primarily the glutamatergic receptor, α-amino-3-hydroxy-5-methyl-4-isoxazole propionic acid (AMPA). The AMPA receptor containing the subunits GluR1, GluR4, and GluR2 are involved in LTP, whereas GluR2, GluR3, and GluR4 are required for the AMPA receptor internalization needed to facilitate LTD (Kessels and Malinow, 2009). N-methyl-d-aspartate (NMDA) receptors at excitatory synapses are also subject to trafficking and significantly decrease in synaptic density during LTD (Peng et al., 2010). In the pyramidal cells of the hippocampus, LTP and LTD bidirectionally regulate dendritic spine growth and retraction, whereas AMPA expression is positively related to the size of the spine head. These dynamic processes are stabilized by concurrent alterations in the expression of synaptic proteins and signaling pathways.

Ketamine blocks NMDA receptors (NMDARs) at concentrations of 2–50 μm. The subsequent suppression of tonic glutamate input to GABAergic interneurons, results in disinhibition of glutamate signaling. This disinhibition and increase in glutamate neurotransmission is mediated by a decrease in GABAergic inhibitory feedback of the pyramidal neurons in layer V of the PFC, a region widely implicated in the development of psychiatric disorders (Homayoun and Moghaddam, 2007). Interestingly, post-mortem studies report reductions in pyramidal cells and GABAergic interneurons in the PFC of depressed individuals (Choudary et al., 2005; Rajkowska et al., 2007). Increases in glutamate will activate ionotropic AMPARs resulting in Na^{2+} influx and subsequent membrane depolarization, induction of signaling cascades and protein synthesis. Certain AMPARs that lack the GluR2 subunit actually result in Ca^{2+} influx (Kessels and Malinow, 2009). Upregulation of AMPA receptor expression following ketamine administration mediates the increased sensitivity to glutamate. It has been suggested that this increased sensitivity or "synaptic scaling" is necessary to maintain stability in synaptic plasticity and increased protein synthesis in the presence of chronic NMDAR blockade (Kavalali and Monteggia, 2012).

Pharmacological inhibition of ketamine's behavioral effects has been achieved using the AMPA receptor antagonist, 2, 3-dihdroxyl-6-nitro-7-sulfamoyl-benzo(f)quinoxaline-2, 3-dione (NBQX), reversing the antidepressant effects of ketamine in the LH paradigm (Maeng et al., 2008; Koike et al., 2011b). Furthermore, co-administration of AMPAR antagonists blocked the effects of ketamine in the FST (Autry et al., 2011). As AMPARs have a clear role in mediating ketamine's effects, a recent study showed the antidepressant-like effect of AMPA administration in the depressive-like WKY rats (Akinfiresoye and Tizabi, 2013). This data indicate that AMPA receptors and indeed the AMPA/NMDA ratio is an important consideration and target in the development of potential therapeutics.

mTOR SIGNALING

Data suggests that the protracted antidepressant-like effects of ketamine are mediated by molecular alterations to the signaling pathway for the mammalian target of rapamycin (mTOR) (see **Figure 1**), a serine/threonine kinase and key component of the insulin-signaling pathway (Li et al., 2010). Two functional mTOR complexes regulate the initiation of protein translation in mammalian cells, mTOR complex 1 (mTORC1) and mTOR complex 2 (mTORC2) (Rosner and Hengstschlager, 2011). A recent post-mortem study implicated decreases in cortical mTOR-signaling kinases in the pathophysiology of MDD (Jernigan et al., 2011). Additionally, rats exposed to CMS exhibit significant reductions in the phosphorylation of several kinases in the mTOR pathway in the amygdala of stressed rats (Chandran et al., 2013).

There is an inverted U-shape associated with ketamine-induced mTOR activation, with higher doses having no effect. In rodents, ketamine administration induced mTOR signaling approximately 30 min after injection. Li and colleagues elucidated some core features of ketamine's mechanism of action, primarily focusing on the alterations in mTOR dependent synapse formation in the PFC of rats (Li et al., 2010). In addition, they reported increased phosphorylation of mTOR, p70 KD ribosomal protein S6 kinase (p70S6K) and eukaryotic initiation factor 4E binding protein 1 (4E-BP1). P70S6K is required to inhibit suppression of eEF2, which prevents protein translation. Simultaneously, the phosphorylation of 4E-BP1 results in the release of eukaryotic translation initiation factor 4E (eIF-4E), thereby triggering the initiation of translation of synaptic proteins. These changes were accompanied by antidepressant-like behavior in the FST and NSF test (Li et al., 2010).

mTOR is ubiquitously expressed and has been found to localize in the cytoplasm of dendrites, where it can initiate the translation of synaptic proteins essential for the induction of LTP (Duman et al., 2012). PSD95, GluR1 and synapsin are upregulated approximately 2 h post-ketamine; this increase is observed for up to 72 h. Similarly, upregulation of Arc, a cytoskeletal protein is observed approximately 1 h post-injection and sustained for up to 6 h (Li et al., 2010). Arc is linked to the induction of early and late phase LTP and memory formation (Panja et al., 2009). A recent study confirmed that ketamine and MK-801 induced increases in immediate early genes, such as Arc, C-fos and Homer1a. Homer1a/Homer1b/PSD-95 signaling is implicated in glutamate induced synaptic plasticity (de Bartolomeis et al., 2013) and may be an interesting marker of plasticity for ketamine-like compounds. Similarly, reductions in the expression of eukaryotic elongation factor 2 (eEF2) is consistently observed in rodents following ketamine administration both in the PFC (Carrier and Kabbaj, 2013) and hippocampus (Autry et al., 2011). Interestingly, females are more sensitive to the behavioral effects of low dose ketamine compared to males; however, females do not exhibit decreases in eEF2 (Carrier and Kabbaj, 2013). Nevertheless, phosphorylation and inhibition of eEF2 may be a useful marker for rapid antidepressants, as increased phosphorylation of eEF2 in the PFC is also reported following chronic fluoxetine treatment in rats (Dagestad et al., 2006).

Pharmacological modulation of different components of the mTOR-signaling pathway (**Figure 1**) has been used to investigate mechanisms underlying the acute and protracted behavioral actions of ketamine. Inhibition of Akt, following blockade of phosphatidylinositol-3-kinase (PI3K) by LY294002, and inhibition of ERK using U0126, prevented ketamine reversal of CMS-induced deficits (Li et al., 2010). The Trk/B inhibitor K252a blocked the effects of ketamine in the TST and the NSF when tested 24 h, but not at 1 h (Koike et al., 2013b). The rapamycin-FKBP12 complex inhibits mTOR signaling when directly bound to mTORC1 (Hoeffer and Klann, 2010). Rapamycin pretreatment inhibited both the molecular and behavioral effects of ketamine on FST, NSF and the LH 24 h post-injection (Li et al., 2010). Furthermore, rapamycin administration did not inhibit the effects of ketamine in the NSF test at 30 min post-injection, but ketamine's effects were completely blocked at 24 h post-injection (Iijima et al., 2012). Thus, it appears that mTOR signaling is clearly associated with the protracted behavioral effects

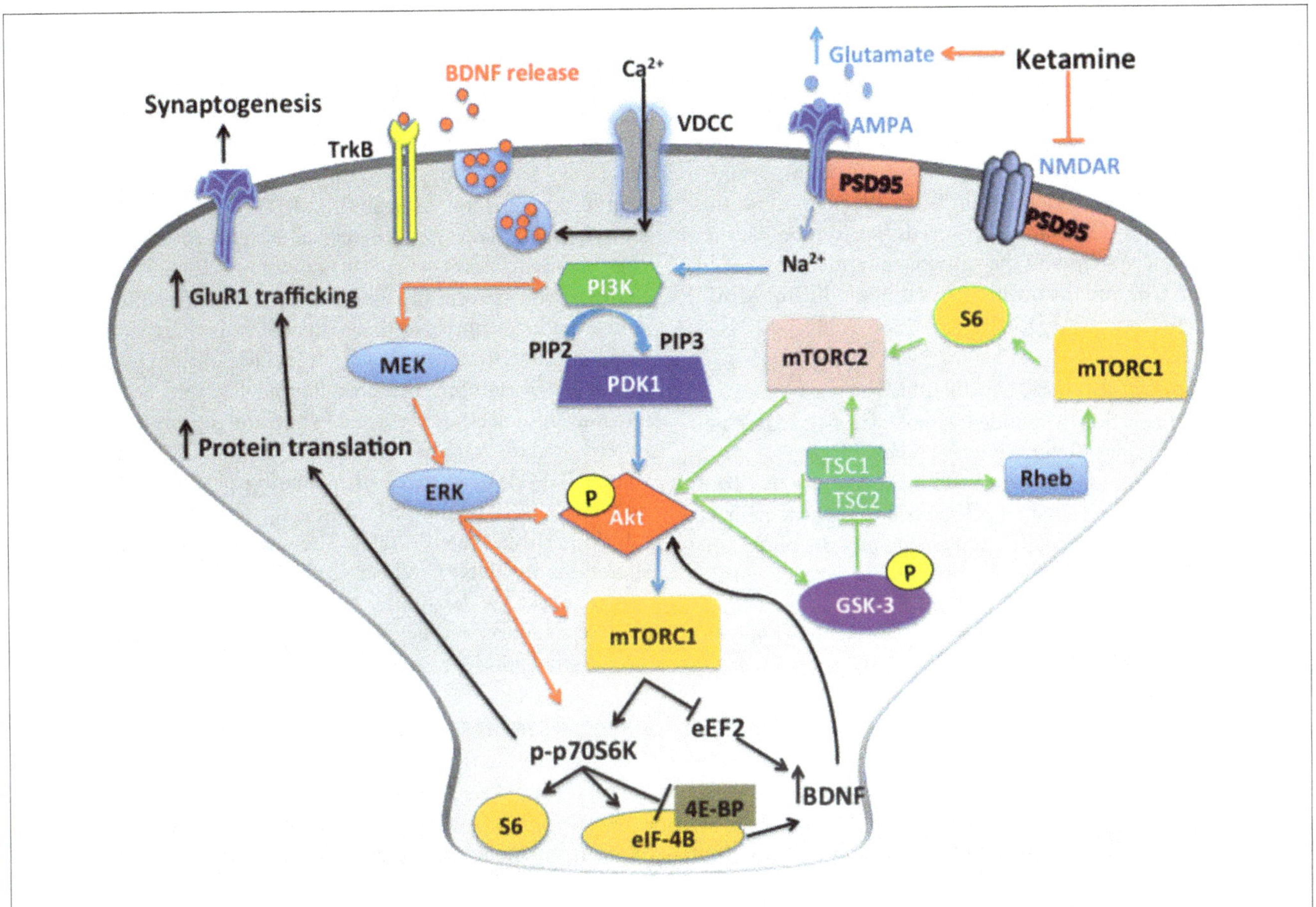

FIGURE 1 | Following blockade of NMDARs, phosphorylation of Akt activates mTOR complex 1 (mTORC1), which results in increased p70S6K phosphorylation and increased protein translation via inhibition of 4E-BP and release of eIF-4B. Glutamate binds AMPARs, which induces depolarization of the membrane, enabling Ca^{2+} influx through VDCCs. This results in BDNF release from synaptic vesicles. The subsequent binding of TrkB receptors induces ERK and Akt signaling. These pathways all converge to increase synaptic protein translation and receptor trafficking to the cell membrane. Additionally, activation of mTORC2 by S6, and inhibition of GSK-3, induces mTORC1 activation via increased Akt phosphorylation. Furthermore, mTORC2 activation induces protein kinase C (PKC) signaling transduction, which regulates actin and other cytoskeletal proteins.

of ketamine measured 24 h later or longer, but other mechanisms may be involved in the immediate effects of ketamine, such as increased AMPAR activation. It is of interest to note that other antidepressants, including 5-HT_{2C} receptor antagonists, citalopram and electro-convulsive seizures (ECS, the equivalent to ECT in rodents) all increase mTORC1 levels (Elfving et al., 2013; Opal et al., 2013). However, the SSRI, sertraline, and the TCA, imipramine, actually have anti-proliferative effects that are mediated by inhibition of mTOR (Lin et al., 2010; Jeon et al., 2011). Furthermore, there is evidence that suggests rapamycin administration alone and the subsequent inhibition of mTOR signaling is capable of inducing antidepressant-like effects in the rat FST (Cleary et al., 2008). Moreover, the effects of long-term modulation of mTOR have yet to be assessed. These data indicate the role of mTOR signaling may be more complex than originally anticipated.

Other drugs have been used to identify neural mechanisms that might account for the antidepressant-like behavioral effects of ketamine. NMDA receptor blockade using MK-801 or CPP reduced immobility in the FST for up to 3 and 24 h, respectively, but neither compound reproduced the protracted effects of ketamine at longer intervals (Autry et al., 2011). The NR2B antagonist RO-25-6981 was suggested to induce mTOR signaling, resulting in similar molecular and behavioral effects as those observed following ketamine administration (Maeng et al., 2008; Li et al., 2010). In addition, the mGlu2/3 receptor antagonists LY341495 and MGS0039 decreased immobility time in the TST. NBQX had a limited effect on these antagonists, whereas rapamycin reversed the behavioral effects of these compounds at 24 h post-treatment, suggesting a role for mTOR signaling but not AMPA in mediating the antidepressant-like effects of mGluR2/3 antagonists (Koike et al., 2011a). The mGluR5 antagonist MPEP induced antidepressant-like effects in the NSF at 30 min and 24 h post-injection (Iijima et al., 2012). The effects at 24 h were blocked by rapamycin and the protein synthesis inhibitor anisomycin but not by the TrkB inhibitor K252a. In addition, the mGluR7 agonist AMN082 produced an antidepressant like effect in the TST 40 min post-injection which was reversed by NBQX pretreatment, suggesting that AMPA mediates the antidepressant effects of this compound (Bradley et al., 2012). Finally, the glycine functional partial agonist GLYX-13 produced an antidepressant-like effect in the FST, NIH and LH tests that extended for 24 h after injection, similar to the effects of ketamine (Burgdorf et al., 2013). These data suggest that when investigating the potential of novel compounds targeting glutamate, both mTOR and AMPA mediation should be assessed. Furthermore, it is important to choose an appropriate rodent strain in which to conduct these assays. For example, CD-1 mice are insensitive to modulation of the glutamatergic system and the subsequent antidepressant-like effects of AMNO82 and the mGluR 7 negative modulator MMPIP (O'Connor and Cryan, 2013).

BRAIN-DERIVED NEUROTROPHIC FACTOR (BDNF)

Chronic administration of antidepressant drugs increases neurotrophins including BDNF (Duman and Monteggia, 2006). BDNF has high affinity for tyrosine kinase receptor B (TrkB), activating a number of signaling pathways that regulate neuronal growth and survival. This pathway also regulates the phosphorylation of cyclic-amp response element binding protein (CREB), which is integral to affective behavior, in addition to learning and memory (Autry and Monteggia, 2012). Post-mortem studies have reported reductions in BDNF and TrkB expression in the hippocampus and PFC of MDD patients and depressed suicides (Krishnan et al., 2007; Castren and Rantamaki, 2010; Yu and Chen, 2011). Rodent models of chronic stress and depression have recapitulated these region-specific changes of BDNF (Duman and Monteggia, 2006; Autry and Monteggia, 2012). At a behavioral level, BDNF administration reduces immobility in the FST (Shirayama et al., 2002; Hoshaw et al., 2005; Deltheil et al., 2008). Additionally, the over-expression of TrkB receptors leads to an antidepressant-like behavioral phenotype in mice (Koponen et al., 2004). BDNF deficient mice are depressive-like in some behavioral tests and fail to respond to conventional antidepressants in the CMS and FST compared to wild type mice (Saarelainen et al., 2003; Monteggia et al., 2007; Ibarguen-Vargas et al., 2009).

Activation of the mTOR pathway by ketamine enhances translation of BDNF in the hippocampus (Garcia et al., 2008a; Autry et al., 2011; Yang et al., 2012). The inhibition of eEF2 and subsequent increase in BDNF translation is proposed to mediate the rapid antidepressant-like effects of ketamine (Monteggia et al., 2013). Equally ketamine is capable of inducing a rapid release of glutamate. Following NMDA receptor blockade, AMPAR activation results in calcium influx via L-type voltage gated calcium channels (VDCC) inducing the release of BDNF from synaptic vesicles (see **Figure 1**). Furthermore, BDNF regulates neuronal mTOR function via Akt and PI3K, creating a positive feedback loop of BDNF production following the activation of mTOR by ketamine (Hay and Sonenberg, 2004; Hoeffer and Klann, 2010).

A single nucleotide polymorphism Val66Met (rs6265) in the BDNF gene has been proposed as a potential impediment to the antidepressant response to ketamine in TRD patients. Val/Val carriers are more sensitive to the antidepressant-effects of ketamine compared to the Val/Met carriers (Laje et al., 2012). However, not all studies have reported a positive correlation of improvement in depressive symptoms with increased BDNF (Machado-Vieira et al., 2009; Rybakowski et al., 2013). It is worth noting that BDNF serum concentrations were significantly lower in bipolar patients that did not respond to ketamine treatment compared to responders at baseline (Rybakowski et al., 2013). Mice that possess this polymorphism did not respond to ketamine and displayed significant impairments in synaptogenesis (Lindholm et al., 2012; Liu et al., 2012). However, at higher doses, repeated dosing or continuous infusion of ketamine, BDNF levels were increased, although this increase was correlated with neurodegeneration and cognitive deficits (Ibla et al., 2009; Goulart et al., 2010). Similarly, humans who chronically abuse ketamine exhibit higher BDNF concentrations compared to healthy controls (Ricci et al., 2011).

As a downstream product of multiple signaling cascades induced by ketamine, the production of BDNF occurs rapidly and may underlie the protracted behavioral response to ketamine. Indeed, acute i.c.v infusion of both BDNF and insulin-like growth factor (IGF-1) are capable of mediating protracted antidepressant like effects in the FST lasting up to 6 days following the infusion (Hoshaw et al., 2008). These data not only indicate that alterations in BDNF levels are most likely involved in the protracted effects of ketamine, but also confirms that rapid and persistent increases in neurotrophins are useful markers of novel rapid-acting antidepressants.

GLYCOGEN SYNTHASE KINASE-3 (GSK-3)

GSK-3 is a serine/threonine protein kinase and a major target for the mood stabilizer lithium (Klein and Melton, 1996; Stambolic et al., 1996). TRD patients are often given a period of antidepressant augmentation treatment with lithium when they fail to response to SSRIs alone (Carvalho et al., 2007; Bauer et al., 2010). Furthermore, studies have shown that GSK-3 is functionally regulated by serotonin modulation, primarily mediated by 5-HT_{1A} autoreceptors and via iPI3K/Akt signaling (Polter et al., 2012). GSK-3$\beta^{\pm}$ heterozygous mice display significant reductions in immobility in the FST (O'Brien et al., 2004). Interestingly mice with a knock-in mutation of GSK-3, which prevents its phosphorylation, do not respond to ketamine treatment in the LH paradigm, suggesting that some of ketamine's potential therapeutic efficacy might be mediated following inhibition of this kinase (Beurel et al., 2011). Furthermore, combination of ketamine and the GSK-3 inhibitor, SB216763, significantly reduced immobility in the FST; at a molecular level, this combination of ketamine and SB216763 amplified the frequency of 5-HT and hypocretin-induced EPSCs and increased spine density in the mPFC. Conversely, it had been shown that ketamine has limited effects on GSK-3 expression in hippocampal synaptosomes (Muller et al., 2013). Moreover, a single dose of ketamine reversed the behavioral effects of CMS, but the GSK-3 inhibitor SB216763 had no effect on CMS-induced behavioral scores (Ma et al., 2013). Further preclinical studies are required to evaluate the role of GSK-3β in the antidepressant-like response to ketamine. A recent assessment of three depressed patients indicates a significant increase in phosphorylated GSK-3β in the plasma of ketamine-treated individuals over the 120-min assessment period (Yang et al., 2013a). Although the inhibition of GSK-3β modulates m-TOR signaling (**Figure 1**) and may potentially augment the effects of antidepressants such as ketamine, it is unclear whether GSK-3 directly mediates the effects of ketamine.

CONCLUSION AND FUTURE DIRECTIONS

The development of ketamine as a rapidly acting antidepressant drug has the potential to revolutionize clinical treatment. Nevertheless, the clinical use of ketamine for depression poses a number of challenges. Ketamine is an hallucinogenic drug subject to abuse and must be given in a controlled setting. The effects of ketamine are short-lasting and can only be sustained by its repeated treatment. A desirable research direction would be to develop other drugs with similar antidepressant effects that are devoid of ketamine's liabilities. However, progress in this area is constrained by uncertainty concerning the critical pharmacological mechanisms underlying the antidepressant effects of ketamine.

Animal models have the potential to translate the pharmacological effects of ketamine that are most critical for its clinical antidepressant effects. A substantial body of literature now indicates that ketamine produces antidepressant-like effects in preclinical tests for antidepressant activity and in animal models of depression. Acute ketamine produces immediate effects on many behavioral tests that are similar to antidepressants. However, the protracted effects of ketamine measured for days after a single administration are not produced by conventional antidepressants. They define a new paradigm for antidepressant drug discovery that is the best temporal correlate with ketamine's clinical activity. Inconsistent findings across laboratories may arise from a disparity in methodology used across studies. The most pertinent variables are that the efficacious dose is dependent on the behavioral task employed, conditions surrounding administration and the time of testing post-administration of ketamine. For example, evidence suggests that the effects of low and seemingly sub-efficacious doses of ketamine are more effective following stress exposure. Behavioral tests with high predictive validity for antidepressant-like effects, such as the FST, are sensitive to acute and chronic ketamine. They can be utilized in conjunction with other tests sensitive only to chronic antidepressant treatment, such as the NSF/SPT, to measure the protracted benefits that are unique to ketamine. Overall, combination of a stress or genetic model of depression/anxiety with behavioral assessment over a 1–2 week period post-treatment with low doses of ketamine will yield the most valid and useful information.

Among the many barriers to translation of ketamine's clinical antidepressant effects across species stand a number of key pharmacological factors. The route of administration of ketamine in preclinical models is by i.p. injection, whereas intravenous infusion is usually employed in clinical trials. Therefore, it may be beneficial for animal studies to employ intravenous infusion where practical. In addition, plasma levels of ketamine monitored in the first 2 h following administration can determine whether the dose/route of administration of ketamine produces comparable bioavailability across species. Given that the half-life of ketamine is short, differing levels of ketamine may account for some variation in the behavioral tests. However, ketamine is no longer present when protracted behavioral effects are measured days after administration. These protracted changes result from rapid and sustained molecular alterations induced following a single treatment with ketamine. In addition, the preservative benzethonium chloride (BCl) is universally used in ketamine preparations both for clinical and preclinical use. Although present in low concentrations, BCl can act synergistically with ketamine to inhibit muscarinic and α7-nicotinic acetylcholine receptors (Durieux and Nietgen, 1997; Coates and Flood, 2001). The extent to which the additive properties of BCl on ketamine-induced modulation of the cholinergic system may affect the antidepressant-like response to ketamine is unknown. In the present review, there was no systematic evidence that positive or negative findings were associated with the source of ketamine in the behavioral studies examined here (**Tables 1, 2**).

The mechanisms underlying ketamine's effects, the simultaneous blockade of NMDA receptors and activation of AMPA receptors, are integral for the induction of the antidepressant response. The long-term consequences of these molecular alterations are likely to mediate ketamine's protracted antidepressant-like effects mediated via increased synaptic plasticity, neuronal survival and maturation. These changes occur within hours of ketamine administration and occur in parallel with both the rapid and protracted behavioral effects in animal models of depression. The rapid modulation of mTOR, its downstream mediators, such as Akt and ERK, and BDNF represent markers of the molecular correlates of the antidepressant effects of ketamine and its ability to modify synaptic plasticity. Novel therapeutics for TRD are likely to modulate these markers in a similar temporal pattern to that of ketamine and can be used to identify better pharmaceutical agents to treat TRD.

ACKNOWLEDGMENTS

This research was supported by USPHS grants R01 MH092412 and R01 MH086599.

REFERENCES

aan het Rot, M., Collins, K. A., Murrough, J. W., Perez, A. M., Reich, D. L., Charney, D. S., et al. (2010). Safety and efficacy of repeated-dose intravenous ketamine for treatment-resistant depression. *Biol. Psychiatry* 67, 139–145. doi: 10.1016/j.biopsych.2009.08.038

Aan Het Rot, M., Zarate, C. A. Jr., Charney, D. S., and Mathew, S. J. (2012). Ketamine for depression: where do we go from here? *Biol. Psychiatry* 72, 537–547. doi: 10.1016/j.biopsych.2012.05.003

Akinfiresoye, L., and Tizabi, Y. (2013). Antidepressant effects of AMPA and ketamine combination: role of hippocampal BDNF, synapsin, and mTOR. *Psychopharmacology (Berl.)* 230, 291–298. doi: 10.1007/s00213-013-3153-2

Autry, A. E., Adachi, M., Nosyreva, E., Na, E. S., Los, M. F., Cheng, P. F., et al. (2011). NMDA receptor blockade at rest triggers rapid behavioural antidepressant responses. *Nature* 475, 91–95. doi: 10.1038/nature10130

Autry, A. E., and Monteggia, L. M. (2012). Brain-derived neurotrophic factor and neuropsychiatric disorders. *Pharmacol. Rev.* 64, 238–258. doi: 10.1124/pr.111.005108

Bauer, M., Adli, M., Bschor, T., Pilhatsch, M., Pfennig, A., Sasse, J., et al. (2010). Lithium's emerging role in the treatment of refractory major depressive episodes: augmentation of antidepressants. *Neuropsychobiology* 62, 36–42. doi: 10.1159/000314308

Bechtholt-Gompf, A. J., Smith, K. L., John, C. S., Kang, H. H., Carlezon, W. A. Jr., Cohen, B. M., et al. (2011). CD-1 and Balb/cJ mice do not show enduring antidepressant-like effects of ketamine in tests of acute antidepressant efficacy. *Psychopharmacology (Berl.)* 215, 689–695. doi: 10.1007/s00213-011-2169-8

Berman, R. M., Cappiello, A., Anand, A., Oren, D. A., Heninger, G. R., Charney, D. S., et al. (2000). Antidepressant effects of ketamine in depressed patients. *Biol. Psychiatry* 47, 351–354. doi: 10.1016/S0006-3223(99)00230-9

Beurel, E., Song, L., and Jope, R. S. (2011). Inhibition of glycogen synthase kinase-3 is necessary for the rapid antidepressant effect of ketamine in mice. *Mol. Psychiatry* 16, 1068–1070. doi: 10.1038/mp.2011.47

Bodnoff, S. R., Suranyi-Cadotte, B., Aitken, D. H., Quirion, R., and Meaney, M. J. (1988). The effects of chronic antidepressant treatment in an animal model of anxiety. *Psychopharmacology (Berl.)* 95, 298–302. doi: 10.1007/BF00181937

Bourin, M. (1997). Animal models of anxiety: are they suitable for predicting drug action in humans? *Pol. J. Pharmacol.* 49,79–84.

Bradley, S. R., Uslaner, J. M., Flick, R. B., Lee, A., Groover, K. M., and Hutson, P. H.

(2012). The mGluR7 allosteric agonist AMN082 produces antidepressant-like effectsbymodulating glutamatergic signaling. *Pharmacol. Biochem. Behav.* 101, 35–40. doi: 10.1016/j.pbb.2011.11.006

Burgdorf, J., Zhang, X. L., Nicholson, K. L., Balster, R. L., Leander, J. D., Stanton,

P. K., et al. (2013). GLYX-13, a NMDA receptor glycine-site functional partial agonist, induces antidepressant-like effects without ketamine-like side effects. *Neuropsychopharmacology* 38, 729–742. doi: 10.1038/npp.2012.246

Caldarone, B. J., George, T. P., Zachariou, V., and Picciotto, M. R. (2000). Gender differences in learned helplessness behavior are influenced by genetic background. *Pharmacol. Biochem. Behav.* 66, 811–817. doi: 10.1016/S0091-3057(00)00271-9

Carrier, N., and Kabbaj, M. (2013). Sex differences in the antidepressant-like effects of ketamine. *Neuropharmacology* 70, 27–34. doi: 10.1016/j.neuropharm.2012.12.009

Carvalho, A. F., Cavalcante, J. L., Castelo, M. S., and Lima, M. C. (2007). Augmentation strategies for treatment-resistant depression: a literature review. *J. Clin. Pharm. Ther.* 32, 415–428. doi: 10.1111/j.1365-2710.2007.00846.x

Castren, E., and Rantamaki, T. (2010). Role of brain-derived neurotrophic factor in the aetiology of depression: implications for pharmacological treatment. *CNS Drugs* 24, 1–7. doi: 10.2165/11530010-000000000-00000

Chandran, A., Iyo, A. H., Jernigan, C. S., Legutko, B., Austin, M. C., and Karolewicz, B. (2013). Reduced phosphorylation of the mTOR signaling pathway components in the amygdala of rats exposed to chronic stress. *Prog. Neuropsychopharmacol. Biol. Psychiatry* 40, 240–245. doi: 10.1016/j.pnpbp.2012.08.001

Choudary, P. V., Molnar, M., Evans, S. J., Tomita, H., Li, J. Z., Vawter, M. P., et al. (2005). Altered cortical glutamatergic and GABAergic signal transmission with glial involvement in depression. *Proc. Natl. Acad. Sci. U.S.A.* 102, 15653–15658. doi: 10.1073/pnas.0507901102

Cleary, C., Linde, J. A., Hiscock, K. M., Hadas, I., Belmaker, R. H., Agam, G., et al. (2008). Antidepressive-like effects of rapamycin in animal models: Implications for mTOR inhibition as a new target for treatment of affective disorders. *Brain Res. Bull.* 76, 469–473. doi: 10.1016/j.brainresbull.2008.03.005

Coates, K. M., and Flood, P. (2001). Ketamine and its preservative, benzethonium chloride, both inhibit human recombinant alpha7 and alpha4beta2 neuronal nicotinic acetylcholine receptors in Xenopus oocytes. *Br. J. Pharmacol.* 134, 871–879. doi: 10.1038/sj.bjp.0704315

Cruz, S. L., Soberanes-Chavez, P., Paez-Martinez, N., and Lopez-Rubalcava, C. (2009). Toluene has antidepressant-like actions in two animal models used for the screening of antidepressant drugs. *Psychopharmacology (Berl.)* 204,279–286. doi: 10.1007/s00213-009-1462-2

Cryan, J. F., Mombereau, C., and Vassout, A. (2005). The tail suspension test as a model for assessing antidepressant activity: review of pharmacological and genetic studies in mice. *Neurosci. Biobehav. Rev.* 29, 571–625. doi: 10.1016/j.neubiorev.2005.03.009

Cryan, J. F., Valentino, R. J., and Lucki, I. (2005). Assessing substrates underlying the behavioral effects of antidepressants using the modified rat forced swimming test. *Neurosci. Biobehav. Rev.* 29, 547–569. doi: 10.1016/j.neubiorev.2005.03.008

Dagestad, G., Kuipers, S. D., Messaoudi, E., and Bramham, C. R. (2006). Chronic fluoxetine induces region-specific changes in translation factor eIF4E and eEF2 activity in the rat brain. *Eur. J. Neurosci.* 23, 2814–2818. doi: 10.1111/j.1460-9568.2006.04817.x

da Silva, F. C., do Carmo de Oliveira Cito, M., da Silva, M. I., Moura, B. A., de Aquino Neto, M. R., et al. (2010). Behavioral alterations and pro-oxidant effect of a single ketamine administration to mice. *Brain Res. Bull.* 83, 9–15. doi: 10.1016/j.brainresbull.2010.05.011

de Bartolomeis, A., Sarappa, C., Buonaguro, E. F., Marmo, F., Eramo, A., Tomasetti, C., et al. (2013). Different effects of the NMDA receptor antagonists ketamine, MK-801, and memantine on postsynaptic density transcripts and their topog-raphy: role of Homer signaling, and implications for novel antipsychotic and pro-cognitive targets in psychosis. *Prog. Neuropsychopharmacol. Biol. Psychiatry* 46C, 1–12. doi: 10.1016/j.pnpbp.2013.06.010

Deltheil, T., Guiard, B. P., Guilloux, J. P., Nicolas, L., Delomenie, C., Reperant, C., et al. (2008). Consequences of changes in BDNF levels on serotonin neurotransmission, 5-HT transporter expression and function: studies in adult mice hippocampus. *Pharmacol. Biochem. Behav.* 90, 174–183. doi: 10.1016/j.pbb.2007.09.018

Diazgranados, N., Ibrahim, L., Brutsche, N. E., Newberg, A., Kronstein, P., Khalife, S., et al. (2010). A randomized add-on trial of an N-methyl-D-aspartate antagonist in treatment-resistant bipolar depression. *Arch. Gen. Psychiatry* 67, 793–802. doi: 10.1001/archgenpsychiatry.2010.90

Dulawa, S. C., and Hen, R. (2005). Recent advances in animal models of chronic antidepressant effects: the novelty-induced hypophagia test. *Neurosci. Biobehav. Rev.* 29, 771–783. doi: 10.1016/j.neubiorev.2005.03.017

Duman, R. S., Li, N., Liu, R. J., Duric, V., and Aghajanian, G. (2012). Signaling pathways underlying the rapid antidepressant actions of ketamine. *Neuropharmacology* 62, 35–41. doi: 10.1016/j.neuropharm.2011.08.044

Duman, R. S., and Monteggia, L. M. (2006). A neurotrophic model for stress-related mood disorders. *Biol. Psychiatry* 59, 1116–1127. doi: 10.1016/j.biopsych.2006.02.013

Durieux, M. E., and Nietgen, G. W. (1997). Synergistic inhibition of muscarinic signaling by ketamine stereoisomers and the preservative benzethonium chloride. *Anesthesiology* 86, 1326–1333. doi: 10.1097/00000542-199706000-00014

Elfving, B., Christensen, T., Ratner, C., Wienecke, J., and Klein, A. B. (2013). Transient activation of mTOR following forced treadmill exercise in rats. *Synapse* 67, 620–625. doi: 10.1002/syn.21668

Engin, E., Treit, D., and Dickson, C. T. (2009). Anxiolytic-and antidepressant-like properties of ketamine in behavioral and neurophysiological animal models. *Neuroscience* 161, 359–369. doi: 10.1016/j.neuroscience.2009.03.038

Fava, M., Rush, A. J., Alpert, J. E., Balasubramani, G. K., Wisniewski, S. R., Carmin, C. N., et al. (2008). Difference in treatment outcome in outpatients with anx-ious versus nonanxious depression: a STAR* D report. *Am. J. Psychiatry* 165, 342–351. doi: 10.1176/appi.ajp.2007.06111868

Garcia, L. S., Comim, C. M., Valvassori, S. S., Reus, G. Z., Barbosa, L. M., Andreazza, A. C., et al. (2008a). Acute administration of ketamine induces antidepressant-like effects in the forced swimming test and increases BDNF levels in the rat hippocampus. *Prog. Neuropsychopharmacol. Biol. Psychiatry* 32, 140–144. doi: 10.1016/j.pnpbp.2007.07.027

Garcia, L. S., Comim, C. M., Valvassori, S. S., Reus, G. Z., Andreazza, A. C., Stertz, L., et al. (2008b). Chronic administration of ketamine elicits antidepressant-like effects in rats without affecting hippocampal brain-derived neurotrophic factor protein levels. *Basic Clin. Pharmacol. Toxicol.* 103, 502–506. doi: 10.1111/j.1742-7843.2008.00210.x

Garcia, L. S., Comim, C. M., Valvassori, S. S., Reus, G. Z., Stertz, L., Kapczinski, F., et al. (2009). Ketamine treatment reverses behavioral and physiological alter-ations induced by chronic mild stress in rats. *Prog. Neuropsychopharmacol. Biol. Psychiatry* 33, 450–455. doi: 10.1016/j.pnpbp.2009.01.004

Ghasemi, M., Raza, M., and Dehpour, A. R. (2010). NMDA receptor antagonists augment antidepressant-like effects of lithium in the mouse forced swimming test. *J. Psychopharmacol.* 24, 585–594. doi: 10.1177/0269881109104845

Gigliucci, V., O'Dowd, G., Casey, S., Egan, D., Gibney, S., and Harkin, A. (2013). Ketamine elicits sustained antidepressant-like activity via a serotonin-dependent mechanism. *Psychopharmacology (Berl.)* 228, 157–166. doi: 10.1007/s00213-013-3024-x

Goulart, B. K., de Lima, M. N., de Farias, C. B., Reolon, G. K., Almeida, V. R., Quevedo, J., et al. (2010). Ketamine impairs recognition mem-ory consolidation and prevents learning-induced increase in hippocampal brain-derived neurotrophic factor levels. *Neuroscience* 167, 969–973. doi: 10.1016/j.neuroscience.2010.03.032

Hay, N., and Sonenberg, N. (2004). Upstream and downstream of mTOR. *Genes Dev.* 18, 1926–1945. doi: 10.1101/gad.1212704

Hayase, T., Yamamoto, Y., and Yamamoto, K. (2006). Behavioral effects of ketamine and toxic interactions with psychostimulants. *BMC Neurosci.* 7:25. doi: 10.1186/1471-2202-7-25

Hoeffer, C. A., and Klann, E. (2010). mTOR signaling: at the crossroads of plasticity, memory and disease. *Trends Neurosci.* 33, 67–75. doi: 10.1016/j.tins.2009. 11.003

Homayoun, H., and Moghaddam, B. (2007). NMDA receptor hypofunction produces opposite effects on prefrontal cortex interneurons and pyrami-dal neurons. *J. Neurosci.* 27, 11496–11500. doi: 10.1523/JNEUROSCI.2213-07.2007

Hoshaw, B. A., Hill, T. I., Crowley, J. J., Malberg, J. E., Khawaja, X., Rosenzweig-Lipson, S., et al. (2008). Antidepressant-like behavioral effects of IGF-I produced by enhanced serotonin transmission. *Eur. J. Pharmacol.* 594, 109–116. doi: 10.1016/j.ejphar.2008.07.023

Hoshaw, B. A., Malberg, J. E., and Lucki, I. (2005). Central administration of IGF-I and BDNF leads to long-lasting antidepressant-like effects. *Brain Res.* 1037, 204–208. doi: 10.1016/j.brainres.2005.01.007

Hoyer, C., Kranaster, L., Janke, C., and Sartorius, A. (2013). Impact of the anesthetic agents ketamine, etomidate, thiopental, and propofol on seizure parameters and seizure quality in electroconvulsive therapy: a retrospective study. *Eur. Arch. Psychiatry Clin. Neurosci.* doi: 10.1007/s00406-013-0420-5. [Epubahead of print].

Ibarguen-Vargas, Y., Surget, A., Vourc'h, P., Leman, S., Andres, C. R., Gardier, A. M., et al. (2009). Deficit in BDNF does not increase vulnerability to stress but dampens antidepressant-like effects in the unpredictable chronic mild stress. *Behav. Brain Res.* 202, 245–251. doi: 10.1016/j.bbr.2009.03.040

Ibla, J. C., Hayashi, H., Bajic, D., and Soriano, S. G. (2009). Prolonged exposure to ketamine increases brain derived neurotrophic factor levels in developing rat brains. *Curr. Drug Saf.* 4, 11–16. doi: 10.2174/15748860978 7354495

Ibrahim, L., Diaz Granados, N., Jolkovsky, L., Brutsche, N., Luckenbaugh, D. A., Herring, W. J., et al. (2012a). A Randomized, placebo-controlled, crossover pilot trial of the oral selective NR2B antagonist MK-0657 in patients with treatment-resistant major depressive disorder. *J. Clin. Psychopharmacol.* 32, 551–557. doi: 10.1097/JCP.0b013e31825d70d6

Ibrahim, L., Diazgranados, N., Franco-Chaves, J., Brutsche, N., Henter, I. D., Kronstein, P., et al. (2012b). Course of improvement in depressive symptoms to a single intravenous infusion of ketamine vs add-on riluzole: results from a 4-week, double-blind, placebo-controlled study. *Neuropsychopharmacology* 37, 1526–1533. doi: 10.1038/npp.2011.338

Ibrahim, L., Diazgranados, N., Luckenbaugh, D. A., Machado-Vieira, R., Baumann, J., Mallinger, A. G., et al. (2011). Rapid decrease in depressive symptoms with an N-methyl-d-aspartate antagonist in ECT-resistant major depression. *Prog. Neuropsychopharmacol. Biol. Psychiatry* 35, 1155–1159. doi: 10.1016/j.pnpbp.2011.03.019

Iijima, M., Fukumoto, K., and Chaki, S. (2012). Acute and sustained effects of a metabotropic glutamate 5 receptor antagonist in the novelty-suppressed feeding test. *Behav. Brain Res.* 235, 287–292. doi: 10.1016/j.bbr.2012.08.016

Irwin, S. A., Iglewicz, A., Nelesen, R. A., Lo, J. Y., Carr, C. H., Romero, S. D., et al. (2013). Daily oral ketamine for the treatment of depression and anxiety in patients receiving hospice care: a 28-day open-label proof-of-concept trial. *J. Palliat. Med.* 16, 958–965. doi: 10.1089/jpm.2012.0617

Jarventausta, K., Chrapek, W., Kampman, O., Tuohimaa, K., Bjorkqvist, M., Hakkinen, H., et al. (2013). Effects of S-ketamine as an anesthetic adjuvant to propofol on treatment response to electroconvulsive therapy in treatment-resistant depression: a randomized pilot study. *J. ECT* 29, 158–161. doi: 10.1097/YCT.0b013e318283b7e9

Jeon, S. H., Kim, S. H., Kim, Y., Kim, Y. S., Lim, Y., Lee, Y. H., et al. (2011). The tricyclic antidepressant imipramine induces autophagic cell death in U-87MG glioma cells. *Biochem. Biophys. Res. Commun.* 413, 311–317. doi: 10.1016/j.bbrc.2011.08.093

Jernigan, C. S., Goswami, D. B., Austin, M. C., Iyo, A. H., Chandran, A., Stockmeier, C. A., et al. (2011). The mTOR signaling pathway in the prefrontal cortex is compromised in major depressive disorder. *Prog. Neuropsychopharmacol. Biol. Psychiatry* 35, 1774–1779. doi: 10.1016/j.pnpbp.2011.05.010

Joffe, R. T., Bagby, R. M., and Levitt, A. (1993). Anxious and nonanxious depres-sion. *Am. J. Psychiatry* 150, 1257–1258.

Kavalali, E. T., and Monteggia, L. M. (2012). Synaptic mechanisms underlying rapid antidepressant action of ketamine. *Am. J. Psychiatry* 169, 1150–1156. doi: 10.1176/appi.ajp.2012.12040531

Kessels, H. W., and Malinow, R. (2009). Synaptic AMPA receptor plasticity and behavior. *Neuron* 61, 340–350. doi: 10.1016/j.neuron.2009.01.015

Kessler, R. C., Chiu, W. T., Demler, O., Merikangas, K. R., and Walters, E. E. (2005). Prevalence, severity, and comorbidity of 12-month DSM-IV disorders in the National Comorbidity Survey Replication. *Arch Gen Psychiatry* 62, 617–627. doi:10.1001/archpsyc.62.6.617

Klein, P. S., and Melton, D. A. (1996). A molecular mechanism for the effect of lithium on development. *Proc. Natl. Acad. Sci. U.S.A.* 93, 8455–8459. doi: 10.1073/pnas.93.16.8455

Koike, H., Iijima, M., and Chaki, S. (2011a). Involvement of the mam-malian target of rapamycin signaling in the antidepressant-like effect of group II metabotropic glutamate receptor antagonists. *Neuropharmacology* 61, 1419–1423. doi: 10.1016/j.neuropharm.2011.08.034

Koike, H., Iijima, M., and Chaki, S. (2011b). Involvement of AMPA receptor in both the rapid and sustained antidepressant-like effects of ketamine in animal models of depression. *Behav. Brain Res.* 224, 107–111. doi: 10.1016/j.bbr.2011.05.035

Koike, H., Iijima, M., and Chaki, S. (2013a). Effects of ketamine and LY341495 on the depressive-like behavior of repeated corticosterone-injected rats. *Pharmacol. Biochem. Behav.* 107, 20–23. doi: 10.1016/j.pbb.2013.03.017

Koike, H., Fukumoto, K., Iijima, M., and Chaki, S. (2013b). Role of BDNF/TrkB signaling in antidepressant-like effects of a group II metabotropic glutamate receptor antagonist in animal models of depression. *Behav. Brain Res.* 238, 48–52. doi: 10.1016/j.bbr.2012.10.023

Koponen, E., Lakso, M., and Castren, E. (2004). Overexpression of the full-length neurotrophin receptor trkB regulates the expression of plasticity-related genes in mouse brain. *Brain Res. Mol. Brain Res.* 130, 81–94. doi: 10.1016/j.molbrainres.2004.07.010

Krishnan, V., Han, M. H., Graham, D. L., Berton, O., Renthal, W., Russo, S. J., et al. (2007). Molecular adaptations underlying susceptibility and resistance to social defeat in brain reward regions. *Cell* 131, 391–404. doi: 10.1016/j.cell.2007.09.018 Laje, G., Lally, N., Mathews, D., Brutsche, N., Chemerinski, A., Akula, N., et al. (2012). Brain-derived neurotrophic factor Val66Met polymorphism and antide-pressant efficacy of ketamine in depressed patients. *Biol. Psychiatry* 72, e27–e28. doi: 10.1016/j.biopsych.2012.05.031

Li, N., Lee, B., Liu, R. J., Banasr, M., Dwyer, J. M., Iwata, M., et al. (2010). mTOR-dependent synapse formation underlies the rapid antidepressant effects of NMDA antagonists. *Science* 329, 959–964. doi: 10.1126/science.1190287

Li, N., Liu, R. J., Dwyer, J. M., Banasr, M., Lee, B., Son, H., et al. (2011). Glutamate N-methyl-D-aspartate receptor antagonists rapidly reverse behav-ioral and synaptic deficits caused by chronic stress exposure. *Biol. Psychiatry* 69, 754–761. doi: 10.1016/j.biopsych.2010.12.015

Lin, C. J., Robert, F., Sukarieh, R., Michnick, S., and Pelletier, J. (2010). The antide-pressant sertraline inhibits translation initiation by curtailing mammalian target of rapamycin signaling. *Cancer Res.* 70, 3199–3208. doi: 10.1158/0008-5472.CAN-09-4072

Lindholm, J. S., Autio, H., Vesa, L., Antila, H., Lindemann, L., Hoener, M. C., et al. (2012). The antidepressant-like effects of glutamatergic drugs ketamine and AMPA receptor potentiator LY 451646 are preserved in bdnf(+)/(-) heterozygous null mice. *Neuropharmacology* 62, 391–397. doi: 10.1016/j.neuropharm.2011.08.015

Liu, R. J., Fuchikami, M., Dwyer, J. M., Lepack, A. E., Duman, R. S., and Aghajanian, G. K. (2013). GSK-3 Inhibition potentiates the synap-togenic and antidepressant-like effects of subthreshold doses of ketamine. *Neuropsychopharmacology* 38, 2268–2277. doi: 10.1038/npp.2013.128

Liu, R. J., Lee, F. S., Li, X. Y., Bambico, F., Duman, R. S., and Aghajanian, G. K. (2012). Brain-derived neurotrophic factor Val66Met allele impairs basal and ketamine-stimulated synaptogenesis in prefrontal cortex. *Biol. Psychiatry* 71, 996–1005. doi: 10.1016/j.biopsych.2011.09.030

Lopez-Rubalcava, C., and Lucki, I. (2000). Strain differences in the behavioral effects of antidepressant drugs in the rat forced swimming test.

Neuropsychopharmacology 22, 191–199. doi: 10.1016/S0893-133X(99)00100-1 Ma, X. C., Dang, Y. H., Jia, M., Ma, R., Wang, F., Wu, J., et al. (2013). Long-lasting antidepressant action of ketamine, but not glycogen synthase kinase-3 inhibitor SB216763, in the chronic mild stress model of mice. *PLoS ONE* 8:e56053. doi: 10.1371/journal.pone.0056053

Machado-Vieira, R., Yuan, P., Brutsche, N., DiazGranados, N., Luckenbaugh, D., Manji, H. K., et al. (2009). Brain-derived neurotrophic factor and initial antide-pressant response to an N-methyl-D-aspartate antagonist. *J. Clin. Psychiatry* 70, 1662–1666. doi: 10.4088/JCP.08m04659

Maeng, S., Zarate, C. A. Jr., Du, J., Schloesser, R. J., McCammon, J., Chen, G., et al. (2008). Cellular mechanisms underlying the antidepressant effects of ketamine: role of alpha-amino-3-hydroxy-5-methylisoxazole-4-propionic acid receptors. *Biol. Psychiatry* 63, 349–352. doi: 10.1016/j.biopsych.2007.05.028

Mantovani, M., Pertile, R., Calixto, J. B., Santos, A. R., and Rodrigues, A. L. (2003). Melatonin exerts an antidepressant-like effect in the tail suspension test in mice: evidence for involvement of N-methyl-D-aspartate receptors and the L-arginine-nitric oxide pathway. *Neurosci. Lett.* 343, 1–4. doi: 10.1016/S0304-3940(03)00306-9

Mathew, S. J., Shah, A., Lapidus, K., Clark, C., Jarun, N., Ostermeyer, B., et al. (2012). Ketamine for treatment-resistant unipolar depression: current evidence. *CNS Drugs* 26, 189–204. doi: 10.2165/11599770-000000000-00000

Monteggia, L. M., Gideons, E., and Kavalali, E. T. (2013). The role of eukary-otic elongation factor 2 kinase in rapid antidepressant action of ketamine. *Biol. Psychiatry* 73, 1199–1203. doi: 10.1016/j.biopsych.2012.09.006

Monteggia, L. M., Luikart, B., Barrot, M., Theobold, D., Malkovska, I., Nef, S., et al. (2007). Brain-derived neurotrophic factor conditional knockouts show gender differences in depression-related behaviors. *Biol. Psychiatry* 61, 187–197. doi: 10.1016/j.biopsych.2006.03.021

Muller, H. K., Wegener, G., Liebenberg, N., Zarate, C. A. Jr., Popoli, M., and Elfving, B. (2013). Ketamine regulates the presynaptic release machinery in the hippocampus. *J. Psychiatr. Res.* 47, 892–899. doi: 10.1016/j.jpsychires.2013.03.008

Murrough, J. W., Iosifescu, D. V., Chang, L. C., Al Jurdi, R. K., Green, C. M., Perez, A. M., et al. (2013). Antidepressant efficacy of ketamine in treatment-resistant major depression: a two-site randomized controlled trial. *Am. J. Psychiatry* 170, 1134–1142. doi: 10.1176/appi.ajp.2013.13030392

O'Brien, W. T., Harper, A. D., Jove, F., Woodgett, J. R., Maretto, S., Piccolo, S., et al. (2004). Glycogen synthase kinase-3beta haploinsufficiency mimics the behavioral and molecular effects of lithium. *J. Neurosci.* 24, 6791–6798. doi: 10.1523/JNEUROSCI.4753-03.2004

O'Connor, R. M., and Cryan, J. F. (2013). The effects of mGlu7 receptor modulation in behavioural models sensitive to antidepressant action in two mouse strains. *Behav. Pharmacol.* 24, 105–113. doi: 10.1097/FBP.0b013e32835efc78

Opal, M. D., Klenotich, S. C., Morais, M., Bessa, J., Winkle, J., Doukas, D., et al. (2013). Serotonin 2C receptor antagonists induce fast-onset antidepressant effects. *Mol. Psychiatry*. doi: 10.1038/mp.2013.144. [Epub ahead of print].

Panja, D., Dagyte, G., Bidinosti, M., Wibrand, K., Kristiansen, A. M., Sonenberg, N., et al. (2009). Novel translational control in Arc-dependent long term potentiation consolidation *in vivo*. *J. Biol. Chem.* 284, 31498–31511. doi: 10.1074/jbc.M109.056077

Parise, E. M., Alcantara, L. F., Warren, B. L., Wright, K. N., Hadad, R., Sial, O. K., et al. (2013). Repeated Ketamine Exposure Induces an Enduring Resilient Phenotype in Adolescent and Adult Rats. *Biol. Psychiatry* 74, 750–759. doi: 10.1016/j.biopsych.2013.04.027

Peng, Y., Zhao, J., Gu, Q. H., Chen, R. Q., Xu, Z., Yan, J. Z., et al. (2010). Distinct trafficking and expression mechanisms underlie LTP and LTD of NMDA receptor-mediated synaptic responses. *Hippocampus* 20, 646–658. doi: 10.1002/hipo.20654

Phelps, L. E., Brutsche, N., Moral, J. R., Luckenbaugh, D. A., Manji, H. K., and Zarate, C. A. Jr. (2009). Family history of alcohol dependence and initial antide-pressant response to an N-methyl-D-aspartate antagonist. *Biol. Psychiatry* 65, 181–184. doi: 10.1016/j.biopsych.2008.09.029

Polter, A. M., Yang, S., Jope, R. S., and Li, X. (2012). Functional significance of glycogen synthase kinase-3 regulation by serotonin. *Cell. Signal.* 24, 265–271. doi: 10.1016/j.cellsig.2011.09.009

Popik, P., Kos, T., Sowa-Kucma, M., and Nowak, G. (2008). Lack of persistent effects of ketamine in rodent models of depression. *Psychopharmacology (Berl.)* 198, 421–430. doi: 10.1007/s00213-008-1158-z

Preskorn, S. H., Baker, B., Kolluri, S., Menniti, F. S., Krams, M., and Landen, J. W. (2008). An innovative design to establish proof of concept of the antidepressant effects of the NR2B subunit selective N-methyl-D-aspartate antagonist, CP-101,606, in patients with treatment-refractory major depressive disorder. *J. Clin. Psychopharmacol.* 28, 631–637. doi: 10.1097/JCP.0b013e3181 8a6cea

Rajkowska, G., O'Dwyer, G., Teleki, Z., Stockmeier, C. A., and Miguel-Hidalgo, J. J. (2007). GABAergic neurons immunoreactive for calcium binding proteins are reduced in the prefrontal cortex in major depression. *Neuropsychopharmacology* 32, 471–482. doi: 10.1038/sj.npp.1301234

Reus, G. Z., Stringari, R. B., Ribeiro, K. F., Ferraro, A. K., Vitto, M. F., Cesconetto, P., et al. (2011). Ketamine plus imipramine treatment induces antidepressant-like behavior and increases CREB and BDNF protein levels and PKA and PKC phosphorylation in rat brain. *Behav. Brain Res.* 221, 166–171. doi: 10.1016/j.bbr.2011.02.024

Rezin, G. T., Goncalves, C. L., Daufenbach, J. F., Fraga, D. B., Santos, P. M., Ferreira, G. K., et al. (2009). Acute administration of ketamine reverses the inhibition of mitochondrial respiratory chain induced by chronic mild stress. *Brain Res. Bull.* 79, 418–421. doi: 10.1016/j.brainresbull.2009.03.010

Ricci, V., Martinotti, G., Gelfo, F., Tonioni, F., Caltagirone, C., Bria, P., et al. (2011). Chronic ketamine use increases serum levels of brain-derived neurotrophic factor. *Psychopharmacology (Berl.)* 215, 143–148. doi: 10.1007/s00213-010-2121-3

Rodgers, R. J., Cao, B. J., Dalvi, A., and Holmes, A. (1997). Animal models of anxiety: an ethological perspective. *Braz. J. Med. Biol. Res.* 30, 289–304. doi: 10.1590/S0100-879X1997000300002

Rosa, A. O., Lin, J., Calixto, J. B., Santos, A. R., and Rodrigues, A. L. (2003). Involvement of NMDA receptors and L-arginine-nitric oxide pathway in the antidepressant-like effects of zinc in mice. *Behav. Brain Res.* 144, 87–93. doi: 10.1016/S0166-4328(03)00069-X

Rosner, M., and Hengstschlager, M. (2011). mTOR protein localization is cell cycle-regulated. *Cell Cycle* 10, 3608–3610. doi: 10.4161/cc.10.20.17855

Rybakowski, J. K., Permoda-Osip, A., Skibinska, M., Adamski, R., and Bartkowska-Sniatkowska, A. (2013). Single ketamine infusion in bipolar depression resistant to antidepressants: are neurotrophins involved? *Hum. Psychopharmacol.* 28, 87–90. doi: 10.1002/hup.2271

Saarelainen, T., Hendolin, P., Lucas, G., Koponen, E., Sairanen, M., MacDonald, E., et al. (2003). Activation of the TrkB neurotrophin receptor is induced by antide-pressant drugs and is required for antidepressant-induced behavioral effects. *J. Neurosci.* 23, 349–357.

Schosser, A., Serretti, A., Souery, D., Mendlewicz, J., Zohar, J., Montgomery, S., et al. (2012). European Group for the Study of Resistant Depression (GSRD)— where have we gone so far: review of clinical and genetic findings. *Eur. Neuropsychopharmacol.* 22, 453–468. doi: 10.1016/j.euroneuro.2012.02.006

Segmiller, F., Ruther, T., Linhardt, A., Padberg, F., Berger, M., Pogarell, O., et al. (2013). Repeated S-ketamine infusions in therapy resistant depression: a case series. *J. Clin. Pharmacol.* 53, 996–998. doi: 10.1002/jcph.122

Seligman, M. E., Weiss, J., Weinraub, M., and Schulman, A. (1980). Coping behavior: learned helplessness, physiological change and learned inactivity. *Behav. Res. Ther.* 18, 459–512. doi: 10.1016/0005-7967(80)90011-X

Shanks, N., and Anisman, H. (1988). Stressor-provoked behavioral changes in six strains of mice. *Behav. Neurosci.* 102, 894–905. doi: 10.1037/0735-7044.102.6.894

Shirayama, Y., Chen, A. C., Nakagawa, S., Russell, D. S., and Duman, R. S. (2002). Brain-derived neurotrophic factor produces antidepressant effects in behavioral models of depression. *J. Neurosci.* 22, 3251–3261.

Solberg, L. C., Baum, A. E., Ahmadiyeh, N., Shimomura, K., Li, R., Turek, F. W., et al. (2004). Sex-and lineage-specific inheritance of depression-like behavior in the rat. *Mamm. Genome* 15, 648–662. doi: 10.1007/s00335-004-2326-z

Souery, D., Oswald, P., Massat, I., Bailer, U., Bollen, J., Demyttenaere, K., et al. (2007). Group for the Study of Resistant, Clinical factors associated with treatment resistance in major depressive disorder: results from a European multicenter study. *J. Clin. Psychiatry* 68, 1062–1070. doi: 10.4088/JCP.v68n0713

Stambolic, V., Ruel, L., and Woodgett, J. R. (1996). Lithium inhibits glycogen synthase kinase-3 activity and mimics wingless signalling in intact cells. *Curr. Biol.* 6, 1664–1668. doi: 10.1016/S0960-9822(02)70790-2

Steru, L., Chermat, R., Thierry, B., and Simon, P. (1985). The tail suspension test: a new method for screening antidepressants in mice. *Psychopharmacology (Berl.)* 85, 367–370. doi: 10.1007/BF00428203

Tejani-Butt, S., Kluczynski, J., and Pare, W. P. (2003). Strain-dependent modification of behavior following antidepressant treatment. *Prog. Neuropsychopharmacol. Biol. Psychiatry* 27, 7–14. doi: 10.1016/S0278-5846(02)00308-1

Tizabi, Y., Bhatti, B. H., Manaye, K. F., Das, J. R., and Akinfiresoye, L. (2012). Antidepressant-like effects of low ketamine dose is associated with increased hippocampal AMPA/NMDA receptor density ratio in female Wistar-Kyoto rats. *Neuroscience* 213, 72–80. doi: 10.1016/j.neuroscience.2012.03.052

Trivedi, M. H., Fava, M., Wisniewski, S. R., Thase, M. E., Quitkin, F., Warden, D., et al. (2006). Medication augmentation after the failure of SSRIs for depression. *N. Engl. J. Med.* 354, 1243–1252. doi: 10.1056/NEJMoa052964

Walker, A. K., Budac, D. P., Bisulco, S., Lee, A. W., Smith, R. A., Beenders, B., et al. (2013). NMDA receptor blockade by ketamine abrogates lipopolysaccharide-induced depressive-like behavior in C57BL/6J Mice. *Neuropsychopharmacology* 38, 1609–1616. doi: 10.1038/npp.2013.71

Wang, X., Chen, Y., Zhou, X., Liu, F., Zhang, T., and Zhang, C. (2012). Effects of propofol and ketamine as combined anesthesia for electroconvulsive therapy in patients with depressive disorder. *J. ECT* 28, 128–132. doi: 10.1097/YCT.0b013e31824d1d02

Wang, X., Yang, Y., Zhou, X., Wu, J., Li, J., Jiang, X., et al. (2011). Propofol pretreatment increases antidepressant-like effects induced by acute administration of ketamine in rats receiving forced swimming test. *Psychiatry Res.* 185, 248–253. doi: 10.1016/j.psychres.2010.04.046

Will, C. C., Aird, F., and Redei, E. E. (2003). Selectively bred Wistar-Kyoto rats: an animal model of depression and hyper-responsiveness to antidepressants. *Mol. Psychiatry* 8, 925–932. doi: 10.1038/sj.mp.4001345

Willner, P. (1997). Validity, reliability and utility of the chronic mild stress model of depression: a 10-year review and evaluation. *Psychopharmacology (Berl.)* 134, 319–329. doi: 10.1007/s002130050456

Willner, P. (2005). Chronic mild stress (CMS) revisited: consistency and behavioural-neurobiological concordance in the effects of CMS. *Neuropsychobiology* 52, 90–110. doi: 10.1159/000087097

Yang, C., Li, X., Wang, N., Xu, S., Yang, J., and Zhou, Z. (2012). Tramadol reinforces antidepressant effects of ketamine with increased levels of brain-derived neurotrophic factor and tropomyosin-related kinase B in rat hippocampus. *Front. Med.* 6, 411–415. doi: 10.1007/s11684-012-0226-2

Yang, C., Zhou, Z. Q., Gao, Z. Q., Shi, J. Y., and Yang, J. J. (2013a). Acute increases in plasma mammalian target of rapamycin, glycogen synthase kinase-3beta, and eukaryotic elongation factor 2 phosphorylation after ketamine treatment in three depressed patients. *Biol. Psychiatry* 73, e35–e36. doi: 10.1016/j.biopsych.2012.07.022a

Yang, C., Hu, Y. M., Zhou, Z. Q., Zhang, G. F., and Yang, J. J. (2013b). Acute administration of ketamine in rats increases hippocampal BDNF and mTOR levels during forced swimming test. *Ups. J. Med. Sci.* 118, 3–8. doi: 10.3109/03009734.2012.724118

Yilmaz, A., Schulz, D., Aksoy, A., and Canbeyli, R. (2002). Prolonged effect of an anesthetic dose of ketamine on behavioral despair. *Pharmacol. Biochem. Behav.* 71, 341–344. doi: 10.1016/S0091-3057(01)00693-1

Yu, H., and Chen, Z. Y. (2011). The role of BDNF in depression on the basis of its location in the neural circuitry. *Acta Pharmacol. Sin.* 32, 3–11. doi: 10.1038/aps.2010.184

Zarate, C. A. Jr., Mathews, D., Ibrahim, L., Chaves, J. F., Marquardt, C., Ukoh, I., et al. (2013). A randomized trial of a low-trapping nonselective N-methyl-d-aspartate channel blocker in major depression. *Biol. Psychiatry* 74, 257–264. doi: 10.1016/j.biopsych.2012.10.019

Zarate, C. A. Jr., Singh, J. B., Carlson, P. J., Brutsche, N. E., Ameli, R., Luckenbaugh, D. A., et al. (2006). A randomized trial of an N-methyl-D-aspartate antagonist in treatment-resistant major depression. *Arch. Gen. Psychiatry* 63, 856–864. doi: 10.1001/archpsyc.63.8.856

Permissions

All chapters in this book were first published in NFTNMI, by Frontiers Media SA; hereby published with permission under the Creative Commons Attribution License or equivalent. Every chapter published in this book has been scrutinized by our experts. Their significance has been extensively debated. The topics covered herein carry significant findings which will fuel the growth of the discipline. They may even be implemented as practical applications or may be referred to as a beginning point for another development.

The contributors of this book come from diverse backgrounds, making this book a truly international effort. This book will bring forth new frontiers with its revolutionizing research information and detailed analysis of the nascent developments around the world.

We would like to thank all the contributing authors for lending their expertise to make the book truly unique. They have played a crucial role in the development of this book. Without their invaluable contributions this book wouldn't have been possible. They have made vital efforts to compile up to date information on the varied aspects of this subject to make this book a valuable addition to the collection of many professionals and students.

This book was conceptualized with the vision of imparting up-to-date information and advanced data in this field. To ensure the same, a matchless editorial board was set up. Every individual on the board went through rigorous rounds of assessment to prove their worth. After which they invested a large part of their time researching and compiling the most relevant data for our readers.

The editorial board has been involved in producing this book since its inception. They have spent rigorous hours researching and exploring the diverse topics which have resulted in the successful publishing of this book. They have passed on their knowledge of decades through this book. To expedite this challenging task, the publisher supported the team at every step. A small team of assistant editors was also appointed to further simplify the editing procedure and attain best results for the readers.

Apart from the editorial board, the designing team has also invested a significant amount of their time in understanding the subject and creating the most relevant covers. They scrutinized every image to scout for the most suitable representation of the subject and create an appropriate cover for the book.

The publishing team has been an ardent support to the editorial, designing and production team. Their endless efforts to recruit the best for this project, has resulted in the accomplishment of this book. They are a veteran in the field of academics and their pool of knowledge is as vast as their experience in printing. Their expertise and guidance has proved useful at every step. Their uncompromising quality standards have made this book an exceptional effort. Their encouragement from time to time has been an inspiration for everyone.

The publisher and the editorial board hope that this book will prove to be a valuable piece of knowledge for researchers, students, practitioners and scholars across the globe.

List of Contributors

Alain M. Gardier
EA 3544 "Pharmacologie des troubles anxio-dépressifs et Neurogenèse", Faculté de Pharmacie, Université Paris-Sud, Chatenay-Malabry, France

Naozumi Araragi and Klaus-Peter Lesch
Division of Molecular Psychiatry, Laboratory of Translational Neuroscience, Department of Psychiatry, Psychosomatics, and Psychotherapy, University of Wuerzburg, Wuerzburg, Germany

Boris Mlinar, Gilda Baccini and Renato Corradetti
Department of NEUROFARBA (Department of Neuroscience, Psychology, Drug Research and Child Health), University of Florence, Florence, Italy

Lise Gutknecht
Department of Neurobiology, Institute of Functional Genomics, National Center for Scientific Research (UMR 5203), INSERM U661, University of Montpellier I and II, Montpellier, France

Indira Mendez-David, Alain M. Gardier and Denis J. David
EA3544, Faculté de Pharmacie, Université Paris-Sud, Châtenay-Malabry, France

Zeina El-Ali and Saadia Kerdine-Römer
INSERM UMR 996, Faculté de Pharmacie, Université Paris-Sud, Châtenay-Malabry, France

René Hen
Department of Neuroscience, Columbia University, NewYork, NY, USA
Department of Psychiatry, Columbia University, NewYork, NY, USA

Emmanuelle Corruble
INSERM U669, Département de Psychiatrie, Hôpital Bicêtre, Assistance Publique Hôpitaux de Paris, Université Paris-Sud, Le Kremlin-Bicêtre, France

Jocelien D. A. Olivier
Department of Women's and Children's Health, Uppsala University, Uppsala, Sweden
Center for Gender Medicine, Karolinska Institutet, Stockholm, Sweden

Christiaan H. Vinkers
Division of Pharmacology, Utrecht Institute for Pharmaceutical Sciences and Rudolf Magnus Institute of Neuroscience, Utrecht University, Utrecht, Netherlands
Department of Psychiatry, Rudolf Magnus Institute of Neuroscience, Utrecht Medical Center, Utrecht, Netherlands

Berend Olivier
Division of Pharmacology, Utrecht Institute for Pharmaceutical Sciences and Rudolf Magnus Institute of Neuroscience, Utrecht University, Utrecht, Netherlands
Department of Psychiatry, Yale University School of Medicine, New Haven, CT, USA

Li-Chun Lin and Etienne Sibille
Department of Psychiatry, Center for Neuroscience, University of Pittsburgh, Pittsburgh, PA, USA

Frederike Schirmbeck and Mathias Zink
Central Institute of Mental Health, Department of Psychiatry and Psychotherapy, Faculty Medicine Mannheim, Heidelberg University, Mannheim, Germany

Tomiki Sumiyoshi
Neurocognition and Pharmacology Laboratory, Department of Neuropsychiatry, University of Toyama Graduate School of Medicine and Pharmaceutical Sciences, Toyama, Japan

Wendy K. Adams
Behavioural Neuroscience Laboratory, Florey Institute for Neuroscience and Mental Health, University of Melbourne, Melbourne, VIC, Australia
Centre for Neuroscience, University of Melbourne, Melbourne, VIC, Australia

Adam L. Halberstadt
Department of Psychiatry, University of California San Diego, La Jolla, CA, USA

Maarten van den Buuse
Behavioural Neuroscience Laboratory, Florey Institute for Neuroscience and Mental Health, University of Melbourne, Melbourne, VIC, Australia
Department of Pharmacology, University of Melbourne, Melbourne, VIC, Australia

Nathan C. Mitchell
Department of Physiology, University of Texas Health Science Center, San Antonio, TX, USA

Georgianna G. Gould
Department of Psychiatry, University of Texas Health Science Center, San Antonio, TX, USA

Corey M. Smolik
Department of Physiology, University of Texas Health Science Center, San Antonio, TX, USA
Department of Pharmacology, University of Texas Health Science Center, San Antonio, TX, USA

Wouter Koek
Department of Psychiatry, University of Texas Health Science Center, San Antonio, TX, USA
Department of Pharmacology, University of Texas Health Science Center, San Antonio, TX, USA

Lynette C. Daws
Department of Physiology, University of Texas Health Science Center, San Antonio, TX, USA
Department of Pharmacology, University of Texas Health Science Center, San Antonio, TX, USA

Allison M. J. Anacker and Andrey E. Ryabinin
Department of Behavioral Neuroscience, Oregon Health & Science University, Portland, OR, USA

Ream Al-Hasani
Basic Research Division, Department of Anesthesiology, Washington University School of Medicine, St. Louis, MO, USA
Department of Anatomy and Neurobiology, Washington University School of Medicine, St. Louis, MO, USA

Jordan G. McCall
Basic Research Division, Department of Anesthesiology, Washington University School of Medicine, St. Louis, MO, USA
Division of Biological and Biomedical Sciences, Washington University School of Medicine, St. Louis, MO, USA

Michael R. Bruchas
Basic Research Division, Department of Anesthesiology, Washington University School of Medicine, St. Louis, MO, USA
Department of Anatomy and Neurobiology, Washington University School of Medicine, St. Louis, MO, USA
Division of Biological and Biomedical Sciences, Washington University School of Medicine, St. Louis, MO, USA
Washington University Pain Center, Washington University School of Medicine, St. Louis, MO, USA

Terence Y. Pang, Xin Du, William A. Catchlove, Thibault Renoir, Andrew J. Lawrence and Anthony J. Hannan
Behavioural Neurosciences Division, Florey Institute of Neuroscience and Mental Health, University of Melbourne, Melbourne, VIC, Australia

Aurélien Bernheim
Center for Psychiatric Neuroscience, Division of Child and Adolescent Psychiatry, Lausanne University Hospital, Lausanne, Switzerland

Olivier Halfon
Division of Child and Adolescent Psychiatry, Lausanne University Hospital, Lausanne, Switzerland

Benjamin Boutrel
Center for Psychiatric Neuroscience, Division of Child and Adolescent Psychiatry, Lausanne University Hospital, Lausanne, Switzerland
Division of Child and Adolescent Psychiatry, Lausanne University Hospital, Lausanne, Switzerland

Thibault Renoir
Melbourne Brain Centre, Florey Institute of Neuroscience and Mental Health, University of Melbourne, Melbourne, VIC, Australia

Kyoko Hasebe and Laura Gray
School of Medicine, Deakin University, Geelong, VIC, Australia

Wissam El-Hage and Vincent Camus
INSERM 930, Faculté de Sciences et Techniques, Université François Rabelais, Tours, France
Centre Hospitalier Régional Universitaire de Tours, Centre Expert Dépression Résistante, Fondation FondaMental, Tours, France

Samuel Leman and Catherine Belzung
INSERM 930, Faculté de Sciences et Techniques, Université François Rabelais, Tours, France

Craig M. Smith, Andrew W. Walker, Ihaia T. Hosken, Cary Zhang and Mouna Haidar
Peptide Neurobiology Laboratory, Neuropeptides Division, The Florey Institute of Neuroscience and Mental Health, The University of Melbourne, VIC, Australia
Florey Department of Neuroscience and Mental Health, The University of Melbourne, VIC, Australia

Berenice E. Chua
Peptide Neurobiology Laboratory, Neuropeptides Division, The Florey Institute of Neuroscience and Mental Health, The University of Melbourne, VIC, Australia

Andrew L. Gundlach
Peptide Neurobiology Laboratory, Neuropeptides Division, The Florey Institute of Neuroscience and Mental Health, The University of Melbourne, VIC, Australia
Florey Department of Neuroscience and Mental Health, The University of Melbourne, VIC, Australia
Department of Anatomy and Neuroscience, The University of Melbourne, VIC, Australia

Caroline A. Browne
Department of Psychiatry, University of Pennsylvania, Philadelphia, PA, USA

Irwin Lucki
Department of Psychiatry, University of Pennsylvania, Philadelphia, PA, USA
Department of Pharmacology, University of Pennsylvania, Philadelphia, PA, USA

Index

www.ingramcontent.com/pod-product-compliance
Lightning Source LLC
LaVergne TN
LVHW060603210926
848485LV00005B/1359